BASIC PRINCIPLES OF CHIROPRACTIC

The Neuroscience Foundation of Clinical Practice

BASIC PRINCIPLES OF CHIROPRACTIC
The Neuroscience Foundation of Clinical Practice

R. C. SCHAFER, DC, FICC

with contributions by
GARY C. JOHNSON, DC and FRANK ZOLLI, DC

Developed by
Associated Chiropractic Academic Press

Published by
THE AMERICAN CHIROPRACTIC ASSOCIATION
1701 Clarendon Boulevard, Arlington, Virginia 22209

USER'S COMMENTS

Users of this manual are encouraged to submit recommended additions, changes, or comments about the subject matter. Comments should be keyed to the specific page, paragraph, and line of the text within the paragraph in which the change or addition is suggested. Reasons should be provided for each comment to assure understanding and complete evaluation. Comments should be forwarded to the author c/o The Associated Chiropractic Academic Press, 5832 Hefner Village Court, Oklahoma City, Oklahoma 73162.

PUBLISHER'S POLICY

This manual has been developed for use as a basic instructional guide. The information contained herein is based on sources believed to be generally correct within the United States. However, because of variances in state statutes, local codes, and court opinions, the publisher assumes no responsibility for the accuracy or scope of the suggestions offered in individual circumstances.

Legal counsel should be consulted for optimal guidance in matters concerning situations having juridical or other medicolegal implications. Questions of ethics and scope of practice should be referred to the Board of Chiropractic Examiners in the state(s) of practice.

The statements expressed herein are either of the author or the authorities cited. The publisher, its contractors, officers, or personnel neither endorse or approve any statements of fact or opinion expressed herein, nor are they responsible for the information presented in these pages.

Library of Congress Catalog Card Number: 86-71160

ISBN: 0-9606618-4-0

Printed in the United States of America

FOREWORD

There is an increasing need for doctors of chiropractic in the United States and abroad that is greater today than ever before. For those who join it, the chiropractic profession offers an opportunity to serve the public, enhance the health and welfare of the people, and enjoy the fulfillment and rewards of professional health-care practice.

The success of the chiropractic profession is based on its distinctive holistic approach, the hands-on spinal and extraspinal techniques, and its focus on neuromuscular conditions associated with joint disorders and spinal subluxations. Thus, a knowledge of the neuromusculoskeletal system is extremely essential in all areas of clinical diagnosis in chiropractic. Furthermore, an understanding of the broad aspects of neurology and clinical neurology, as they apply to chiropractic principles and therapeutic procedures, is necessary to the practice of chiropractic.

I feel that this textbook, *Basic Principles of Chiropractic: The Neuroscience Foundation of Clinical Practice*, is one of the most comprehensive. It provides practitioners and students with enlightening reading enjoyment as well as a valued source manual that will supply continuous use for concise correlated information that encompasses the foundation of chiropractic principles and philosophy.

As a member of the Editorial Board of Review of this book, I found the manuscript's comprehensive references to integrate the latest neurologic findings with the chiropractic clinical principles originally envisioned by its founding father, Dr. D. D. Palmer. Of most interest is the elaborative emphasis on the subluxation complex with its neurologic and muscular manifestations.

With the support and encouragement of Dr. E. Maylon Drake, president, and Dr. Matthew M. Givrad, executive vice-president, of the Los Angeles College of Chiropractic, I was able to work continuously with the author. In addition, I would like to take this opportunity to thank Dr. Schafer and Drs. Zolli and Johnson, and all others who contributed to this writing and bringing this much needed text to the chiropractic profession.

—Tuan A. Tran, PhD
Vice-president, Institutional Studies
Los Angeles College of Chiropractic
Whittier, California

PREFACE

This book is not designed to replace standard manuals concerning the study of human anatomy, physiology, pathology, and neurodiagnosis. Rather, its purpose is to serve as a helpful companion of such references by reviewing basic neurologic principles and showing how they are applied effectively within the practice of chiropractic.

The text is composed of three general parts and evolves from general perspectives to those more specific and practical within clinical application. Part I, consisting of two chapters, introduces the basic neurologic principles of chiropractic. Chapter 1, authored by Dr. Frank Zolli of New York Chiropractic College, describes the historical influences on the science of chiropractic, the basic principles of the profession, and how these principles meet the health needs of society. Chapter 2 gives a summary of the general principles and terminology of clinical neurology. The objective of this chapter is to establish a basic framework for understanding the general anatomy and physiology by which the human nervous system operates.

Part II consists of two chapters that describe the longitudinal and horizontal neurologic systems and their components, with emphasis on their architecture and general functions. The topics within Chapter 3 pertain to the longitudinal neurologic systems; viz, the sensory, motor, cognitive, visceral, vascular, and cerebrospinal fluid systems. Topics within Chapter 4 describe the horizontal neurologic systems; viz, the supratentorial, posterior fossa, spinal, and peripheral levels. This knowledge of the longitudinal and horizontal levels will form a two-dimensional architectural grid that enables the clinician to deduce the anatomical site of any neurologic lesion.

The six chapters within Part III concern applied neurology within the clinical scene and offer a third dimension to the architectural grid established in Part II. To set the tone for the core material of this book, Chapter 5 is an introductory summary of clinical neurology within chiropractic, authored by Dr. Gary Johnson of Logan College of Chiropractic.

Chapters 6 and 7 focus attention on the causes and effects of spinal subluxations. Chapter 6 outlines the general causes and potential effects of the subluxation complex that serve as the basis for practical applications within chiropractic practice. On the foundation established in Chapter 6 and preceding chapters, Chapter 7 describes the specific potentialities of the subluxation complex known today such as those occurring at or near the intervertebral foramen and the remote manifestations commonly associated with a spinal subluxation complex. The effects of root irritation, compression, or traction and related spinal cord deficits, axoplasmic flow disturbances, associated circulatory changes, and cerebrospinal fluid flow alterations are a few of the major topics of this chapter.

Chapters 8 and 9 are directed to the clinical disorders of the sensory and motor system most frequently seen in clinical practice. In Chapter 8, emphasis is placed on those sensory mechanisms underlying common diagnostic approaches, pain, and circulatory/thermal regulation. In Chapter 9, the emphasis is on motor disturbances as expressed through specific static and dynamic neuromusculoskeletal mechanisms.

Within pioneer chiropractic, almost as much attention was given to the treatment of complaints stemming from visceral dysfunction as from somatic disorders. During the last 20 years, however, the emphasis within research has been on explaining why chiropractic health care obtains results in many disorders derived basically from structural faults. Without discounting the significant facts obtained in understanding human biomechanics and its role within clinical chiropractic, the topics of Chapter 10 delineate those viscerosensory and visceromotor mechanisms and disorders of the autonomic system that are so often encountered within clinical practice. Chapter 10 also describes the basic role of reflexology in chiropractic health care. The book concludes with a comprehensive index to aid the reader in quickly locating specific topics.

The author's appreciation is extended to the many chiropractic colleges and professional authorities who contributed their suggestions and experiences to the development of this manual. The overtones of the Editorial Review Board have been extremely helpful during development of the manuscript. It is hoped that the readership will recognize the fact that the demanding professional roles of these highly respected authorities offer little personal time—yet they have volunteered to contribute many hours in reviewing the prepublication manuscript of this book for the sole purpose of helping to maintain a high grade of professional communications. Their continuing self-sacrifice should be applauded. Please review their names, which are listed on the title page.

—RCS

ACKNOWLEDGMENTS

Cooperating Individuals

Howard A. Balduc, DC
Wanda Becher
Gerald M. Brassard, DC, FICC, FACC
Arnold E. Cianciulli, DC, MS, FICC, FACC
Ronald L. Harris, DC, FICC
Paul A. Jaskoviak, DC, FICC
John F. Kirby, MSc, PhD
Mary Jane Newcomb, DC, MA, PhD
Ravid Raphael, BA, DC, DABCO
Neil Stern, DC, FICC
Tuan A. Tran, PhD
Howard Vernon, DC, FCCS
Lawrence Wald, DC
Harry L. Wallace, DC

Cooperating Chiropractic Colleges

Canadian Memorial Chiropractic College
Cleveland Chiropractic College
Los Angeles College of Chiropractic
New York Chiropractic College
Northwestern College of Chiropractic
Palmer College of Chiropractic
Parker College of Chiropractic
Texas Chiropractic College
Western States Chiropractic College

Cooperating Organizations

American Chiropractic Association
Associated Chiropractic Academic Press
Behavioral Research Foundation

Illustration and Photography Credits

Unless credited to other sources, all drawings, photographs, and tables incorporated in this book have been published with the permission of the Associated Chiropractic Academic Press (ACAP).

Note: When various apparatus and products are shown or described in this book as a general example of what is being used in the field, the use of such illustrations should not be construed to be an endorsement of any particular instrument, modality, product, or procedure.

CONTENTS

PART III: CLINICAL NEUROLOGY

Part I: Introduction

Chapter 1

An Introduction to the Principles of Chiropractic

Frank Zolli, DC
Director, Clinical Science Center, New York Chiropractic College

Chiropractic is that branch of the healing arts which is composed of a distinct philosophy, art, and science. Art and science may lead the practitioner to answer *how* and *where* to treat a patient, but it is the principles of chiropractic philosophy that give purpose to the adjustment. The principles of chiropractic answer the question *Why?*

NATURE AND SCIENCE

It has long been recognized that nature is much smarter than man. However, this fact has somehow been lost in the wake of the technologic advances that have engulfed man. This is not to say that progress should not be achieved, nor is it an argument for the maintenance of the status quo. A prime characteristic of life is the ability of an organism to change and adapt to its environment. This adaptation mechanism is a basic component of chiropractic thought. However, as happens in any changes that occur, there are benefits and liabilities that are the direct result of these changes.

Science that exists for the sake of science, with little or no attention to the sociologic complications of its actions, may produce change. It may even produce progress, but at what cost? A world that is enhanced by nuclear power but unable to deal efficiently with the potential of a nuclear disaster is a world of fear and confusion. Perhaps if science could be sensitive to the community of people that it serves, the progress it achieves will be better integrated in the day-to-day living of the public.

Likewise, other institutions must meet the challenge of confronting technologic change and incorporating it into our daily living. Church and state should grow and evaluate its positions regarding those ideas that have long been the core of its policies. Change that is essential to an organism must also be essential to the system within which the organism exists; otherwise, there is conflict.

Chiropractic Has Grown on a Foundation of Principles

Enter chiropractic. Since its inception it has been a primary target of organized allopathic criticism. Largely because of this allopathic discrimination, the chiropractic profession has been ignored by large segments of the general population and chiropractic has been the recipient of unjust legislative and economic practices.

Despite these circumstances, chiropractic has continued to grow. It is now the largest, drugless healing profession in the world. It has survived despite the internal quarrels amongst chiropractors. The reason that chiropractic has survived is simple. It is a philosophy, art, and science dedicated to helping humanity improve by establishing the optimum relationship between structure and function.

Science is a common bond among all branches of the healing arts. The art of chiropractic, diagnosis and technique, is influenced by the current knowledge of the basic sciences. The more information these subjects produce, the more diagnostic and clinical skills will be enhanced. And finally, philosophy. Chiropractic has prevailed because it is greater than any chiropractor.

Chiropractic principles can withstand the attacks of allopathic denigration or the debate of chiropractors who interpret them in different ways. These principles lend a certain perspective to chiropractic care. That is, doctors and patients are part of a magical experience called *life;* an experience that can be filled with joy and sadness, health or disease, happiness or pain. It is an experience that can at times be filled with questions which appear to have no answers. It is for these reasons that chiropractic philosophy is the strength of the profession. Chiropractic principles have provided chiropractors with the strength and flexibility to survive and grow.

Historical Perspectives

In order to grow, one must appreciate the history that is part of this profession. The exact origin of therapeutic manipulation, however, has never been determined. There is evidence that it has been practiced for thousands of years by many different cultures and civilizations. Among these people to whom some form of manipulative healing is ascribed are the Japanese, Egyptians, Tibetans, Syrians, Balylonians, Tahitians, Incas of South America, and the Indians of North America. Each of these people is said to have practiced manipulation at a time in history when global communication was limited. Yet, each of these people performed similar treatments in an effort to alleviate sickness. It may be inherent in man's nature to attempt to heal from within. At the very least, it is an idea that is similar among the different people that populate the earth.

The different viewpoints in the healing arts today have many roots in history. In some primitive societies, it was believed that the cause of disease could be found in some outside influence that entered the victim, and thus rose the belief in hexes, evil forces and demons. Some societies thought to blame afflictions on the "will of the gods." Other societies looked upon disease as an abstraction of the soul from its body.

From these two general points of view, evolved the various theories that supported the "within" and "without" philosophies. The conflict has been passed down throughout the ages. It is still a point of contention among today's health-care practitioners. It should be noted at this point that there is an intermingling of fact and fiction in the roots of healing. Much of what has been passed down historically is a mixture of science and religion. In a simple world, people looked for simple answers to explain the complex questions and phenomena they could not understand. They found their answers in the gods. Through the actions of the gods, people were able to project the wonders of the universe. By attempting to understand the nature of some of the gods, a pattern of thought that could determine attitudes regarding health was developed.

THE GREEK INFLUENCE

Although the roots of healing and the inherent philosophical differences are prehistoric, there is a definite starting point to the conflict. Two Greek deities, Hygeia and Asclepius, by their very natures, represent the difference in health care attitudes.

The goddess Hygeia watched over the health of Athens. She was identified with Athena, the goddess of reason. Although Hygeia was associated with health, she was not actually involved in treating the sick. Instead, she was the guardian of health who symbolized the belief that people could remain well if they lived according to reason.

According to Greek legend, Asclepius was the first physician. He was the son of Apollo and the nymph Coronis and was taught the art of healing by the centaur Chiron. He gained fame by mastering the curative powers of plants, as well as ability with the use of his knife. His fame was so great that he eventually ascended to the position as *the god of medicine*.

In ancient sculpture, Asclepius is seen standing, dressed in a long cloak, with a bare breast. His usual attribute is a club-like staff with a serpent coiled around it. This staff, with its single serpent is the only true symbol of medicine. The caduceus, with its winged staff and intertwined serpents, which is frequently used in this country to represent traditional medicine, is without medical relevance since it truly represents the magic wand of Hermes (Mercury), the messenger of the gods and patron of trade. The wand symbolically represents the rhythmic ever-spiraling upward and change in polarity of the two serpents (the opposites of nature), represented in ancient Chinese lore as yin and yang.

Because of Asclepius' powers, Hygeia was relegated to a subservient role in his retinue, most probably as his daughter. Here she was joined by her sister, Panakeia, who because of her knowledge of drugs from plants and the earth became omnipotent as a healing goddess.

Hippocrates

The unification of both deities seemed to take place in the person of Hippocrates. For Hippocrates, rational living and fitness to the environment were essential tenets of his health care philosophy. He complimented this philosophy with the clinical application of mild remedies to assist nature in the healing of the sick.

Besides his views, there were two other schools of thought during the lifetime of Hippocrates. There existed priest-doctors, dedicated to the god of medicine and the serpent cult. These doctors based their treatments upon bathing, fasting, drugs, and suggestion. They also performed surgery under the influence of sleeping potions and hypnotic suggestion.

Hippocrates served as chief physician and teacher at the Coan school, located on the island of Cos. To Hippocrates, disease was not the result of the ravages of an indwelling demon, but rather, a condition of disharmony in a person's body: a battle between the disease and the self-healing tendency of the body, the *vis medicae naturae*. Hippocrates believed that the sick body triggers natural forces to restore equilibrium and restore good health.

Hippocrates founded his teachings on the firm belief that, while the cause of disease could be found either outside or inside the victim, "it is our natures that are the physicians of our diseases." The knowledge of his time was limited; therefore, the corrective mechanisms were not known, but the basic idea was understood. At this time in history, it should be noted that neither the thermometer nor the stethoscope had been invented. The more advanced diagnostic equipment employed today had not yet been developed. Despite this, Hippocrates proved to be an unparalleled diagnostician. To achieve this diagnostic acumen, Hippocrates used his powers of observation and logical reasoning. Writing of epilepsy, which was then thought of as a sacred disease, he said, "it is no more sacred than any other disease, but has a natural cause and its supposed divine origin is due to man's inexperience." He had an uncanny ability to foretell the course of a malady, laying more stress on prognosis than diagnosis. Therefore, the emphasis of treatment at the Coan school was on the patient.

Implicit in his writings is that both health and disease are under control of natural laws and reflect the influence exerted by the environment and the way of life. In one of his works, *Air, Water, Places*, which today would be classified as a treatise on ecology, he noted the effects of food, occupation, and, especially, climate in causing disease. In aphorisms, he reminded his students not to meddle with, nor hinder, nature's attempt toward recovery.

Hippocrates usually confined his treatment to assisting nature with mild remedies. Once the treatment was administered, the patient, through his physiology, reacted in his own individual way against the disease. Therefore, health was thought to depend on a state of equilibrium among the various internal factors that govern the operations of the body and the mind. This equilibrium was believed to be reached only when man lives in harmony with his external environment.

Disease was considered by Hippocrates to be an infringement upon natural laws. Time and again, he stated that the life and lifestyle of the patient were implicated in the disease process and that the cause is to be found in the combination of circumstances rather than in the simple direct effect of some external agency.

Hippocrates was a proponent of rational living, a point of view that links him with the rules attributed to Hygeia. Hippocrates believed that disease would ensue when changes in conditions are too rapid or too violent to allow the adaptive mechanisms to come into play. Changes that occur, whether they be seasonal or environmental, are best when they are done moderately and gradually.

From a broad perspective, this Hippocratic view is as true and accurate today as when it was first espoused. Any profound change in social patterns will influence the health of nations and the incidence of disease in their populations. The sickness of an individual is not easily separated from the sickness of society. In our lifetime, perhaps the best example to support this point of view can be found in the Vietnam conflict. Can anyone deny that the stresses and frustrations caused by this debacle contributed to illness in this country?

The health of populations is affected not only by medical practices employed in any given era, but also from social, technical and economic factors. What will be the effect of women's liberation or the refinement of food products or economic recessions and depressions? Only time will lend a clue to what degree society will endure in terms of sickness and disease as a response to these changes.

Hippocrates believed that every practitioner of medicine "was to be skilled in nature and strive to know what man is in relation to food, drink, and occupation, and what effect each of these has on the other." He also recognized the importance of the spine and spinal manipulation. He said, "Get knowledge of the spine, for it is the requisite for many diseases."

Euryphon

The other school of thought that existed in this time period was the Cnidian school. This school had been influenced by Egyptian and Mesopotamian cultures and emphasized the treatment of the disease rather than the patient. Euryphon was the chief physician and teacher. As Hippocrates had influenced the Coan school, so too did Euryphon influence the Cnidian attitudes toward treatment.

Cnidian physicians aimed at exact diagnosis, classification, and specific therapy. A broad spectrum approach that emphasized lifestyle and environment as affecting a patient's health was inconsistent with his belief. Euryphon believed that definite events occurred which affected an individual. These events, once directed towards an individual, were believed to transform a healthy person to a sick patient. Euryphon's approach promoted a *specific cause* for each disease. He believed that the Hippocratic approach was too philosophical when compared to his more practical method.

Herodicus and Serapion

Other great healers of the period gained fame because of their ability to treat the sick, and as such, have influenced patient care to this day. Herodicus, the first great drugless healer, achieved wide fame in curing diseases by correcting abnormalities of the spine. He refrained from using drugs and tonics and utilized manual manipulation and therapeutic exercise in treating his patients.

Serapion taught a timeless lesson to all students of healing, past and present. There are no two patients alike, he believed, and because of this, we must depend on experience alone in our treatment of the sick. Anatomy, physiology, and pathology might deviate from those standards taught students of healing. Therefore, he thought that the best method in treating patients is by combining book knowledge with intuition guided by observation. Intuitive skill is inborn, but it needs experience and practice to make it functional.

Galen

After Hippocrates, the most distinguished physician of antiquity was Galen: the founder of experimental physiology. Despite the limited resources of accumulated knowledge, his anatomical investigations were quite complete and accurate. He dissected animals, describing what he saw and attempting to relate his findings to his knowledge of human anatomy.

Among other things, Galen taught the proper position and relations of the vertebrae and the spinal column. He advised his students to "Look to the nervous system as the key to maximum health." This statement is perhaps based on his studies where he sectioned the spinal cord at various levels and observed the resulting sensory and motor disturbances.

Galen described the heart and its three layers of fibers, although he hesitated to call the tissues muscle. This reluctance was due to his observation that heart muscle is characteristically different from other, ordinary muscle. He also recorded that section of the heart's nerve supply was not followed by cessation of its activities.

The founder of experimental physiology also had a philosophical side to him. Galen was a firm believer in a supreme creator of the universe in all its parts. He claimed that God's purpose could be elicited in great detail from examination of His work. To this end, he set himself to prove that the body organs are in such perfect relation to the functions to which they minister that it is impossible to imagine any better arrangement.

Galen was a tremendous teacher who achieved wide fame in medical education. He knew of insensible perspiration. He ligatured the recurrent laryngeal nerve. He advocated the examination of urine in certain diseases, the value of specific foods, the critical days in fever, the significance of the pulse, the character of the arteries, and the nature of parasitic worms.

Historic Influence on Modern Thought

There have been other physicians and teachers who contributed to health history. Many of the accomplishments of these people have been improved upon by the technologic advances that have since occurred, but this brief recount of history illustrates the origins of health attitudes and the basic differences that pervade the healing arts. The controversy is deep rooted in history, yet as contemporary as each new day.

The broad spectrum approach maintains that there is a correlation between the state of one's health and environmental factors. The specific etiology theory maintains that there is a specific cause that creates a disease condition. The difference in the two is underscored by the lack of resolve that has lingered through the ages. From Hygeia and Asclepius, to Hippocrates and Euryphon, to the chiropractic and the allopathic physician, the controversy has never changed. On the one hand, there is an attempt by physicians to control nature by living within its confines reasonably; while on the other hand, there is the attempt by other physicians to control nature by the imposition of pills, potions, and surgery.

TODAY'S CHALLENGES

Modern chiropractic is in a unique position. It finds itself compelled to maintain the principles and philosophy that have enabled it to become the largest drugless healing profession in the world; yet, it must remain contemporary in thought to treat effectively those patients in need of chiropractic care. The dilemma that confronts chiropractic is: How can chiropractors be successful in the 20th century, utilizing principles that seem, to say the least, outdated? How can sophisticated human beings accept the principles and practice of healing the sick that have been passed down through the ages?

The reason chiropractors can apply such dated principles is that they have endured and consistently achieved more results that any modern wonder drug. Each year new pills and drugs are put on the market in a seemingly endless parade of futility. Yet, the principles that have maintained the chiropractic profession have remained unaltered. Why? Because they are true to the tenets of nature and the rational approach in treating the sick.

The chiropractic profession has grown since 1895, but a large segment of the population is still ignorant of the concept of health and the services provided by chiropractors. This ignorance is a reflection of the health attitudes that have been pushed on society by the medical establishment and the pharmaceutical industry.

The Effect of Commercial Promotion

There are seemingly endless advertisements on television and radio and in magazines and newspapers that promote the use of medications to relieve the suffering of the multitudes. The result is that more and more members of society are being taught (conditioned) to depend on chemical compounds for meeting the ordinary problems of everyday life.

An adjunctive movement that downplays individuality and undermines personal ability is produced by the commercialism of a variety of products. According to these advertisements, in order to be attractive or desirable one must wear a certain brand of clothes or cologne. These same ads imply that if it were not for the use of a certain toothpaste or breath mints there would be no relationships between men and women. It seems society is being programmed on all levels to accept outside assistance to achieve any type of well being.

The medical establishment, which has long criticized the chiropractic profession for being unscientific and too philosophical, labors under the pretense that being scientific and aphilosophical yields better clinical results. In general, this is not true. In this lifetime, one in four members of society will have to undergo some form of psychotherapy. Life expectancy past the age of 40 has not significantly increased in several decades; and the quality of life, due to stress and frustration, is questionable. Each year, a larger portion of income is spent on medical care and the quest for health. These facts have not only been accepted as a way of life, but people continually contribute to their growth by insisting on living in a way that is incompatible with the principles of good health.

The spell that has been cast on society by traditional medicine is awesome. It has been and continues to be reinforced on a daily basis, and with each passing day, the power of traditional medicine grows. In truth, the *power* of a doctor is based neither on science, as some would have us believe, nor on philosophy, but on faith. A doctor, any doctor, is the personification of the intelligence and skill that unites a patient with health. Because these qualities are possessed by those individuals trained in schools of healing, patients must have faith in their doctors. This kind of faith is reminiscent of ancient times when doctors were considered elite members of a priesthood. Allopathic physicians produce new therapies and surgical feats, disguise their alterations of established procedures in mystical and impressive language, then wait for the recognition and accolades of the masses.

Chiropractors, in their effort to survive, have been overwhelmed by the deluge of medical propaganda. They, too, can be accused of utilizing "mystical" power, although for a different reason. There is not enough patient education on an individual basis to allow access to the knowledge essential to their health. Because of this, effort should be made to effectively counteract the large scale public relations, for any chiropractor is a patient who has responded favorably to treatment.

If, in the course of treatment, the patient has been educated about chiropractic, he will become *health conscious*. This awareness will enable the patient to be sensitive to his own needs, as well as the health requirements for other people in his life. A skeptical person who feels he might benefit from chiropractic care will be more comforted by a satisfied patient who can share a personal experience of chiropractic rather than any form of media advertising. A person-to-person recommendation is the highest form of advertising.

Sensationalistic advertising, which has become a common method of exposing the public to chiropractic, cheapens the profession and falls short of educating patients. An occasional lecture does not fortify the idea of rational living and the necessity of chiropractic care. Chiropractors have always been credited with being able to relate to and speak with patients. This process of communication is essential to the growth of chiropractic. Unfortunately, it appears to some that the current trend seems to be similar to the allopathic approach: administer treatment and forget about lengthy communication with patients.

Social Consequences

People can accept the limitations of their physical ability. They cannot accept the limitations of society. Newspapers are packed with stories about the atrocities of modern civilization. There are stories about war, murder, rape, poverty. People live in the land of freedom and opportunity, yet their thoughts are continually being directed toward the disagreeable events of life. Constant exposure to negative situations is detrimental to an individual's health. Even more detrimental is the accompanying frustration that is caused by being unable in most instances to change such situations.

The problems of society are caused by people. A doctor cannot cure the ills of society by treating society. A doctor can only be responsible for utilizing his skills in the best interest of his patients. This is the focus of a true healer. A true healer treats patients on an individual basis, providing them with the opportunity to achieve health. When this is achieved, their health is a reflection of their lives; and in this way, they can more fully contribute to society.

How is it that society pursues health through faith in drugs and science, while alternate forms of healing are looked upon with scorn and ridicule? There are several factors that directly influenced this present state of affairs.

The Effects of Blind Faith

The American public has been led to believe the "breakthroughs" that have occurred in science have been the key to achieving the high standard of health enjoyed in this country. They do not consider that the life expectancy in some European countries which do not have the benefits of living in such an advanced society is greater than our own. The American citizen in encouraged to believe that money can create drugs for the cure of heart disease, cancer, and mental health. There is insufficient effort made to recognize the factors that contribute to the high incidence of these conditions. There is even less effort made to control the indiscretions of daily life that limit the occurrence of such conditions. Perhaps these conditions, which are directly linked to the irresponsibility of individuals, are caused by their orientation regarding health. This irresponsibility can best be described as *blind faith.*

The blind faith factor has caused intelligent people to believe what allopathic doctors say regarding their health. This same faith that elevates doctors above the status of mere mortals is also given to the "magic" of drugs. Why monitor one's health status if it can easily be restored with the application of some magic tonic?

The word *miracle* is often attributed to the effect of a new drug. This new-found "miracle" then becomes the source of anticipated comfort and experienced hope to the masses. There are few individuals who understand how the "miracle" drug might work. Even fewer who understand its potential side effects. But as long as some fantastic attribute is attached to the drug, people will believe what they *want* to believe. Thus, the sophistication that society pretends to possess is as illusory as the curative power of the drugs they seek. Men still find it easier to believe in miracles and mysterious forces rather than trust in rational processes. Men today want miracles just as much as they did in the past. Although it is true that faith in the healing power of ancient gods has decreased, faith (and other emotionally based beliefs) still maintains more power than rational thought in human beings.

Aside from the oath that bears reference to his name, most people know nothing of Hippocrates. They do not know he was a physician of considerable skill, able to achieve remarkable results with his patients long before the modern scientific era. By empirically manipulating the psychologic, physiologic and, social factors that affected a person's health, he achieved the reputation as the greatest healer of antiquity. His observations and writings are the cornerstone of healing. He possessed keen insight into the human condition and transformed his thoughts into timeless writings that have been passed down through the ages.

Most people regard the fame of Hippocrates with his affiliation with traditional medicine. They do not realize that, more than anything else, Hippocrates represents a concept in healing: The concept that man must live in harmony with his environment, and when in a state of disharmony, the physician is to intervene in the most natural way. Yet this tradition has been obscured in the last century. It is consistent with the chiropractic concept of health, but seemingly in opposition to the germ theory and limited-causality concept of traditional medicine.

The Holistic vs the Traditional Approach

Harmony with nature, without and within ourselves, is an intuitively attractive idea. To live in accordance with the natural forces of life and in harmony with one's environment has been a recurring philosophical theme. Today, this quest has been all but forgotten because most people find it easier to achieve health by depending on doctors and outside agents rather than attempting to live wisely, in harmony with nature.

There are examples of entire cultures that have pursued health by following their natural instincts. Oriental and holistic practitioners treat the imbalance and allow the body to heal itself from within. The focus of these practitioners is not the disease. Instead, the focus is the patient as he is related to society, the environment, and himself. These healers benefit from the fact that their practices are a combination of a philosophy and clinical experience. The Oriental is mindful of yin and yang, the balance and harmony of the opposites of nature.

The holistic healer maintains an intuitive clinical sense and a deep respect for the natural healing power of the body as it relates to all environmental factors. The drawback to these approaches is that they are incongruous with the beliefs and attitude of today's society. Man today has time to do all things but heal himself. He will allow investment time to yield a profit, he will allow young athletes time to reach their athletic potential, and he will allow time for everything else but his homeostatic mechanisms to synchronize with his lifestyle.

Enter traditional medicine. The major benefit of traditional medicine is that it buys time by treating the disease. If in the time bought from medicine the imbalance that is the source of the disease is not corrected, sickness will occur again. The unfortunate side effect of this transitory feeling of health is that not only does it afford the time to find the source of the disease, it also enables the individual to get back into the routine that has contributed to this decline in health. Regardless, health has been restored and fate has been side-stepped. Society continues to live this illusion.

Pain, a by-product of disease, is a reminder that there is an imbalance in our lives. The end point of life is death, but this is nothing more than a natural cycle that has been established by nature. The important aspect of this cycle is not that we die, but rather, the quality of life we live. This is the focus of a true healer: treating patients on an individual basis, so their health is a reflection of their lives, and, in this way, they can more fully contribute to society.

Traditional medicine does not maintain the approach just discussed, yet it is the most dominant branch of the healing arts. Again we are faced with the question, why? The answer is not easily discerned, nor is it confined to one field of learning. The answer has its roots in philosophy, its cause in sociology, and its effect in the distortion of the truth.

AN EPIDEMIOGRAPHIC PERSPECTIVE

As man and civilization "advanced," the needs of society expanded at a tremendous rate. The need to mechanize the processes of manufacturing gave birth to one of the most significant movements in history of man: the industrial revolution. The effect of this revolution spread, at first, throughout Europe, and then eventually covered almost the entire world.

The Role of Poor Hygiene

England prospered through the technologic advances that characterized the movement, but it also suffered the ill side effects that manifested themselves in the destruction of human values. In time, it became obvious that disease and physical frailty were common among the poor. The disadvantaged populations of manufacturing towns became infested with disease. Now the quest for happiness was no longer a life of harmony with nature, but instead, survival. Since the factors that accompanied disease were inevitably the same (want, dirt, and pollution), it was believed that health could be restored by bringing back to the multitudes pure air, pure water, pure food and pleasant surroundings. With this in mind, civic organizations undertook the task of health restoration. Their common sense approach was successful and the quality of health of the English working class was greatly improved. As the quality of life increased, the disease rate decreased.

The same story was seen in Munich, Germany, when it experienced a significant decrease in the incidence of typhoid that was directly attributed to having water brought into the city from the surrounding mountains and having the city sewage diluted. Anti-filth campaigns were waged in Spain during the early part of the 19th century, and the result was that Barcelona did not experience further outbreaks of yellow fever.

Perhaps the best example of the multicausal origin of disease could best be found in the case of the renowned scientist, Rudolph Virchow. He was appointed to study an epidemic that was raging throughout the industrial district of Upper Silesia. In a minority report, Virchow traced the origin of the epidemic to unfavorable meteorological conditions! A famine had occurred because heavy rains had ruined the year's crops. Furthermore, the following winter had been extremely severe, forcing the poor to huddle together in their homes, cold and hungry. It was then that the typhus epidemic had broken out, first spreading through the poor population, and eventually reaching the wealthier class. From this experience, Virchow proposed the theory that poverty is the breeder of disease and that it was the responsibility of the physician to support social reforms that would reconstruct society in a pattern more favorable to health. According to Virchow, the treatment of individual cases is only a small aspect of medicine; more important is the control of crowd disease, which demands social and possibly political action.

The Role of Acquired Resistance

There is also evidence to indicate that a certain amount of natural resistance has been established and has contributed to the control of disease and infection. The mortality rate in North America and Europe from tuberculosis has been steadily on the decline since the turn of the 19th century. No drug therapy was available during this time, vaccination was not practiced, and those therapeutic procedures available were of limited value and reached only a small percentage of the population.

The same holds true for measles. The incidence of measles was on the decline before the measles vaccine was introduced. Statistical evidence confirms that the disease is much less a problem today then it was several years ago. This decrease has been attributed to the measles vaccine, while the decreased incidence of measles should be credited to man's natural resistance. Populations will build a natural immunity to a disease process if they are exposed to the disease over a period of time.

Because the decrease in the death rate appeared obvious to everyone after 1900, traditional medicine and the germ theory in particular have been given the credit for the improvement of the general health of the public. This is an injustice. An even greater injustice is the present dáy belief that the control of diseases can be attributed to the widespread use of antibacterial drugs. In truth, the mortality of many infections had begun to recede in Europe and North America long before the specific methods of therapy were introduced and the germ theory of disease was such a popular concept. This is not to negate the positive contributions science and medicine have made to health of mankind. Scientific medicine has greatly helped deal with the negative side effects of urban and industrial civilization.

Pasteur

Louis Pasteur, one of the most renowned scientists of all time, was able to influence society on many planes due to his varied scientific accomplishments. He disproved the theory of spontaneous generation. He proved that microorganisms cause fermentation and disease. He originated and was the first to use vaccines for chicken pox, cholera, anthrax, and rabies. Through his work, he was able to save the wine and silk industries in France. When Pasteur proposed his *germ theory of disease*, he did not envision a simple connection between germs and disease. He was cognizant that other factors also contributed to the occurrence of a disease process. The simplistic outlook has been the result of a lack of education on the part of patients and their miseducation by physicians. The oversimplification is that *germs cause disease:* to treat the disease, kill the germs by using drugs.

The Role of Cleanliness and Social Reform

Some medical breakthroughs were the result of plain old common sense combined with an acute faculty of observation.

Semmelweis

Ignaz Semmelweis, a Hungarian obstetrician, noted that the death rate seemed to be higher in certain clinics where medical students and physicians came directly to the ward from the morgue or autopsy rooms. Upon witnessing the autopsy of a pathologist who had died of an infectious process that developed after a dissection wound, he observed and noted the pathologic changes that had occurred as a result of the infection were similar to those of a woman who had died of puerperal fever. Semmelweis concluded the infectious nature of puerperal fever and instituted certain practices intended to prevent the spread of infection. On the wards he supervised, all hands had to be cleaned before a patient was examined and the rooms had to be regularly cleaned. The result was the mortality in his service immediately dropped. He published his views, but they were met with strong opposition by the medical establishment.

Lister

Joseph Lord Lister noted the similarity between wound infections and certain fermentative and putrefactive changes, which Pasteur had already proved were caused by microorganisms. He concluded that wound infections were caused by microbes. With this in mind, he started protecting wounds with dressings saturated with a solution of phenol. He also developed operating room procedures calculated to destroy microorganisms.

Misdirected Credit

Traditional medicine, combining the works of Pasteur and the observations of Semmelweis and Lister, have been able to produce some preventive measures against disease. There have been other accomplishments that are a credit to the medical profession and a definite boon to the health of man, but to credit medicine with stemming the tide of infectious disease during the past century is an error.

By the time scientists entered the battle at the beginning of the 20th century, social reformers had already reduced the effects of poor nutrition and infectious disease. As Rene DuBos, an eminent scientist, has pointed out, the introduction of easy-to-launder, inexpensive cotton undergarments and transparent glass that brought light into the most humble dwelling have contributed more to the control of infection that all the drugs and medical practices combined. The accolades given scientific medicine in its control of infectious disease should be rightfully shared with social reformers whose efforts laid the groundwork for the overall improvement of health experienced by man. The trends of improvement extend throughout history. It has been established in society by reformers, and medical science has not significantly altered them.

THE NEED FOR AN INFORMED PUBLIC

The public should be informed about the events that have helped shape the currently accepted beliefs regarding health. The public should be made aware of the chiropractic concept of health. They must be made to realize that the breakthroughs that have influenced the health of society have not been achieved through the work of science alone.

Medical research continues its attempts at finding the causes of a myriad of diseases. With all the research that is taking place in laboratories, few have been looking at our society or environment. There has never been a prescription written to provide relief for a patient suffering from poverty, decaying housing, or social alienation. However, these problems are rarely addressed as being causal factors in disease. As a society, we are overfed and undernourished. We eat to excess, drink to excess, and overindulge. We work and play at a staggering rate, yet there is a residual frustration in our lives. No longer are we obsessed with death and disease. Man has become civilized to a point where threats of physical danger are usually no longer a priority, widespread nutritional deficiencies are a thing of the past in civilized cultures, and the bacterial diseases have been held in check to a great extent by medical science.

The newest threats come in the form of vascular disease, cancer, and mental disease. The unfortunate fact is that today, we must deal not only with those diseases caused by our lifestyles, but we have yet to conquer the diseases of days gone by. Because people have been made to believe the best way to safeguard their health is to support the development of new drugs, they have lost their perspective of what constitutes good health. There is overwhelming evidence that our most prevalent diseases are directly related to our lifestyles, but still the rational approach to health is held in deference to the long awaited medical miracle.

Modern medical science has frequently proven itself inadequate in treating its patients. The public, many of whom have had some bad experience with an allopath, is aware of the problem and is actively searching for a viable alternative to traditional medicine. Now with proper re-education and competent, ethical care, chiropractors have an opportunity to prove to the public that such an alternative does exist. The chiropractic profession, long the second-class citizen of the healing arts, now has the opportunity to take its place as the leader in the field of health.

Semantics

The misconceptions regarding health have been transmitted to public attitudes concerning doctors. For instance, consider the definition of the word *doctor*, which comes from the Latin root meaning *teacher*. Rare today is the doctor who will instruct patients about the maintenance of their health. *Dorland's Medical Dictionary* defines a doctor as a practitioner of the healing arts; one who has received a degree from a college of medicine, osteopathy, or veterinary medicine; licensed to practice by a state.

Another example of our altered conception can be seen by looking at the word *physician*. It is derived from the Greek word meaning *nature*, yet nowhere in the modern interpretation of the word *physician* is there any reference made toward nature. To Hippocrates, every practitioner of medicine "was to be skilled in nature and must know what man is in relation to food, drink, and occupation, and what effect each of these has on the other."

Today, *Dorland's Medical Dictionary* defines a physician as follows: an authorized practitioner of medicine, as one graduated from a college of medicine or osteopathy and licensed by the appropriate state board. The focus of a physician is no longer geared towards clinical ability, but rather, the recognition of the appropriate societal authorities.

Because of the defensive posture assumed by most doctors, no longer is there a correlation between daily activities and interactions of patients with an effective treatment plan intended to help the patient in the most holistic manner. Instead, doctors recommend advice only as it relates to their specialty. No longer is the compassionate treatment of the sick the apparent primary concern of the physician. Seemingly, the primary concern is the establishment and maintenance of reputation.

In view of the distortion one can establish by looking at the words *doctor* and *physician*, let us examine the word medicine. According to *Dorland's Medical Dictionary*, medicine is: any drug or remedy; the art and science of the diagnosis and treatment of disease and the maintenance of health; the treatment of disease by other than surgical means. The definition of remedy is: anything that cures, palliates, or prevents disease.

The definition of *allopathy* is: a term applied to that system of therapeutics in which diseases are treated by producing a condition incompatible with or antagonistic to the condition to be cured or alleviated.

One of the more interesting definitions is assigned to *surgery*, which is: that branch of medicine which treats disease, injuries and deformities by manual or operative methods. The roots of the word surgeon are from the Greek words *cheir*, meaning hands, and *ergon*, meaning work. It seems that by definition, the focus of a chiropractor and a surgeon are similar; the difference lies in their clinical orientation.

The following definition of chiropractic is a combination of the thoughts of two great pioneer chiropractors, B.J. Palmer and Willard Carver:

> Chiropractic is a philosophy, science and art. It is the science that teaches health in anatomical relation and disease in disrelation. It is the philosophy of things natural, and the art of adjusting the segments of the spine by hand, for the correction of disease.

It is amazing how the term medicine has become synonymous with the allopathic physician. It is clear, by definition, that chiropractic can be considered generic medicine. It is even more clear by clinical results that chiropractic is the practice of medicine in its purest form; viz, the art and science of the diagnosis and treatment of disease and the maintenance of health; the treatment of disease by other than surgical means. Although chiropractic is not, nor will probably ever be, associated with drug therapy, it is *a remedy*. It is also a distinct *art* and *science* that employs diagnosis as an indicator of how a patient might best be treated, whether exclusively within the realm of chiropractic or by another branch of the healing arts.

Chiropractors, acting in the best interest of their patients, should never forget the ancient law of healing, ie, *Salus aegroti suprema lex*, the welfare of the ailing is the supreme law. Adherence to such a mandate can only be achieved when one is secure in the belief of his abilities and the principles of his profession.

It is obvious that there have been an abundance of radical anti-chiropractic positions expressed in the past, and all too many have been ignorant of the services performed by chiropractors. Traditional medicine can ill afford to allow us the opportunity to succeed where they have failed. In this regard, they would do well to follow the advice of the noted physician John Mennell: "... under certain circumstances I think you are justified in asking a well-trained manipulator, whoever he might be, to treat your patient for that specific complaint, just as you would ask a pharmacist to make up a prescription... Do not deprive your patient of relief from pain because of your prejudice."

Scope of Practice

The definition of chiropractic given previously covers the spectrum of what chiropractic is. It is the combined effort of the ideas of two men who in their own ways shaped the future of chiropractic. Their legacy is an emerging profession that must unify its efforts in order to prevail. This unification can begin by acknowledging that, despite our educated interpretations, the principles of chiropractic are the same for all chiropractors.

Society has imposed certain restrictions on all the health-care professions. Thus, each state has its own rules and regulations regarding the scope of practice allowed chiropractors. The blame for such a situation existing rests not with chiropractic, but with chiropractors.

From the beginning, chiropractic has been a controversial profession. The different points of view that existed among pioneer chiropractors linger to this day. The differences are not clinical or philosophical but seem to be egotistic in nature. The quality of a chiropractor was determined by whose policies the chiropractor adhered to, not by his ability to treat the sick. Just as chiropractic pioneers were unable to blend their differences to form a strong unified profession, today's practitioners are equally unwilling. It seems ludicrous to maintain differences that are based upon egotism when the principles of the profession are the same for all chiropractors.

If chiropractic is to advance, unity is essential. Chiropractors should apply their principles to the condition of the profession. The healing power of the body comes from within the body. The chiropractic profession must heal itself from within the ranks of chiropractors. The common bond, chiropractic principles, is alive and well and helping sick people to get well. It is time for the profession to get well.

There are a variety of techniques available to chiropractors. It is up to the individual doctor to decide which forms of analysis and technics he can comfortably and wisely use. It is up to the individual chiropractor to decide the parameters within which he can comfortably and effectively practice chiropractic. There must be mutual respect between chiropractors. There is no need for animosity within the profession when the profession must endure adversity from outside sources. There is, however, a need for meaningful research and debate.

Chiropractic is a concept that supersedes the bias of individual chiropractors. Chiropractic will endure, not only because of the efforts of chiropractors, but also, in spite of them.

A cure can be effected only at the prerogative of nature. Each individual has the potential to heal, but whether or not this potential is realized is the result of the doctor's skill at facilitating the healing process and the body's willingness to respond. Whether the doctor be a chiropractor, allopath, osteopath, or surgeon, the ultimate healing ability still rests with the patient.

Education in the Healing Arts

The chiropractic profession has received certain benefits from its relationship with the allopathic profession. Due to the prominent position traditional medicine has maintained in society, the education of allopathic physicians was more scrutinized than any other branch of healing arts. During the 18th and 19th centuries, almost any man in America could become a doctor if he could afford the tuition fees or had family contacts for arranging to serve as an apprentice to an established practitioner. Not even a high school education was needed, and it was possible to become a doctor in 6 months of study.

Through the years, the conditions that determined the future of healing have been altered. In 1910, a relatively unknown high school teacher named Alexander Flexnor published Bulletin #4 for the Carnegie Foundation for the Advancement of Teaching titled, *Medical Education in the United States and Canada.* The effect was to revolutionize medicine as a science, while the practice of the art would be relegated to a secondary role.

The immediate impact of the Flexnor report was to close many of the substandard medical schools of the day, leaving the field to those better equipped, staffed, and organized. Overproduction of poorly trained and ill-educated physicians was sharply curtailed, and the standards of medical licensure and practice improved. The long-term effect of the Flexnor report and the ensuing battle over which direction the education of medical doctors would go, has produced highly trained technicians, many of whom do not exhibit the sensitivity or compassion to be called *doctors* in the true sense of the word.

In truth, Flexnor won his battle to standardize medical education and improve the scientific background of the medical doctor, but this increase in science has been achieved at the expense of the art that is clinical medicine. The sophistication of medical education has been copied by the chiropractic profession. So, too, have the inherent drawbacks. Overall, this trend has had a positive effect on chiropractic, but the drawbacks need to be eliminated by both professions.

The greatest benefit the allopathic profession has bestowed on chiropractic is adversity. Although it has slowed our growth, it has caused chiropractors to concentrate their skills in treating their patients and measuring up to the challenge of survival. The staying power of the chiropractic profession is found in its principles and philosophy. It is these very principles that will correct the deficiencies of chiropractic education and insure the continued growth of chiropractic.

PRINCIPLES

Before discussing the principles of chiropractic philosophy, it should be pointed out that any philosophy rests on a foundation of metaphysical concepts. A health-care philosophy serves to give purpose and direction to and reinforcement for selected clinical practices and procedures. The basis of clinical practice must be founded on a thorough knowledge of anatomy, physiology, and biomechanics.

Historic Principles of Chiropractic

The historic principles that follow are listed out of respect for our chiropractic heritage. When our knowledge of the subjects related to the human body was limited, it was these principles that enabled chiropractors to treat the sick.

1. *The Major Premise.* A universal intelligence is in all matter and continually gives to it all its properties and actions, thus maintaining it in existence.
2. *The Chiropractic Meaning of Life.* The expression of this intelligence through matter is the chiropractic meaning of life.
3. *The Union of Intelligence and Matter.* Life is necessarily the union of intelligence and matter.
4. *The Triune of Life.* Life is a trinity having three necessary united factors; viz, intelligence, force, and matter.
5. *The Perfection of the Triune.* In order to have 100% life, there must be 100% intelligence, 100% force, and 100% matter.
6. *The Principle of Time.* There is no process that does not require time.
7. *The Amount of Intelligence in Matter.* The amount of intelligence for any given amount of matter is 100% and is always proportional to its requirements.
8. *The Function of Intelligence.* The function of intelligence is to create force.
9. *The Amount of Force Created by Intelligence.* The amount of force necessary is that which unites intelligence and matter.
10. *The Function of Force.* The function of force is to unite intelligence and matter.
11. *The Character of Universal Forces.* The forces of universal intelligence are manifested by physical laws, are unserving and unadaptive, and have no solicitude for the structures in which they work.
12. *Interference with Transmission of Universal Forces.* There can be interference with transmission of universal forces.
13. *The Function of Matter.* The function of matter is to express force.
14. *Universal Life.* Force is manifested by motion in matter; all matter has motion, therefore there is universal life in all matter.
15. *No Motion Without the Effort of Force.* Matter can have no motion without the application of force by intelligence.

16. *Intelligence in Both Organic and Inorganic Matter.* Universal intelligence gives force to both organic and inorganic matter.

17. *Cause and Effect.* Every effect has a cause, and every cause has an effect.

18. *Evidence of Life.* The signs of life are evidence of the intelligence of life.

19. *Organic Matter.* The material of the body of a "living thing" is organized matter.

20. *Innate Intelligence.* A "living thing" has an inborn intelligence within its body, called innate intelligence.

21. *The Mission of Innate Intelligence.* The mission of innate intelligence is to maintain the material of the body of the "living thing" in active organization.

22. *The Amount of Innate Intelligence.* There is 100% of innate intelligence in every "living thing," the requisite amount, proportional to its organization.

23. *The Function of Innate Intelligence.* The function of innate intelligence is to adapt universal forces and matter for use in the body, so that all parts of the body will have coordinated action for mutual benefit.

24. *The Limits of Adaptation.* Innate intelligence adapts forces and matter for the body as long as it can do so without breaking a universal law, or innate intelligence is limited by the limitation of matter.

25. *The Character of Innate Forces.* The forces of innate intelligence never injure or destroy the structures in which they work.

26. *Comparison of Universal or Innate Forces.* In order to carry on the universal cycle of life, universal forces are destructive and innate forces constructive in regard to matter.

27. *The Normality of Innate Forces.* Innate intelligence is always normal, and its function is always normal.

28. *The Conductors of Innate Forces.* The forces of innate intelligence operate through or over the nervous system in animal bodies.

29. *The Interference with Innate Forces.* There can be interference with the transmission of innate forces.

30. *The Cause of Disease.* Interference with the transmission of innate forces causes the incoordination of disease.

31. *Subluxations.* Interference with transmission in the body is always directly or indirectly due to subluxation in the spinal column.

32. *The Principle of Coordination.* Coordination is the principle of harmonious action of all the parts of an organism, in fulfilling their offices and purposes.

33. *The Law of Demand and Supply.* The law of demand and supply is existent in the body in its ideal state: wherein the "clearing house" is the brain; innate, the virtuous "banker"; brain cells, the "clerks"; and nerve cells, the "messengers."

The preceding principles are a reflection of chiropractic history. The language of many of these principles can today be translated into a common language between branches of the healing arts. Why? Because the basic knowledge common to the healing arts is the same.

The Tangible vs the Intangible

In healing, there has been an acknowledgment that there is a force of power that supersedes the doctor and the patient. In ancient times, physicians invoked the gods to intervene on behalf of their patients and restore health. Nowadays, this faith has been directed towards science. Religion, like philosophy, is removed from science. As the world became more scientific and specialized, subjects that seemed incompatible with the progressive nature of science were relegated to an insignificant role in education. Science produced results and phenomena that people could see, hear, or touch. Religion and philosophy could make no such claim; therefore, they were placed in a position of secondary importance.

Science taught society how to achieve results for immediate gratification, but did little to answer questions regarding the purpose of life. If there is a purpose to life, what is it? Science has its part in the scheme of life (eg, its manifestations through form), but it can give only a mechanical theory as an answer to this complex question.

Because so much emphasis has been placed on the power of science and the skill and education of doctors, many authorities believe that both doctors and patients have lost their perspective regarding health. The prevalent attitude is that the doctor has the power to cure and the patient has no power at all. In reality, the doctor-patient relationship should benefit from the arrangement. The patient gives the doctor the opportunity to practice skills taught in school. The doctor affords the patient a chance to regain health. Each day the master plan of the universe unfolds, and each day doctors and patients assume their roles in this adventure.

Rational thought can give no other conclusion than that the intelligence that maintains order in the universe is the source of healing. There is no disgrace in a doctor acknowledging a power superior to his own. This acknowledgment of a force or power pervading the universe should serve as a reminder that the skill of a physician just facilitates the healing process; it does not create the process. It should also be remembered that because the source of healing is universal in nature, it is not the property of any one branch of the healing arts. A cure can best be effected by practicing within the natural confines of our ability.

In recognition of this subservience and limited ability, certain scientific laws have been defined. Man is unable to control the universe. He may have some control on the events that occur on this planet; but aside from this power, his influence is limited. The universe continually unfolds at its own pace, without the intervention of man. This being the case, man is not as important as he perceives himself to be. He is but another creature, another aspect of life that moves in time. The progression of time continually occurs on all levels of life, from the amoeba to the cerebrum of man. From the most active of organisms to the most stationary objects, life unfolds. Although each new adventure seems important within the context of the world in which it occurs, it is minor in regard to the universal plan.

Pertinent Concepts of Science and Philosophy

To accept a role as a viable part of life lends a new and different perspective to daily routine. There are certain laws that have been proposed by science that are applicable to philosophy. The first law states that *energy can be neither created nor destroyed; it can only change form.* Each person, at one time or another, is said to be in his own little world. That is because each person's existence is a little world, and we each tend to center ourselves in it.

At the beginning of time, there was an X amount of energy dispersed throughout existence. The potential of everything that initially manifested or that could be manifested had to exist of this energy. With this in mind, consider that each human being is energy and maintains a place in the universal plan. Consider that the goal of each human being is to learn and experience as much as possible before undergoing the period of transition known as death. Although death marks the end of life as we perceive it, according to science it is nothing more than a state that will enable that which was at one time a physically manifested human life to change into another form. Many conjecture that this transition being what it is, life does not end with death; it simply changes.

A second law of science states that *for every action, there is an equal and opposite reaction.* Thus, the laws of science confirm the philosophical concepts of harmony in nature. Ancients referred to this as the *law of compensation;* the Hindus call it *karma.* Hermetic philosophy holds that there is a necessity for being able to experience a variety of emotions, because there will naturally occur a balance in their dispersion.

Life is also rhythmic in nature. No life is made up of only pain, nor is a life exclusively made up of happiness. The Chinese say that yin swings to yang and then back again, just as night follows day and spring follows winter.

One function of a chiropractor is to remember this concept of balanced swings in polarity of nature. For example, a patient usually presents with some degree of pain. To treat patients on a daily basis and focus only on their pain is a frustrating and emotionally draining experience. Likewise, to tell a patient to learn from their pain is not conducive to building a practice. But to treat patients with sensitivity and empathy and not lose sight of the fact that these painful situations are finite in nature take the pressure of making an instantaneous correction away from the chiropractor and allows him to practice the art of healing fully.

Also, to tell a patient that his pain is part of the universal plan would rarely comfort him. Although that might well be the case, it is not in the best interest of the patient to tell him this when he is in distress. A chiropractor has no more insight into the universal plan than any other person. Chiropractors might be more sensitive to it, but they do not possess an in-depth knowledge of it. Chiropractors can best play their role in the universal plan by applying their science, art, and philosophy to their patients. In this way, they will facilitate healing. If through corrected health care the quality of life that a person is experiencing improves, he can better function—whether or not he is cognizant of his role.

THE GOAL OF CHIROPRACTIC HEALTH CARE

The essential element of chiropractic health care is enabling the patient to affect his internal homeostatic mechanisms and thereby achieve or maintain health. In order for this to be done, the inherent recuperative powers of the body must be influenced. Inherent growth, maintenance, and recuperative powers are collectively called *innate intelligence.*

There is a normal physiologic balance within an individual, a balance that has been functional since conception. It has determined the sequence that the new life developed, giving attention, when appropriate, to the nervous system, heart, blood vessels, bones, and muscle. It has been able to adjust itself to the needs of the individual without the benefit of outside intervention. It is a function of the chiropractor, when homeostasis is thrown into a state of imbalance, to utilize his skill and knowledge to reinstate normal balance and tone to the body so it can properly function and administer to the needs of the individual.

Why is it that innate intelligence functioned so accurately in the womb, but once in society, it must be aided by doctors? The answer is simple. In a natural setting, life progresses in a natural sequence, uninhibited by any devices of man. Society is far from a natural setting. Instead, it breeds situations that can easily tax and overcome an individual's normal physiologic resistance and necessitate some form of external intervention.

Universal intelligence maintains order in the universe, and it maintains order within every individual, animal, plant, and mineral. Unfortunately, society is maintained by "educated" intelligence. Educated intelligence and its materialistic viewpoints have helped to pervert natural instincts regarding health and have distorted the basic values that are conducive to peaceful, healthful living. This situation has taken many years to evolve, and there is no direct answer to the dilemma. The only significant contribution that can be made in changing these attitudes is to treat and train individuals effectively so they can, in turn, make a greater positive contribution to society. There is little chance that society will ever improve itself to a point where there is no need for doctors, but a situation can be realized where the role of a doctor is seen as being adjunctive to a patient's health as opposed to being the source of a patient's health.

A most humanistic description of innate intelligence has been provided by Buckminster Fuller. He wrote:

> I am 78—and at my age I find that I have now taken in more than 1,000 tons of water, food, and air, the chemistry of which is temporarily employed for different lengths of time as hair, skin, flesh, bone, blood, etc, then progressively discarded. Then I lost 70 pounds and I said, "Who was that 70 pounds?—because here I am." The 70 pounds I got rid of was ten times the flesh and bone inventory at which I had weighed in 1895.
>
> I am certain I am not the avoirdupois of the most recent meals that I have eaten, some of which will become my hair, only to be cut off twice a month. This lost 70 pounds of organic chemistry wasn't me, nor are any of the remaining presently associated atoms "me." We have been making great error in identifying "me" and

> "you" as these truly transient and ergo, sensorially, detectable chemistries... There have been quite a number of weighings of people as they died. Many cancer-doomed paupers have been willing to have their beds placed on scales. The only difference manifest between weight before and after death is that caused by air exhaled from the lungs or urine that has been passed. Whatever life is, it doesn't weigh anything.

Like electricity, innate intelligence does not have weight, but its manifestations are so evident that it cannot be ignored with respect to the maintenance of health in an individual. Nor can it be questioned with respect to the ability to marshal the recuperative powers inherent in the body.

Unlike universal intelligence, whose power is dispersed throughout the cosmos, innate intelligence is concentrated within structure—reaching its highest forms within living cells. Innate intelligence is linked with universal intelligence but is subordinate to it and does not possess the same resources. Not possessing the same resources and being under the influence of universal laws, it lends to each life an aura of mortality.

It is the purpose of innate intelligence to maintain a functioning life. When the body malfunctions, the inherent recuperative powers of the body are stimulated and initiate the natural healing processes that enable the body to restrain and eliminate the disease state. These recuperative powers are manifested through tissue which is finite in ability; ie, they are governed by the laws of manifest nature. Each time a patient is treated, there is no guarantee that a response in the form of healing will take place.

There is a finite quality to everything that concerns being human. This does not exclude a doctor's knowledge and ability but does include a patient's capability to heal. When one considers how many times a human heart beats in a lifetime, how fast a neural impulse travels, or how many cells make up the brain, there is a sense of awe and respect for the power and majesty of life. No machine on earth possesses the qualities of the human body, and no machine on earth is as cognizant of its mortality.

Each person lives an undetermined amount of time. Each person will change continually during this period of time. Doctors can only strive to help their patients stay functional and productive throughout life.

How long is life? There is no correct answer to this question. There are, however, many theories about the factors that affect life.

Time and the Healing Process

In a world inundated with fast-food franchises, split-second computers, and technology that spans continents in a matter of milliseconds, it is difficult for doctors and patients to accept that all things, especially the healing process, takes time. In a society that is dominated by material and financial compensations, it is no wonder that we have little patience for the necessity of *time* in the natural healing process of the body. In general, people would rather sacrifice their health than their money or possessions.

When the body is not functioning at its maximum, it should not be expected to, nor can it, achieve normal productivity. Whether or not there is a conscious acknowledgment of a patient's ill health on the part of the doctor or the patient, the body's inability to perform will reinforce the fact that the patient is ill.

Patients must be educated that their health did not change in a matter of minutes, but instead has continually and progressively developed into a state that has necessitated external intervention. The human body was not created to endure and tolerate prolonged pain, although it can if the need arises. Pain is meant to be an acute signal that there is a detrimental situation within the body. It now becomes the goal of the doctor-patient relationship to correct the imbalance and restore health to the degree possible under the circumstances.

The patient who presents to an office after trauma exhibits a direct cause-effect relationship to a problem. Granted, the time factor that is required to enable the patient to feel better is unknown. However, when the patient understands the cause of the problem and its morphogenesis, he is likely to be more tolerant of the healing process and its required time. Unfortunately, such a direct cause-effect relationship cannot be made with the ill-postured patient who comes in with a chronic low-back condition. The patient's body is a reflection of a life that has been less than the person's ideal dreams and expectations. But through the skill of the chiropractor and the cooperation of the patient, a healing process can now be initiated that will alleviate the musculoskeletal conditions present and enable the patient to face the challenges of life from a position of better health as opposed to progressive disease.

There are factors that influence the amount of time required in the healing process. Among them are the skill of the chiropractor, the attitude and cooperation of the patient, and the stresses placed upon the patient. Because a chiropractor can only be responsible for his skill, it is unfair to project a specific amount of time to alleviate a patient's condition. It is equally unfair for a patient to expect that a doctor's skill is the only determinant in their condition.

Time is a universal concept that has been given parameters by man. To this end, man finds himself controlled by time. There is no such thing as a second, minute, hour, day, week, month, or year. These are man made parameters, devised to control or at least to give some order to daily living. In this effort to measure and control time, man has become controlled. Many people are distressed because they mark birthdays not as significant days to commemorate accomplishments, but as periods of meditation to ponder acts and things not achieved.

BIOSPHERE
↕
SOCIETY—NATION
↕
CULTURE—SUBCULTURE
↕
COMMUNITY
↕
FAMILY
↕
TWO—PERSON
↕

PERSON (Experience and Behavior)

↕
NERVOUS SYSTEM
↕
ORGANS/ORGAN SYSTEM
↕
TISSUES
↕
CELLS
↕
ORGANELLES
↕
MOLECULES
↕
ATOMS
↕
SUBATOMIC PARTICLES

Figure 1.1. Systems hierarchy; levels of organization. The entire model can best be seen by stacking the component parts vertically. The larger, more complex components of the model are placed higher than the smaller, less complex parts of the chain (adapted from Reiser/Rosen: *Medicine as an Experience*).

A Biopsychosocial Model

It was Hippocrates who stressed that man should be studied in his entirety and in relation to his environment. Chiropractic has long attempted to focus not only on individual patients but on their interaction within their personal environment. A precise definition of this interaction can be seen when one considers the biopsychosocial model of a patient (Fig. 1.1).

An appraisal of this model indicates that there are two distinct components within it. Those levels under the box marked "PERSON" are a definition of how a patient and his or her components are affectively treated with chiropractic care. The reaction is based upon the stimulation of the CNS, and it affects all parts of the body. Thus, although chiropractic is well known for its treatment of musculoskeletal problems, its influences within the body cannot be confined by conventional definitions or commonly held misconceptions.

Once a patient has been effectively treated, the patient is better able to relate to his environment. Therefore, those levels that supersede the box marked "PERSON" indicate the complex environment of which man is a part. In the continuity of natural systems, every unit, at the same time, is a part and a whole. The factors that affect each level of the model can be seen if one views the stacked model in the shape of a series of boxes (Fig. 1.2)

Chiropractic has long emphasized ecology, both personal and environmental, as a method of treating the public's health needs. Overall health reflects a high level of intra- and inter-systemic harmony, and disruption can be initiated at any level. Whether or not this disruption is contained or expands to other levels depends on the capacity of the system to adapt and react to change. The human body is an integrated organism. There is no part of the body that does not affect the functioning of other parts. Chiropractors work on the whole person by affecting changes primarily in the spine and neuromusculoskeletal system.

People are complex. Situations affect different people in different ways, but the result is that people basically want to be happy and comfortable.

Even situations that occur of an unpleasant nature can be better tolerated in a healthy body. A body that is functioning optimally will maintain a positive attitude. This attitude, although initiated at one level of the biopsychosocial model, can then be reflected throughout the organism. By treating each individual patient whose disorder belongs to a system, the entire system can be affected.

By acknowledging the need of coordination in maintaining the welfare of the organism and therefore the system, there is an inherent need on the part of the practitioner for astute observation and diagnosis. For years the healing arts have viewed the study of disease to be science, while the treatment of a patient has been considered an art. Applying the biopsychosocial model to this statement proves it false. Unless the two entities, study (observation) and treatment, are exclusive, they cannot be considered separately. If a given state of disease is manifest in a patient, it is evident because it affects that person. The treatment of an individual is an attempt to alleviate the patient's problem, and it grants the patient an opportunity to contribute to his welfare and the welfare of any other person in his environment.

The Chiropractic Approach

The effective application of chiropractic principles in clinical practice is the unique characteristic that separates the chiropractor from the allopath. It is this blending of science and philosophy that allows the chiropractor to approach patients with a human quality that has never been consistently duplicated by any other profession.

The chiropractic approach is undiluted with the pretense of scientific jargon that separates the patient, a person, from the doctor, another person. A chiropractor who is enthusiastic about his work shares this enthusiasm with his patients. In turn, patients share their lives with their chiropractor, and the result is a doctor-patient relationship that is dynamic. And it is only right that the chiropractor-patient relationship be dynamic, because this microcosmic relationship is an accurate description of the chiropractic profession.

The work of chiropractic pioneers established chiropractic as a profession. The tradition that has been handed down to the profession today is a challenge. Chiropractors, often the victims of intolerance, must be tolerant. The theories and methods that have laid the basis for this great profession might today be better understood in a language common to all members of the healing arts. With the current knowledge that has been accumulated in anatomy, physiology, and biomechanics, perhaps there are more effective techniques today than there were when chiropractic was new. The leverage of chiropractic lies in the fact that it can incorporate this new body of information into the profession without compromising its basic principles that are so essential to clinical practice. In fact, the information that is currently in vogue can only strengthen the chiropractic approach to healing.

Intraprofessional Harmony

Theories, by their very nature are subject to change. Principles are not. Chiropractic works. This has been proven time and again by countless pioneer chiropractors who successfully treated the sick. Their methods were different from each other and different

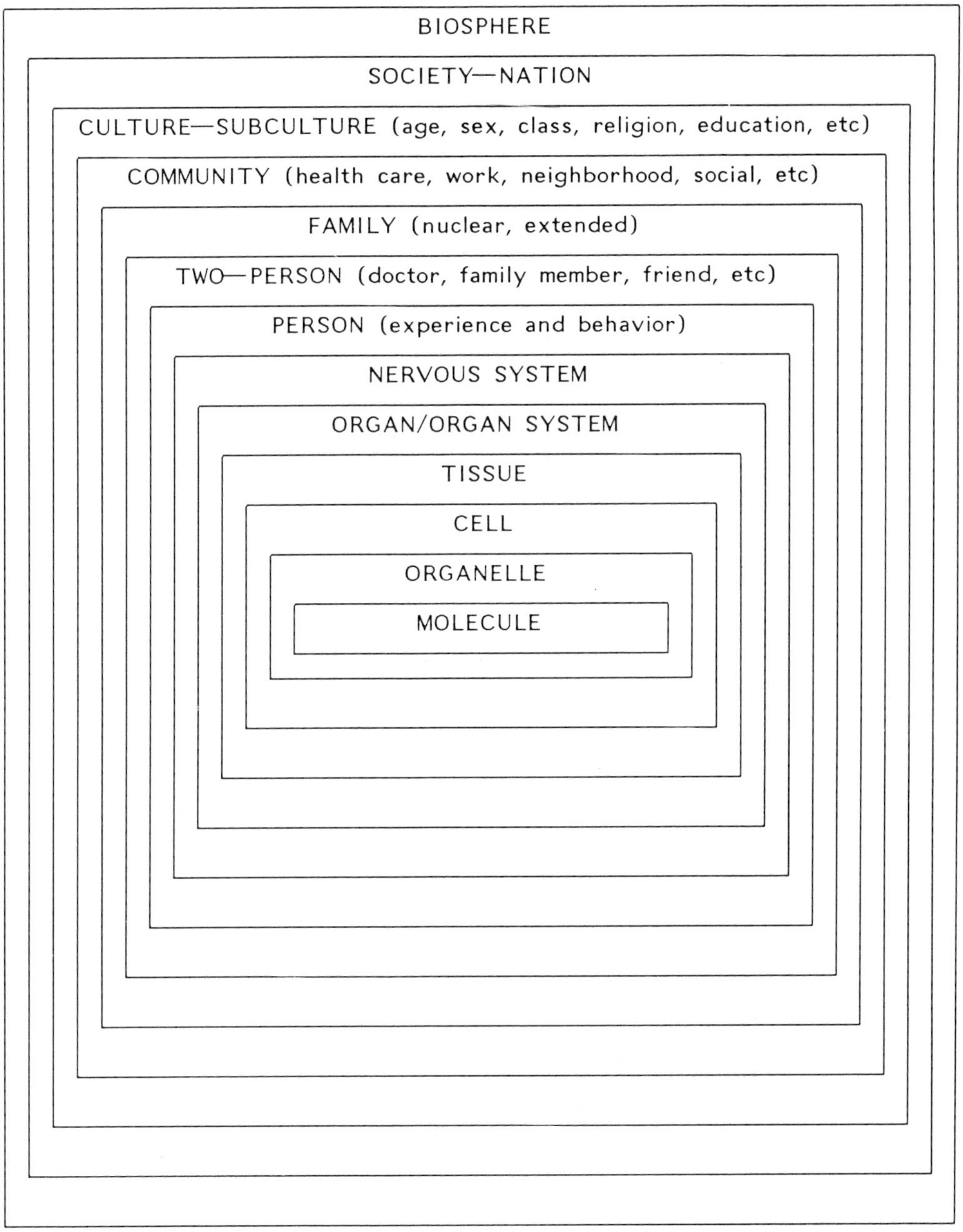

Figure 1.2. The solid square is comprised of individual boxes that are distinct yet support one another. If any part of the box were to be eliminated, the entire structure would be weakened. Each component, is a distinct whole, yet a part of the entire structure. By existing in this fashion, the component parts create a "solid" environment (adapted from Reiser/Rosen: *Medicine as an Experience*).

from the methods commonly used today, but these methods produced results that were unusual at the time. In similar fashion, chiropractors embrace new techniques and are learning new approaches today. Some of these will stand the test of time, some will be refined or replaced, but all of them, to be considered chiropractic, must be consistent with the principles of chiropractic.

Education and its infatuation with scientific dogma has deprived the doctor of a most powerful ally: one's humanity. The ability to possess knowledge and skill yet maintain faith in the intuitive ability of human instincts is rare. All too often a patient lauds a physician's skill, but finds him lacking as a human being. A doctor cannot be lacking either in technical skill and knowledge or in humanism because the combination of the two is what makes a doctor. Technical skill alone makes a technician. Despite any title he might possess, the shortsighted, limited scope with which a patient is viewed can only be the observation of a technician. Combining this technical skill with sensitivity and empathy transforms the *technician* into a *doctor*.

Concluding Remarks

Part of chiropractic art is being a *doctor*. This art can only be realized when a physician has enough confidence and skill so as not to be threatened by a patient's question or to be unsympathetic to a patient's needs. More than anything else, a doctor needs to be *human* in his approach to patients.

Chiropractic is a philosophy, art, and science. Art and science are subject to change. As these components relate to chiropractic, they have changed and will continue to change so as to strengthen the principles of chiropractic philosophy.

The triune of philosophy, art, and science must be kept in perspective if chiropractic is to continue to grow. The health of society depends on this. The future of chiropractic demands it.

Bibliography

Calder R: *Medicine and Man.* New York, New American Library, 1962.

De Baz P: *The Story of Medicine.* New York, Philosophical Library, 1974.

DeGiacomo FP: *Man's Greatest Gift to Man.* Old Bethpage, NY, LSR Learning Associates, 1978.

Dorland's Medical Dictionary, ed 22. Philadelphia, W.B. Saunders, 1977.

Dubos R: *Mirage of Health.* New York, Harper Bros, 1971.

Flexner A: *Medical Education in the United States and Canada.* New York, Carnegie Foundation, 1910.

Fuller BJ, Fuller BF: *Physician or Magician: The Myths and Realities of Patient Care.* New York, McGraw-Hill, 1978.

Garland J: *The Story of Medicine.* Boston, Houghton-Mifflin, 1949.

Garrison FH: *History of Medicine.* Philadelphia, W.B. Saunders, 1906.

Haggard H: *The Doctor in History.* Oxford, CN, Yale University Press, 1934.

Lapatra J: *Healing.* New York, McGraw-Hill, 1978.

Lepore MJ: *Death of the Clinician, Requiem or Reveille?* Springfield, IL, Charles C. Thomas, 1982.

Ligeros K: *How Ancient Healing Governs Modern Therapeutics.* New York, G.P. Putman's Sons, 1937.

Magraw RM, Magraw DB: *Ferment in Medicine.* Philadelphia, W.B. Saunders, 1966.

Mendelsohn RS: *Confessions of a Medical Heretic.* Chicago, Contemporary Books, 1979.

Palmer DD: *Textbook of the Science, Art and Philosophy of Chiropractic.* Portland, OR, Portland Printing House, 1910.

Schafer RC: The historic roots of chiropractic philosophy. In Schafer RC: *Chiropractic Health Care,* ed 3. Des Moines, IA, The Foundation for Chiropractic Education and Research, 1979.

Silverman M, Lee PR: *Pills, Profits, and Politics.* Berkeley, CA, University of California Press, 1974.

Stephenson RW: *Chiropractic Textbook.* Davenport, IA, Palmer Chiropractic College, 1948.

Zolli F: *Chiropractic Concepts in Healing.* Old Brookville, NY, New York Chiropractic College, 1984.

Chapter 2

General Principles of Clinical Neurology

The nervous system and the endocrine system work as partners to provide the majority of functional control for body processes. Guyton, the renowned physiologist, describes the basic function of the nervous system to be the controlling factor for rapid activities such are necessary for muscle contraction, rapidly changing visceral events, and the rate of endocrine secretions. The dominant action of the nervous system over the physical processes of the body is called *neurarchy*. In contrast to the nervous system, the endocrine system principally regulates the metabolic functions of the body and controls prolonged physiologic activities.

It is obvious that a detailed knowledge of neural anatomy, physiology, the electric activity of the nervous system, and even its basic neuropathologic processes cannot be described in one chapter. However, the brief descriptions that follow will serve as reminders of the fundamental processes involved, and more detail will be added in subsequent chapters as the need arises.

OVERVIEW

The demanding role of the nervous system of the human body can be appreciated by recognizing that during every minute of life the nervous system must receive thousands of signals from a countless variety of sensory organs, integrate the data, prepare necessary responses, and effect the responses via a multitude of motor and/or autonomic efferent mechanisms. Thus, a specialized network of nerve tissue permeates the body in such a manner that some parts receive and respond to stimuli from the external or internal environments, some parts transmit signals to and from integrating and coordinating centers, and some parts conduct messages from centers peripherally to muscles, vessels, or glands to effect an action.

As an aid in understanding the structural roles involved, physiologists McNaught/Callander portray the general design of the body as consisting of synchronized *master tissues* and *vegetative systems*. The quick-acting master tissues specialize in receiving messages from the external and internal environments and reacting to them (eg, nerve and muscle tissues). Specialized peripheral receptors such as the telereceptors and contact receptors are impressed by stimuli from the external environment, while deep proprioceptors in muscles and joints and the interoceptors and chemoreceptors of the viscera are impressed by stimuli arising within the internal environment.

The slower-acting vegetative systems (eg, digestive, respiratory, circulatory, excretory systems) provide the basic utilities of life necessary for cellular nutrition, growth, or repair and the removal of waste products. These systems are largely regulated by the sympathetic and parasympathetic divisions of the autonomic nervous system, whose activities are modified, balanced, and integrated by centers within the central nervous system (CNS) to meet the constantly changing needs of the body.

The Evolution of Neurologic Theory

The early roots of neurology in the history of health science are extremely cloudy, but bits and pieces have been found by historians and reported by Singer, Majno, and others.

Early Foundations

During the 4th century BC, Plato believed that health disturbances were the effect of disturbed basic elements within the body, which he labeled air, earth, fire, and water. Aristotle taught that the center of sensations of the body was within the heart. He believed that the heart received ripples from the periphery and referred them through blood vessels. Although the School of Hippocrates later placed the center of consciousness in the brain, the subject remained controversial until the 3rd century BC when teachers at the learning center of Alexandria distinguished nerves from tendons and blood vessels, and some motor and sensory functions within peripheral nerves were established.

The early Greeks taught that nerve functions were accomplished by the movement of "humors" within the body, and this belief prevailed until the 17th century in most Western countries. Claudium Galen, in the 2nd century AD, accepted the general principles established at Alexandria and added knowledge about the spinal cord that was so detailed it remained unchanged until the 19th century. Galen was also the first to teach the proper positions and relationships of the vertebrae to the spinal column and the significance of the pulse and the arteries.

During the 19th century, physiologists began applying the new knowledge of electricity to neural function and muscle contraction, and action potentials were established in nerves and muscles in the 1800s. Most of the data collected at this time were manifestations following severed nerves. Schwann described nerve fibers and cells in 1839, but the segmental structure of nerve fibers and demyelination processes were not defined by Ranvier until the 1870s.

The all-or-nothing principle of neuromuscular excitability was not firmly established until 1871 by Bowditch for heart muscle, until 1909 by Lucas for skeletal muscle, and until 1922 by Adrian/Forbes for nerves. It should be pointed out that D. D. Palmer established the basic principles of chiropractic in the 1890s, in the middle of these rudimentary findings.

Contemporary Developments

With the development of the vacuum tube in the 1920s, neurologic data expanded rapidly because measurements could be made in millisecond and microvolt ranges. The modern views of the relationship between neural structure and function were established during the period between 1900 and 1920, as were concepts of chemical actions at the junctions between excitable cells, but the compound action potential of nerve tissue was not proved until 1937. The ionic basis of the action potential in single nerve fibers was established in 1952. With the development of the electron microscope during the 1950s, the investigation of intricate neurologic morphology began.

Most of the facts proved during this century evolved from theories established many decades before. In reviewing the history of neuroscience, it is amazing to see how often the speculations of scientists with disciplined imaginations, who had to base their theories primarily on empiric experiences, proved quite accurate once technology advanced to the point where their hypotheses could be proved. The science of chiropractic is no exception to this pattern. The lack of theoretical explanations has never been a problem. The challenge has been to formulate hypotheses in such a manner that they can be tested and to develop the means to do so under controlled conditions.

Scientific Theories and Principles of Chiropractic

As a science, chiropractic and other licensed health-care professions are based upon facts demonstrated within the basic sciences; and as healing arts, many procedures are based on empiric evidence and scientific theories and principles that await indisputable confirmation.

In discussing the evolution of neurology and the concept of chiropractic, Haldeman/Hammerich show how chiropractic concepts have evolved in parallel with increasing knowledge of neurologic anatomy and physiology. Likewise in osteopathy, Denslow explains that much is known, much is unknown, and much is controversial about the osteopathic lesion (subluxation). The same is true for chemotherapy.

Basic Principles

Most authorities will agree with Vear when he states that the scope of chiropractic practice is inexorably tied to the biologic concept that relates structure to function and how that concept relates to health and disease.

Although not limited to these by far, it can be stated that the core of the chiropractic approach is built upon three related scientific principles that have been published within the ACA booklet *Chiropractic State of the Art* for many years. They are listed below with slight modification to be current with terminology in use today.

1. *Disease may be caused by disturbances of the nervous system.* While many factors impair health, disturbances of the nervous system are among the most important factors of disease etiology. The nervous system coordinates cellular activities for adaptation to external or internal change. Agents and conditions that irritate the nervous system, and to which the body cannot successfully adapt, produce changes in the pattern of nerve impulses deviating from the norm. Thus originate many functional disturbances, which, if left unchecked, can lead to disease processes.

2. *Disturbances of the nervous system may be caused by derangements of musculoskeletal structures.* Off-centerings (subluxations) and fixations of vertebral and pelvic segments represent common mechanical clinical findings. Extended abnormal involvement of the nervous system may result from disturbances, strains, and stresses arising within the musculoskeletal system due to an individual's attempt to maintain various static and dynamic postures. The mechanical lesion (subluxation) is a common result of gravitational strains, asymmetrical activities and efforts, developmental defects, or other mechanical, chemical, or psychic irritations of the nervous system.

3. *Disturbances of the nervous system may cause or aggravate disease processes in various parts or functions of the body.* Vertebral and pelvic subluxations may be involved in common functional disorders of a visceral and vasomotor nature and at times may produce phenomena that relate to the special organs. Under predisposing circumstances, almost any component of the nervous system may directly or indirectly cause reactions within any other component by means of reflex mediation. The conjunction of independent causes of bodily dysfunction may jointly have more serious debilitating effects than a singular cause might have separately. A subluxation complex may contribute to the "triggering" or exacerbating of certain types of neurovascular and neurovisceral instabilities, and correction of the lesion(s) is often an imperative toward effective total management of the case.

Clinical Efficiency

Support of the efficacy of chiropractic theory and practice within the scientific community has grown steadily in recent years. Janse, Biederman, and Weiant, among others, reinforce their discussions on this topic with numerous quotations from American and European medical doctors.

In discussing the scientific basis for chiropractic, Inglis and associates report in their well-documented monograph that chiropractic theory has been confirmed to be sometimes more effective than medical treatment in many cases. Brunarski comes to the same conclusion after reviewing a large number of clinical trials, and points out that bias against manipulation may have missed important differences in treatment effectiveness. More recently, Rupert and associates describe the results of chiropractic adjustments in a controlled clinical trial conducted in Egypt. Many similar studies are being planned today.

Wayne has documented the effects of a subluxation on the functional efficiency of the body, and Haldeman has emphasized the importance of nerve pressure, afferent input from paraspinal structure, protective reflexes, and the somatovisceral reflex. Similar concepts are reported by Lövgren.

In writing of the theory of manipulative medicine, Pinkenburg stated that current evidence strongly suggests that sensory afferent impulses may play an important role in the maintenance of dynamic equilibrium of the human body in its environment. Overstress of muscles, tendons, and ligaments brings about a change in patterns of afferent nerve impulses that are fired from their nociceptors and mechanoceptors and transmitted to the central nervous system (CNS). It can be hypothesized that, as a result of these changes, stress develops that affects not only the body's dynamic equilibrium with the forces of gravity but also possible visceral dysfunction, and, in turn, visceral disorders influence the body's dynamic equilibrium.

In reviewing musculoskeletal factors in chronic disease, Thorpe points out that many chronic diseases can be helped by manipulative therapy. He concludes that because the spinal segments are extremely sensitive, and since they are interrelated with the viscera and muscles, they affect body reflexes in cases where chronic disease exists.

The efficiency of chiropractic care in mental/emotional disturbances has also been documented. The most notable of these are from Quigley, in reference to patients at the Clear View Sanitarium; the many writings of H. S. Schwartz, especially his analysis of 350 mental patients treated by chiropractors; and Mears' paper on cervical spine distortion. Guze, Homewood, Kimmel, and Sulzer have also reported favorably on the role of chiropractic in structural psychotherapy and somatopsychic disorders.

Neurologic Aspects of Homeostasis

Homeostasis is defined in *Taber's Cyclopedic Medical Dictionary* as "the state of equilibrium of the internal environment of the body that is maintained by dynamic processes of feedback and regulation." *Stedman's Medical Dictionary* defines homeostasis as "the state of equilibrium (balance between opposing pressures) in the body with respect to various functions and to the chemical composition of the fluids and tissues." *Dorland's Medical Dictionary* simply defines it as "a tendency to stability in the normal physiologic states of the organism." Hoag explains that the term *homeostasis* should not suggest a fixed state of physiologic balance, but rather, a state of dynamic equilibrium. He also explains how the musculoskeletal system is important in its maintenance.

The restoration of homeostasis was written about extensively in early chiropractic literature, and it still is today, especially by those who emphasize *systemic* (primarily autonomic) *balancing*. Frequent examples are seen within the current literature of those who apply acupuncture, applied kinesiology, or the principles of Bennett's neurovascular reflexes.

The term is infrequently used in medical literature except by physiologists. For example, Guyton refers to the process throughout his text whenever he describes a functional control system or mechanism. Pottenger felt that the diencephalon was the central control center for homeostasis, as it seemed to be a major receiving and distributing center for nerve impulses that arise in any and all parts of the body.

The necessity of homeostasis to maintain health is often referred to in the writings of chiropractic educators Harper, Janse, Vernor, and D. D. Palmer, but the subject is rarely indexed. It can be assumed that the many references to *innate intelligence* within pioneer chiropractic literature were reflections of homeostatic processes. Homewood also makes this assumption. Jacquet refers to homeostasis in terms of bioenergetics and explains what Lowen calls "the inner language of the body."

Strang is one of many current chiropractic educators who states without hesitation that "Chiropractic rationale begins with the law of biology known as homeostasis," and he offers considerable text to relate its importance to diagnosis and case management within chiropractic. He explains that (1) homeostasis enables the body to stay in balance in an ever-changing environment, (2) the nervous system is the prime controller of homeostasis, and (3) faulty musculoskeletal relationships can cause dysfunction in the nervous system. In addition, he quotes the following which is attributed to Janse: "Normal integrated neurological conduct equals homeostasis and health, and disturbed neurological conduct results in pathophysiology, disintegration of homeostasis, and eventually the intrusion of disease."

Neurologic Aspects of Immunogenesis

It has been strongly felt by most chiropractic practitioners that periodic chiropractic adjustments, even when the patient is in a healthy state, will do much to enhance the patient's resistance to adverse forces. While allopathy has placed great emphasis on the ability of environmental pathogens to attack a host, chiropractic's approach has been directed to the ability of a host to ward off most such attacks if a healthy homeostasis exists. Obviously, both viewpoints are worthy of consideration—being opposite sides of the same coin.

Some microorganisms are highly virulent and severely attack even the most apparently healthy individual. The AIDS virus is a current example. On the other hand, we do not live within a sterile environment. We are constantly exposed to large quantities of potentially dangerous bacteria, viruses, fungi, chemicals, etc, within the air we breath and the food we ingest without noticeable effect. Streptococci can be shown in the nasopharynx of most everyone, yet it is obvious that few people manifest clinical "strep throat."

The conclusion can easily be drawn that assisting the patient's *vis medicatrix naturae* has always been the objective of mainstream chiropractic. Evidence to confirm the efficiency of chiropractic care in this area of preventive health is essentially empiric so far, yet it is based upon some rational scientific principles.

Several years ago, Zhigalina pointed out that the vagus nerve is considered the efferent path for the effect of the CNS on immunologic reactions. Stimulation of the vagus produces an increase in the titer of antibodies, a rise in leukocytes, an increase in phagocytic activity, a decrease in serum protein, and a redistribution of its fraction. He also explains how vagal stimulation is capable of raising the immunologic reaction of the organism and may be used in applied immunology. In this same text, Gordienko and associates state that antigens have the ability to excite peripheral receptors, to cause transformation of these excitations into propagated impulses, and to cause well-defined changes of the biopotentials in the sensory nerve. It was also found that different oscillation of potentials was obtained with different antigens, and it appeared that certain antigens in contact with skin receptors choose their excitation, which is transmitted by the nerves and may play a decisive role in the organization of the defensive processes of the organism against the initial infection.

Although many of Gordienko's experiments added great credibility to chiropractic hypotheses, one in particular should be described: A rabbit's ear was prepared by isolating the blood circulation but leaving the innervation intact. An antigen was introduced intracutaneously, and this lead to the production of specific agglutins when the antigen contacted the skin receptors for ½—1 minute. Because the blood circulation had been restricted, these results attest to the possibility of the *reflex production* of specific agglutinins on the intracutaneous introduction of an antigen. Gondienko's group also showed that skin receptors of the immunized animals react to specific antigens for a longer duration and often more powerfully. The change in reaction proved again that immunogenesis is ensured above all by stimulation of the nervous system and initiation of its reflex mechanisms.

It has long been held empirically within chiropractic that even subclinical states of malnutrition have an adverse effect upon the nervous system. In this context, the relationship between nutrition and infection established by Faulk and associates, among others, is significant. They determined that nutrition and infection interact in two ways: (1) malnourished people are more prone to infection and (2) infection may predispose malnutrition.

Pain Control by Spinal Manipulation

As most patients enter a chiropractor's office with a complaint of pain, the relief of pain has always been a common goal in chiropractic therapeutics. The excellent results achieved have generally been attributed to the reduction of nerve irritation, muscle spasm, edema, and circulatory stasis. However, Vernon and associates have recently expanded our view by showing, under controlled conditions, that plasma levels of ß-endorphins (intrinsic opiate-like compounds) are increased after chiropractic spinal adjustments. These and other effects of chiropractic adjustments will be described in following chapters.

BASIC NEUROEMBRYOLOGY

A brief review of neural embryology is helpful to appreciate the fact that the location of structures in the adult reflect an orderly development from their primitive states.

The origin and development of the nervous system is a gradual process of cell division, migration, remodeling, and specialization, which results in neural circuits requiring cell-to-cell recognition. The mechanisms responsible for this cell-to-cell recognition remain relatively unknown as compared to the sequence of events that occur.

The CNS at birth has completed most of its early stages of cell division, migration, and specialization. Most of the neural circuitry has been laid down. Neuroblasts are continuing to divide only in limited brain regions, according to Bishop. Most mammals, therefore, have a nearly full complement of neurons at birth. Nonetheless, the functional capabilities of the CNS of the newborn have little resemblance to those of the adult. Postnatal maturation must proceed in the proper sequence and at the proper rate if CNS development deficits in the adult are to be avoided.

The Neural Tube

During the 3rd week of development, the embryonic disk consists of two rapidly differentiating layers and a thickened area (primitive streak) from which the notochord is an extension. Ectoderm covering the folds of the notochord soon fold inward to form the lateral grooves of the primitive neural tube. It is from this basic structure that the entire CNS develops. The cells lining the neural tube become the nerve tissue of the brain and spinal cord. The canal itself becomes distended with fluid to form the ventricles of the brain and central canal of the spinal cord.

Longitudinal Differentiation

The ectodermal neural tube is formed between the 18th and 25th day of gestation. During the first stage of differentiation, the distended body of the neural tube begins to constrict to form three primary vesicles: the cephalad forebrain (prosencephalon), midbrain (mesencephalon), and caudad hindbrain (rhombencephalon). See Figure 2.1.

During the second stage, the forepart of the tube constricts and becomes the telencephalon (cerebral hemisphere area) and diencephalon (thalamus and hypothalamus area), and the hindpart constricts and becomes the metencephalon (midbrain and cerebellum area) and myelencephalon (medulla area). Even before the neural tube closes, the tail of the body of the neural tube begins to develop into the spinal cord. These subdivisions are the precursors of the four major anatomical levels in the adult (Table 2.1).

Transverse Differentiation

During the stages of longitudinal differentiation, transverse differentiation also occurs. The *alar plate* develops on the dorsal aspect (sensory functions), mesodermal tissues grow into the neural tube and form blood vessels, and the *basal plate* forms on the ventral aspect (motor functions). These transverse divisions later become the major longitudinal functional systems in the adult (ie, the sensory, motor, visceral, vascular, consciousness, and cerebrospinal fluid systems). See Figure 2.2.

Peripheral Differentiation

Cells continue to divide and split away from the neural tube as it closes to form two columns (neural crests) along the junction between the surface ectoderm and the neural tube. Cells within these crests multiply, migrate laterally, and differentiate to form the dorsal root ganglia (cell bodies of sensory neurons), autonomic ganglia (cell bodies of visceral neurons), Schwann cells for myelination and its neurilemma, and outgrowths of the neural tube (axons and dendrites). The neural crest also gives rise to the adrenal medulla.

As development progresses, the cells within the dorsal root ganglia send axons peripherally throughout the embryo and centrally into the alar plate as a CNS connection. Connections between peripheral structures and the CNS are also made by outgrowths of axons from neurons in the basal plate. The cell bodies within the autonomic ganglia project motor axons to and receive sensory axons from the viscera.

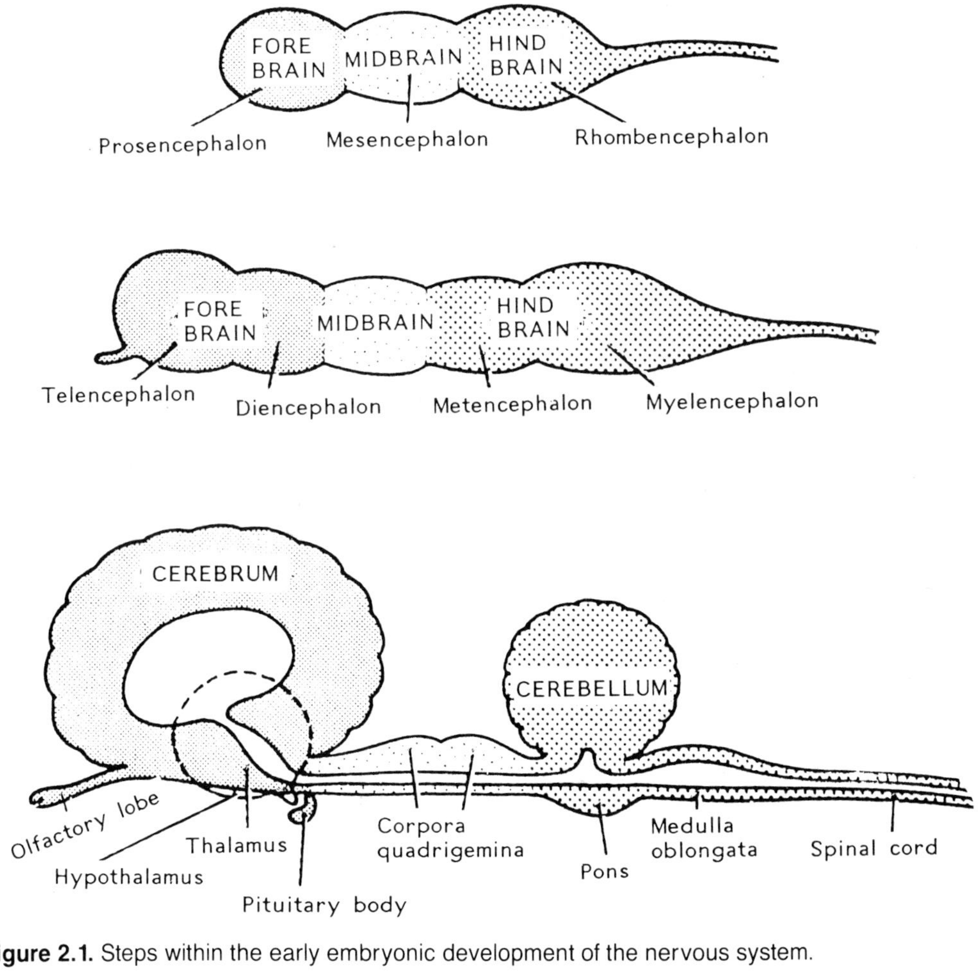

Figure 2.1. Steps within the early embryonic development of the nervous system.

Table 2.1. Progression of Major Structures from the Neural Tube

Prosencephalon (Forebrain)	Telencephalon →	Rhinencephalon Basal ganglia Cerebral cortex Lateral ventricles	Supratentorial level
	Diencephalon →	Epithalamus Thalamus Hypothalamus Optic nerves Neurohypophysis Pineal gland Third ventricle	
Mesencephalon (Midbrain)	Mesencephalon	Midbrain	Posterior fossa level
Rhombencephalon (Hindbrain)	Metencephalon Myelencephalon	Cerebellum Pons Medulla oblongata Fourth ventricle	
Neural tube tail →		Spinal cord and central canal	Spinal level
Neural crest →		Peripheral nerves and ganglia	Peripheral level

Werner's studies suggest that the influence of nerves upon the morphology of peripheral tissues is an intrinsic mechanism of different types of neurons rather than being dependent on influences from the CNS. Sensory neurons subserving different functions have uniquely different influences on the morphology of muscle cells than do gamma motor neurons. The quantity of varying axoplasmic flow along the axons to their terminals appears to be a regulating factor.

Somites

Embryonic mesoderm that lies adjacent to the neural tube becomes segmented into cell masses (somites) as the end of the neural tube closes, later differentiating into:

1. A ventromedial portion *(sclerotome)* that gives rise to the cartilage and bone of the spinal column and base of the skull. This portion also incorporates the notochord, whose remnant becomes the nucleus pulposis of the intervertebral discs.
2. A dorsomedial portion *(myotome)* that differentiates into primordial muscle cells that migrate peripherally to form all striated skeletal muscle of the body except that of the branchial arches.
3. A lateral portion *(dermatome)* that gives rise to cells that migrate peripherally to form the connective tissue layer of the skin (Fig. 2.3).

Distally growing motor axons appose with peripherally growing sensory axons of the dorsal root ganglia to form a spinal or cranial nerve that innervates the somite at the same level. Nerves formed in this manner are mixed nerves; ie, they contain both motor and sensory fibers. In such nerves, sensory axons from CNS cells supply dermatomal and endodermal derivatives, and the motor axons from CNS cells innervate myotomal derivatives and autonomic ganglia. It is in this manner that the innervation patterns of peripheral nerves are established. This is an important fact to remember during the diagnosis of the origin of pain.

BASIC NEUROCYTOLOGY

The Neuron

A neuron is a nerve cell, the structural and function unit of the nervous system that initiates and conducts electrochemical impulse activity (Fig. 2.4). Its basic parts are the main cell body (perikaryon), containing typical organelles for metabolism (eg, mitochondria, lysosomes, Golgi apparatus, and endoplasmic reticulum) and a large nucleus with a conspicuous nucleolus; a single axon process, which may extend from a few millimeters to several feet in length, which conducts impulses away from the cell body; and one or more shorter dendrite processes (eg, unipolar, bipolar, multipolar), which conduct impulses toward the cell body. These processes are protoplasmic outgrowths from the primitive cell body. They range in length from almost nil to several feet in length.

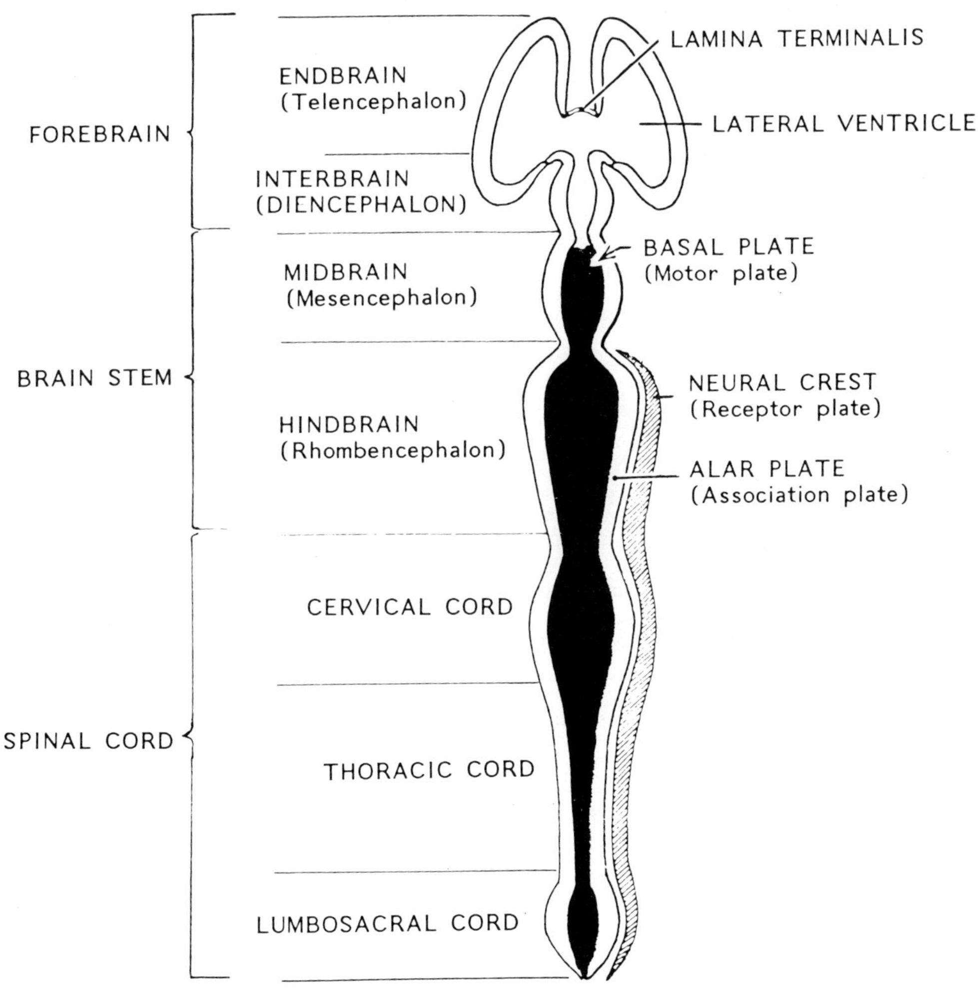

Figure 2.2. Basic longitudinal and transverse differentiation of the nervous system during early embryonic development.

Basic Considerations

The length of neuron processes is sometimes quite remarkable. For example, some motor axons extend as far as from the lumbar segments to the intrinsic muscles of the foot. But this is not maximum. Prichard points out that some dorsal root ganglion cells conveying lower extremity joint position have one process in the terminal joint of a toe and another in the cuneate nucleus of the superior aspect of the cervical cord.

Besides their sometimes extraordinary length, central and peripheral neuron processes are often highly branched, the number varying according to their function. For example, the number of muscle fibers innervated by a motor unit may range from 2000:1 for a weight-lifting muscle (eg, biceps, gastrocnemius) to 12:1 in muscles that perform fine movements (eg, extraocular, facial, and intrinsic finger muscles). A single dorsal root ganglion cell may be related to hundreds of light pressure, deep pressure, thermal, and pain receptors over a large area of skin or to a single mechanoreceptor in a joint or one muscle spindle.

Like other cells of the body, neurons are covered by a plasma membrane and use metabolic energy to sustain an inner negative transmembrane electric potential difference during the resting state. Unlike most other body cells, neurons do not undergo periodic division and replication, and they are specialized for rapid and precise signaling of large quantities of information over considerable distances in many cases. In addition, their shape and size varies considerably depending upon their location within the nervous system (Fig. 2.5) and nerve cell cytoplasm is heavy laden with concentrations of Nissl bodies, neurofilaments (Fig. 2.6), and neurotubules. The latter appear to function in cytoplasmic transport mechanisms. The root of the axon, the *hillock*, is normally devoid of Nissl bodies.

Terminology

Afferent neurons conduct impulses toward the CNS; *efferent* neurons conduct impulses away from the CNS. Sensory neurons conduct afferent impulses that give rise to sensations. The cell bodies of *upper motor*

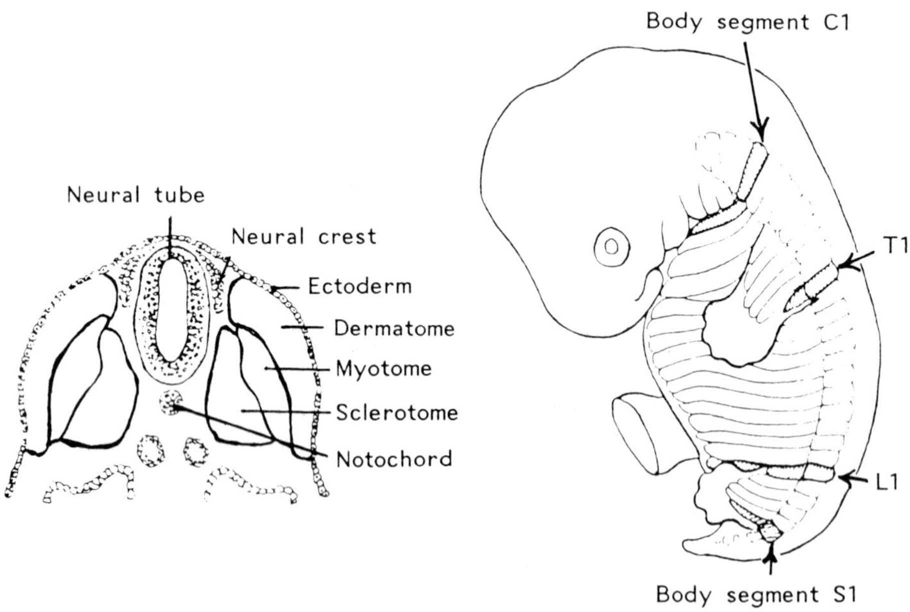

Figure 2.3. *Left,* schematic of transverse section of 1-month old embryo, showing the early formation of dermatome, myotome, and sclerotome from somites. *Right,* early embryo, depicting segmentation in terms of mesodermal somites (myotomes).

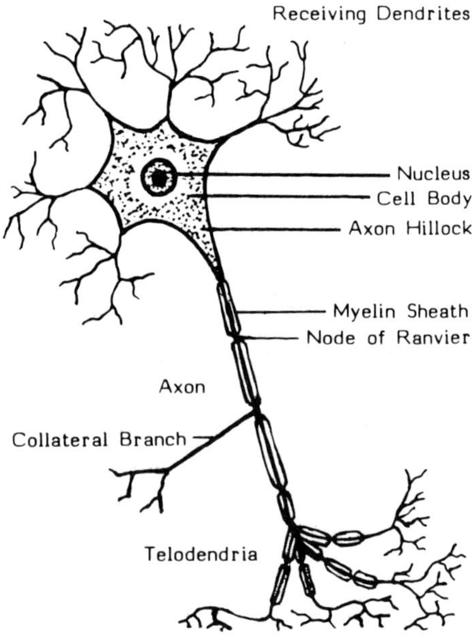

Figure 2.4. Schematic of a multipolar peripheral motor neuron.

neurons lie in the motor area of the cerebral cortex and their axons conduct efferent impulses down the spinal cord to synapse with lower motor neurons. The cells bodies of *lower motor neurons* lie within the anterior gray columns of the spinal cord, their axon terminals innervate striated muscle, and their impulses initiate muscle contraction. The axon of a *commissural neuron* crosses to the opposite side of the brain or spinal cord. An *associative neuron* mediates impulses between neurons, often between a sensory and motor neuron. The cell body of a *preganglionic neuron* lies within the CNS, and its axon ends within an autonomic ganglion. A *postganglionic neuron* has its cell body in an autonomic ganglion, and its axon terminates in smooth muscle of viscera, the heart, or a gland. *Inhibitory neurons* have the effect of lessening activity of the cells innervated, and *excitatory neurons* activate function of the cells supplied.

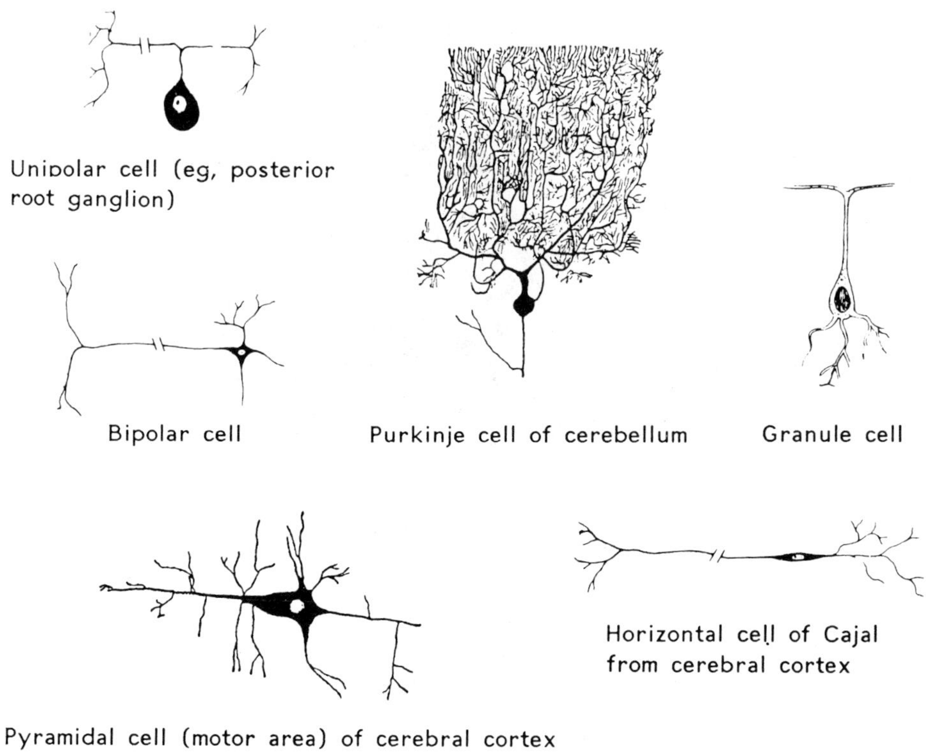

Figure 2.5. Neurons vary considerably in size and shape according to their location and function.

Neuroglia

Neuroglia, sometimes called glia, is the collection of glue-like nonneuronal cellular elements that surround cranial and spinal ganglia of the central and peripheral nervous systems. Neuroglia primarily consists of oligodendroglia cells, astrocytes, ependymal cells, microglia cells, and connective-tissue elements. The Schwann cells around peripheral nerve fibers function in a similar manner to the oligodendroglia cells of the CNS. Only a few decades ago, neuroglia was believed to serve only as supporting cells between neurons and their supplying blood vessels, but it is now known to have important metabolic functions.

Microglia cells and connective-tissue elements are derived from mesoderm that originally surrounded the neural tube. All other neuroglia cells are of ectodermal origin (cells of primitive neuroectoderm that lined the neural tube).

Astrocytes, Ependymal Cells, and Microglia

Astrocytes are large neuroglia cells, which are sometimes called macroglia or spider cells (Fig. 2.7). Their function appears to be in selectively transporting substances between capillaries and the neurons of the CNS.

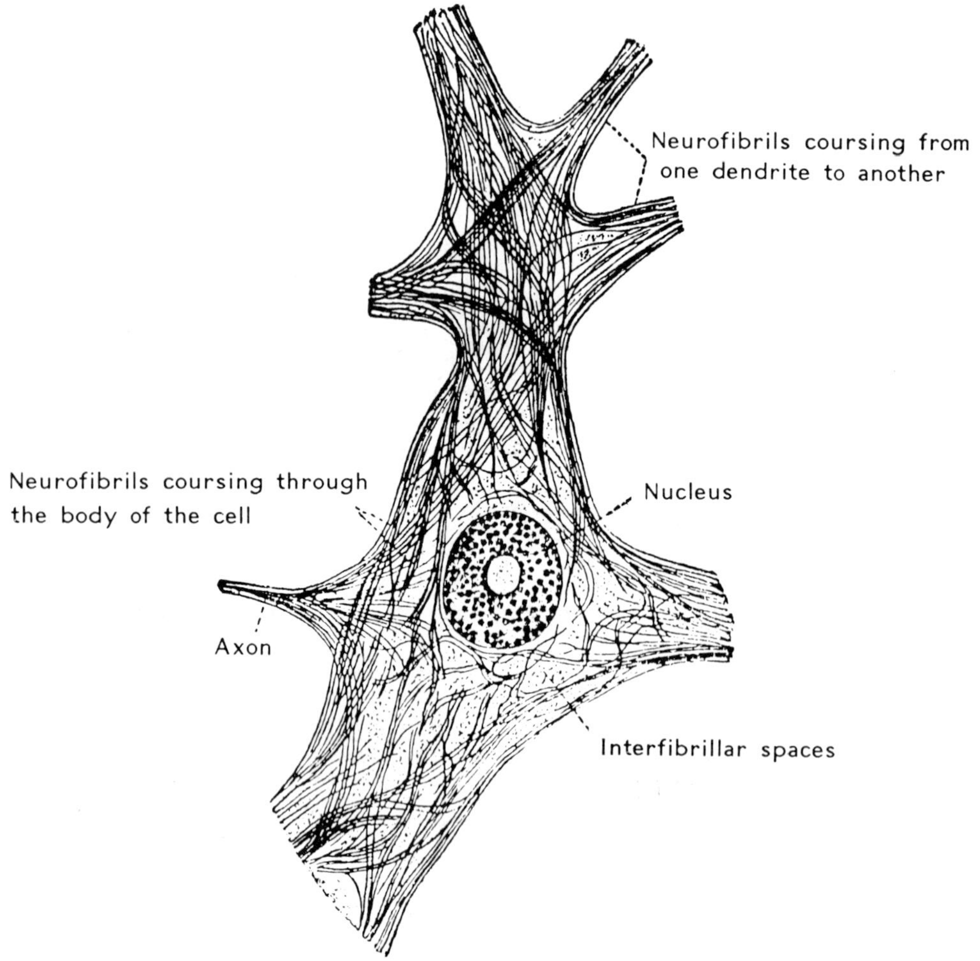

Figure 2.6. Showing neurofibrils in a cell from the anterior gray column of the spinal column.

Ependymal cells form the membrane lining the central canal of the spinal cord and the ventricles of the brain. Their function appears to be in serving as a selective barrier between cerebrospinal fluid and brain tissue.

Microglia (mesoglia) are seen in small numbers that are widely scattered throughout the CNS. They are small neuroglia cells that may proliferate rapidly and become phagocytic to remove damaged tissue or foreign organisms. Thus, they are often considered elements of the reticuloendothelial system.

Oligodendroglia, Schwann Cells, and Myelination

The *oligodendroglia cells* of the CNS have a variable number of veil-like processes that wrap around individual axons to form the myelin sheath. Thus, they are predominant in white matter of the CNS. In the peripheral nervous system, *Schwann cells* are responsible for forming the insulating sheaths of myelin (a protein-lipid substance).

The plasma membrane of a Schwann cell twirls about a segment of the axon and tightens to squeeze out the cytoplasm; then the apposing surfaces of the membranes become fused (Fig. 2.8). The final thickness of a myelin sheath is generally proportional to axon length and diameter. A single Schwann cell is responsible for the myelination of only a certain length of axon, which varies in length according to the axon's thickness, and each segment is separated by a minute gap (internode) called a *node of Ranvier*. In contrast, a single oligodendroglia cell may myelinate several adjacent axons in the CNS.

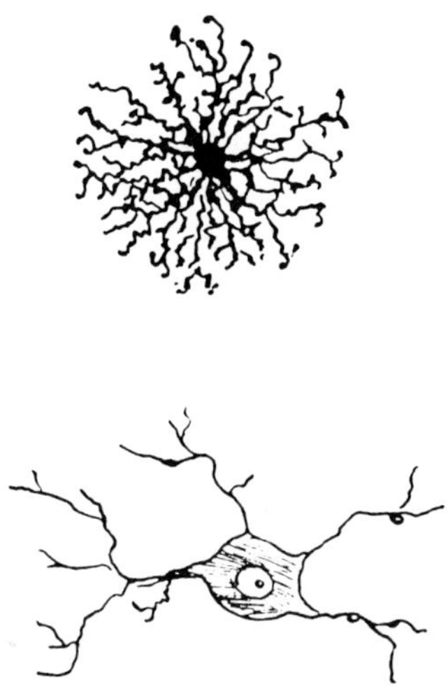

Figure 2.7. Neuroglia cells; *upper,* an astrocyte; *bottom,* an oligodendroglia cell.

Myelination does not occur around the perikaryon, its hillock, or its dendrites. Thus, where there are large concentrations of nerve cell bodies such as at the cerebral cortex, basal ganglia of the brain stem, much of the thalamic area, and the anterior horns of the spinal cord, these cell bodies constitute the gray matter of the CNS. Thus, the gray matter contains the cell bodies and synapses where the adjusting of sensory to motor neurons takes place, forming the major collecting and distributing stations. The white matter of the CNS is formed by the relatively large myelinated and fine unmyelinated fibers that are grouped together into the nerves and tracts of the brain and spinal cord.

Many peripheral nerves have an inseparable myelin sheath and a neurilemma (Fig. 2.9), both of which are products of Schwann cells. The neurilemma is a thin membrane

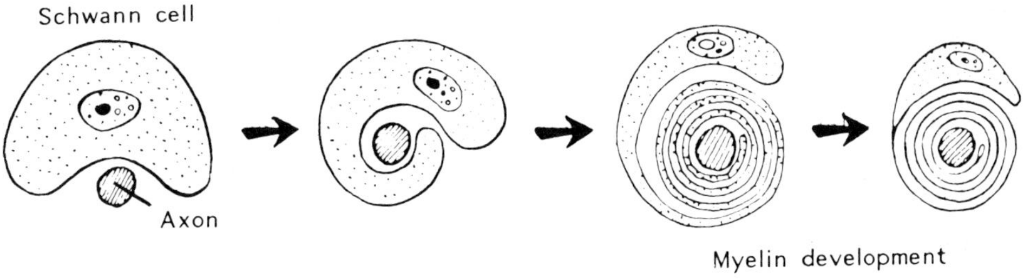

Figure 2.8. The progressive steps of a Schwann cell during myelination.

that enwraps the spiraling layers of myelin. Nerve fibers located within the white matter of the brain and spinal cord have a myelin sheath but no neurilemma. In contrast, postganglionic autonomic fibers have a neurilemma but no myelin sheath.

Impulse conduction within an axon travels at a much more rapid rate in myelinated fibers than in unmyelinated fibers. This is because the multiple layers of regularly-arranged concentric rings of lipid molecules of Schwann cell membrane (which is free of cytoplasm) is an excellent electric insulator. Thus, neurons that must convey impulses rapidly to and from the CNS are heavily myelinated. In contrast, the postganglionic fibers in the sympathetic nervous system have no apparent myelin sheath and viscerosensory nerves have only a thin coating.

Chusid points out that myelination of the spinal cord begins about midfetal life but is not complete in some tracts until another 20 years later. The oldest tracts myelinate first; the pyramidal tracts myelinate later, especially during the 1st and 2nd year of life.

Connective Tissue

All parts of the neuron are encased in a membrane that acts as a boundary between its biochemical contents and that of the surrounding medium. The peripheral nerves are richly surrounded by connective tissue. Each myelinated nerve is surrounded by collagenous *endoneurium*, groups of fibers are bound by *perineurium*, and these groups form a nerve trunk that is covered by a thick sheath of *epineurium* (Fig. 2.10). These three sheaths of connective tissue are analogous to the pia, arachnoid, and dura maters of the CNS and are continuous with them at the spinal root level. A similar system is seen in muscle tissue. Each cylindrical muscle fiber is covered with a specialized layer of sarcolemma that covers a peripheral longitudinal layer of nuclei and cylindrical myofibrils, and sarcolemma insulates each fiber from adjacent fibers so that nervous excitation of one fiber does not affect its neighbors.

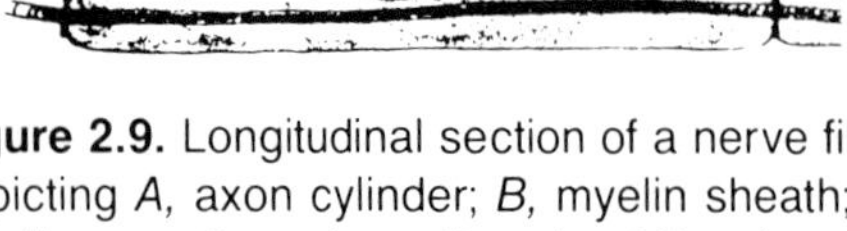

Figure 2.9. Longitudinal section of a nerve fiber depicting *A*, axon cylinder; *B*, myelin sheath; *C*, neurilemma; *D*, nucleus; *E*, node of Ranvier.

Except for the surrounding meninges, the parenchyma of the CNS is sparse in terms of gross connective tissue except for that around the larger blood vessels. It is for this reason that scar tissue formation is rarely a significant consequence of CNS infection.

Electric Changes in Axons

The electric activity of the nervous system has given the investigator a means of studying the functioning nervous system, but it is not likened to an electric current flowing over a wire. It is a process of progressive ionic changes whose electric signs constitute the action potential. Rather than think of nerve fibers as electric extension cords, some physiologists feel it would be better to think of them as living, squirming, moving streams through which a peristaltic-like flow of electrochemical supplies is driven from the cell body.

The Functional Parts

Each functioning neuron consists of the four specialized functional parts previously described: the receiving dendrites, the nerve

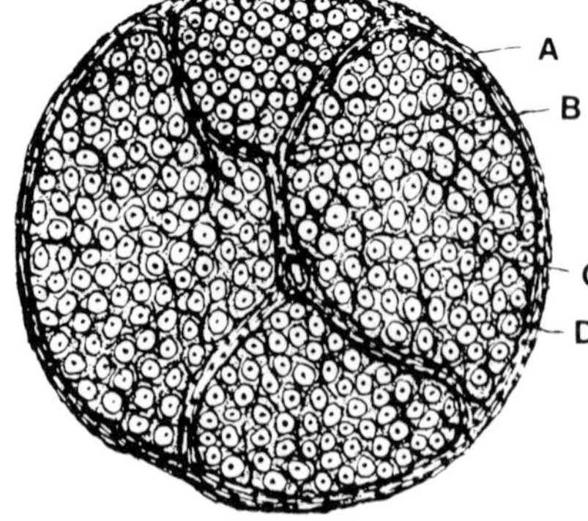

Figure 2.10. Transverse section of a nerve. *A*, epineurium; *B*, perineurium; *C*, endoneurium; *D*, section of a single fiber.

cell body, the axon, and its transmitting area. The terminal transmitting area consists of several synaptic knobs (end feet), which, according to Guyton, may range in number from a few to more than 100,000. The general arrangement of neurons depends to a large extent on the connections that they establish with each other for functional purposes.

The Reception Area. Once a neuron is stimulated, which is usually at its receptor organs, excitation develops by graded depolarization that travels over the dendrites and nerve cell body.

The Cell Body. The perikaryon serves as the metabolic center of activity. Impulses are initiated by an ionic change in the cell's cytoplasm following an influx of sodium, which produces a polarity reversal so that the inner cell is briefly positive compared with the negative cell exterior. If an electric connection is made between the inside and outside of a neuron, the cell acts as a battery, and an electric current is initiated. This process continues along the axon. The speed of the impulse varies in proportion to the fiber's diameter: faster in large-diameter fibers, slower in small-diameter axons. Some human nerves conduct impulses at a rate exceeding 200 miles/hour.

The Axon. Action potentials are produced and conducted along the axon if its initial segment is sufficiently depolarized. Efferent nerve impulses are produced in the axon near the nerve cell body at an unmyelinated low-threshold dendrite area, and they are transmitted in an all-or-none manner in both velocity and magnitude by an *action potential.*

The Transmitting Terminals. The terminals of an axon contain multiple, tiny, mitochondria-containing vesicles that serve as a reservoir for biochemical neurotransmitters. Various synonyms are used to describe these end organs such as boutons, end feet, presynaptic terminals, synaptic knobs, or terminal knobs.

The Impulse Flow

Although the electrochemical processes underlying the production of changes in potential are not established beyond dispute, there is little doubt that there is only one type of nerve impulse and that this is universal to the nervous system. It has also been known for some time that it is the nerve itself and not the stimulus that provides the energy for transmission of the impulse. Brazier explains that the traveling impulse within a nerve is a progression of ionic changes that derive their energy for their transmission from the metabolic activity of the nerve itself and not from the stimulus. The stimulus only serves as a "trigger" to initiate the mechanisms involved.

Each point at which an impulse reaches becomes electrically negative to the inactive regions on each side of it as the wave of activity passes along the neuron. Although all nerve impulses are considered identical in character, they vary considerably in frequency, velocity, and length of train.

An action potential initiated in the fingertip, for example, will spread up its axon to the dorsal root ganglion in the cervical spinal cord, ascend to the brain stem via one or more central axons, and then communicate with cerebral centers via other fibers. This process *(neuronal propagation)* is what allows the nervous system to transmit information from one area of the body to another.

Impulse Progression. The propagated action potential along a nerve is primarily dependent on the different concentrations of sodium and potassium ions on the two sides of the semipermeable membrane covering the nerve fiber. According to the *membrane theory,* the "pores" of this surface membrane are permeable to potassium and impermeable to sodium when resting. The resting (polarized) state, in which the inside of the membrane is negatively charged and the outside of the membrane is positively charged, is the result of electrochemical processes in the neurons and serves as a potential source of energy (Fig. 2.11).

When a neuron is excited electrically or chemically, electrochemical changes occur at the point of stimulation that depolarize the membrane so that its resting permeability is altered. Its electric status is reversed so that the inside of the membrane becomes positively charged and the outside of the membrane becomes negatively charged. Because of this change in polarity, the self-propagated current flows from the stimulated (active) area on the neuron to the adjacent inactive area largely by sodium and potassium ion concentration changes. This area, in turn, becomes the new active area to excite the next area. After passage of a nerve impulse, repolarization and ionic balance during the *refractory period* are quickly restored so that another impulse can be received. In myelinated nerves, the active region "triggers" the resting area ahead only at the nodes of Ranvier, where myelin is absent; ie, the nerve impulse is propagated from node to node (refer to Fig. 2.11).

Wavelengths. As the impulse travels along a nerve, the length of the traveling region of activity that shows a potential change from its resting state is called the *wavelength*. The wavelengths of fine fibers measure only a few millimeters, but those of large fibers may be 5—6 centimeters in length.

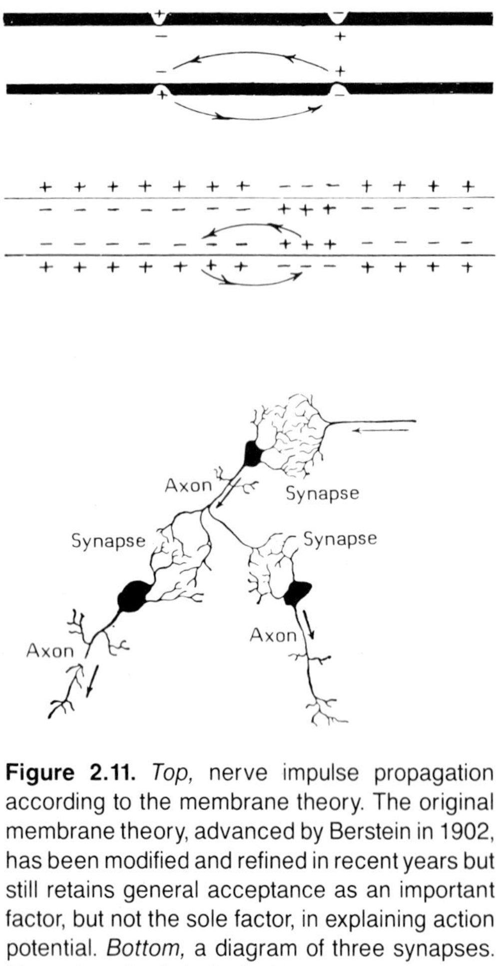

Figure 2.11. *Top,* nerve impulse propagation according to the membrane theory. The original membrane theory, advanced by Berstein in 1902, has been modified and refined in recent years but still retains general acceptance as an important factor, but not the sole factor, in explaining action potential. *Bottom,* a diagram of three synapses. Nerve impulse is indicated by arrows.

Excitable and Nonexcitable Periods. Three distinct periods should be noted when action currents within nerves are studied: (1) the normal period, (2) an absolute refractory period, and (3) a relative refractory period.

• *The absolute refractory period.* This is a short period following stimulation during which the nerve fiber is not excitable, making it impossible for a fiber to respond continuously to stimuli. Thus, there is a rhythmic discharge of nervous waves (impulses) from receptor to nerve fiber rather than a continuous flow. Small nerve fibers have longer refractory periods than do large fibers.

• *The relative refractory period.* The intensity of a stimulus at the receptor end of a fiber must reach threshold value before it can excite the neuron. During the relative refractory period, the stimulus must be stronger than during the normal resting period. The smaller the fiber, the higher the threshold value of the stimulus must be to produce excitation.

Impulse Frequency, Speed, and Strength. The frequency of impulses usually varies directly with the strength of the stimulus. Velocity of conduction, as described previously, varies with the diameter of the neuron's axis cylinder; ie, thicker fibers conduct more rapidly than finer fibers. Although the strength of the electric charge of a neuron varies according to its size, all neurons are governed by the *all-or-none law*, which states that fibers give a maximum response to a stimulus or no response at all; ie, a stimulus above threshold value will not increase the strength of a single fiber's electric charge.

The largest and fastest fibers in most peripheral nerves are those that bring messages to the CNS about skeletal muscle tension and position. Motor neurons to skeletal muscle are almost as large. The prominence of these types of fibers reflects the adaptive utility of rapid movement. Sensory data from cutaneous structures and viscera travel centrally much slower. Autonomic efferent fibers to smooth muscles and glands are even smaller and slower compared to those of somatic neurons.

Impulse Spread. The nervous system as a whole is bound together by connecting pathways. Some of these are long well-defined fiber bundles that are connected in a manner to enhance uniform and definite responses to stimulation. Other pathways are diffuse, poorly integrated, and not well adapted to conduct impulses over long distances.

Neuronal impulses have many pathways open to them. The varying resistance offered at available synapses usually prevents a wide diffusion, and the formation of pathways reenforces this limitation. Nevertheless, an unusually strong stimulus may produce a great impulse spread throughout the gray mater. If this happens, a barrage of efferent impulses may be sent to large groups of muscles (eg, gross contractions, convulsions). Typical examples of this are often seen in the spreading of impulses that occurs readily in infants in comparison to that in the adult. Conditions that may cause marked contractions in an infant commonly produce only a mild reaction in an adult (eg, gooseflesh).

Because they are junction points in the communication system of neuronal impulses, synapses play an important role in selecting and processing neuronal messages. They determine the directions of signal spread and the ease or difficulty of impulse transmission, which allows signal blocking or amplification. They also determine the quantity of connections; ie, changing the impulse of one or a few neurons to impulses within multiple neurons, changing impulses from multiple neurons to impulses within one or a few connecting neurons, or causing highly intricate impulse patterns in successive neurons.

Convergence of Impulses. Impulses arising from many receptors may converge upon one nerve fiber (effector mechanism), which becomes the *final common path* for all the impulse activity (Fig. 2.12). Thus, stimulation of many receptors will produce a more vigorous response than the stimulation of only a few receptors. The energy of one impulse is added to the energy of other impulses activated at the same time when all have more or less open pathways to a common effector.

The Synaptic Chemical Transmitters. The transmitting pole of the axon ends in branching terminal telodendria with unmyelinated tips. Chemical transmitters are synthesized by enzymes manufactured in the cell body and transferred along the axon by the active oxygen-dependent axoplasmic transport system. These chemicals are then stored until needed in the axon terminals within small vesicles.

When the energy impulse reaches the terminals (by sodium entering the fiber and potassium leaving it), a chemical transmitter substance (excitatory or inhibitory) is liberated into the synapse in proportion to the magnitude of the impulse, diffuses across the synaptic space, and chemically affects the receptor sites at the postsynaptic dendrites or effector cell(s). It is likely that neural impulses accelerate on-going transmitter secretory processes, rather than initiate them from a completely inactive state.

Prichard explains that calcium must be present in the extracellular fluid around the synapse for transmitter release to occur. Current theory holds that depolarization of a presynaptic terminal causes calcium to enter the terminal vesicles from extracellular fluid. This leads to a release of large numbers of transmitter molecules into the synaptic cleft, across which they diffuse and contact excitatory or inhibitory receptors on the postsynaptic surface of the receiving membrane. Thus, the same chemical transmitter (eg, norepinephrine) may have an excitatory or inhibitory effect, depending upon the net effect of the receptors stimulated. To add to the complexity, some receiving membranes reach their maximum effect in 1—2 milliseconds, others in 200—300 milliseconds. In addition, some synaptic effects last for a fraction of a second, others for several hours. Some transmitters increase the firing rate of neurons, while others *(modulators)* have no effect on firing rates but change the connecting neuron's sensitivity to other transmitter substances.

About 30 different transmitter substances have been isolated to date. A list of major transmitters is shown in Table 2.2.

The Somatic Neural Communication Chain. Each presynaptic neuron communicates with many postsynaptic neurons, and

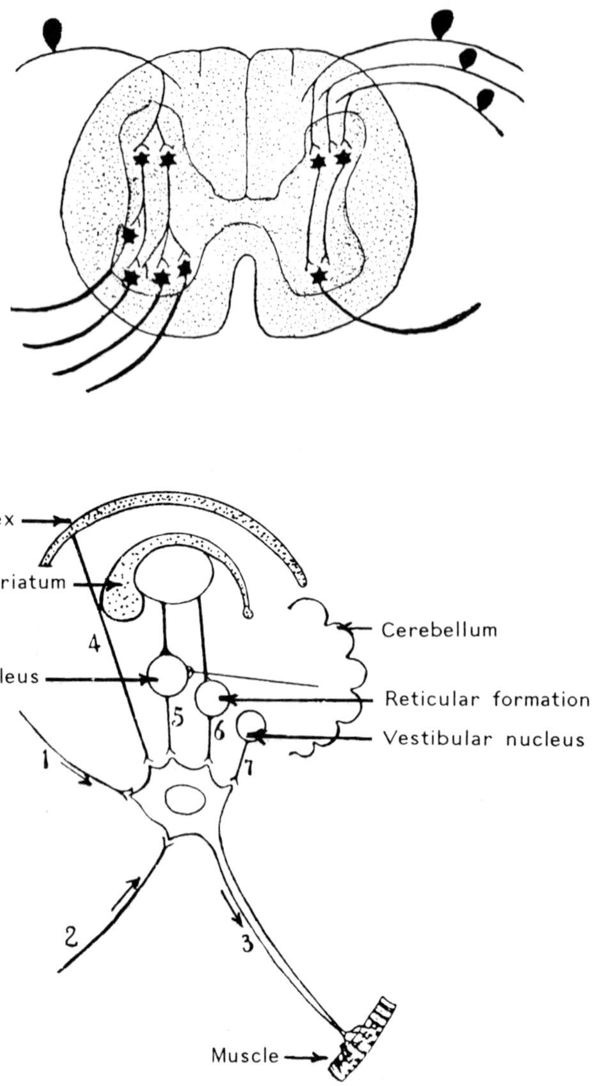

Figure 2.12. *Top,* cross section of the spinal cord depicting a spreading reflex on the left and a converging reflex on the right. *Bottom,* convergence of various paths upon an anterior horn cell: afferent fibers from periphery, *1* and *2;* final common path motor neuron, *3;* corticospinal fiber, *4;* rubrospinal fiber, *5;* reticulospinal fiber, *6;* and vestibulospinal fiber, *7.*

Table 2.2. Major Synaptic Transmitter Substances

Name	Primary Location(s) of Originating Neurons	Usual Action
Acetylcholine	Basal ganglia, other parts of the brain, terminals of recurrent nerve in the anterior horns of the spinal cord	Excitatory, except possibly at some peripheral parasympathetic synapses
Dopamine	Substantia nigra, essentially those fibers that terminate in the striatal portion of the basal ganglia	Inhibitory
Enkephalins and endorphins	Terminals in the thalamus, hypothalamus, brain stem, and spinal cord	Excite secondary inhibitory systems
Epinephrine	Brain stem hypothalamus	Inhibitory
Gamma aminobutyric acid (GABA)	Neurons that terminate in the spinal cord, cerebellum, basal ganglia, and other areas	Inhibitory
Glutamic acid	Terminals of various sensory pathways	Excitatory
Glycine	Neurons that terminate in the spinal cord	Inhibitory
Norepinephrine	Brain stem, hypothalamus	Inhibitory
Serotonin	Median raphe of brain stem that terminate in the brain, hypothalamus, and dorsal horns of spinal cord	Inhibitory (especially pain and anxiety-producing impulses)
Substance P	Pain fibers terminating in the substantia gelatinosa of the spinal cord	Excitatory

each neuron in the chain repeats this excitation generation, conduction, and transmission process until the last neuron in the chain releases its transmitter substance at the effector (eg, a neuromuscular junction). This communication is usually considered to be unidirectional, but some authorities believe a reverse flow occurs in such disorders as fasciculations, myokymia, causalgia, and phantom-limb phenomena.

Somatic Effector Impulse Variables. A muscle reacts in proportion to the quantity of fibers activated and the frequency of impulse bombardment. A neural impulse, to be adequate for muscle contraction, must consist of several appropriate variables. These include sufficient stimulus intensity, frequency of impulse bombardment, rate of wave rise, and duration to fire the contractile elements within the muscle fibers.

Chemical Synaptic Inhibition and Extrication

As synaptic function is based on a carefully controlled integration of chemical influences, a slight chemical imbalance (eg, from certain medications, nutritional and electrolytic imbalances) may produce a distinct effect upon synaptic transmission in terms of noxious systemic and behavioral effects. Impulse transmission among billions of neurons, many of which have thousands of transmitter-releasing terminals, is one reason the nervous system is the most complex tissue in the animal kingdom.

Action potential transmission at the synapse is not in the all-or-none fashion. It may be inhibited or amplified according to the specific type of transmitter substance produced. Inhibitory factors can also be produced presynaptically in the axon or produced centrally by hypoxia or drugs. Synapses are more readily fatigued than are nerve fibers, and they are more readily affected by anesthetics and other drugs (eg, nicotine).

When stimulated, some fibers (cholinergic) liberate an acetylcholine substance; other fibers (adrenergic) liberate epinephrine. These neurotransmitters are the two major substances liberated at synapses, but more have been isolated and many more are suspected. The cholinergic fibers include all preganglionic fibers, all postganglionic parasympathetic fibers, postganglionic sympathetic fibers to the sweat glands, and efferent fibers to skeletal muscle. The adrenergic fibers include nearly all postganglionic sympathetic fibers except those supplying the sweat glands.

A hypersensitive synaptic response to stimuli often follows the depression of higher inhibition centers, where even slight stimulation may be interpreted as pain and mild sounds are perceived as loud noises. While in this condition systemically, an individual is highly susceptible to suggestion—beneficial or detrimental.

Electric Transmission

It has recently been shown that some nerves communicate with each other by electric rather than chemical transmission at synapses. The mechanism is probably due to linkage of cytoplasmic bridges between end feet and receptor membranes. The transmission usually has an excitatory effect, but for reasons unknown, it may be inhibitory in some situations.

Unlike chemical transmission, Pappas shows that electric synaptic transmission may be bidirectional; thus, either side may be pre- or post-synaptic at different times. While it has been shown that electric transmission is also faster than chemical transmission, further studies are necessary to determine the exact scope, distribution, and mechanisms involved in humans.

Axoplasmic Flow

During impulse activity, materials are transported from the cell body's endoplasmic reticulum, microtubules, and neurofilaments along the axon via its gel-like *axoplasm* that is continuously synthesized in the cell body. This axoplasmic flow moves materials slowly up and down the fibers during impulse activity.

Investigations, still in their infancy, have isolated three major types of axoplasmic transport: *fast, slow, and retrograde.* The exact mechanisms are unknown, but certain facts have been demonstrated. For example, fast transport seems to move polypeptides, proteins, and particulate matter at a rate of 400mm/day. This rate depends on tissue temperature and oxygen and ATP concentrations; age and fiber function or size are not factors. It is thought that protein filaments bind to the transported material and creep along the axon by attaching to successive locations on the longitudinally oriented microtubules. If a neuron becomes ischemic, electric excitability and fast transport fail in about 15 minutes.

Slow transport moves at a rate of 1—3mm/day and appears to be linked to the transient binding of mitochondria to the same protein filaments involved in fast transport. Axon mitochondria have been observed to have a constant to-and-from movement with a net distalward drift.

Retrograde transport has most of the properties of fast transport except its rate is about 200mm/day. It is postulated that it may be the mechanism for the centripetal movement of certain viruses and toxins (eg, rabies, tetanus).

Interneuron Communication

There are four basic ways in which neurons are functionally linked together: (1) one receptor neuron may be linked with one connector neuron that communicates with one effector neuron (Fig. 2.13). This is a rare occurrence. (2) One receptor neuron may be linked to one connector neuron that relays messages to several effector neurons. (3) Several receptor neurons may be linked to one connector neuron that communicates with one effector neuron. (4) Several re-

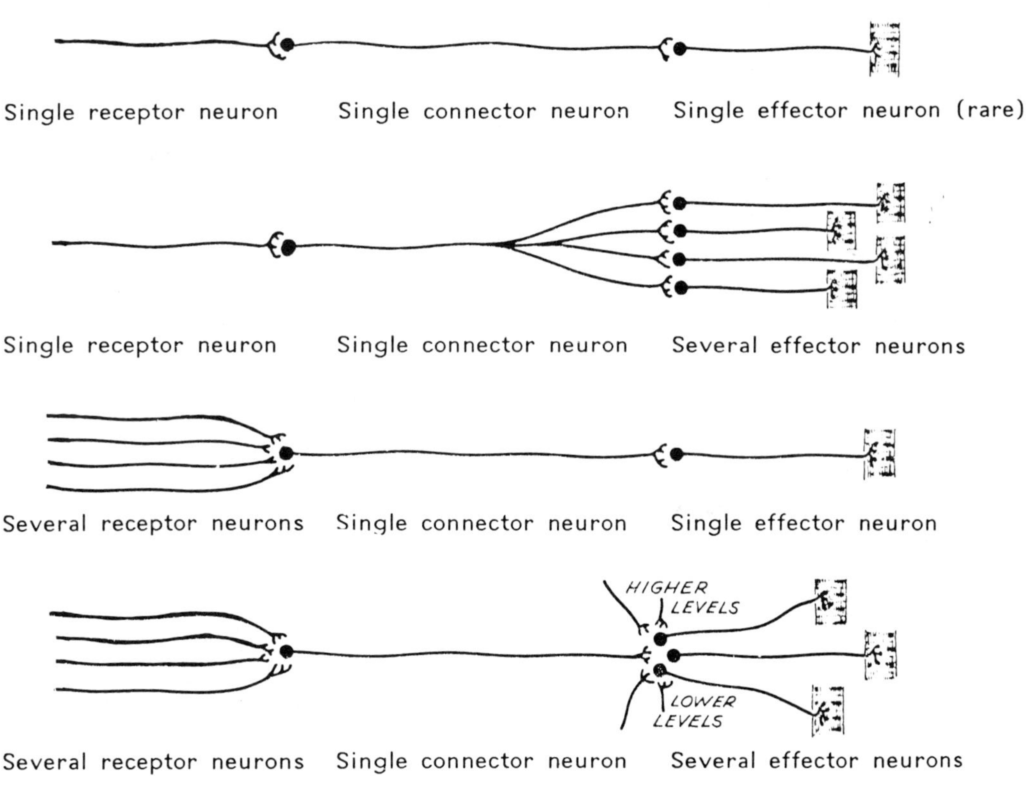

Figure 2.13. The four basic types of neuron receptor-connector-effector arrangement. Not shown in the above diagrams are the collateral branches. Most axons give off one or more collaterals.

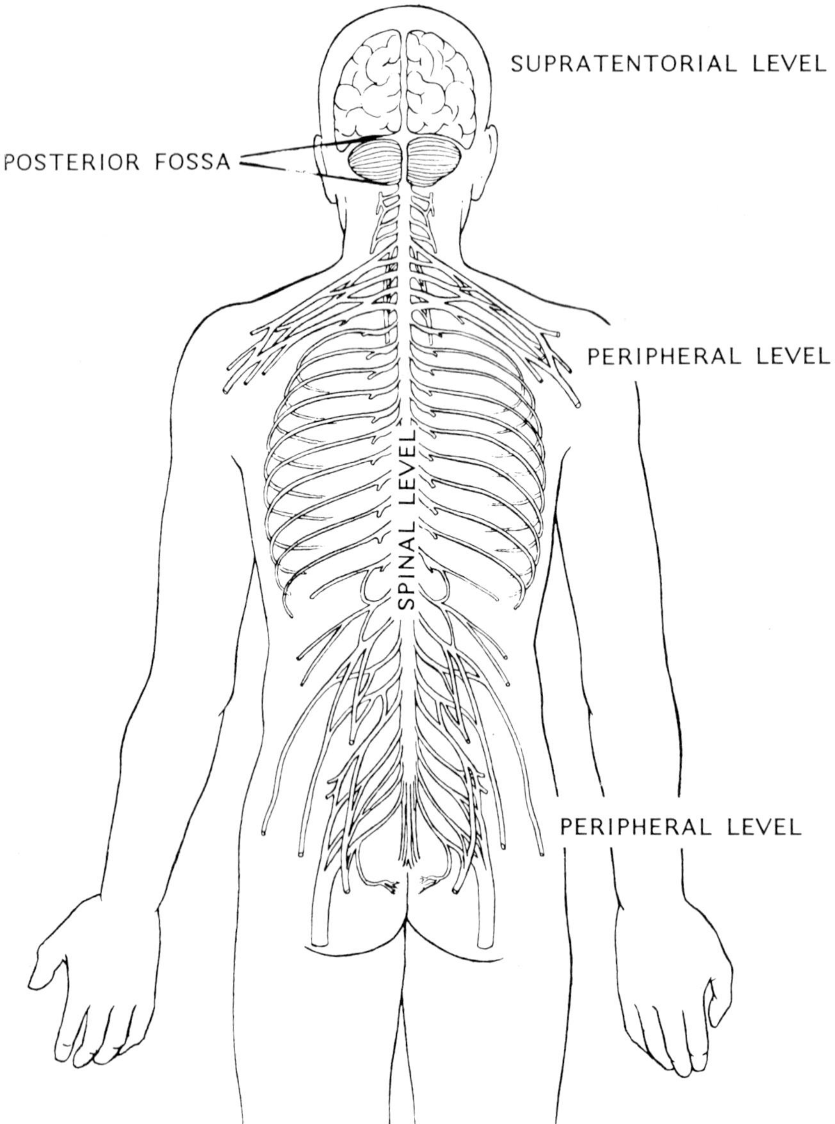

Figure 2.14. Levels of the neuraxis.

ceptor neurons may be linked to one connector neuron that relays messages to several higher and/or lower effector neurons.

The dendrite tree of a single neuron's cell body may consist of hundreds of synapses communicating from multiple sources, and its axon may send off collaterals to form synapses with many other neurons, gland cells, or muscle cells. Some axons (eg, Golgi Type I) extend far from the cell body to conduct messages within the CNS, while other axons (eg, Golgi Type II) end near or within the dendritic field of the neuron. Daube/Sandok feel that these latter axons are probably more involved in data processing than data conduction.

GROSS NEUROLOGIC AREAS AND LEVELS

The basic concerns of neurologic diagnosis are to determine if there is a lesion involving the nervous system; if so, where is it located; what is its nature; and how can the condition be best corrected? To determine the anatomical location from which the neurologic signs and symptoms are initiated, the nervous system can be analyzed from the standpoint of arbitrary levels and longitudinal systems and whether the lesion is unilateral, midline, bilateral, or diffuse.

The levels of the neuraxis, as classified in this manual, are shown in Figure 2.14. These levels are not exact anatomical divisions; rather, they are bounded areas that are useful during neurologic diagnosis. They are:

1. *The supratentorial level*, which consists of the cerebral hemispheres and parts of cranial nerves I and II.
2. *The posterior fossa level*, which is composed of the cerebellum, brain stem, and portions of cranial nerves III—XII.
3. *The spinal level*, which includes the spinal cord and parts of the nerve roots contained in or near the intervertebral foramen.
4. *The peripheral level*, which consists of parts of both cranial and peripheral nerves that are located outside the cranial vault and vertebral column, and the structures innervated by these nerves.

Basic Considerations

Nerve Composition

A longitudinal section of a peripheral nerve is shown in Figure 2.15. A bundle of these fibers enclosed in a tubular sheath is called a *funiculus*. A nerve may consist of a single funiculus or of many funiculi collected into larger bundles. This cable grouping is practical in that it affords a variety of different types of nerve fibers a common vascular supply, but it also allows common susceptibility to local mechanical, metabolic, and thermal conditions. An interesting characteristic of fascicular structure is its constant rearrangement in the longitudinal dimension; ie, fibers destined to branch from a main nerve trunk in the same branch are concentrated in the same fascicle or in adjacent ones well before the branch point.

It has been previously described that each myelinated nerve is surrounded by collagenous *endoneurium*, intrafascicular connective tissue, which serves to bind the fibers together into funiculi. Endoneurium consists primarily of collagen and fibroblasts that invest axons and related Schwann cells and are usually separated from them by basal membrane (laminae). Each myelinated fiber occupies a tubule that is formed by endoneurium, and several unmyelinated fibers may be enveloped by the same chain of Schwann cells located in one endoneurial tubule.

Groups of funiculi are bound by *perineurium* to form a tubular sheath, and these groups form a nerve trunk that is covered by a thick sheath of *epineurium* (refer to Fig. 2.10). The pathway of a group or bundle of nerve fibers within the spinal cord or brain that constitutes an anatomical or functional unit is called a *tract*.

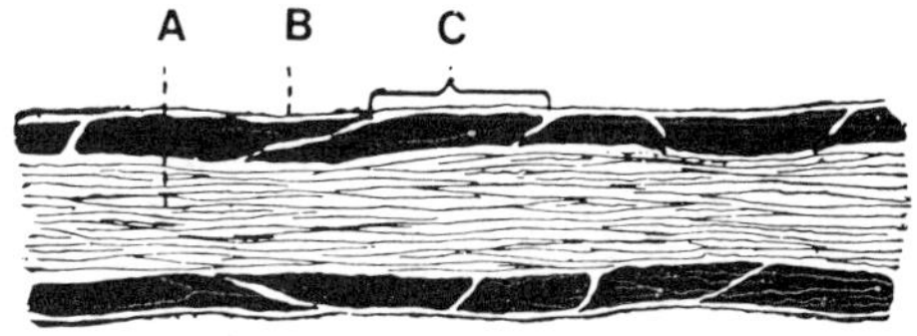

Figure 2.15. Longitudinal section through a nerve fiber. *A*, fibrils of axis cylinder; *B*, neurilemma; *C*, segment of Lantermann.

Perineurium is composed of connective-tissue elements mixed with a concentric lamellae of flattened polygonal cells that serve as the primary barrier to diffusion of many types of substances through nerve. Olsson states that vascular permeability within the perineurium is sharply limited compared to all other tissues except the CNS. It is also worthy to note that current theory holds that a system similar to the blood-brain barrier seen in the brain appears to exist in peripheral nerves.

Epineurium, in contrast to perineurium, is a loose connective tissue that does not firmly adhere to adjacent structures. Thus, the mobility of a nerve is limited mainly by its tethering branches and attached blood vessels. The capillaries supplying a nerve penetrate the perineurium and either run parallel with the fibers, which is typical, or form short transverse connecting vessels. Fine nerve fibers (vasomotor) accompany these capillaries and play a vital role in neuronal health and during therapy.

Considerably more than 75% of a nerve is composed of nonnervous substance. About 50% consists of areolar connective tissue, blood, and lymph. More than 25% is myelin.

Nerves branch frequently throughout their courses, and these branches often meet with one another or with the branches of other nerves. Yet, each fiber always remains distinct. A nerve, therefore, is merely an association of individual fibers that function independently of one another. Most nerves are mixed nerves; ie, they contain both sensory and motor fibers of widely different sizes.

Like branches of a tree, nerve-cell processes and their collateral branches decreasingly taper in size as they extend peripherally, becoming smaller in diameter than their parent trunks. This characteristic is important to remember because nerve conduction velocity is directly proportional to the diameter of the axon.

Ganglions, Nuclei, and Nerve Centers

Ganglions are collections of nerve cells outside the CNS. They appear in the course of the cranial and spinal nerves and form the ganglia of the autonomic nervous system. They are generally considered as being located peripheral to the CNS, but some large collections of nerve cells in the brain are called *ganglia* (eg, the basal ganglia) by some rather than as nuclei.

Nuclei are collections of nerve cells within the CNS, the fibers of which go to form one anatomical nerve or a tract within the brain or cord; eg, the nucleus of the facial nerve.

Nerve centers are groups of neurons and synapses regulating a certain function. They may be either nuclei or ganglions, as these terms refer to an *anatomical* entity. The term *center* refers to a *functional* entity. For example, the rate of respiration is regulated by a center in the medulla oblongata, and odor is interpreted by a center in the cerebrum. The center is in communication with the organ by means of nerve fibers and end organs that are adapted to receive and transmit specific impulses.

The fibers that connect centers with the organs they control do not usually extend all the way to the organs; they end in masses of gray matter, which serve as *relay stations*. They form synapses here with other neurons that transmit their impulses onward, possibly to one or more other relay stations or directly to the organs. There may be a large number of relay stations involved. In such a series, the neuron first to be stimulated is called the *neuron of the first order*, and the succeeding neurons are called neurons of the second, third, and fourth order, etc.

The Brain as a Whole

The brain is the largest and most complex mass of nervous tissue in the body. It comprises five connected parts: the cerebral hemispheres, the midbrain, the cerebellum, the pons, and the medulla oblongata (Fig. 2.16).

During embryonic life, the cerebral hemispheres, their commissures, and the 1st, 2nd, and 3rd ventricles are developed from the forebrain. The corpora quadrigemina, the central peduncles, and the cerebral aqueduct are developed from the midbrain. The medulla, pons, cerebellum, and 4th ventricle are developed from the hindbrain.

The weight of the adult brain is about 48.6 oz in the male and about 44 oz in the female. The weight of the brain is an indication of growth, which in early life depends on the enlargement of the cells and their processes, the myelination of certain nerve fibers, and an increase in the amount of neuroglia. The brain grows rapidly up to the 5th year of age and, in general, ceases to grow much beyond the 20th year. In advanced age, the brain gradually loses weight.

The development of the brain is not only a matter of growth but also a matter of forming new pathways; ie, new synapses and a permanent modification of the synapses that are functionally active during various forms of mental activity. The nature of brain tissue and the use to which it is put determine to some extent the length of time during which development may continue. It appears that mental activity keeps the brain active and capable of development, just as exercising a muscle tends to prevent atrophy or loss of function. This point has been commonly neglected in geriatric care, where the mentally healthy elderly are often treated socially as children.

The Skull

The brain (Fig. 2.17) appears firm in illustrations and upon dissection after being injected with a formalin solution. This firmness, however, is not present in vivo. In the living body, the brain is soft but still main-

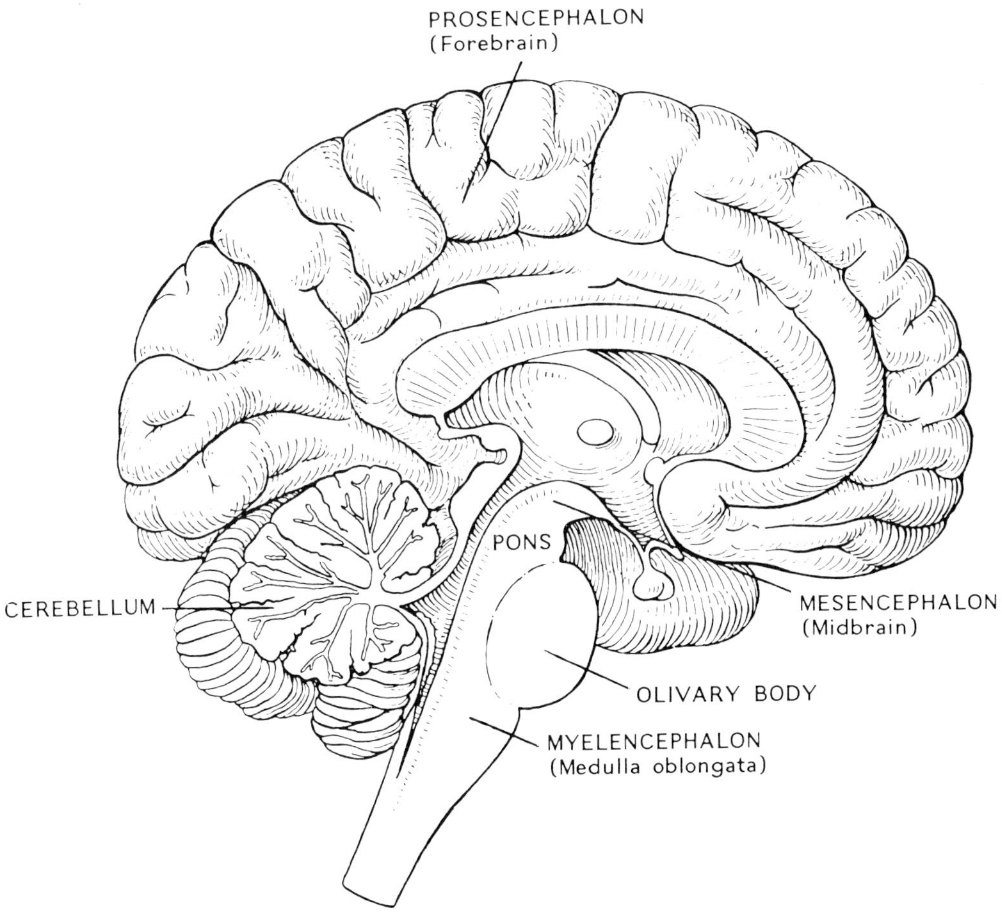

Figure 2.16. Diagram illustrating the gross divisions of the central nervous system.

tains a certain degree of cohesiveness. Because of its soft consistency, it requires dependable protection against mechanical compression.

Nilsson reminds us that a protective shielding is furnished by the bone-lined cranial cavity. The individual bones forming the cranial vault are the paired temporal and parietal and the single frontal, ethmoid, sphenoid, and occipital bones (Fig. 2.18). Firmly adherent to the external cranial wall, except under its floor, is the scalp. This structure is composed of the skin, the tela subcutanea, the galea aponeurotica, the subaponeurotic soft tissue, and the external periosteum of the bones forming the roof and sides of the cranium.

On the inner cranial wall is the internal periosteum (also referred to by some as the external layer of the cranial dura matter), while next to it is the shallow subdural space containing a small amount of fluid. Then follows the arachnoid meninx and the subarachnoid cerebrospinal fluid. The innermost meninx is the pia mater, which lines the surface of the brain.

Besides the classic brain-protecting structures and elements of the scalp, cranium, meninges, and cerebrospinal fluid, other structures help as shock absorbers to protect the brain. These include joint fat, ligaments, discs, muscles, and the spinal curves that soften or entirely obliterate most sharp jars from harming the brain during body movements.

The Fontanels and Sutures

The anterior and larger fontanel remains about the same size for the first year of life,

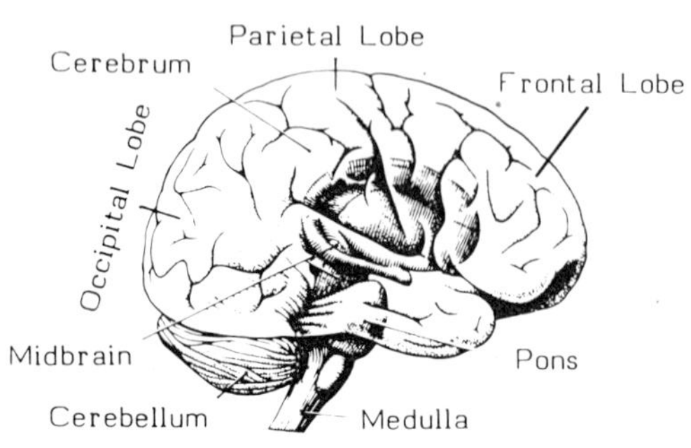

Figure 2.17. Lateral schematic of the brain.

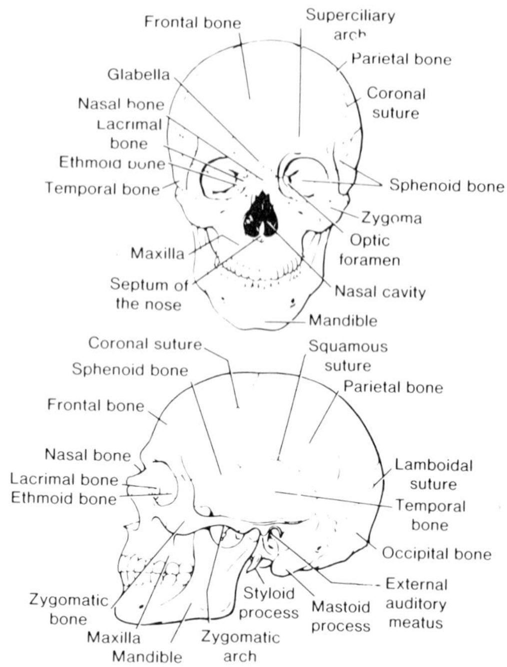

Figure 2.18. Bones of the cranium.

then diminishes and closes about the 12th month. The posterior fontanel closes in about 6 weeks. In rickets, hydrocephalus, hereditary syphilis, and cretinism, the fontanels and sutures remain open after the normal time for closure.

Normal skull measurements and proportions depend upon the proper sequential closing of the sutures, and most all abnormal head shapes are the result of premature closure. Growth always occurs in a direction perpendicular to the line of the suture, thus inspection and palpation allow us to determine the suture(s) at fault. If one suture closes prematurely, growth occurs in the remaining open sutures in compensation and this results in deformity.

The Meninges

The brain and spinal cord are enclosed within three membranes. They are, from without inward, the dura mater, arachnoid mater, and pia mater.

Dura Mater

The dura mater is a dense membrane of fibrous connective tissue that contains many blood vessels. The cranial and spinal portions of the dura differ, but they form one complete membrane. The cranial dura is arranged in two layers that are closely connected except where they separate to form sinuses for the passage of venous blood (viz, the intracranial venous sinuses). The outer (endosteal) layer adheres to the cranial bones and forms a part of their internal periosteum. These layers are separated from the bone of the skull by the *epidural space*. The inner (meningeal) layer covers the brain and sends numerous prolongations inward for the support and protection of the different lobes of the brain. These projections also form sinuses that return the blood from the brain and form sheaths for the nerves that pass from the skull.

In two areas, the dura mater folds into the cranial cavity to form a fibrous barrier: (1) the *falx cerebri*, located between the cerebral hemispheres; (2) the *tentorium cerebelli*, demarcating the superior limit of the posterior fossa (Fig. 2.19). Two similar folds of dura should be noted: (1) the slight *falx cerebelli*, which attaches to the internal occipital crest and (2) the *diaphragma sellae*, which forms a tentorium for the hypophysis cerebri. Beneath the dura mater lies the *subdural space*.

The spinal dura mater forms a loose sheath around the spinal cord. It consists of an extension of only the inner layer of cranial dura. The outer layer ceases at the foramen magnum, and its role is taken by the periosteal lining of the vertebral canal. Outside the spinal dura is the epidural space, which contains venous plexuses and fat. Between the spinal dura and the arachnoid maters is a potential space (subdural cavity) that contains only enough fluid to moisten their contiguous structures.

Arachnoid Mater

The arachnoid mater is a delicate filamentous serous membrane placed between the dura and pia maters. The cranial portion loosely invests the brain, and, except for the longitudinal fissure, it passes over the

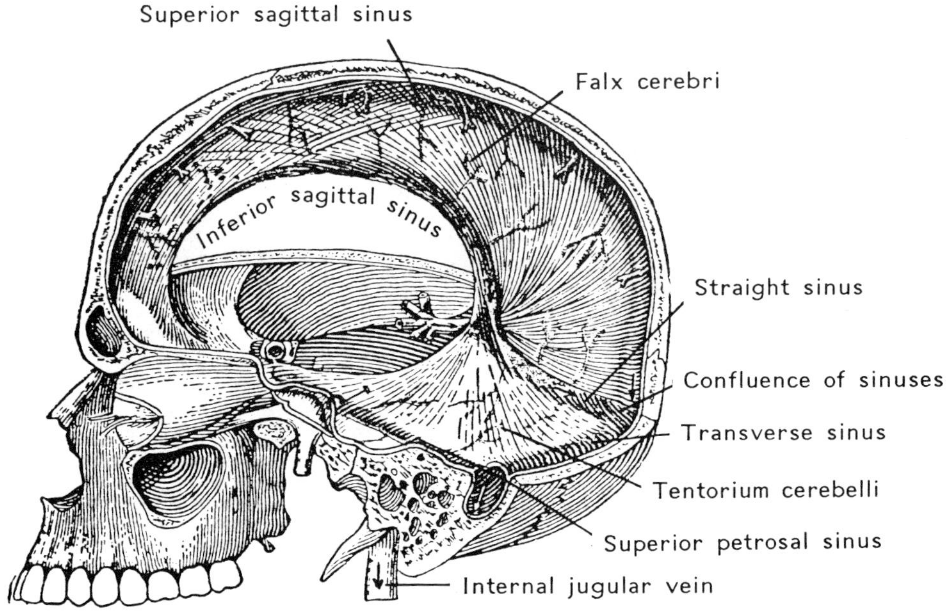

Figure 2.19. Schematic of the falx cerebri and tentorium.

various convolutions and sulci and does not dip into them. The cavity (subarachnoid space) between the arachnoid and the pia maters is occupied by spongy connective tissue and intercommunicating channels. It surrounds the entire brain and spinal cord and is filled with cerebrospinal fluid. Small tufts of arachnoid villi (Pacchionian granulations) invaginate into the dural venous sinuses, especially along the dorsal convexity of the cerebral hemispheres, parallel to the interhemispheric (longitudinal) fissure (Fig. 2.20).

The spinal portion of arachnoid is tubular, loosely surrounds the spinal cord, and contains cerebrospinal fluid.

Pia Mater

The pia mater is the innermost layer of meningeal coverings. It is a vascular membrane, composed of a single cell layer of cells derived from mesoderm, consisting of a plexus of blood vessels held together by fine areolar connective tissue. The cranial portion closely invests the surface of the brain and dips into the convolutions.

The spinal portion of pia mater is thicker and less vascular than the cranial aspect. It is closely adherent to the entire surface of the spinal cord and sends a process into the ventral fissure. To stabilize the spinal cord within the vertebral column, dentate ligaments extend on either side between the origins of the spinal nerves, pierce the arachnoid, and insert into the dura. While the dural sac and subarachnoid space ends at the S2 level, the pia mater continues downward from the end of the spinal cord as a filamentous membrane (filum terminale) to join the dural sac at the S2 level and then attaches caudally to the posterior surface of the coccyx (sacrococcygeal ligament).

The Ventricular System

The ventricular system consists of the dura, arachnoid, and pia maters; the epidural, subdural, and subarachnoid spaces; and the cerebrospinal fluid (CSF). It exists at the supratentorial, posterior fossa, and spinal levels.

CSF is colorless, alkaline, and has a normal specific gravity of 1.005—1.008. It circulates through the ventricles and the subarachnoid space and consists chiefly of water; a large amount of carbon dioxide; some glucose, salts similar to those found in plasma, and lymphocytes; and traces of protein and pituitary hormones.

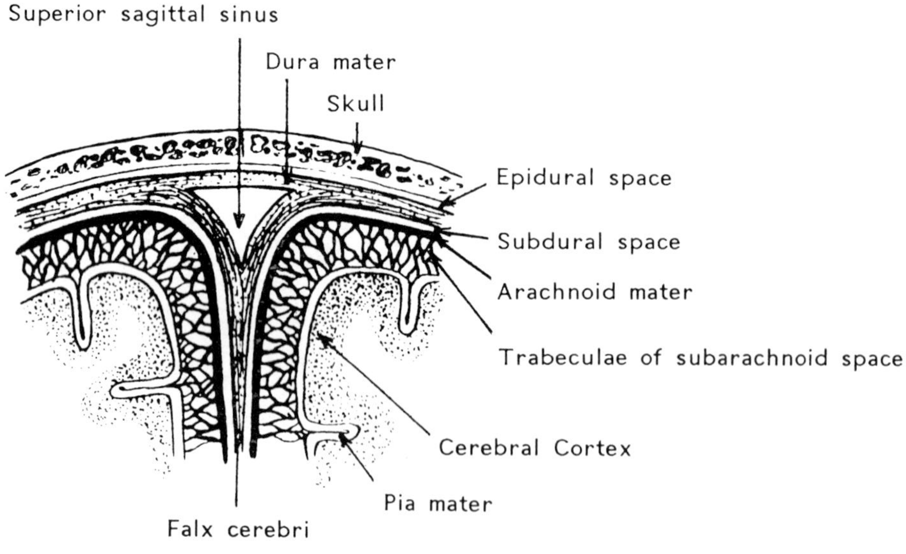

Figure 2.20. Coronal section of the meninges near the superior sagittal sinus.

Major purposes of CSF are to keep the inner and outer surfaces of the brain and spinal cord moist, to lubricate them, to compensate for fluctuations in cranial blood volume in an attempt to maintain a cranial fluid content constant, to serve as an exchange medium of metabolic substances between nerve cells and CSF, and to serve as a protective hydrolic cushioning and buffering mechanism to disperse forces applied against the cranium or that travel upward in the spine from the lower extremities (eg, during gait, jumps).

The meningeal membranes and spaces filled with CSF form a pad enclosing the brain and spinal cord on all sides. CSF is secreted and diffused from blood by the epithelial cells that surround the choroid plexus of the ventricles. After filling the lateral ventricles, it escapes via the foramen of Monro into the 3rd ventricle and then through the aqueduct into the 4th ventricle (Fig. 2.21). From the 4th ventricle, CSF passes through the median foramen of Magendie and the two lateral foramina of Luschka, into the subarachnoid spaces, and reaches the cisterna magna. CSF fluid from the cisterna magna also bathes the peripheral parts of the brain in contact with the ventricular system. The subarachnoid space communicates with the interior of the brain via the ventricular system.

CSF fluid also travels along the course of certain cranial nerves, especially the olfactory nerve. This loophole allows the entry of infection from the nasal cavities to the cerebral cavity.

From the subarachnoid spaces, CSF is absorbed into the blood stream through the villi of the arachnoid mater that project into the superior sagittal sinus. A small amount passes into the perineural lymphatics of the cranial and spinal nerves.

The Major Cranial Blood Vessels

The brain is supplied by two pairs of major arteries: anteriorly by the *internal carotid* and posteriorly by the *vertebral*. Many of

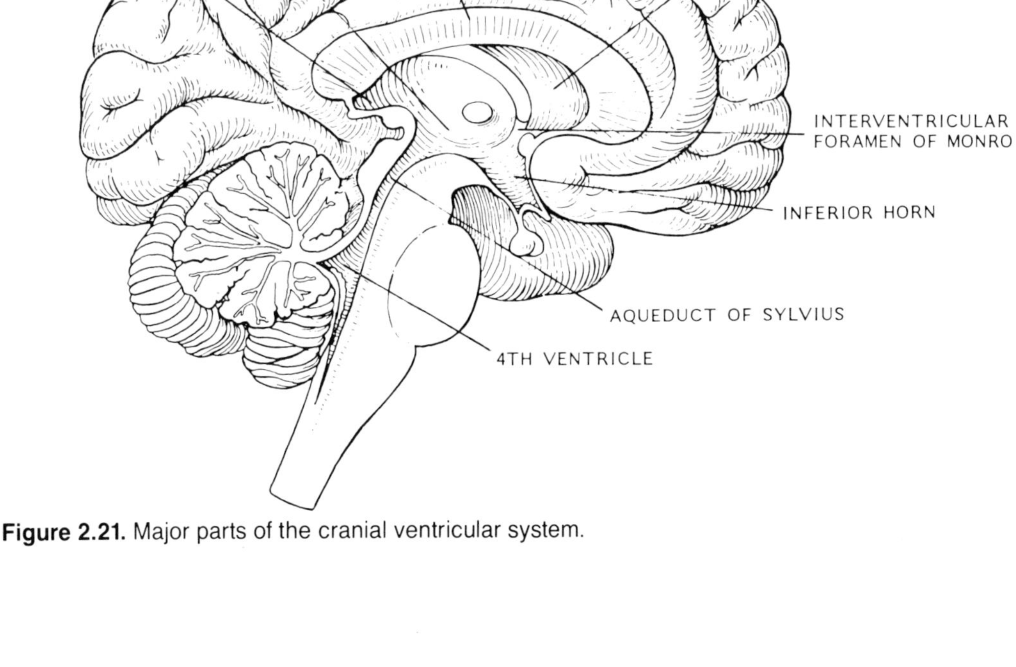

Figure 2.21. Major parts of the cranial ventricular system.

the major arterial channels can be seen on the undersurface of the brain beneath the arachnoid mater (Fig. 2.22).

The Internal Carotid Arteries

The internal carotids ascend the anterolateral neck and pierce the dura mater medial to the anterior clinoid processes, which they groove. They immediately give off (1) the *ophthalamic arteries*, which run below the optic nerve through the optic canal and (2) the *posterior communicating arteries*, which run posteriorly, medial to cranial nerve III, to join with the *posterior cerebral artery*. They then ascend with the optic nerve and end as the *anterior* and *middle cerebral arteries*. After running medially above the optic nerve, the anterior cerebral arteries are joined together by the *anterior communicating artery*. Then they continue in the midline between the two hemispheres to supply the medial surfaces of the cerebrum. The middle cerebral artery runs laterally in the stem of the lateral cerebral sulcus, coursing between the temporal and frontal lobes to emerge upon the surface of the insula (island of Reil), where its branches supply the lateral surface of the hemisphere. A series of anastomotic channels lying at the base of the brain, known as the cerebral arterial *circle of Willis*, permits communication between the carotid and vertebral systems.

The Vertebrobasilar System

The vertebral arteries ascend through the cervical transverse processes and pierce the dura matter behind the occipital condyle and the margin of the foramen magnum, which they groove. They then project forward to the inferior edge of the pons where they join together to form the *basilar artery*, whose branches solely supply the caudal structures of the brain (viz, the occipital lobe, cerebellum, undersurface of temporal lobe, thalamus, midbrain, medulla, and portions of the superior spinal cord).

The basilar artery ascends the midline bony slope from the inferior edge of the pons to its upper edge, where it terminates in a T-shaped bifurcation, above cranial nerves III and IV, to form the right and left posterior cerebral arteries. Before this occurs, three

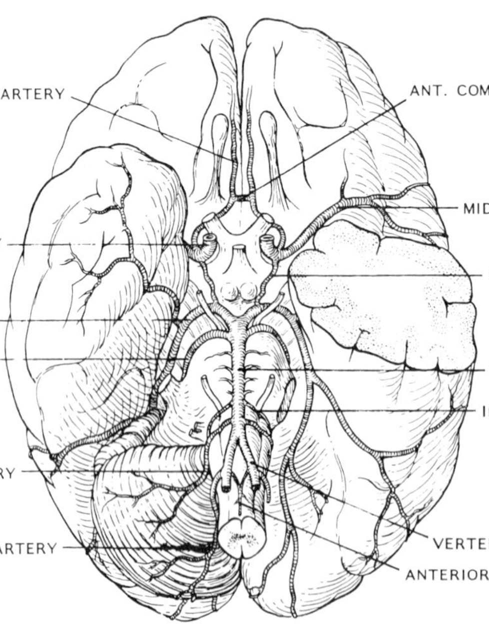

Figure 2.22. The arterial supply of the brain as viewed from its base.

pairs of arteries branch horizontally from the basilar artery:

• The first and largest branches of the vertebral arteries are the *posterior inferior cerebellar arteries.* During their course to the cerebellum, they loop around or among cranial nerves IX, X, and XI.

• Next, two other smaller paired branches proceed horizontally from the basilar artery: (1) the *anterior inferior cerebellar arteries* (that pass above, below, or between cranial nerves VII and VIII), which project labyrinthine branches to the inner ear, and (2) the *superior cerebellar arteries.*

Venous Drainage of the Brain

The veins within the skull roughly follow the arterial courses. They meet at enlarged channels (venous sinuses) contained within the two layers of dura mater. The two major sinuses are the *superior* and *inferior sagittal sinuses* that run medially between the cerebri in the falx cerebri, merge in the occipital region to form the confluence of sinuses that drains into the *transverse* and *sigmoid sinuses* and then exits the skull through the jugular foramina as the *internal jugular veins.*

The Supratentorial Level

On each side of the cranial vault, the floor of the skull is separated into three fossae (anterior, middle, and posterior). See Figure 2.23. The rigid tentorium cerebelli, which lies

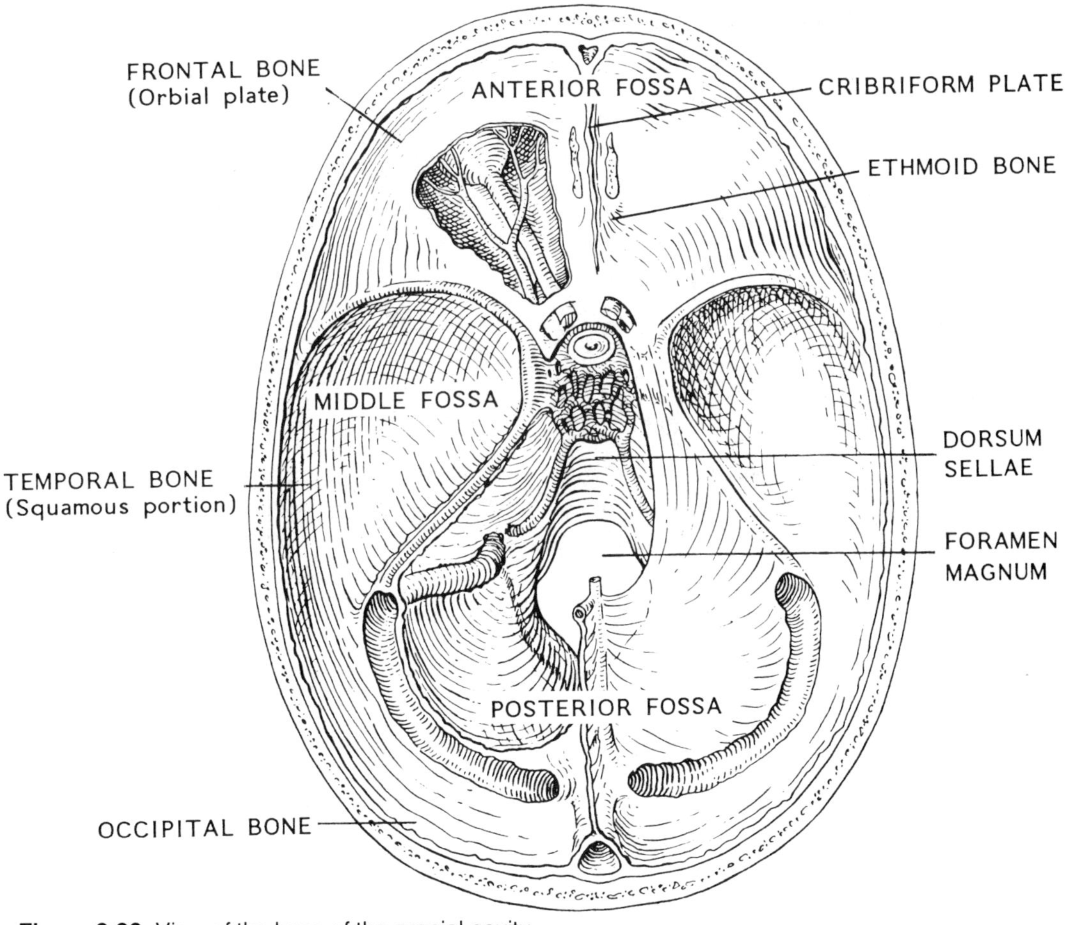

Figure 2.23. View of the base of the cranial cavity.

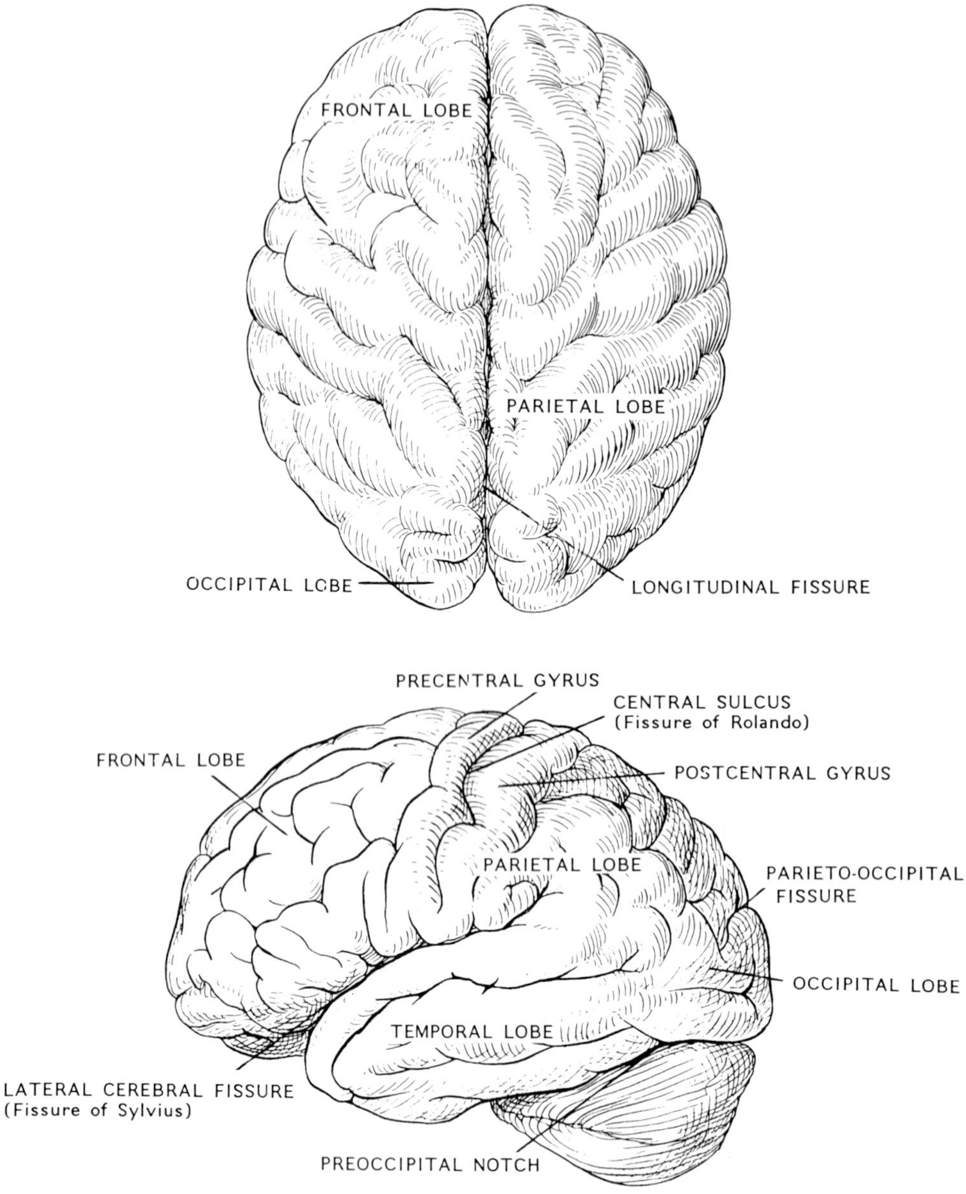

Figure 2.24. Superior and lateral views of the cerebral hemispheres.

nearly horizontal and attaches to the petrous ridges laterally and the occiput posteriorly, divides the posterior fossa from the anterior and middle fossae.

The structures of the nervous system situated above the tentorium cerebelli are those of the *supratentorial level*, all of which are derivatives of the primitive telencephalon and diencephalon. The major structures at this level are the cerebral hemispheres, the diencephalon, and portions of the olfactory and optic cranial nerves.

The Cerebrum

All lobes of the brain and portions of the brain stem partake in the *consciousness system*, which is concerned with maintaining wakefulness, awareness, and sleep states. The supratentorial level is also concerned with such faculties as cognition, imagination, intelligence, language, memory, olfaction, perception, vision, and volition. The cerebrum serves are the primary center for memory, motor response patterns, will power, and sensory discrimination.

The two cerebral hemispheres are separated by the *longitudinal fissure*, and each hemisphere has a convoluted surface. These convolutions have the effect of increasing the amount of cerebral gray matter, which contains a network of intricate layers of interconnecting neuron cell bodies. They number in the thousands of millions, and each cell communicates synaptically with hundreds of others. Depending upon the authority used, 75%—90% of all neuron cell bodies are located in the cerebral cortex. At the bottom of the longitudinal fissure are association and commissural neurons (corpus callosum) that link the different lobes of each hemisphere and link the two hemispheres with each other.

On the surface of the cerebrum, various folds *(gyri)* are separated from one another by grooves *(sulci)*, the more prominent of which are the *fissures*—which serve as landmarks to separate each hemisphere into frontal, parietal, temporal, and occipital lobes (Fig. 2.24). A *central fissure* separates the frontal lobe from the parietal lobe. Anterior to this fissure lies the motor and premotor cortices; posterior, the sensory and sensory cortical areas. The limbic lobe, which processes data concerning memory and emotions, is located near the medial surface of a hemisphere.

The large tracts running to and from the cerebral cortex can be classified into three major groups: the commissures, projection fibers, and association fibers.

The Commissures. The commissures are numerous nerve fibers that connect neurons of the two cerebral hemispheres, crossing from one side to the other and then to subcortical areas. Each cerebral hemisphere exerts its primary intersegmental control over the contralateral side of the body. Thus, lesions at this level are associated with a loss of function on the opposite side of the body (eg, numbness, paralysis).

The Projection Fibers. Projection fibers connect subcortical cell stations with the cortex. Many, but not all, afferent fibers reaching the cortex have their cell bodies in specific stations in the thalamus. In contrast, efferent fibers from the cortex may end in the thalamus, brain stem, or spinal cord. Projection fibers communicate with the cortex in a fan-like manner (Fig. 2.25) and project to the cortex in a spatial pattern so that body parts are generally represented with the foot at the superior aspect of the central fissure and the head at the temporal lobe (Fig. 2.26). These primary receiving areas, however, are not the only stations of afferent pathways to the cortex.

The Association Fibers. Association fibers connect cells within the primary sensory and motors areas with other primary, secondary, and general intercommunicating sensory and motor fibers within the same hemisphere. It is by this design that protective sensory and motor responses can be quickly coordinated; eg, the head is automatically turned toward the direction of a noise or diverted from a bright light, and other appropriate somatic and endocrine actions are taken. This system, which is thought to be able to interconnect an impulse entering a single fiber indirectly with any other neuron of the body, entails 100 times as many neurons within the cortical layers as ever leave it.

The Diencephalon

The supratentorial diencephalon is that area of transition located between the cerebrum and the structures of the posterior fossa. The major structures of the diencephalon include the optic pathway, thalamus, hypothalamus, pineal body, pituitary gland, and 3rd ventricle. Each area of the cerebral cortex is closely connected to a corresponding but smaller area in the thalamus, and activation of one area causes a reciprocal activation of the other area.

Cranial Nerves I and II

The olfactory nerves (cranial I) are located at the floor of each frontal lobe, and the optic nerves (cranial II) develop as outgrowths of primitive diencephalon. The origins of cranial nerves are shown in Figure 2.27.

The Posterior Fossa Level

Portions of the nervous system located below the tentorium cerebelli but above the

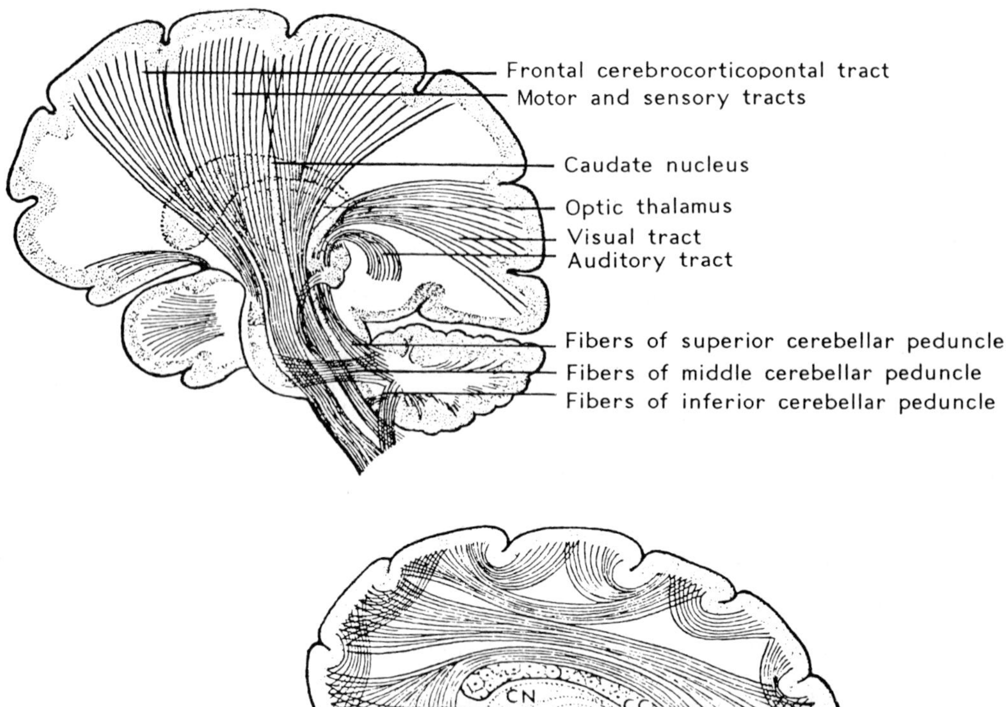

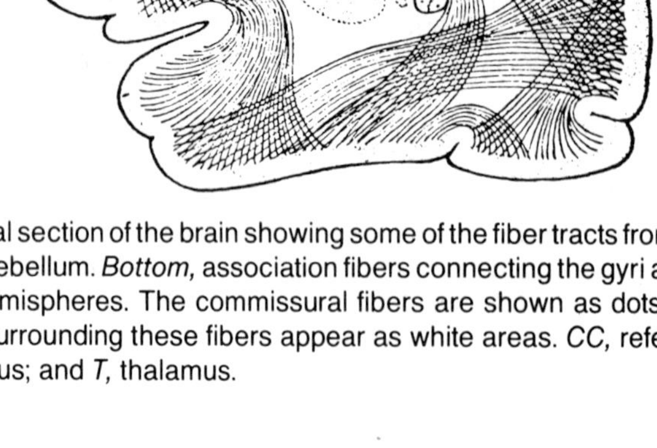

Figure 2.25. *Top,* dorsoventral section of the brain showing some of the fiber tracts from the spinal cord to the cerebral cortex and cerebellum. *Bottom,* association fibers connecting the gyri and commissural fibers connecting the two hemispheres. The commissural fibers are shown as dots as they are cut across; the myelin sheaths surrounding these fibers appear as white areas. *CC,* refers to the corpus callosum; *CN,* caudate nucleus; and *T,* thalamus.

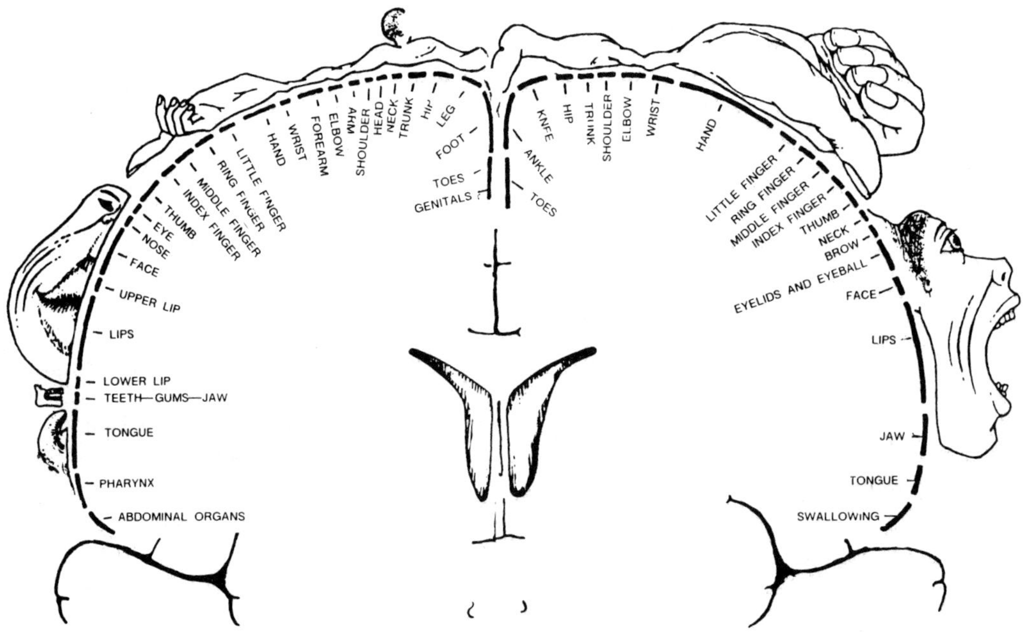

Figure 2.26. *Left,* sensory representation of the body in the postcentral gyrus. *Right,* motor representation of the body in the precentral gyrus. These homunculus-like designs help to visualize the order and comparative size of body centers as portrayed along the cerebral cortex.

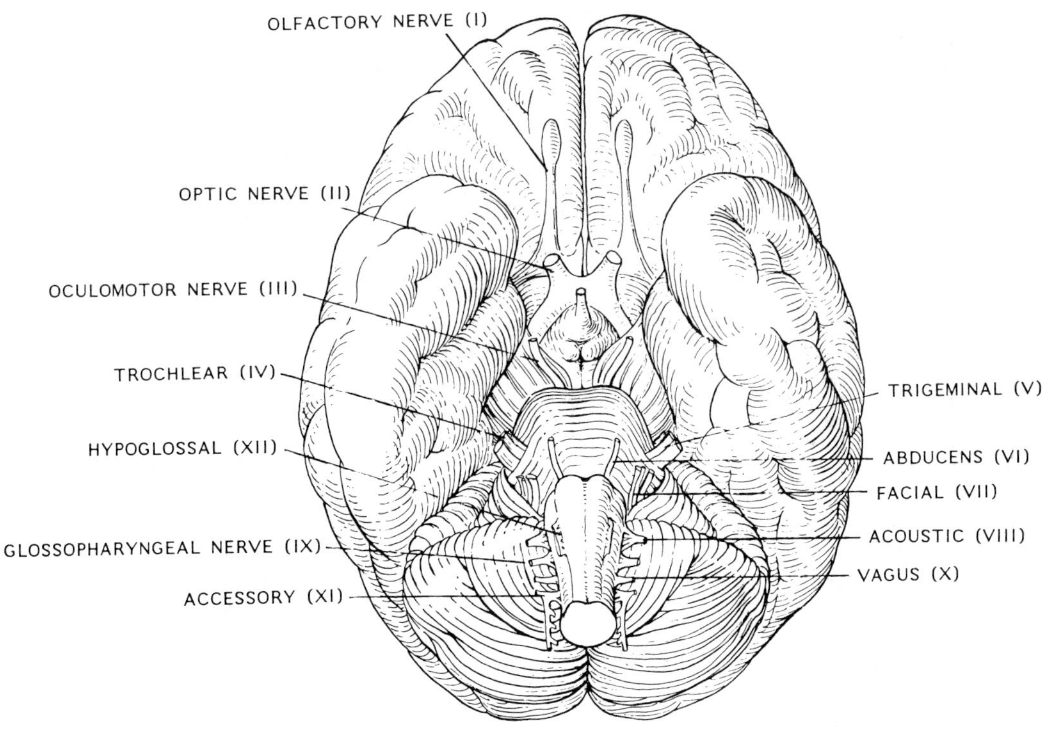

Figure 2.27. Basilar view of the origins of the cranial nerves.

foramen magnum comprise the structures at the *posterior fossa level*, which are derivatives of primitive mesencephalon, metencephalon, and myelencephalon. The major structures at this level are the cerebellum, midbrain, pons, medulla, and portions of cranial nerves III—XII contained within the skull.

The majority of what is called *subconscious* activity is coordinated and controlled in the posterior fossa area. Typical examples are blood pressure, respiration rate, body temperature, balance, and emotional patterns.

The term *brain stem* is a generalized term that refers to all structures of the brain except the cerebral and cerebellar hemispheres such as the medulla oblongata, midbrain, and pons. The lower 10 cranial nerves arise from the brain stem (refer to Fig. 2.27). The cerebellum, whose surface is highly convoluted with folds (folia), is a metencephalic derivation. It consists of two hemispheres and a midline vermis.

In many respects, the brain stem can be considered as the superior aspect of the spinal cord. As such, lesions in this area usually manifest as segmental and intersegmental disturbances. The segmental nerves of the brain stem are the cranial nerves, and brain stem lesions alter cranial nerve function as spinal cord lesions alter spinal nerve function. It should be noted, however, that the brain stem is an area where nerve tracts cross or have previously crossed to the contralateral side. Thus, if a posterior fossa lesion involves an intersegmental pathway, it will cause a loss of intersegmental function on the opposite side of the body. An extensive posterior fossa lesion may also affect consciousness (eg, coma).

The Longitudinal Systems

The major longitudinal systems, as classified in this manual, include the

- Cerebrospinal fluid system
- Consciousness system
- Motor system
- Sensory system
- Vascular system
- Visceral system.

Lesions within these systems may occur at one or more of the horizontal levels previously described; viz, the supratentorial, posterior fossa, spinal, and peripheral levels. Symptoms of dysfunction usually arise as altered states of consciousness, incoordination, numbness, pain, paralysis, pressure, tingling, or weakness.

The Sensory System

The afferent system receives information from the external and internal environments and transmits it to the CNS where it is processed and integrated. The major structures of the somatosensory system, from the peripheral to the central, include the receptor organs, the special sensory organs (eg, for vision, hearing, taste, smell, balance), their afferent fibers, the dorsal root ganglia, the posterior roots, the ascending tracts of the spinal cord and brain stem, portions of the thalamus, the thalamocortical radiations, and their endings in the sensory and sensory association cortex of the parietal lobe.

The Motor System

The efferent system, which is present at all major levels, governs the activity of the somatic muscles. Its major structures, from the central to the peripheral, include the motor and premotor cortices of the frontal lobe, the descending tracts that transverse the internal capsule, the cerebral peduncles and medullary pyramids, other centers in the brain stem, the descending tracts of the spinal cord, the anterior roots, the efferent fibers, and their endings within the surface membrane of skeletal muscle. The cerebellum, basal ganglia, and related pathways are also included in this system.

The Visceral System

The visceral system, which is also present at all major levels, consists of afferent and efferent neural structures that innervate the vegetative organs and homeostatic mechanisms (Fig. 2.28). Its major structures, from

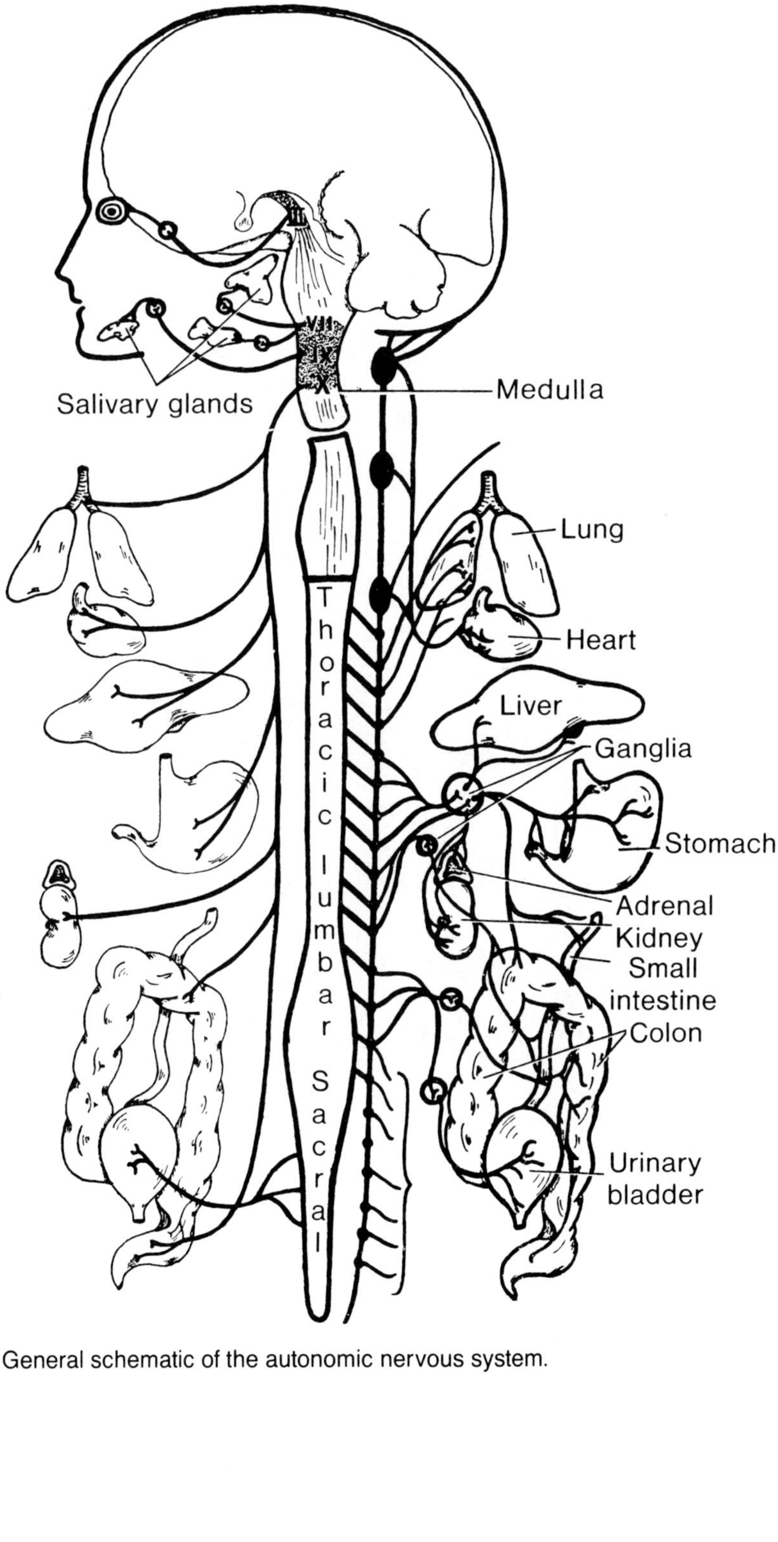

Figure 2.28. General schematic of the autonomic nervous system.

the central to the peripheral, include supratentorial areas within the limbic lobe and hypothalamus, posterior fossa fibers of certain cranial nerves and the reticular formation, ascending and descending tracts within the brain stem and spinal cord, many ganglia and plexuses, the autonomic nerves, and their peripheral effectors and receptors.

The autonomic nervous system is responsible for the innervation of the smooth muscle of the viscera, heart, glands, and vessels. It is divided into a thoracolumbar sympathetic division and a craniosacral parasympathetic division, and these systems are generally interdependent and antagonistic in the function of their effectors.

The sympathetic system is composed of a ganglionated trunk located lateral to the vertebral column that is connected to spinal cord centers via the *rami communicantes* through the spinal nerves and to the viscera via the splanchnic nerves and various abdominal ganglia. The sympathetic ganglia are also connected to each other by fibers (gangliated cords). In the thoracolumbar sympathetic system, myelinated fibers communicate with the spinal cord via the white ramus (Fig. 2.29). The efferent fibers leaving these ganglia (gray ramus) are essentially unmyelinated, and greatly exceed the number of preganglionic fibers. Thus, the result of excitation is quite diffuse.

The parasympathetic system consists of certain nerve fibers of some cranial and the middle sacral nerves. Cranial preganglionic fibers pass from the CNS through ventral roots but they synapse in ganglia (eg, ciliary, sphenopalatine, otic, submaxillary, sublingual) in or near the organs they innervate. Thus, the result of their excitation is more

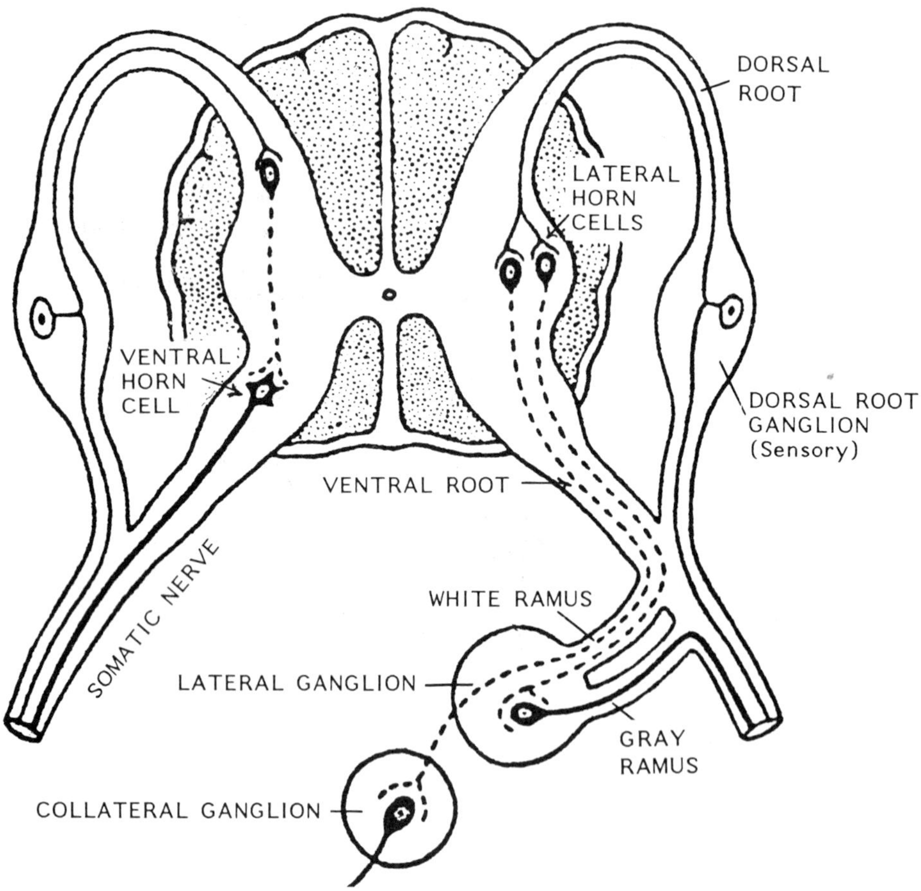

Figure 2.29. Autonomic afferent and efferent pathways in and near the spinal cord.

localized. Sacral fibers collect to form the pelvic nerve, which proceeds to the pelvic plexus and from which postganglionic fibers are distributed to the pelvic organs.

The Spinal Levels

Those portions of the CNS located below the foramen magnum are the spinal levels, which are surrounded by the vertebral column and sacrum. The major structures are the caudal edge of the medulla, the spinal cord, and the origins of the spinal nerves. The spinal cord proper consists of cell bodies and fiber tracts. Cervical and lumbosacral enlargements are exhibited in the spinal cord and are related to the innervation of the upper and lower extremities. Cross sections through these enlarged areas show a relative increase in gray matter.

The spinal cord is much shorter than the vertebral canal; it ends at or near the L1 vertebral level. Thus, for most of its length, a cord segment is not on the same level as its corresponding vertebral segment. Below the L1 level, the collection of descending nerve roots within the lumbosacral canal is the *cauda equina.*

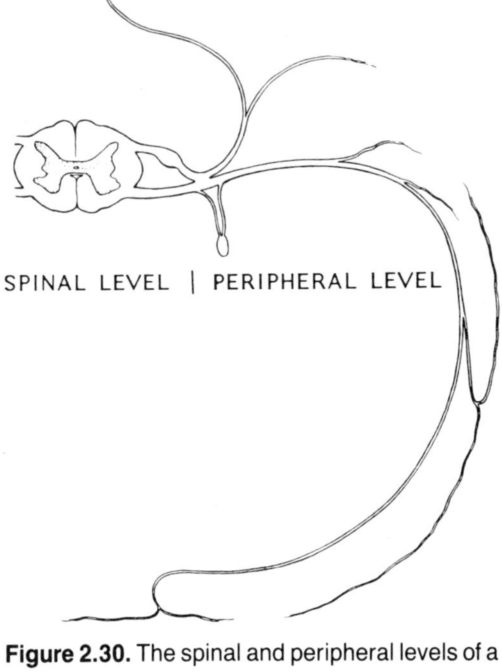

Figure 2.30. The spinal and peripheral levels of a thoracic nerve.

Bilaterally attached to the spinal cord, by anterior (motor) and posterior (sensory) nerve roots, are the 31 pairs of spinal nerves. Two exceptions to this arrangement are that C1 has only a motor root and the 1st coccyxgeal nerve (and possibly S5) has only a sensory root. As the anterior and posterior roots leave the spinal cord, they join near the intervertebral foramen (IVF) and then branch again into anterior and posterior divisions as they enter the peripheral level (Fig. 2.30).

The axons of motor neurons emerge from the cord through the anterior roots to innervate voluntary muscle. They have large cell bodies that are located in the anterior gray matter of the spinal column. In contrast, cell bodies of the sensory neurons are situated in the dorsal ganglia, exterior to the CNS, and their axons enter the cord via the posterior roots and terminate in the posterior horns. Interneurons, of varying length, lie wholly within the cord. Fibers connecting the autonomic ganglia are not considered to be interneurons.

The spinal levels transmit information to and from segmental and higher central centers. Thus, a lesion at a spinal level may alter peripheral function at that level and intersegmental function below that level.

The Peripheral Levels

The peripheral levels of the nervous system include all the nervous tissue located outside the CNS; thus, the peripheral and cranial nerves and their branches. This includes the afferent and efferent somatic nerves, the autonomic ganglia and nerves, the sensory receptors, and the motor end organs.

Each pair of spinal nerve that emerges from the CNS represents a specific spinal cord segment. On their initial route to peripheral structures, nerve fibers of the larger anterior division in some areas gather in certain distributing areas (plexuses) such as the *brachial plexus,* which serves the upper extremities, and the *lumbosacral plexus,* which serves the lower extremities.

MICRONEUROPATHOLOGIC REACTIONS: GENERAL CONSIDERATIONS

Basic Considerations

Any one of the various cellular elements of the nervous system may undergo physical change as the result of trauma or dysfunction. Such structural changes may reflect damage produced by a pathologic process or the reaction to it. Pathologic changes may also be primarily functional with little change in structure. Such changes at the spinal and peripheral levels are a primary concern within chiropractic and serve as the basis for many adjustive and reflex therapeutic approaches.

In many pathologic conditions, the various cells react in concert and their reflected clinical features are nonspecific. For example, CNS neuronal loss is invariably accompanied by loss of astrocytes and microglia at the site. At other times, specific changes occur that show or suggest a particular disease entity.

Cerebral Edema

Cerebral edema may be caused by a large variety of factors. It is the direct effect of fluid accumulating in the brain, especially in its white matter, and may be diffuse around or localized within a focus of injured tissue. Astrocytes, myelin lamellae, perivascular spaces, and extracellular spaces may be swollen, depending upon the pathophysiologic mechanisms involved.

Neuronal Pathology

Ischemic Cell Changes

Oxygen may be deprived from a nerve cell by anoxia, lack of circulating blood, vasospasm, embolism, lack of metabolic substrates, or the presence of poisons that block oxidative metabolism.

When oxygen is deprived from a nerve cell, oxidative metabolism ceases. The immediate physiologic change is an acute swelling of the neuron. Subsequently, in a matter of hours (8—12), irreversible changes occur: the neuron becomes shrunken, the cytoplasm becomes diffusely eosinophilic, the nucleus becomes pyknotic, and the outline of the cell body becomes sharply angular. Complete dissolution of the cell follows these morphologic changes.

Central Chromatolysis

This is an *axonal reaction* that often occurs especially in large motor cells within the anterior horns of the cord or motor nuclei of the brain when their axons are damaged proximally. The cell bodies swell, their Nissl bodies dissolve, and the nucleus migrates peripherally. This process starts in 2 or 3 days after injury and reaches maximum in 2—4 weeks. However, unlike the results of ischemia, central chromatolysis is reversible within a few months if the cause has been removed.

Wallerian Degeneration

In contrast to ischemic effects and central chromatolysis, Wallerian degeneration begins at the distal aspect of the axon after its cell body has been separated from the axon by trauma or disease. As an axon is nourished primarily by axoplasmic flow from the cell body, a severed axon cannot survive. The neurofibrils disappear rapidly, then the cylinder of the fiber breaks up into short fragments, and finally the fragments are dissolved (apparently digested by chemicals from its myelin envelope).

The process of Wallerian degenerative is not identical in the peripheral and central nervous systems: (1) Although Wallerian degeneration occurs within a few weeks within peripheral nerves, the process may take several months when CNS neurons are severed. (2) Axon regeneration is possible in a peripheral nerve if the cell body and the Schwann cells in the endoneurium are not destroyed, but such regeneration is unlikely in the CNS. In damaged peripheral nerves, the Schwann cells along the length of the degenerating fiber form myelinated tubes when they fragment, providing a cellular chain (framework) to receive axonal sprouts growing distally. As there is no basement membrane or collagen sheaths in the CNS and oligodendroglia do not proliferate like Schwann cells, this identical process cannot occur. However, recent evidence has shown some instances of CNS axonal regeneration.

Wallerian degeneration does not usually extend postsynaptically. There are, however, two important exceptions to this rule: (1) muscle atrophy follows the separation of a somatic efferent, and (2) certain CNS pathways can be affected by *transneuronal degeneration*. Why this occurs has not been determined, but it is thought that presynaptic fibers exert some type of postsynaptic trophic influence.

Storage (Balloon) Cells

Many metabolic diseases affecting the nervous system are associated with an accumulation of substances. Tay-Sachs disease (lipid storage disease) is a typical example. As the substances accumulate, the cytoplasm of the involved cell bodies become severely swollen, and the nucleus and Nissl bodies are forced to a corner of the angular cell. The cause can only be identified by biochemical (usually postmortem) identification of the accumulating material.

Inclusion Bodies

Inclusion bodies are discrete deposits within nerve cells whose presence often identifies a specific type of disease process. For example, they appear in the cytoplasm as Lafora bodies in myoclonus epilepsy, Lewy bodies in Parkinson's disease, Negri bodies in rabies, and Pick bodies in Pick's disease. They also appear in the nucleus as Cowdry type A inclusions in various viral infections.

Neurofibrillary Degeneration

Neurofibrillary degeneration is a process in which masses of neurofibrils become clumped within the cytoplasm of CNS cells. It is a type of neuronal degeneration that is closely related to advanced age but is especially prominent in clinical dementia (Alzheimer's neurofibrillary degeneration). Senile plaques are usually associated, which consist of a central core of amyloid deposits surrounded by a ring of degenerated axons, astrocytes, and microglia.

Oligodendroglia and Schwann Cell Pathology

Oligodendroglia and the myelin sheaths they create in the CNS are highly sensitive to injury, and when damaged, their nuclei rapidly fragment and dissolve. In demyelinating (myelinoclastic) diseases (eg, multiple sclerosis), the myelin appears to be attacked by some unknown substance that breaks the myelin into its component lipids, after which they are absorbed. Rarer myelin diseases are the genetic dysmyelinating (leukodystrophy) disorders, where the myelin is defectively formed and unstable due to a metabolic error.

Disease processes affecting Schwann cells are associated with segmental myelin breakdown and loss (demyelination). If the process is severe, the axon becomes affected and Wallerian degeneration occurs. In certain rare genetic disorders of peripheral nerves (hypertrophic neuropathy), nerve fibers undergo repetitious demyelination and remyelination. Each episode leaves a thin film of scar tissue in concentric layers, the axons thus progressively become larger and firmer until they are destroyed, and then only the connective tissue remains.

Microglia Pathology

Microglia react in a predictable manner in most diseases of the CNS. Microglia cells near the site of irritation greatly multiply, and their nuclei elongate to form *rod cells*. The process may be halted here in low-grade disorders such as chronic syphilitic encephalitis (general paresis). If necrosis continues, the cells become phagocytic and engulf necrotic debris and damaged neuron fragments in the area involved.

Astrocyte Proliferation

Astrocytosis (gliosis), the effect of almost any injury of the CNS, is the formation of scar-like changes within injured neural tissue. During the reaction, astrocytes greatly increase in number and progressively form longer and thicker processes that form a dense network within and around the injured area.

In certain CNS diseases, especially metabolic disturbances, the nuclei of astrocytes undergo morphologic changes. Alzheimer's disease and hepatic failure are typical examples. In certain CNS viral diseases, intranuclear inclusion bodies may develop within astrocytes.

When noxious stimuli are present (eg, infection) in the ventricular system, ependymal cells are readily destroyed, subependymal astrocytes proliferate, ependymal granulations develop, and the tissue becomes infiltrated with leukocytes.

NEURONAL ELECTRONEUROPHYSIOLOGY

The function of a normal neuron is the initiation and transmission of impulses. This is an electrochemical process manifested as changes in electric potential. The metabolic activities of the neuron are only indirectly involved.

Basic Considerations

All nerve and muscle cells have various electric potentials. In nerve fibers, these include resting (inactive) potentials, active potentials, and various local potentials (viz, generator, electrotonic, synaptic).

Membrane Potentials

In living tissues, current is caused by the movement of charged ions, and it can flow through the low-resistant neuronal membrane as the result of an applied voltage or a change in membrane conductance. The difference in the electric charge between the inside and outside of the cell is the *membrane potential.* When a nerve cell is inactive, its baseline level is its *resting potential* and determined primarily by potassium ion concentrations.

The cytoplasm of a neuron is a highly conductive electrolytic solution, and any change in the potential of one part produces an equal change in the potential at all other points. Thus, any local change in membrane potential will produce a flow of current throughout the cell by initiating an action potential. When impulse activity exists, *action potentials* are produced and operate according to the all-or-none principle in the neuron, spread to all parts of the cell, and are determined primarily by sodium ions.

Local Potentials

Localized changes in membrane potential that are the reaction to a stimulus are called *local potentials.* All local potentials are *graded potentials* (ie, their amplitudes are proportional to the size of the stimulus); thus, their strength is proportional to the strength of the stimulus. Unlike action potentials, local potentials remain localized in the area of the cell irritated, can be summated and integrated within single neurons, and *do not* operate according to the all-or-none principle.

Local potentials are generated by (1) electrotonic potentials (a flow of electric current) and (2) changes in the characteristics of resting receptor membranes or synapses.

Electrotonic Potentials. Action potentials are initiated by an electrotonic potential, and these decremental potentials can be initiated by action, synaptic, or receptor potentials. Electrotonic potentials are the result of a voltage change, while action, synaptic, and receptor potentials are due to membrane changes.

Receptor (Generator) Potentials. Receptors are specialized to respond to certain types of stimuli (eg, light, sound, touch, heat, etc). Once stimulated, they generate local electrotonic potentials that, in turn, initiate action potentials (Fig. 2.31). It should be noted that sufficient depolarization from any origin anywhere on the axon can initiate an action potential. However, in sensory neurons, it is usually started at a membrane (receptor) distal to the cell body; in motor neurons, it is usually started by synaptic potentials near the axon hillock (generator). It takes about 30 millivolts of excitatory postsynaptic potential to elicit an action potential in a nerve cell body but only 11 millivolts to achieve an action potential at the hillock area.

Synaptic Potentials. These are changes in potentials that occur in postsynaptic cell membranes in response to chemical or electronic message transmission produced presynaptically. They usually involve an electrochemical and chemoelectric conversion process; ie, (1) a presynaptic electric signal, (2) a synaptic chemical signal, and (3) a postsynaptic electric signal.

Resting Potential

Extracellular fluid contains positively charged ions (anions) of sodium, potassium, and calcium, and negatively charged ions of chloride (cations). Intracellular fluid contains many negatively charged indiffusible ions, which are derived from protein. If a voltage is applied, these anions and cations move towards a pole with an opposite charge.

A nerve or muscle cell's resting potential is in the range of -70 to -90 millivolts. The sensitivity to neuronal membrane becomes greater as the voltage becomes more negative and less sensitive as the voltage rises. Resting potential is determined by two factors:

1. *Cell permeability.* The membrane of a cell is semipermeable; ie, it is permeable to some ions but not others. When at rest, the molecular arrangement within the neuronal membrane allows almost free flow to the small potassium ions but inhibits the diffusion of the larger sodium and calcium ions. An ion (eg, potassium) has a *high conductance* if it can move through a membrane easily. Thus, in terms of neuronal membrane:

- *Potassium* has a high internal ionic concentration (about 140 mEq/L), low external concentration (about 4 mEq/L), and high permeability during rest.
- *Sodium* has a low internal ionic concentration (about 14 mEq/L), high external concentration (about 142 mEq/L), and low permeability during rest. Increasing the sodium concentration of the resting external medium increases the amplitude of the action spike; and, conversely, lowering the sodium concentration reduces the amplitude following stimulation.
- *Chloride* has a low ionic internal concentration (about 8 mEq/L), high external concentration (about 108 mEq/L), and moderate passive permeability during rest.

2. *Energy-dependent mechanisms.* Certain dynamic energy-dependent metabolic mechanisms are contained within cell membrane that move ions from one side of the membrane to another so that their interior and exterior concentrations are altered.

A neuron's inactive potential is stable as long as there are adequate supplies of oxygen and glucose. However, active transport ceases and resting potential cannot be maintained if something (eg, anoxia, cold) interferes with the cell's energy-producing system or if an enzyme block occurs.

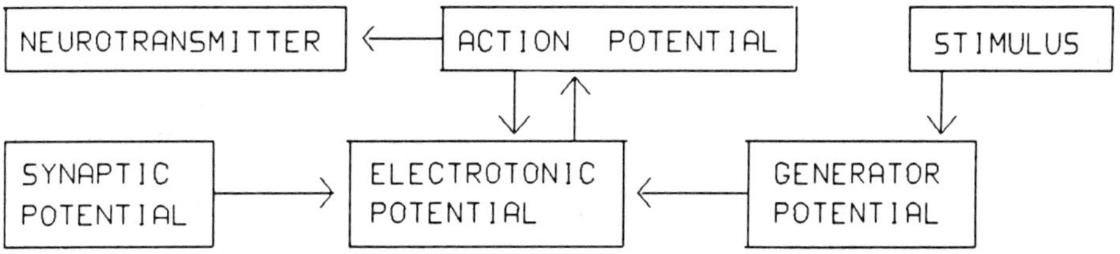

Figure 2.31. Initiation of electric potentials in the nervous system. Arrows indicate potentials that may be initiated by each source. From the above, it can be seen that a disruption of a neuron's receptor potential, resting potential, action potential, or synaptic potential will result in altered neuronal function.

The steady resting potential of a neuron is presently thought to be a balance struck among (1) ion leakage that reduces concentration gradients, (2) ion pumping that increases concentration gradients, and (3) the cell's internal negative charge that repels anions and attracts cations.

The Sodium Pump

Nerve cells obtain energy from oxygen and glucose through glycolytic pathways, the Krebs cycle, and the electron transport system—all of which provide the energy necessary for neuronal function in the form of adenosine triphosphate (ATP). ATP, provided by the mitochondria, is important during resting potential for the system *(active transport)* that moves potassium into and sodium out of the nerve cell. This hypothetical mechanism within the neuronal membrane *(sodium pump)* allows this movement against their concentration gradients, and it is not confined to nerve cells.

The movement of ions across a permeable membrane occurs freely by diffusion if the electrochemical gradient does not oppose it. In the recovery phase following an action potential, the outward flow of sodium has to be forced against a gradient. This is the basis for the "sodium pump" theory, and the energy to maintain this pump is thought to be derived from metabolic processes within the nerve. Prichard states that it is thought to consume 20% of the entire energy requirements of the animal body.

It is known that the result of active transport through the cell membrane is an unequal concentration of ions on opposite sides of the membrane. Consequently, there is a small continuous efflux of potassium ions and an influx of sodium ions, but these ions are transferred back through the membrane by the sodium pump to maintain a dynamic steady resting state rather than a true state of equilibrium. As a large number of positive sodium ions are pumped to the exterior, this leaves a large number of nondiffusible negatively charged ions internally (eg, protein ions, phosphate ions, etc). Thus, the interior surface of the resting membrane becomes negative and the exterior surface becomes positive in charge.

The sodium pump appears to be a membrane enzyme that is capable of splitting ATP and using the energy released to move potassium and sodium ions through the membrane against their concentration gradients. This system is also thought to be a "coupling system" in that, if either ion is removed from the system, the remaining ion is not transported well.

A hypothetical sodium/calcium countertransport pump, a chloride pump, and an ATP-requiring calcium pump have been brought forth in addition to the ATP-requiring sodium/potassium pump. Absolute proof of the existence of such pumps has not been established, but the theories explain most experimental findings.

Local Effects

Local effects are the result of a shift of membrane potential within a specific area of the cell due to a hyperpolarizing or depolarizing stimulus. This may be an effect of: (1) A local change in applied voltage from some source (eg, electrotonic potential). It is in this manner that an action potential is initiated. (2) A local change in membrane permeability to one or more ions. This occurs in response to neurotransmitters (synaptic potential) or external stimuli (receptor potential) and is the mechanism by which signals are transmitted to or from the neuron.

Neuronal Summation

It was previously mentioned that all local potentials are graded potentials. These changes in amplitude rise and fall occur over several milliseconds, far outlasting the stimulation time. If a second local stimulus is applied to a neuron before the effect of one has subsided, the result is a larger local potential. Thus, local potentials can be *summated.* It is in this manner that individual stimuli that are below threshold can be increased in value collectively to produce an action potential.

Temporal summation is achieved because local potential changes initiated close to each other in time are additive. *Spatial summation* is achieved in border zones when local potential changes are initiated at different sites. Thus, through temporal and spatial summation, the cell body can integrate stimuli from different sources that converge on an area of cell membrane.

Neuronal Accommodation

Changes occur in the ionic conductivity of neuronal membrane whenever a local stimulus is applied for more than a few milliseconds. These changes tend to restore the membrane to its inactive baseline potential even if the stimulation is continued. This phenomenon *(accommodation)* can occur if a stimulus is increased slowly, and the effect is no change in membrane potential (Fig. 2.32).

Action Potentials

A neuron's inactive potential can be changed by either the membrane becoming less negative outside (depolarization) or more negative inside (hyperpolarization). Rapid transient changes occur in response to electrical, mechanical, or chemical stimuli; while prolonged changes, which may last for many minutes, result from anoxia or effects that change the concentration of ions on either side of the membrane.

Excitability

A neuron's minimal level of excitability is determined by its threshold, which may be reached either by a single sufficient stimulus or by summation. The term *threshold* is used in two senses. First, it refers to the voltage required to induce an action potential such as when extrinsic stimulation is applied and recorded. Second, it is used to describe the relative state of membrane potential. For example, the closer the membrane potential is to threshold, the easier it is to fire; the farther the membrane potential is from threshold, the more difficult it is to fire.

The first portion of the membrane potential change is that of the local potential. The rapidly rising phase of the action potential occurs at threshold as an effect of the influx of positive ions (sodium and some calcium). During long intervals between action potentials, the sodium pump continually transports internal sodium to the exterior.

Under typical conditions, the threshold of a neuron for excitation is -59 millivolts, representing a postsynaptic excitatory potential of +11 millivolts; ie, 11 millivolts more positive than a neuron's average resting potential of -70 millivolts. Once the threshold is reached, the membrane becomes suddenly more permeable to sodium, which is thought to be related to a change in the binding of calcium in the membrane. This shifts the membrane potential toward the equilibrium potential of sodium rather than that of potassium. The polarity of the membrane is reversed by this depolarization, and a flow of current occurs as many sodium ions and some calcium ions flow inwardly and the abundant potassium ions, subsequently, flow outwardly. This change in conductance results in the *action potential.*

At the phase when sodium conductance is high internally, a stimulus applied at this time will have no effect; ie, action potentials, unlike local potentials, cannot be summated.

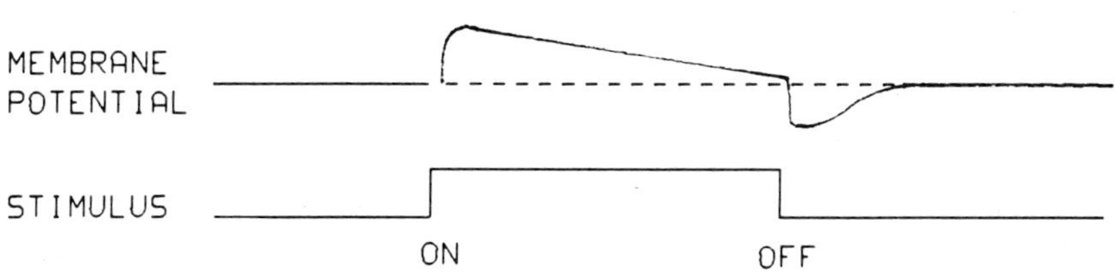

Figure 2.32. Accommodation of neuronal membrane potential to an applied on—off stimulus of constant strength.

This period of complete unresponsiveness (absolute refractory period) is followed by the relative refractory period, as sodium conductance begins to return to its resting equilibrium, where a greater stimulus will produce a smaller action potential.

Propagation

Besides the horizontal current produced by the flow of positive sodium ions through an area of depolarized membrane, there is also a longitudinal current (electrotonus), which, unlike the action potential, has no refractory period. It flows on the interior and exterior surfaces of the membrane and tends to depolarize the areas surrounding the action potential. This depolarization (an electrotonic potential) is usually sufficient to shift the membrane potential to threshold and produce an action potential in the adjacent area of membrane. In this manner, the action potential progresses away from the site of initial stimulation along the axon. The potential is prevented from reversing backward into an area just depolarized because of the refractory period. That is, after passage of a nerve impulse, repolarization and ionic balance during the refractory period are quickly restored so that another impulse can be received.

There are several other theories regarding the electric propagation of the nerve impulse. However, all recognize a decrease in resistance across the membrane as a crucial event for the impulse to pass. The degree of resistance may be regarded as an index of the membrane's permeability to certain ions. However, unlike a membrane's resistance, the capacitance of nerve membrane does not change appreciably during the passage of an impulse.

The conduction rate of the action potential is determined by (1) the diameter of the axon (ie, the larger the axon, the lower the resistance), (2) the quantity of current necessary to produce depolarization in adjacent membrane, and (3) whether the axon is myelinated. In myelinated nerves, the active region "triggers" the resting area ahead only at the nodes of Ranvier, where myelin is absent; ie, the nerve impulse is propagated from node to node in a leaping manner *(salatory transmission)*. Refer to Figure 2.11. This occurs because an action potential at one node produces sufficient longitudinal current to depolarize the next node.

Conductances carrying the inward flowing depolarizing sodium and calcium currents of the action potential are different from each other and different from those carrying the outward flowing repolarizing potassium current. Because they are separate, they can be stopped medically by certain drugs called "blockers."

Facilitation

After repetition of a reflex act, its establishment becomes increasingly easy, and, within limits, the reaction time lessens. This type of facilitation is the basis of habit formation. The term *facilitation* is also used to describe the state of a neuron that has been summated to some degree below its firing threshold at which point meager stimuli from some source can easily excite the neuron.

Reaction Time

The time elapsing between the application of a stimulus and the beginning of a response is the *reaction time*. Reaction time varies in different individuals and in the same individual under different conditions. The most commonly involved factors are:

- The strength of the stimulus. The stronger the stimulus, the more prompt the response.
- The nature of the stimulus (eg, the response to sound is more prompt than that to light).
- The number of synapses through which the impulses must pass; ie, a greater number delays to some extent the reaction time. The time it takes an impulse to be transmitted through a synaptic center primarily depends on the strength of the stimulus and the physiologic state of the synapse (ie, normal, hyporeactive, hyperreactive).

Synaptic Transmission

The membrane depolarization caused by an action potential on presynaptic terminals causes the vesicles to empty, and the quantity of neurotransmitter released at a presynaptic vesicle is directly proportional to the change in membrane potential (ie, its amplitude). Calcium flows into the terminals when the depolarization alters its conductance, and this appears to trigger the release of the neurotransmitter, which diffuses across the synaptic cleft. Sodium and magnesium ions are also involved in this triggering process. The neurotransmitter extruded into the cleft excites or inhibits the subsequent neuron depending upon the type of receptor contacted.

Once an excitatory neurotransmitter contacts the specialized cells of the postsynaptic membrane, the membrane's permeability is altered, the local potential is changed, ionic conductance is altered, sodium ions enter the cell, and a flow of current is produced. This phase of sodium permeability lasts for 1—2 milliseconds, but the potential may persist for about 15 milliseconds until the sodium pump becomes effective in re-establishing the resting potential.

The synaptic potential, like a receptor potential, is a graded response that initiates a local electrotonic potential. The neurotransmitter may also act on a second chemical messenger in the postsynaptic membrane to create a longer change in permeability via an effect on the sodium pump.

Synaptic Inhibition

With a few exceptions, each neuron releases the same type of transmitter substance at all its terminals (Dale-Feldberg law) and that substance will have either an excitatory or inhibitory influence on all associated postsynaptic receptors relative to their properties and local hormonal influences. As postsynaptic effects are receptor dependent, a neuron releasing the same transmitter may cause an inhibitory effect on some connecting neurons and an excitatory effect on other connecting neurons.

Some axon end feet within the CNS release inhibitory transmitters. Common examples are the amino acid glycine and GABA (gamma aminobutyric acid). Inhibitory neurons tend to block unimportant signals and thus allow transmission of selected messages (eg, to centers that otherwise would be subjected to a continuous bombardment of impulses from receptors located throughout the body). Inhibition can also occur if mechanisms produce a postsynaptic hyperpolarization that moves the membrane potential farther from its threshold.

Presynaptic Inhibition

Because the release of a neurotransmitter is a graded response governed by the amplitude of the action potential at the vesicle, changes in membrane potential at the terminal will modify synaptic transmission. This is typically seen where some terminals synapse directly on others that they can partially depolarize and thus inhibit release when they are acted upon by an action potential. The most common occurrence is seen in peripheral synapses of sensory paths. The result (presynaptic inhibition), therefore, is a smaller release, and this effect is usually of a longer duration (eg, 0.5 sec) than is postsynaptic inhibition (eg, 10—15 milliseconds). The same timeframe is true for excitation.

Postsynaptic Summation

When either peripheral or central impulses from several sources act on single cells, synaptic potentials will summate both spatially and temporally.

A single end foot has been computed to cause an excitatory postsynaptic potential of about 1 millivolt or less. As the usual threshold for excitation is 10 or more millivolts, a minimum of ten end feet firing simultaneously anywhere on a receptive membrane of a nerve cell, even at widely separated areas, is necessary to produce an action potential. This is an example of *postsynaptic spatial summation*, and it occurs because a potential change at any single point within the cytoplasm will cause the potential to change throughout the cytoplasm. In addition, as each end foot can fire at intervals about 1 millisecond apart and its postsynaptic effect may last up to 15 milliseconds, a rapidly firing end foot will have a summed postsynaptic effect. This is an example of *postsynaptic temporal summation*. Through either spatial or temporal summation, it can be seen that potentials derived from presynaptic, synaptic, or postsynaptic excitatory and inhibitory mechanisms of identical value will cancel each other.

CLINICAL APPLICATIONS

Symptoms of neurologic dysfunction may reflect a degenerative, a neoplastic, a vascular, an inflammatory, a toxic or metabolic, or a traumatic disorder. *Degenerative disorders* are characterized by gradual but widespread neuronal damage that manifest as diffuse, chronic, progressive diseases. As any cell within the nervous system can undergo neoplastic changes, *neoplastic disorders* feature one or more gradually enlarging masses of proliferating cells. The type of neoplasm is named after the predominant cell type (eg, astrocytoma, oligodendroglioma, Schwannoma). *Vascular disorders* are invariably associated with acute symptoms and signs that may be focal or diffuse, depending upon cause and site (eg, hemorrhage, anoxia, encephalopathy). *Inflammatory disorders* usually exhibit progressive subacute symptoms that may be focal (eg, abscess) or diffuse (eg, encephalitis, meningitis). *Toxic* or *metabolic disorders* are characterized by widespread neural dysfunction exhibiting diffuse signs and symptoms that may arise as an acute, a subacute, or a chronic process. *Traumatic disorders* affecting the nervous system as usually focal and have an acute onset, reflecting the offending agent and the area of tissue damaged. However, delayed effects may produce signs and symptoms pointing to a pattern of progressive degeneration.

Importance of Normal Findings

In nerve, muscle, or gross static and dynamic analyses or any other diagnostic procedure, a clinician may use a normal finding to eliminate certain disorders during the differential diagnosis process. When properly interpreted, however, a normal value may also aid in differentiating among possible diagnoses that yield normal values with different frequencies in occurrence. Gorry and associates suggest a simple method that has the examiner estimate the probability of various diagnoses and then combine these estimates with the anticipated frequency of negative results for each disorder under consideration. Thus, from a clinical standpoint aside from the medicolegal factor involved, the recording and appraisal of a normal finding can be just as important as that of an abnormal finding.

Applied Neuroembryology

Developing cells change their response to metabolic injury as they grow, and the embryo changes metabolically as it develops. Although developmental patterns are determined primarily by genetics and latent genetic defects may be precipitated by noxious agents (eg, anoxia, hypoglycemia, drugs, radiation, toxins), different agents may produce different types of malformations at the same stage of development.

Most gross embryologic malformations such as meningocele and meningomyelocele are rarely seen in the chiropractic office. However, various anomalies not obvious externally are often shown in roentgenography for another reason (eg, spina bifida occulta, hemivertebrae, etc). Aside from such developmental defects, knowledge of neuroembryology is helpful in localizing the site of neural damage and in recognizing various patterns of pain.

Daube/Sandok explain that because the nervous system and the skin both derive from ectoderm, a genetically determined disorder of one system may affect the other. This is often seen in the neurocutaneous syndromes and ectodermal dysplasias. For example, in *Sturge-Weber syndrome*, meningeal angioma and cortical calcification manifest in the nervous system and a port-wine nevus manifests on the face. In *tubercular sclerosis*, cortical giant cell tumors, gliomas, and periventricular tumors arise in the nervous system and depigmented patches, subungual fibromas, and adenoma sebaceum appear in the skin. In *von Recklinghausen's disease*, schwannomas and gliomas appear in the nervous system and neurofibromas and café-au-lait spots arise in the skin.

The CNS and the retina of the eye are also closely related embryologically, and developmental syndromes often manifest both CNS and retinal signs. Typical examples are the retinal tumors associated with neuroectodermal dysplasia and the cherry-red macula spot of Tay-Sachs disease.

Pathoanatomical Correlations

Rarely do patients enter a doctor's office with a singular complaint. They invariably mention a few symptoms that are a priority concern to them, and, upon questioning, will reveal several associated concerns. The clinician will then use inductive and deductive reasoning to arrive at an initial picture that will be constantly altered, refined, and reorganized according to the findings of subsequent examinations and patient progress. With knowledge of the neuroanatomy and neurophysiology of the various parts of the nervous system, neurologic signs and symptoms can be related to specific areas of distress within the nervous system in most instances.

Topographic Localization

The term *localization* means determining the location along various pathways where function is interrupted. It becomes precise when one or more areas where both segmental and intersegmental functions are altered in one or more systems and they can be identified.

During the diagnostic process, the topographic localization of a neural deficit is arrived at by two basic steps (dimensional viewpoints):

1. By relating a patient's symptoms and signs to one of the six major longitudinal functional subsystems of the nervous system that are described in this chapter and Chapter 3; viz, the sensory, motor, visceral, vascular, consciousness, and cerebrovascular systems.

2. By localizing the lesion at one of the four well-defined horizontal levels of the nervous system described in this chapter and Chapter 4; viz, the supratentorial, posterior fossa, spinal, and peripheral levels. These levels are the points at which the function of each longitudinal system can be integrated and modified.

The cerebral cortex is not required for the total perception of sensation but is for its finer discrimination. Total loss of the cerebral cortex causes a "vegetative" existence. Even if large areas of the somesthetic cortex are destroyed, for example, the patient will still be able to perceive when an object touches the skin. However, the blindfolded patient will be unable to distinguish the shape, size, and other characteristics of the stimulus. Two-point discrimination will also be impaired. Likewise, destruction of the frontal lobes does not destroy a patient's ability to think. However, it does impair the patient's ability to think in abstract terms. Thus, these points (differentiation and abstraction), along with others, are commonly utilized during diagnosis to help localize the anatomical location of a lesion.

Diffuse vs Focal Lesions

If the responsible lesion is *diffuse* (involving bilateral, usually symmetrical, areas but not extending across the midline), its anatomical level(s) should be noted. A diffuse lesion may involve a single level or be distributed over multiple levels. If the lesion is *focal* (well-circumscribed), its anatomical level should be noted as well as whether it is located on the left, right, or midline of the body. Note that a focal lesion may involve the midline *and* contiguous structures bilaterally. The term *multifocal* refers to lesions involving more than one circumscribed area or several noncontiguous structures.

The history of a neurologic disorder's onset and progress is usually extremely helpful in its diagnosis. Diffuse disorders may be acute, subacute, or chronic. Diffuse vascular disorders (eg, hemorrhage, anoxia) are usually acute; inflammatory disorders (eg, meningitis, encephalitis), subacute; and degenerative disorders, chronic. Toxic and metabolic disorders are usually diffuse; their timeframes will depend upon the specific toxin or metabolite involved.

Almost all progressive focal lesions are space-occupying lesions (eg, hemorrhages, abscesses, tumors), and the specific type of mass determines its course. Focal vascular disorders (eg, hematoma, infarct) are usually acute; inflammatory disorders (eg, abscess), subacute; and neoplasms, chronic. Traumatic disorders usually manifest in an acute manner, but their specific localization and course are determined by their site, severity, and the complications involved.

Transient Physiologic Disorders

Neurologic disorders with a history of transient episodes, lasting from seconds to hours, are often seen in chiropractic practice. Their cause can generally be attributed to temporary neuronal hyper- or hypo-activity, and a few typical examples will be described in this section. Symptom manifestation will vary depending upon which specific sensory or motor cells are involved; eg, twitchings, hyperesthesia, photophobia, abnormal behavior, muscle weakness, numbness, or tingling.

Potassium Imbalance

A neuron's *resting potential* is primarily determined on the internal and external concentrations of potassium. For example, an increase in extracellular potassium will produce a resting potential closer to threshold (ie, a partially depolarized neuron); thus, the cell will become so sensitive that it will fire upon normally subthreshold stimuli. In near-threshold levels of extracellular potassium, the cell may fire spontaneously. This may be the direct cause of idiopathic pain or the convulsions associated with transient hypoxia. In very high levels of extracellular potassium with an extremely low concentration gradient, however, firing function is invariably lost.

A reduction of extracellular potassium will hyperpolarize the resting potential, and the neuron will become less excitable because the membrane potential is farther from threshold value. This effect is commonly seen when strong diuretics are prescribed (eg, for hypertension, obesity, PMS) and is typical of hypokalemic periodic paralysis and some renal diseases.

Sodium Imbalance

A neuron's *action potential* is primarily determined on the internal and external concentrations of sodium. Imbalances can be an effect of alterations in sodium conductance or ion concentration. For example, a membrane cannot conduct an action potential if (1) sodium concentration cannot be increased or (2) conductance is increased far beyond normal. Minor structural changes may produce an especially porous membrane that will cause increased sodium conductance, and the effect will be a partially depolarized (excitable) cell. However, if the leakage is severe, conduction will become blocked.

Calcium Imbalance

A reduction in extracellular calcium causes decreased concentration gradients for both potassium and sodium. Thus, calcium serves as a membrane stabilizer. In hypocalcemia, for example, it is common to see increased neuronal excitability and sometimes spontaneous activity because of the reduced resting potential. This state will usually manifest as paresthesias or involuntary muscular twitching. However, an opposite effect may be seen because an extremely low calcium level will block synaptic transmission.

An increase in extracellular calcium, rarely demonstrable overtly when mild or moderate, has the opposite effect. That is, action potential will be blocked, but synaptic transmission will be enhanced.

Drug Reactions

Certain drugs may alter normal function of the axon or synapse (presynaptically or postsynaptically). Local anesthetics usually prevent changes in sodium conductance within the axon's membrane to the degree that action potentials become blocked. At the synapse, transmitter release may be inhibited or postsynaptic receptors may be blocked by certain drugs.

Nerve Fatigue

The effects of chronic pain on the nervous system brings about changes in the nervous system similar to those produced by prolonged muscular effort. Prolonged pain, however, is not the only mechanism that can cause such an effect. The onset of clinical fatigue appears to be favored by poor health, postural stress, chronic aches and discomforts, mental/emotional conflicts, and periods of intensively prolonged concentration or eyestrain. Work done under compulsion (eg, a sense of duty) results in nervous system fatigue more readily than when interest and motivation are high. Worry and fear have long been known to cause effects within the autonomic nervous system. It is for this reason that indigestion, palpitation, hyperhidrosis, constipation, and vasomotor headaches are commonly associated with neurasthenic conditions.

Similar effects as those seen in neuronal fatigue occur at synapses as the result of the accumulation of circulating metabolic waste products or fatigue-producing substances developed within the brain and in toxicosis. They are also seen in some psychic disturbances such as depression and after prolonged concentration. The higher cerebral centers are most easily and quickly affected. It is thought by many authorities that it is for this reason that young children "go stale" quickly unless their mental training is properly balanced by rest and recreation. The same effect is likely seen in adult "burnout."

It is often stated that change of activity is equivalent to rest. It is questioned whether this is true of mental activity, but it may be true of muscular activity. The explanation offered by Kimber and associates is that when nervous stimuli are altered, new pathways and groups of muscles are called into play. For example, a person who is tired of inside work may go outside and walk, because the fresh air, changed environment, and different thoughts serve as new stimuli, travel different CNS paths, and throw into activity different groups of muscles.

The fatigue of nerve cells resulting from typical daily activities is normally repaired by a night's sleep. However, if overly demanding activities are continued day after day for an extended period, the effects of fatigue accumulate and a pathologic state is likely to result. This is more apt to happen if mental conflicts add their quota. If monotony is also added (a situation where the same neurons are activated by similar stimuli), abnormal states variously known as brain fag, burnout, neurasthenia, or a nervous breakdown are likely to develop. Depression or exhaustion of the higher CNS centers is usually the starting point of such a condition.

If motivation or will-power is weakened, the power of concentration lessened, and the mental faculties impaired, the imagination is likely to substitute morbid ideas, fears, and phobias that under ordinary circumstances would not arise, or, if they did, they would be quickly dismissed or reasoned away.

Neural Regeneration

After pressure injuries or toxic neuropathy, peripheral nerves have great recuperative potential. Unfortunately, expectations are usually disappointing following trauma or severe pathology.

Because the cell body is essential for the nutrition of the whole cell, it follows that if the processes of a neuron are severed by trauma or disease, they will die from malnutrition. If, for instance, a postganglionic spinal nerve is cut, all portions distal to the cut will die because the processes have separated from their cell bodies in the ganglion or spinal cord. The affected axis cylinder fragments, the axon breaks up, and Schwann cells proliferate to form digestive chambers. The fibers and the medullary sheath degenerate and are absorbed, and, in time, an endoneurial tubule (band of Buengner) exists that is completely filled with Schwann cells. Endoneurial tubes do not degenerate as axons and myelin do after injury. Because they are filled with proliferated Schwann cells, they remain available for entry by regenerating axons.

Segments of the proximal axons develop sprouts that tend to grow along the course of the degenerated distal segments. This appears to be a random process that is guided somewhat by the endoneurial tubules. Some succeed in uniting with healthy segments if they enter a tubule and others do not. If nerve compression is relieved, additional sprouts are encouraged to grow.

A destroyed CNS nerve, in contrast, does not necessarily mean that function cannot be restored to a considerable extent. Illis explains that previously unused or little used pathways may become effective through neuromuscular education following degeneration of major connections.

Pressure Neuropathy

Prichard points out that nerves are richly supplied with anastamoses in the longitudinal direction. This allows nerves to be entirely freed from surrounding tissues for lengths up to several centimeters without altering their function. "What nerves cannot stand is pressure and stretching; these lead rapidly to functional deterioration, which eventually becomes irreversible and ends in physical degeneration if the pathologic condition is not relieved." It is for this reason that a surgeon cannot stretch a cut nerve to fill a widely separated gap. Approximation must be achieved by relocating the nerve's course, thus sacrificing some small branches, or by a nerve graft.

Pressure on a nerve interferes with the circulation to the neuronal membrane and with its axoplasmic flow. It is theoretically possible that pressure, if severe enough, can directly block conduction, but this would be a rare circumstance. A local block can occur within a few minutes after pressure is applied, but this is the effect of total ischemia. Even in cases of chronic partial ischemia, conduction is reduced as it passes through the affected area. In such situations, the adverse effects of any degree of ischemia may be cumulative and eventually lead to a complete conduction block.

Interference with axoplasmic flow by direct pressure or the associated ischemia will also produce functional failure in a matter of hours. If this pressure is removed, recovery will occur quite rapidly depending upon how fast the effects of the metabolic damage can be repaired. If the pressure is not removed, more serious peripheral degeneration effects occur in the neuron.

Traumatic Neuropathy

The connective tissue ends of a sharply severed nerve readily unite by cicatrical tissue while the fibers fragment and are absorbed. Before healthy fibers can unite during the regeneration process, they must, in some manner, pass over or around the intervening scar tissue. If they cannot, they may form a tangled mass of neural and connective-tissue elements (neuroma).

In most traumatic situations, there is often considerable local edema and tissue reactions around the injured neurons to offer pressure complications besides the typical processes of Wallerian degeneration.

Toxic Neuropathy

The last stages of toxic neuropathy resemble the typical Wallerian degeneration that follows nerve trauma except that the changes are scattered along the length of the nerve rather than being concentrated at a focal area. Various complexities arise if the disease process is specific for myelin, axons, or nerve cells.

Bibliography

Adams RD, Victor M: *Principles of Neurology*, ed 2. New York, McGraw-Hill, 1981.

Adrian ED: Sensory mechanisms: introduction. In Field J, Magoun HW (eds): *Handbook of Physiology*. Washington, DC, American Physiological Society, vol 1, 1959.

Adrian ED: The all-or-none principle in nerve. *Journal of Physiology*, 47:460-474, 1914.

Afifi AK, Bergmann RA: *Basic Neuroscience*. Baltimore, Urban & Schwarzenberg, 1980.

American Chiropractic Association: *Chiropractic State of the Art*. Arlington, VA, 1984, pp 8-9.

Baker AB (ed): *Clinical Neurology*, ed 2. New York, Harper & Brothers, Hoeber Medical Division, 1962.

Basmajian JV (ed): *Grant's Method of Anatomy*, ed 9. Baltimore, Williams & Wilkins, 1975, pp 39-49, 479-492.

Bennett MVL: Electrical transmission: A functional analysis and comparison with chemical transmission. In Brookhart JM, Mountcastle VB (eds): *Handbook of Physiology*. Baltimore, Williams & Wilkins, pp 357-358.

Biederman F: *The Fundamentals of Chiropractic from the Perspective of a Medical Doctor*. Heidelberg, Haug, 1968.

Bishop B: Neural plasticity. *Physical Therapy*, part 1, 62(8):132-134; part 2, 62(9):1275-1282, 1982.

Bittner H, Harper WD, Homewood AE, Janse J, Weiant CW: Chiropractic of today. *ACA Journal of Chiropractic*, 7(11):S81-88, 1973.

Brazier MAB: *Electrical Activity of the Nervous System*, ed 4. Baltimore, Williams & Wilkins, 1977, pp 1-91.

Brunarski DJ: Clinical trials of spinal manipulation: A critical appraisal and review of the literature. *Journal of Manipulative and Physiological Therapeutics*, 7(4):343-347, December 1984.

Bullock TH: The neuron doctrine and electrophysiology. *Science*, 129:17, 1959.

Burke DC, Murray DD: *Handbook of Spinal Cord Medicine*. London, Macmillan, 1975, pp 1-12.

Chusid JG: *Correlative Neuroanatomy & Functional Neurology*, ed 19. Los Altos, CA, Lange Medical, 1985, pp 82-86, 322-337, 473-492.

Clark RG: *Manter and Gatz's Essentials of Clinical Neuroanatomy and Neurophysiology*, ed 5. Philadelphia, F.A. Davis, 1975.

Coers C, Woolf AL: *Innervation of Muscle*. Springfield, IL, Charles C. Thomas, 1959.

Curtis DR, Eccles JC: Synaptic action during and after repetitive stimulation. *Journal of Physiology* (British), 150:374, 1960.

Daube JR, Sandok BA: *Medical Neurosciences*. Boston, Little, Brown, 1978, pp 2-4, 8-21, 24-44, 46-67, 68-89.

Eccles JC: The synapse. *Scientific American*, 212(1): 56, 1965.

Everett NB: *Functional Neuroanatomy*, ed 6. Philadelphia, Lea & Febiger, 1971.

Faulk WP, Demaeyer EM, Davies AJ: Some effects of malnutrition on the immune response in man. *American Journal of Clinical Nutrition*, 27:638-646, 1974.

Gardner EB: The neurophysiological basis of motor learning: a review. *Journal of the American Physical Therapy Association*, 47:1115, 1967.

Glynn IM, Karlish SJD: The sodium pump. *Annual Review of Physiology*, 37:13-55, 1975.

Gordienko AN (ed): *Control of Immunogenesis by the Nervous System*. Washington, DC, US Department of Commerce, 1958, pp 22-33, 45-52, 53-58.

Gorry GA, Pauker SG, Schwartz WB: The diagnostic importance of the normal finding. *New England Journal of Medicine*, 298:486-489, 1978.

Granit R: *The Basis of Motor Control*. New York, Academic Press, 1970.

Guyton AC: *Textbook of Medical Physiology*, ed 6. Philadelphia, W.B. Saunders, 1981, pp 560-576.

Guze H: The role of chiropractic in an integrative psychotherapy. In Schwartz HS (ed): *Mental Health and Chiropractic, A Multidisciplinary Approach*. New Hyde Park, NY, Sessions, 1973, pp 148-154.

Haldeman S, Hammerich K: The evolution of neurology and the concept of chiropractic. *ACA Journal of Chiropractic*, 7(8):S57-63, 1973.

Haldeman S: Interactions between the somatic and visceral nervous systems. *ACA Journal of Chiropractic*, V:57-64, August 1971.

Haldeman S: Neurophysiological concept of importance to chiropractors. *Journal of the Canadian Chiropractic Association*, 18(3):6, 1974.

Harper WD: *Anything Can Cause Anything*, ed 3. Seabrook, TX, published by author, 1974.

Haymaker W (ed): *Bing's Local Diagnosis in Neurological Diseases*, ed 14. St. Louis, C.V. Mosby, 1956.

Hensinger RN, MacEwen GD: Congenital anomalies of the spine. In Rothman RH, Simeone FA (eds): *The Spine*. Philadelphia, W.B. Saunders, 1975, vol I.

Hoag JM: The musculoskeletal system: A major factor in maintaining homeostasis. *Journal of the American Osteopathic Association*, 78:562, 1979.

Homewood AE: Chiropractic and emotional disorders. In Schwartz HS (ed): *Mental Health and Chiropractic, A Multidisciplinary Approach*. New Hyde Park, NY, Sessions, 1973, pp 94-106.

Homewood AE: *The Neurodynamics of the Vertebral Subluxation*, ed 3. Place of publication not shown, published by author, 1981, pp 21, 250.

Hubbard JI: *The Peripheral Nervous System*. New York, Plenum, 1974.

Illis LS: Regeneration in the central nervous system. *Lancet*, 1:1035-1037, 1973.

Inglis BD, Fraser B, Penfold BR: The scientific basis for chiropractic. In Inglis BD, Fraser B, Penfold BR (eds): *Chiropractic in New Zealand*. Davenport, IA, Palmer College of Chiropractic, 1979, pp 200-226.

Iversen LL; The chemistry of the brain. *Scientific American*, 24(3):134, 1979.

Jacobson E: *Tension in Medicine*. Springfield, IL, Charles C. Thomas, 1967.

Jacquet P: Bioenergetic analysis and chiropractic: Theoretical considerations and practical application. *Annals of the Swiss Chiropractors' Association*, 7:208-218, 1981.

Janse J: *Principles and Practice of Chiropractic*. Lombard, IL, National College of Chiropractic, 1976, pp 47-48.

Jaskoviak PA, Schafer RC: *Applied Physiotherapy: Practical Applications Within Clinical Chiropractic*. Arlington, VA, American Chiropractic Association, 1986, pp 3, 16.

Jewett DL, Rayner MD: *Basic Concepts of Neuronal Function*. Boston, Little, Brown, 1983.

Kandel ER: Small systems of neurons. *Scientific American*, 24(3):66, 1979.

Katz B: *Nerve, Muscle, and Synapse*. New York, McGraw-Hill, 1966.

Kimber DC, Gray CE, Stackpole CE: *Textbook of Anatomy and Physiology*, ed 11. New York, Macmillan, pp 186-268.

Kimmel EH: Psychophysiological aspects of the subluxation. In Schwartz HS (ed): *Mental Health and Chiropractic, A Multidisciplinary Approach*. New Hyde Park, NY, Sessions, 1973, pp 135-147.

Kuffler SW, Nichols JG: *From Neuron to Brain*. Sunderland, MA, Sinauer Associates, 1976.
Kupfermann I: Modulatory actions of neurotransmitters. *Annual Review of Neuroscience*, 2:447, 1979.
Kuntz A: *The Autonomic Nervous System*. Philadelphia, Lea & Febiger, 1953.
Leach RA: *The Chiropractic Theories*, ed 2. Baltimore, Williams & Wilkins, 1986.
Levi-Montalcini R, Calissano P: The nerve growth factor. *Scientific American*, 240(6):68, 1979.
Lövgren PW. Principles of treatment in chiropractic. *Scandinavian Journal of Rehabilitation Medicine*, 11(4):157-162, 1979.
Majno G: *The Healing Hand*. Cambridge, MA, Harvard University Press, 1975.
McLennon H: *Synaptic Transmission*. Philadelphia, W.B. Saunders, 1963.
McNaught AB, Callander R: *Illustrated Physiology*, ed 4. New York, Churchill Livingstone, 1983, pp 20-21, 204-209, 211, 213, 219.
Mears D: Mental disease and cervical spine distortion. *ACA Journal of Chiropractic*, 2(9), September 1965.
Nelson WA: Function vs structure. *ACA Journal of Chiropractic*, IV:7-8, February 1970.
Noback CR, Demarest RJ: *The Nervous System: Introduction and Review*. New York, McGraw-Hill, 1972.
Ochs S: Axoplasmic transport—a basis for neural pathology. In Dyck PJ, Thomas PK, Lambert EH (eds): *Peripheral Neuropathy*. Philadelphia, W.B. Saunders, Chapter 12.
Offner F: The excitable membrane. *Biophysical Journal*, 12:1583-1629, 1972.
Olsson Y: Vascular permeability in the peripheral nervous system. In Dyck PJ, Thomas PK, Lambert EH (eds): *Peripheral Neuropathy*. Philadelphia, W.B. Saunders, 1975, Chapter 10.
Palmer DD: *Textbook of the Science, Art and Philosophy of Chiropractic*. Portland, OR, Portland Printing House, 1910.
Pappas GD: Junctions between cells. In Weissman G, Claiborne R (eds): *Cell Membrane: Biochemistry, Cell Biology, and Pathology*. New York, HP Publications, 1975, Chapter 9.
Parke WW: Applied anatomy of the spine. In Rothman RH, Simeone FA (eds): *The Spine*. Philadelphia, W.B. Saunders, 1975, vol I, pp 28-31.
Patton HD, et al: *Introduction to Basic Neurology*. Philadelphia, W.B. Saunders, 1976.
Peele TL: *The Neuroanatomic Basis for Clinical Neurology*, ed 2. New York, McGraw-Hill, 1961.
Pinkenburg C: A basis for the theory of manipulative medicine. *Journal of Manipulative and Physiological Therapeutics*, 3(2):81-85, June 1980.
Pottenger FM: *Symptoms of Visceral Disease*, ed 6. St. Louis, C.V. Mosby, 1949, pp 74-76.
Prichard JW: Nerve. In Albright JA, Brand RA (eds): *The Scientific Basis of Orthopaedics*. New York, Appleton-Century-Crofts, 1979, pp 385-408.
Quigley WH: *Case Histories of Mental Illness Under Chiropractic Care*. Davenport, IA, Clear View Sanitarium, 1954, 1968.
Quigley WH: Physiological psychology of chiropractic in mental disorders. In Schwartz HS (ed): *Mental Health and Chiropractic, A Multidisciplinary Approach*. New Hyde Park, NY, Sessions, 1973, pp 107-119.
Rupert RL, Wagnon R, Thompson P, Moh TE: Chiropractic adjustments: Results of a controlled clinical trial in Egypt. *ICA Review*, pp 58-60, Winter 1985.
Schwartz HS (ed): *Mental Health and Chiropractic, A Multidisciplinary Approach*. New Hyde Park, NY, Sessions, 1973.
Schwartz HS: Foundations of chiropractic psychosomatics. *Journal of the National Chiropractic Association*, June 1949.
Schwartz HS: Preliminary analysis of 350 mental patients records treated by chiropractors. *Journal of the National Chiropractic Association*, November 1949.
Shepherd GM: Microcircuits in the nervous system. *Scientific American*, 238(2): 92, 1978.
Singer M: The influence of the nervous system on the regeneration of body parts. *Osteopathic Annals*, 3(7): 217-219, 1975.
Singer SJ: *A Short History of Anatomy and Physiology from the Greeks to Harvey*. New York, Dover Press, 1957.
Speransky AD: *A Basis for the Theory of Medicine;* translated by C.P. Dutt. New York, International Publishers, 1943.
Stedman's Medical Dictionary, ed 24. Baltimore, Williams & Wilkins, 1984.
Stevens CF: The neuron. *Scientific American*, 24(3): 54, 1979.
Strang VV: *Essential Principles of Chiropractic*. Davenport, IA, Palmer College of Chiropractic, 1984, pp 48-58.
Sulzer JL: Chiropractic healing as psychotherapy. In Schwartz HS (ed): *Mental Health and Chiropractic, A Multidisciplinary Approach*. New Hyde Park, NY, Sessions, 1973, pp 155-160.
Thomas CL (ed): *Taber's Cyclopedic Medical Dictionary*, ed 14. Philadelphia, F.A. Davis, 1981.
Thorpe RG: Musculoskeletal factors in chronic disease. *Osteopathic Annals*, 3(1): 7-10, 1975.
Vear HC: An assessment of chiropractic scope of practice. In Coyle BA, Martinez DP: *Proceedings of the Second Conference on Current Topics in Chiropractic: Reviews of the Literature*, May 4-5, 1985. Sunnyvale, CA, Palmer College of Chiropractic—West, 1985, p C1-2.
Verner JR: *The Science and Logic of Chiropractic*, ed 4. Englewood, NJ, published by author, 1950.
Vernon HT, Dhami MSI, Howley TP, Annett R: Spinal manipulation and beta-endorphin: A controlled study of the effect of a spinal manipulation on plasma beta-endorphin levels in normal males. *Journal of Manipulative and Physiological Therapeutics*, 9: 115-123, 1986.
Wayne KM: Disturbances of the nervous system as related to chiropractic. *Journal of the Canadian Chiropractic Association*, 13(2):20-23, 1969.
Werner JK: Trophic influence of nerves on the development and maintenance of sensory receptors. *American Journal of Physical Medicine*, 53(3): 127-142, 1974.
Weiant CW: *Rational Bateriology*. New York, New York Institute of Chiropractic, 1953.
Zhigalina LI: The role of non-specific stimulation of the nervous system in certain immunological reactions. In Gordienko AN (ed): *Control of Immunogenesis by the Nervous System*. Washington, DC, US Department of Commerce, 1958, pp 110-124.

Part II: The Neurologic Systems

Chapter 3

The Longitudinal Neurologic Systems

This chapter succinctly describes the basic structure and function of the six major longitudinal systems; viz, the sensory, motor, visceral, vascular, consciousness, and cerebrospinal fluid systems.

As we begin this chapter, it might be well for the reader to subjectively grasp the significance of the motor and sensory systems as far as possible. One exercise in this is to imagine that you had become unconscious and someone has placed you in a remote dark empty cellar, far beyond any source of environmental sound. The first thing you realize is that you are a total sensory and motor paralytic from the neck down. You are unable to move even a fingertip because your motor system is not functioning. Because there is no feeling, you do not know whether you are recumbent or tied in a chair. Your vision is normal, but there is no light. Your hearing is normal, but there is no sound. Your taste buds are functional, but there is nothing to eat or drink. Your olfactory organs are functional, but there are no detectable odors. There is little left except thought and memory.

After a time in this predicament, thoughts undoubtedly arise such as, "I wish I had really looked at the beauty of the world when I had a chance. I wish I had listened to the music of the masters and even the birds in my backyard when I had a chance. I gulped down so many delicious meals. I had a beautiful garden, but I rarely took time to appreciate its design and fragrance. I even failed to take time to appreciate the texture of my own clothes. I was in such a hurry to go nowhere that was more important. I missed so much."

OVERVIEW

The human nervous system is a marvel in organizing and adapting to internal and external environmental changes: (1) The receptors and afferent neurons of the visceral and somatic input systems are necessary to detect internal and external environmental changes. (2) The visceral efferent neurons and the muscles of the motor output system must be stimulated if action is to be taken. (3) The integrative system serves as intermediary stations via a complex arrangement of interneurons whose synapses control impulse strength and signal direction from the sensory system to the motor system.

The visceral (autonomic, vegetative) system is organized in a manner that is similar to the somatic system, but there are some important differences. Both visceral and somatic systems have longitudinal afferent sensory and efferent motor components. These fibers interact at each horizontal level of the axial nervous system to provide the various reflex mechanisms necessary to maintain *homeostasis:* See Table 3.1.

The visceral system is far more independent from consciousness than is the somatic system. Three mechanisms especially provide this independence: (1) All somatic reflexes are mediated in the CNS; visceral reflexes can also occur in the periphery. (2) Many viscera are directly regulated by circulating hormones, but their respective glands are under neural control. (3) Visceral receptors do not require external stimuli; eg, glands function without external control or conscious awareness.

Disorders within a longitudinal system may occur at any one or more of the horizontal levels; viz, the supratentorial, posterior fossa, spinal, and peripheral levels. When dysfunction occurs, symptoms usually arise as pain, pressure, tingling, numbness, weakness, paralysis, incoordination, nausea, dizziness, or altered states of consciousness.

THE SENSORY SYSTEM

The CNS derives information to determine its functions in voluntary and involuntary behavior via data from the body's internal and external media. The following review of the sensory system is designed to underscore how such environmental information is detected and translated by receptors, transmitted to the CNS, integrated, and perceived by conscious and subconscious faculties.

Daube/Sandok classify afferent (sensory) impulses according to their origin and specificity. See Table 3.2.

Basic Types of Sensory Perception

The perception of sensation can be superficial, deep, or combined, and this may occur consciously, unconsciously, or both.

• *Superficial sensation* includes such afferent signals as touch, pain, warmth, cold, two-point discrimination, weight differentiation (barognosis), and graphesthesia. This group would also include the special sensations of vision, smell, hearing, and taste.

• *Deep sensation* includes the afferent signals of deep pressure, jointposition and movement, equilibrium, deep pain, and vibration (pallesthesia). This group would also include the unconscious perception of such physiologic sensory input as muscle length and tension, arterial blood pressure, central venous pressure, lung inflation, cranial blood temperature, blood and CSF pH, blood oxygen and carbon dioxide levels, and plasma osmotic pressure.

• *Combined sensations* include (a) *stereognosis*, the ability to recognize familiar objects placed on the hand; and (b) *topognosis*, the ability to localize and perceive cutaneous stimuli.

Classic literature often uses Head's two groups in classifying cutaneous sensibility.

• *Protopathic.* These essentially comprise the crude, poorly localized sensations perceived at the thalamic level such as simple touch, pain, and severe changes in tempera-

Table 3.1. Levels of the Autonomic Nervous System and Major Structures

Level	Major Structures Involved
Peripheral	Receptors, ganglia, effectors.
Spinal	Preganglionic sympathetic and parasympathetic neurons.
Posterior fossa	Reticular formation and preganglionic parasympathetic neurons; eg, respiration, cardiovascular control.
Supratentorial	Hypothalamus and limbic system: anterior hypothalamus, parasympathetic; posterior hypothalamus, sympathetic. Data are also transmitted to the thalamus and cerebral cortex.

ture. Following nerve injury, protopathic sensations return rapidly (7—10 weeks) during regeneration.

• *Epicritic.* These include sensations requiring cerebral participation for fine discrimination such as light touch, mild—moderate temperature changes, two-point discrimination, barognosis, and graphesthesia. Epicritic sensations return slowly (1—2 years) during regeneration or do not return at all.

Sensory Neuron Levels

The function of the transducer-like receptor organs is to convert chemical, mechanical, photic, and thermal stimuli into neuronal potentials that can be transmitted to and within the CNS by specific pathways so that they can be perceived, interpreted, and integrated. This process is usually (but not always) conducted, processed, and utilized over three orders of neurons: primary, secondary, and tertiary (refer to Fig. 2.13).

Primary Neurons

The dendrites of peripheral sensory neurons receive impulses from sensory receptors, and their unipolar cell bodies lie outside the CNS in a spinal root ganglion. There are no synapses in a posterior (dorsal) spinal ganglion. Each ganglion cell has a single nerve process (dendraxon) that divides so that the distal branch innervates the receptor and the proximal branch enters the CNS via a posterior root of the spinal cord or brain stem and then through the posterolateral sulcus at the *posterior root entry zone*

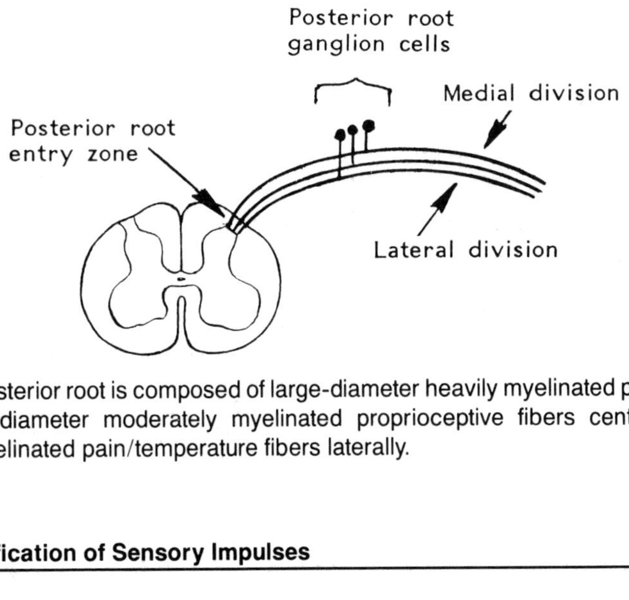

Figure 3.1. The posterior root is composed of large-diameter heavily myelinated proprioceptive fibers medially, medium-diameter moderately myelinated proprioceptive fibers centrally, and smaller-diameter thinly myelinated pain/temperature fibers laterally.

Table 3.2. Classification of Sensory Impulses

Type		Origin
General somatic afferent	*(GSA)*	Joints, skin, striated muscle.
Special somatic afferent	*(SSA)*	Equilibrium, hearing, vision.
General visceral afferent	*(GVA)*	Smooth muscle and viscera (essentially unconscious perception).
Special visceral afferent	*(SVA)*	Smell, taste.

(Fig. 3.1). The proximal axons of a primary neuron may synapse immediately with secondary neurons in the CNS or ascend within a tract (usually a white matter fasciculus) for a considerable distance before they synapse. See Figure 3.2 and Table 3.3.

Secondary Neurons

The axons of primary sensory neurons synapse close to the cell bodies of secondary neurons that lie within the posterior gray matter of the spinal cord or an analogous area of the brain stem (derivatives of the embryonic alar plate; refer to Fig. 2.2). The axons of secondary sensory neurons cross the midline (decussate) in their cephalad course and then ascend to the brain stem to end in specific sensory nuclei of the thalamus, where they synapse with the cell bodies of tertiary sensory neurons. The crude recognition of general somatic information enters consciousness at this level.

Tertiary Neurons

The axons projecting from the cell bodies of the tertiary sensory neurons of the thalamus extend to the somesthetic area of the sensory cortex via the thalamocortical radiation (refer to Fig. 2.25). Auditory and visual fibers extend to the temporal and occipital

Table 3.3. Primary Sensory Pathways

Pathway	Primary function
Posterior (dorsal) columns:	
Fasciculus gracilis	Conscious proprioception, tactile discrimination, stereognosis, barognosis, vibration
Fasciculus cuneatus	Conscious proprioception
Posterior (dorsal) spinocerebellar tract	Unconscious proprioception
Anterior (ventral) spinocerebellar tract	Unconscious proprioception
Lateral spinothalamic tract	Pain, temperature
Anterior (ventral) spinothalamic tract	Simple touch

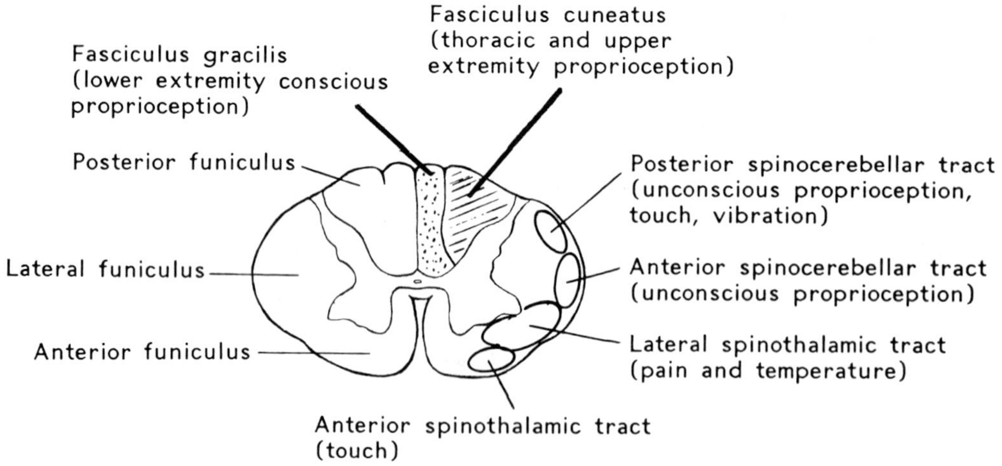

Figure 3.2. Horizontal section of the upper cervical cord showing the location of major ascending sensory tracts and their relationship within the funiculi.

lobes, respectively. However, the primary area of the cortex involved for somatic sensory impulses is in the postcentral gyrus of the parietal lobe and distributed in a homunculus-like manner (Fig. 3.3). It is at this level where the finer, more discriminative, aspects of somatic sensory perception occur.

Receptors: General Considerations

It was described in the previous chapter that whenever a stimulus of adequate threshold acts upon a receptor, the receptor organ depolarizes and a graded generator potential initiates. If this is strong enough, an electrotonic potential is produced that induces a train of centralward action potentials of uniform amplitude.

Receptor Adaptation

Because all action potentials are of the same amplitude, the intensity of stimulation is coded by the quantity of neurons activated and the frequency (modulation) of the dis-

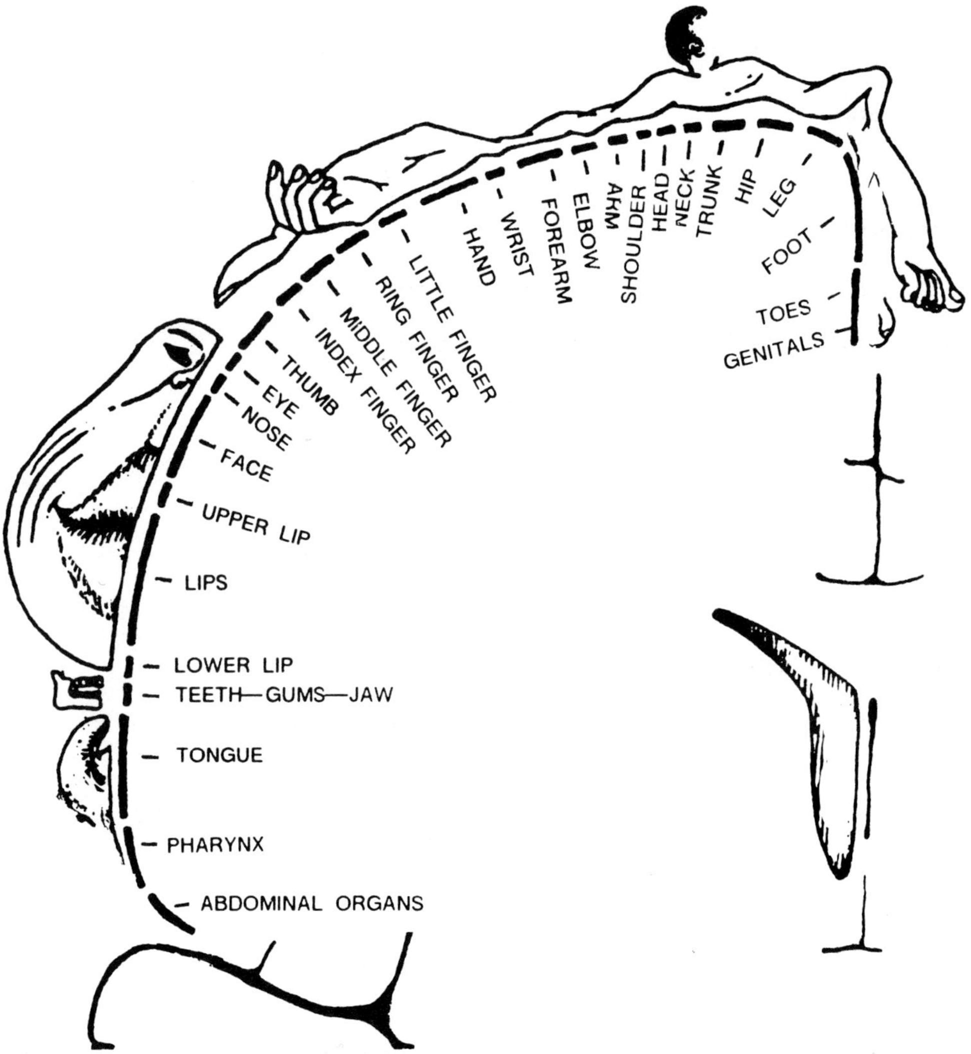

Figure 3.3. Sensory representation of the body in the postcentral gyrus. This homunculus-like design helps to visualize the order and comparative size of body centers as portrayed along the cerebral cortex. Redrawn from Penfield/Rasmussen.

Table 3.4. Peripheral Nerve (Mixed) Fiber Types

Fiber class	Fiber diameter (microns)	Conduction velocity (ųsec)	Function	Sen. type
Striated Muscle Afferents				
A-alpha	12—20	70—120	Muscle spindle primaries; viz, annulospiral endings	Ia
	12—20	70—120	Golgi tendon organs	Ib
A-beta	6—12	30—70	Touch, pressure, vibration, muscle spindle secondaries (eg, flow spray endings)	II
A-delta	2—6	4—30	Fast pain, temperature, pressure	III
Joint Afferents				
A-alpha	12—20	70—120	Joint receptors	Ia
Cutaneous Afferents				
A-alpha	6—12	30—70	Paccinian corpuscles, touch receptors	
A-delta	2—6	4—30	Fast pain, temperature, pressure	III
C	<2	0.5—2	Slow pain, temperature, crude touch, some mechanoreceptors	IV
Visceral Afferents				
A	2—12	4—70	Various visceral receptors	
C	<2	0.2—2	Various visceral receptors	
Striated Muscle Efferents				
Alpha	12—20	70—120	To extrafusal skeletal muscle, from alpha motor neurons	
Gamma	2—8	10—50	To intrafusal muscle spindles from gamma motor neurons	
Visceral Efferents				
B	<3	3—30	Preganglionic autonomic	
C	<1	0.5—2	Postganglionic autonomic	

charges. The axonal discharge frequency is high initially but gradually decreases (adapts) when receptor stimulation is sustained. If a sensory receptor is repetitively stimulated, successively smaller generator potentials are produced (receptor fatigue).

Recovery depends on the type of receptor stimulated. Some receptors (eg, tonic) adapt slowly and respond variably according to the strength of the stimuli applied; other receptors (eg, phasic) adapt quickly and initiate impulses almost continuously.

Receptor Specificity

Sensory receptors are specialized cells that detect particular environmental changes. There are various types of receptor organs and each is more sensitive to one or more types of stimuli but not sensitive to other types. This specificity is determined by the location of the receptor organ and the organ's general structural and chemical composition (surface membrane, organelles).

Hirschy describes five general types of sensory receptors: (1) *mechanoreceptors*, which detect mechanical deformation of the receptors or cells adjacent to the receptors; (2) *chemoreceptors*, which detect tastes, odors, arterial oxygen levels, osmolarity of body fluids, CO_2 concentrations, and other factors that make up body chemistry; (3) *thermoreceptors*, which detect changes in temperature, with some receptors detecting cold and others warmth; (4) *electromagnetic receptors (visual)*, which detect light on the retina; and last but not least, the (5) *nociceptors*, which detect painful damage in the tissues, whether it be of a physical or chemical nature. All sensory receptors initiate impulses from their sites to the spinal cord via Type I—IV sensory afferent fibers (Table 3.4).

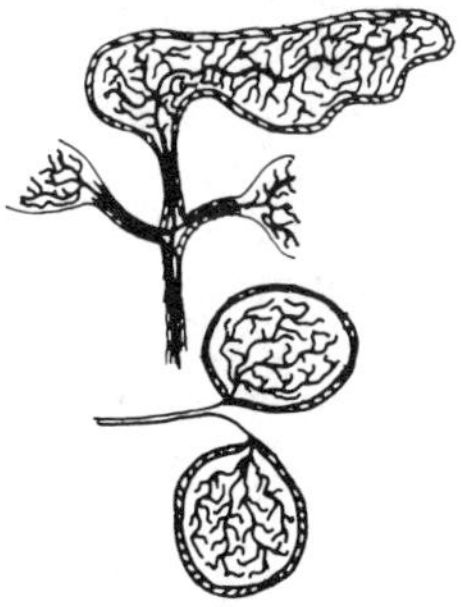

Figure 3.4. Two types of sensory receptor end organs: *Left,* a flower-spray Ruffini end organ. These slowly responding receptors located in joint capsules and the midlayer of skin signal messages of joint position and possibly of heat. *Right,* a Golgi-Mazzoni corpusle, a small flower-spray pressuresensitive organ containing an afferent neuron. They are found near joint capsules.

Sensory receptors can also be described from other viewpoints. For example, a *teleceptor* is any sensory receptor that is sensitive to distant stimuli such as those for sight, hearing, smell, and, to some extent, temperature. *Exteroceptors* include the teleceptors and those receptive to mechanical, electromagnetic, and chemical contact (eg, retinal receptors, Merkel's and Meissner's corpuscles, Krause's end bulbs). They are primarily affected by changes in the external environment. *Proprioceptors* relay input from muscle spindles, Golgi tendon organs, pacinian corpuscles, labyrinthine receptors, and the soft tissues of joints to offer data about posture, position, stretch, and compression. *Interoceptors* are sensitive to changes within blood vessels, respiration, and the viscera. These latter types also convey signals of hunger, thirst, nausea, and sexual sensations. Special interoceptors convey smell and taste sensations.

Skin receptors concerned with touch, pressure, or pain function as both somesthetic exteroceptors and as proprioceptors. They initiate many of the basic inborn protective reflexes such as grasp reflexes, withdrawal reflexes, and placement reactions.

Golgi tendon organs and muscle spindles transmit changes in muscle length, contraction, and tension, and the specialized receptors in the eye and ear are quite specific for type of stimuli to which they will respond. Such specialization, however, is not true of most receptors found in or near the skin. The stimuli from touch or pressure, for example, may excite bare nerve endings, hair follicle endings, Krause's end-bulbs, Meissner's corpuscles, Merkel's discs, Pacinian corpuscles, or Ruffini's corpuscles. See Figures 3.4 and 3.5. Pacinian corpuscles are also activated by vibration, Krause's end-bulbs by cold, and Ruffini's corpuscles by heat. While bare nerve endings are commonly thought of as the primary receptors of noxious stimuli (pain), they have also been shown to react to temperature, light touch, and deep pressure stimuli. Thus, while it was once thought that receptors were quite specific, it is now known that they have considerable overlap in function.

A few joint-related receptors are insensitive to movement but discharge in proportion to the joint angle. There is no position in which all joint receptors are silent.

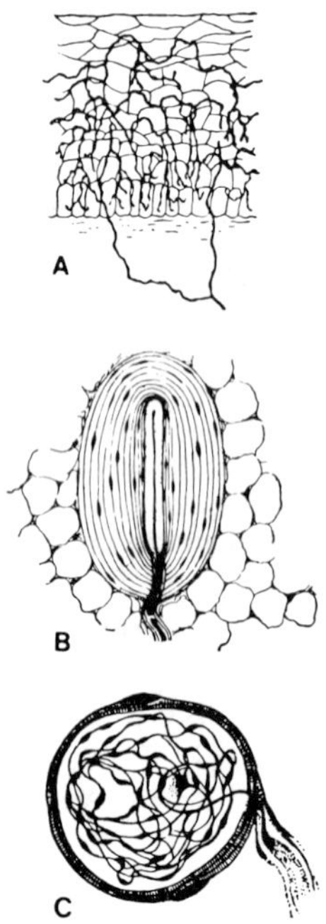

Figure 3.5. *A,* an end organ with diffuse sensory nerve fiber terminations in stratified squamous epithelium. Two types of surface receptors, composed of a lamellated capsule enclosing a sensory nerve twig, are shown. *B,* a Pacinian corpuscle, a rapidly responding receptor sited in the deep layer of skin and near tendons and joints. They are highly sensitive to movement, pressure, and vibration stimuli. *C,* a Meissner corpuscle, involving many terminals, found just beneath the dermis. They send patterned signals of touch necessary for precise discrimination and integrative processing.

Balance Recovery

Besides those receptors involved in receiving impressions from the surface and in maintaining the erect posture against gravity, there are other postural mechanisms concerned with sustaining body equilibrium. These are necessary to keep the body in the correct position during complex motor activities. For example, when the body is thrown off balance (eg, from a stumble or blow), compensatory movements beyond conscious control are made to restore normal posture. These reflex movements receive their sensory input from inner-ear proprioceptors, stretch receptors of the cervical musculature, other joint and muscle proprioceptors, the sensory organs of touch (especially of the plantar surfaces of the feet), and visual stimulation. The orientation of visual impressions is important in maintaining erect posture by establishing relationships to objects about the individual.

Labyrinthine Receptors

Inner ear sensory organs contribute stimuli to postural tone through impulses arising when the neck is moved. Small particles of calcium (otoliths) are suspended within the fluid of the semicircular canals. When the head is tilted, the otoliths drift from one part of the canal's wall to another. As these floating otoliths touch the sides of the canal's walls, they press against a few of the many hair-like sensory nerve receptors that line the canal's walls. This slight pressure stimulates impulses that ultimately produce a sensation of position and a reflex righting of the head relative to gravitational pull (Fig. 3.6).

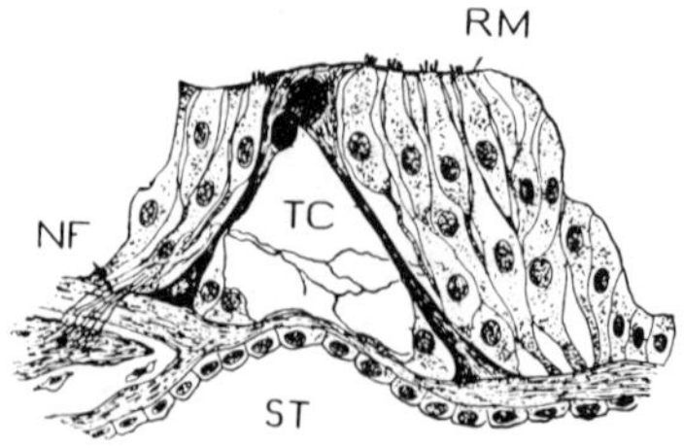

Figure 3.6. Schematic section of the organ of Corti: *TC,* tunnel of Corti; *ST,* scala tympani; *RM,* reticular membrane; *NF,* nerve fibers.

Only slight stimulation is necessary to evoke the reflexes necessary to maintain the body erect. Equilibrium reflexes evoked by stimulation of the semicircular canals dominate all other righting reflexes. Once these reflexes are lost (eg, pathology), one must rely solely on muscle and tendon proprioceptors, visual stimuli, and cutaneous touch and pressure to maintain an erect position.

Cervical Receptors

With the head erect, the labyrinths are placed in an optimum position to act synergistically with the neck reflexes, and these in turn react with other existing proprioceptive and exeroceptive impulses to supply a symmetric distribution of tone in proper quantities to postural muscles. Specifically, neck righting reflexes are evoked from impulses arising in joint receptors of the neck to produce contraction to align the body with the head. A typical spinal proprioception pathway is shown in Figure 3.7.

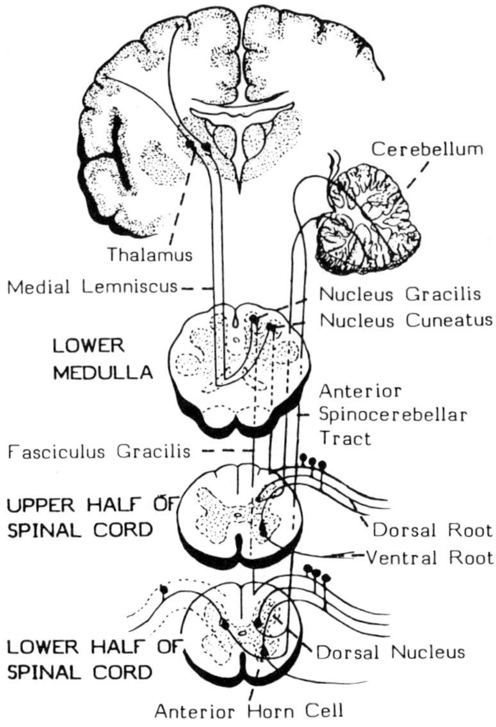

Figure 3.7. A typical proprioception pathway.

The cervical muscles are richly supplied with proprioceptors, and the atlanto-occipital and atlantoaxial joints are especially endowed with receptors. These facts, besides the specialized proprioception receptors of the inner ear, make head position important in maintaining structural balance. Almost all movements are started with a head movement in the direction desired, and only a slight poorly directed head movement during a complicated movement is necessary to throw the entire body out of alignment. In contrast, cervical reflexes appear to be dominant on the upper limbs, while labyrinthine reflexes appear to be dominant on the lower limbs.

It is not unlikely that proprioceptive impulses combined with the interacting postural reflexes of good body mechanics play a role in the maintenance of good health and optimal performance. Conversely, the maladjustment of nervous impulses within the CNS as a result of pressure, irritation, or poor posture may be a causative factor in the production of poor health and hindered performance by contributing to dysfunction from the subtle yet persistent stress involved.

Joint Receptors for Pain

Wyke, Newton, and others point out that articular capsules are richly supplied with nociceptors. See Table 3.5.

Three systems of innervation are described by Rossi: (1) a coarse system in the loose areolar tissues; (2) a fine network with numerous terminations in the histiocytic cell layer; and (3) an extremely delicate network intermeshed within the fine network that is closely attached to the capillaries, connective tissue, and histiocytes.

Clinicians realize that joint pain that is not associated with what is commonly thought of as acute sprain or strain often presents a history that contains mention of working in unusual postures just prior to the onset of pain. Painting a ceiling, lifting an object in an awkward position, prolonged ironing, and the chores of spring gardening are typical examples. Until recently, it was thought that the origins of such syndromes were primarily myogenic. Recent studies, however, have added a distinctly neurogenic component in such postural stresses.

Table 3.5. Joint Receptors*

Type	I	II	III	IV
Resembles	Ruffini corpuscles	Pacinian corpuscles	Golgi end-organs	
Location	Outer layers of joint capsule, grape-like clusters (3—8)	Sparsely found in deep layers of joint capsule and in fat pads, grape-like clusters (2—4)	Joint ligaments, grape-like clusters (2—3)	Joint capsule (except synovia), joint ligaments, fat pads, periosteum; absent in articular fibrocartilage
Endings	Encapsulated	Thickly encapsulated	Thinly encapsulated	Free nerve endings, plexus
Fiber type and size	Myelinated, small (6ɥ—9ɥ)	Myelinated, medium (9ɥ—12ɥ)	Myelinated, large (13ɥ—17ɥ)	Myelinated and unmyelinated, variable size (92ɥ—2ɥ)
Threshold	Very low	Low	High	High
Conduction	Slow	Medium	Rapid	Slow
Adaptation	Slow	Rapid	Very slow	Nonadapting
Action	Mechanoreceptor	Dynamic mechanoreceptor	Dynamic mechanoreceptor	Nociceptor
Function	Signals static position of joint, speed and direction of joint movement; constantly firing; aids in regulating postural tone and muscle tone during joint motion.	Signals only rapid changes in movement: acceleration, deceleration; helps to initiate momentum; does not signal joint velocity, amplitude or direction.	Signals direction of movement; guards against excessive joint movement by regulating muscle tone (braking mechanism).	Signal noxious changes: mechanical or chemical.

*Adapted from data of Kessler/Hertling and Wyke.

If a blindfolded person maintains a limb in an asymmetrical posture for some time, it is typically misplaced in the direction of previous asymmetry when an attempt is made to restore it to a symmetrical position. This effect, called *apostural persistence*, is thought to be caused by adaptation in joint receptors or muscular forces such as are involved, for example, after contraction. In studies conducted by Howard/Anstis, the after-effects of holding the head to one side were compared with the after-effects of holding it straight while straining against a torque. After-effects in the self-perceived position of the head were evident in only the former condition and were found to be reduced when the head was in the opposite direction to that in which it was adapted. It was thus concluded that postural persistence is a function of adaptation in joint receptors, at least in moderate loading.

Major Pathways

Pain and Temperature Mechanisms

In contrast to other sensory systems, there is no central *pain* center that serves as a *localized* receiving center for nociceptive impulses. Peripheral nociceptive information is complexly modified in the CNS by neurotransmitters, synaptic relays, motor and sympathetic reflex linkage, and antinociceptive modulating and integrating mechanisms. All pain is mediated by the nervous system, yet only some pain originates from neuropathology.

The major structures involved in the detection and transmission of painful stimuli are the first-order neurons and posterior root, the lateral spinothalamic tract of the spinal cord, the thalamus, parietal cortex, and the prefrontal cortex. It should be noted, however, that lesions in these structures greatly modify pain (+/-), but they rarely abolish it. From a clinical standpoint, the major pathways are those that convey sensations of pain/temperature, touch, proprioception, and discrimination.

Receptors. Pain receptors are the most primitive of all neuroreceptors, and reflex responses to painful stimuli appear early during embryogeny. The primary locations for pain receptors are the (1) skin and subcutaneous tissues, (2) periosteum, (3) vascular walls, (4) joint structures (eg, capsules, para-articular soft tissues), (5) falx and tentorium of the cranial vault, and (6) deep tissues diffusely distributed throughout the body.

The parenchyma of the heart, lungs, abdominal and pelvic organs and the brain itself does *not* contain receptors for pain. The same is true for osseous tissue. However, the walls of associated arteries, the dura and visceral capsules, surrounding peritoneal and pleural membranes, and periosteum do. It is for this reason that almost any parenchymal lesion that produces inflammation, swelling, or severe contraction will cause pain if nearby bare nerve endings are stimulated.

It should be noted that the overstimulation of almost any receptor can give rise to pain. Whether this is do to a normal response in nonnociceptors or an effect on neighboring bare nerve ending is unclear. Prichard states that excessive receptor stimulation causes cells in any tissue to release, by cell rupture or increased permeability, substances (eg, bradykinin) that are not ordinarily present in extracellular fluid. Such substances are thought to act on bare nerve ending in the area in a manner similar to transmitter substances on postsynaptic membranes so that action potentials are initiated in nociceptor fibers.

Primary Tracts. Spinal cord impulses conveying pain and temperature signals appear to travel the same major course:

1. Proximal axons from the posterior root ganglia enter the spinal cord at the lateral aspect of the posterior root entry zone (refer to Fig. 3.2) into the substantia gelatinosa, divide into branches that ascend and descend longitudinally in the *posterolateral fasciculus* (Lissauer's tract) for 1—3 segments, and then leave the fasciculus to synapse with cells of secondary neurons in the posterior gray horn of the spinal cord.

2. These secondary neurons either synapse locally or cross through the anterior white commissure to the contralateral side and ascend in the *lateral spinothalamic tract* (refer to Fig. 3.2) in a route that is determined by fiber origin (ie, sacral, lumbar,

thoracic, cervical). See Figure 3.8. These axons extend up the cord and through the medulla, pons, and midbrain (spinal lemniscus) to synapse with cells of the *anterior (ventral) posterolateral nucleus* of the thalamus.

3. Third-order axons arising from the thalamus (thalamocortical fibers) extend to their respective terminations (refer to Fig. 3.3) in the *postcentral gyrus* of the parietal lobe of the cerebral cortex. The conscious perception of pain apparently results when spinothalamic stimuli activate certain anterior posterolateral thalamic or cortical neurons, or both. Although the crude perception of pain occurs at the thalamic level, the localization of pain and associated psychic elements of somatic pain require functionally active thalamocortical fibers.

The points shown in Figure 3.9 describe the course of the major pathway for pain/temperature impulses, but it should also be recognized that collateral fibers are given off at various levels of the neuraxis during this ascending course. One important level is in the brain stem where synapses are made with neurons of the centrally located reticular formation that provide data to the ascending activating system. These neuronal connections, whose signals are widely dispersed to the cortex, are important in maintaining an alert state of consciousness. This process will be explained later in this chapter.

Cranial vs Spinal Pain-Conducting Neurons. The pathways for pain described above are essentially those of structures located below the foramen magnum. Painful stimuli from the face, for example, are conducted primarily by the trigeminal (cranial V) nerve, which has its primary sensory cell bodies in the semilunar (gasserian) ganglion. Proximal axons enter the brain stem in the pontine region, descend ipsilaterally to the upper cervical cord, synapse with second-order neurons, cross to the contralateral side, and then ascend to the anterior posteromedial nucleus of the thalamus. It is for this slightly divergent course taken by nerves entering the CNS above and below the foramen magnum that lesions in the lower part of the brain stem may alter pain perception in the face ipsilaterally and in the lower body contralaterally.

Localization of Pain. The manifestations of pain/temperature-pathway lesions vary according to which level the neuraxis is involved:

1. *Peripheral level.* Lesions of the peripheral neuraxis can cause either an increase or

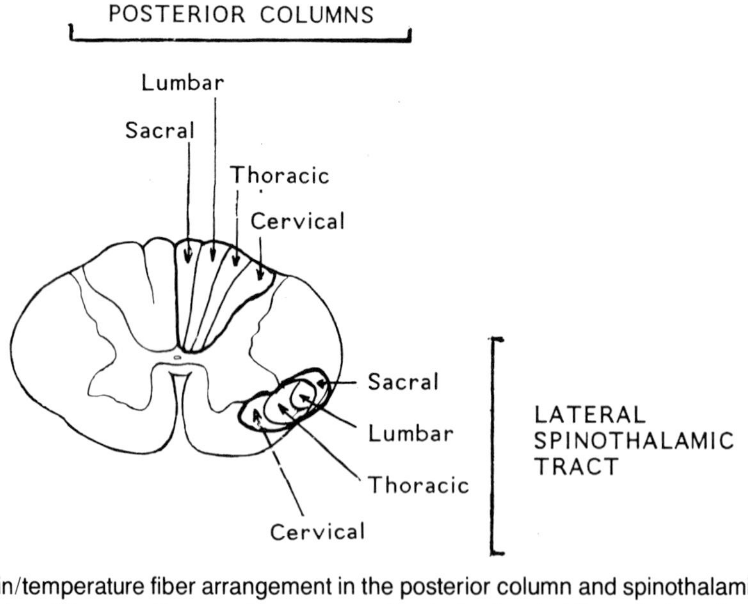

Figure 3.8. Pain/temperature fiber arrangement in the posterior column and spinothalamic tract. The presence and size of these pathways will vary according to the level of the spinal cord considered.

decrease in local pain/temperature perception, depending upon whether the involved neurons or their synapses are in a state of hypersensitivity or if transmission is blocked.

2. *Spinal level.* Lesions involving the lateral spinothalamic tract produce contralateral pain/temperature loss at and below the level of the lesion.

3. *Posterior fossa level.* Lesions in the posterior fossa produce contralateral pain/temperature loss at and below the level of the lesion and possibly an ipsilateral deficit in the face.

4. *Supratentorial level.* Lesions of the higher CNS seldom cause painful syndromes unless pain-sensitive structures (eg, the dura, arteries, periosteum) are involved; rather, they frequently exhibit poor contralateral pain-localization and temperature-discrimination deficits.

Conscious Proprioception and Tactile Discrimination

Proprioception refers to the inborn kinesthetic awareness of body posture, position, movement, weight, pressure, tension, changes in equilibrium, resistance of external objects, and the associated stereotyped response patterns. This awareness is the result of impulses generated in afferent receptors located within muscles, tendons, joints, skin, viscera, middle ears, and eyes. The responsive reflex patterns consist of highly coordinated movements of numerous muscle groups and joints that must be precisely regulated and timed as to sequence, speed, intensity, and duration.

Sensory data from the musculoskeletal system is necessary to direct and control motor function. This is accomplished through conscious and unconscious input. The primary course of conscious proprioception is as follows:

1. Peripheral neurons conveying conscious proprioception data have their cell bodies in the posterior ganglia. The distal processes extend to receptors in striated muscle, tendons, and joints. The proximal axons enter the medial division of the posterior root entry zone of the spinal cord, and ascend in a posterior column without synapsing. In the posterior white matter, fibers from the upper extremity and trunk constitute the *fasciculus cuneatus;* thus, this tract is prominent in the cervical and upper thoracic cord but not found in the lower cord; while fibers from the pelvis and lower extremity comprise the *fasciculus gracilis* (refer to Fig. 3.2). The first-

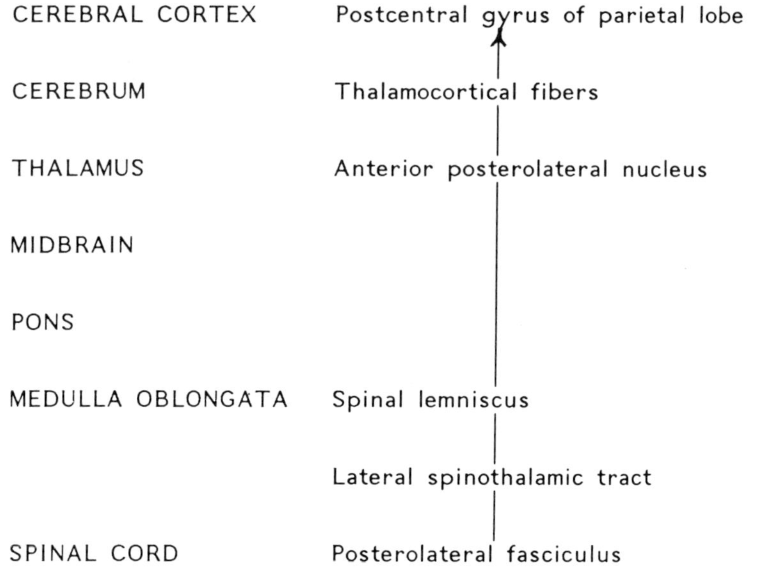

Figure 3.9. Pathway of lateral spinothalamic pathway, conveying pain and temperature signals.

order neurons ascending in the fasciculi cuneatus and gracilis terminate in the cuneatus and gracilis nuclei of the lower medulla oblongata and synapse with second-order neurons.

2. These secondary neurons cross to the opposite side as *internal arcuate fibers*, ascend to the thalamus as the *medial lemniscus*, terminate in the *anterior posterolateral nucleus*, and synapse with third-order neurons (Fig. 3.10).

3. Third-order thalamocortical axons arise from the posterolateral nucleus, extend via the posterior limb of the internal capsule, and then terminate in the somesthetic area of the postcentral gyrus of the parietal lobe in a homunculus-like manner (refer to Fig. 3.3).

Lesions within this pathway manifest as a loss of two-point discrimination and conscious joint position, atopognosia, asterognosis, and possibly as ataxia if the lesion is bilateral.

Unconscious Proprioception

From 40%—60% of nerve fibers supplying a muscle is sensory in function. Some of these afferent fibers are concerned with pain, but most are concerned with proprioception to register muscle fiber contraction or stretch. This is invariably an *unconscious* process, yet it plays a vital part in controlling muscular force and timing. The complete process is a combined effect from afferent fibers from muscles, tendons, and joints. These sensory muscle fibers originate from sites on perimysium, endomysium, capillaries, or in interstitial fat. Other sensory fibers originate from receptors concerned purely with pressure. These are abundant in joint tissues and offer *conscious* information as to limb position.

The primary course of unconscious proprioception impulses is as follows:

1. Peripheral neurons conveying unconscious proprioception data have their first-order neuron cell bodies in the posterior root ganglia. The distal processes extend peripherally to receptors located primarily in muscle spindles and Golgi tendon organs. The proximal axons enter the medial division of the posterior root entry zone of the spinal cord. From here, two primary courses are taken: (a) Some of the fibers from muscle spindles pass directly through the posterior gray matter to the anterior gray matter, comprising the afferent limb of the *stretch reflex*, which will be described later in this chapter. (b) Other fibers ascend as either the *anterior* or *posterior* spinocerebellar tracts so that the cerebellum can modify the

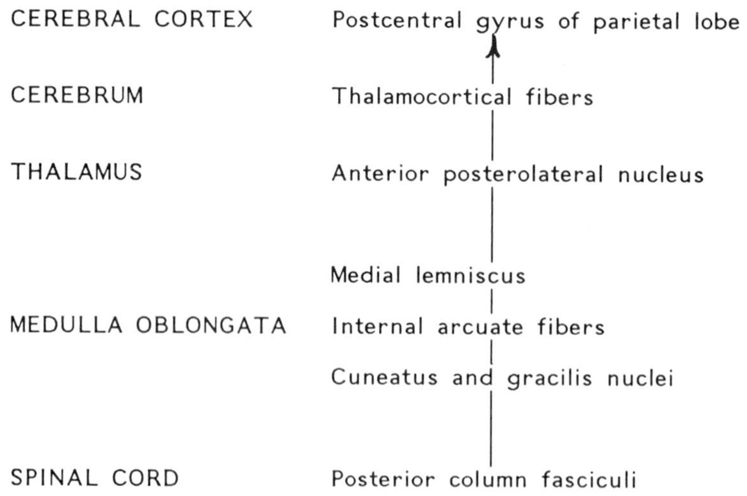

Figure 3.10. Pathway of the posterior column (medial lemniscus) pathway, conveying conscious proprioception and tactile discrimination signals.

unconscious afferent impulses to assure smooth, well-coordinated motion by cerebellar-efferent directives.

2. *The anterior spinocerebellar pathway.* First-order neurons entering the spinal cord at the lumbar and sacral levels convey signals from the pelvis and lower extremities. They synapse at the level of entry in the posterior gray horn, second-order neurons remain uncrossed or cross to the opposite side of the cord, ascend through the spinal cord, medulla, and pons in the lateral fasciculus as the *anterior spinocerebellar tract,* and most fibers project to the cerebellum via a circular route as the *superior cerebellar peduncle* (brachium conjunctivum). To offer a means for bilateral input, some fibers at the posterior fossa level re-cross to the ipsilateral side before they are projected to the cerebellum.

3. *The posterior spinocerebellar pathway.* First-order neurons entering the spinal cord at the thoracic level convey signals from the thorax and abdomen. They synapse at the level of entry, if they enter the CNS between T1 and L1, in the *nucleus dorsalis of Clarke* (Clarke's column) of the posterior gray horn. Second-order neurons enter the ipsilateral lateral funiculus and ascend the spinal cord as the *posterior spinocerebellar tract,* and then project to the cerebellum as the *inferior cerebellar peduncle* (restiform body). See Figure 3.11. This course changes somewhat above T1 and below L1 segments:

- Fibers carrying unconscious proprioception signals that enter the CNS above T1 ascend in the posterior columns to the lower medulla's representation of Clarke's column (*the lateral cuneate nucleus*). Here they synapse with second-order neurons (*the cuneocerebellar tract*) that run with posterior spinocerebellar fibers of the ipsilateral *inferior cerebellar peduncle* to the cerebellum.
- Similar fibers entering the CNS below L1 ascend in the posterior columns until they reach a point where they can enter Clarke's column. They then synapse there with second-order neurons that ascend as the *posterior spinocerebellar tract.*

Lesions within pathways for unconscious proprioception messages manifest primarily as motor incoordination in the extremities (eg, past pointing, ataxia). However, rarely are such pathways involved singularly. Spinocerebellar tract deficits usually play a part in a larger clinical picture of cord injury or pathology.

Touch

The perception of touch can be divided into two general types: (1) *simple touch,*

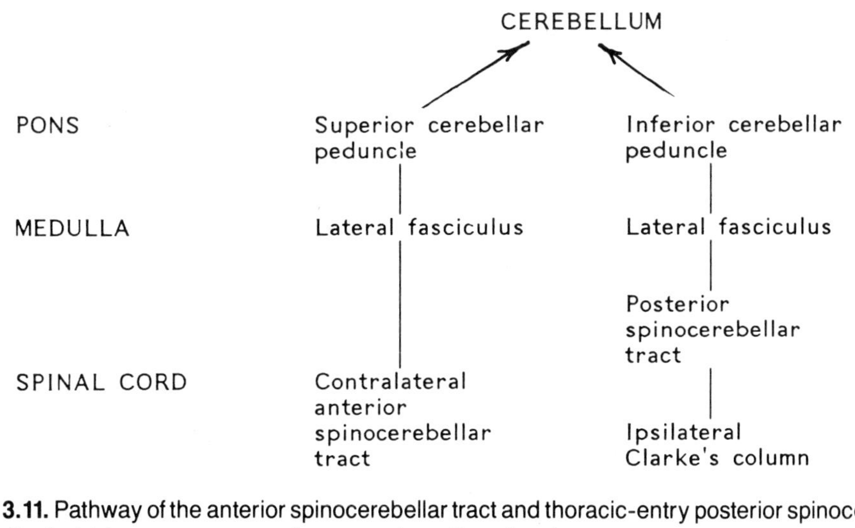

Figure 3.11. Pathway of the anterior spinocerebellar tract and thoracic-entry posterior spinocerebellar tract, both of which convey unconscious proprioception signals.

which is the crude perception of localized cutaneous pressure; and (2) *tactile discrimination*, which perceives the depth and quality of the pressure as well as the approximate shape and size of the stimulus as modified by the recall of associated past experiences.

It has been previously described that fibers conveying tactile discrimination signals for stereognostic perception ascend in the posterior column as the *fasciculus gracilis* with those conveying conscious proprioception data. Some fibers carrying messages of simple touch may also take this route. Other fibers conveying touch signals extend cephalad as the *anterior spinothalamic tract.*

The primary course of touch signals via the anterior spinothalamic tract is as follows:

1. Peripheral neurons conveying touch signals have their cell bodies in the posterior root ganglia. They project myelinated processes distally to receptors in the skin, around hair follicles, and in subcutaneous tissues. The proximal axons pass through the posterior root, enter the posterior root entry zone of the spinal cord, ascend and descend for several segments, and then synapse with second-order neurons near the core of the posterior gray horn.
2. These secondary neurons cross to the opposite side in the anterior white commissure, turn upward and ascend the cord as the *anterior spinothalamic tract*, and terminate in the *anterior posterolateral nucleus* of the thalamus, where they synapse with third-order neurons.
3. At the level of the pons and above, the course is the same as that taken by those of the fasciculus gracilis. Third-order thalamocortical axons arise from the posterolateral nucleus, extend via the posterior limb of the internal capsule, and then terminate in the somesthetic area of the postcentral gyrus of the parietal lobe in an homunculus-like manner (refer to Fig. 3.3).

Pathways of Other Sensations

The tracts conveying visceral signals will be described later in this chapter. The pathways for vision, hearing, equilibrium, taste, and smell will be described in Chapter 4.

Clinical Considerations

The diagnosis of neurologic diseases can often be frustrating because of the transient nature of many symptoms and signs. Besides frequent symptomatic peaks and valleys, neurologic symptoms may mimic a large variety of organic and functional disturbances. In general, the objective of the neurologic examination is to evaluate disturbances of motion, sensation, reflexes, skills, neuronutrition, and the general psyche.

The basic equipment usually required for evaluating the sensory system are a wisp of cotton or camel's hair brush, a pin or pinwheel, tubes of hot and cold water, a tuning fork (C128), olfactory solutions, taste test solutions, an ophthalmoscope, a penlight, a skin pencil, eye and color charts, and objects to test stereognosis objects. Common accessory equipment includes devices to detect localized areas of skin resistance and skin temperature variations.

The most common features associated with diseases of the sensory system are headache, vomiting, spinal and extremity pain, paresthesia, anesthesia, tinnitus, vertigo, deafness, and visual disturbances. Less common afferent nerve lesions take the form of sudden behavioral changes, disorders of memory and thinking, disturbances of consciousness, and hallucinations.

To experience any sensation, it is necessary that: (1) the sensory receptors are intact, (2) the sense-conveying fibers are normal, (3) the sense-interpreting centers are active, and (4) the associative centers of consciousness are intact.

Common terms used clinically to describe sensory perceptions are listed in Table 3.6.

Localization: General Principles

Correlating the patient's signs and symptoms of sensory dysfunction with the specific anatomical pathway level involved will be a distinct aid in determining the site of the lesion. *Supratentorial lesions*, for example, exhibit contralateral sensory deficits. In *posterior fossa lesions*, the primary signs will be contralateral sensory features in the trunk and extremities and, possibly, ipsilater-

Table 3.6. Common Terms Used to Describe Abnormal Sensory Perceptions

Term	Description
Acroesthesia	Abnormal sensitivity, especially pain, of the extremities.
Acroparesthesia	Numbness, prickling, or tingling sensations of the distal extremities (eg, fingers and toes).
Allesthesia	A single stimulation that is perceived as being displaced across the midline to a homologous region; ie, perceived contralaterally. This is sometimes referred to as *allochiria* or *allochesthesia.*
Alliesthesia	The perception of an external stimulus as being pleasant at one time and unpleasant at another.
Analgesia	Complete loss of normal pain sensibility.
Anesthesia	Complete loss of sensation. *Dissociated anesthesia* is the loss of some forms of cutaneous sensibility (usually pain/temperature) with the preservation of others (eg, tactile).
Astereognosis	Inability to recognize familiar objects by touch even if anesthesia is not present; usually indicates a lesion in the parietal cortex of the cerebrum.
Atopognosis	Inability to localize tactile stimuli without visual aid.
Baragnosis	Inability to distinguish objects of different weight without the aid of vision; usually indicates a lesion in the parietal cortex of the cerebrum.
Causalgia	Intense burning pain accompanied by trophic skin changes due to autonomic nerve fiber injury. The median or posterior tibial nerve is usually involved.
Colic	A nondiagnostic term that refers to any symptom complex whose major feature is acute paroxysmal pain.
Dysesthesia	Impaired sensitivity; a painful sensation from a stimulus that is normally not painful; formication.
Formication	False perception of insects crawling upon the skin; a common effect of cocaine withdrawal.
Hyperalgesia	Increased sensibility to pain-provoking stimuli; also called *hyperalgia.*
Hyperaphia	Excessive sensitivity to touch stimuli.
Hyperesthesia	Excessive sensitivity to any sensory stimulus; often restricted to increased tactile sensibility.
Hypoesthesia	Diminished sensation, especially tactile. This is often referred to as *hypesthesia.*

Table 3.6, continued

Term	Description
Neuralgia	Severe sharp pain along the course of a nerve; typically a functional disorder from nerve trunk pressure, faulty nerve nutrition, toxicosis, neuritis, or hysteria. This is sometimes referred to as *neurodynia.*
Paresthesia	Any disagreeable sensation such as numbness, tingling, prickling, or formication; usually restricted to abnormal nonpainful sensory aberrations.
Phantom pain	A projection of the sensation of pain to a part of the body that has been lost (eg, amputated). It is due to the stimulation of pain fibers that previously innervated the lost part.
Sensory displacement	When two stimuli are applied simultaneously, one is well localized while the other is displaced toward it.
Sensory extinction	When two stimuli are applied simultaneously, one is well localized while the other is perceived poorly or not at all.
Synesthesia	Two sensations are perceived from a single stimulus, one of which is well localized while the other is perceived contralaterally or in an area in which there is dysesthesia or burning pain. This is sometimes referred to as *synchiria.*

al sensory loss in the face. In *spinal cord lesions*, signs and symptoms manifest as sensory loss at the lesion level, with a varying degree of loss at all levels below the level of the lesion. In *peripheral nerve* or *nerve root lesions*, manifestations occur in a segmental manner and involve all peripheral sensory functions (often including pain). See Table 3.7.

The sensation of light touch is commonly measured clinically with a wisp of cotton, pressure by using thumb pressure, pain with a blunted pin, and two-point discrimination by using calipers. These and other sensory tests will be described in Chapter 8.

Supratentorial Level Lesions

All major sensory pathways have decussated once they reach the supratentorial level; thus, lesions at this level generally manifest as extensive contralateral sensory loss. Two important syndromes that are initiated at this level are described below.

Thalamic Syndrome. If a lesion involves the sensory fibers of the thalamus, all somatic afferent sensations will be lost in the contralateral half of the body (Fig. 3.12). The pain is usually persistent with associated outbursts of poorly localized pain. The character of the pain may be described as highly distressing burning, drawing, pulling, swelling, or tension sensations. Homonymous hemianopsia will be part of the clinical picture if that portion of the thalamus related to the optic nerve is involved. Ataxia, hyperkinesia, inability to discriminate tactile and joint signals, paresthesia, and weakness are also typical components of the syndrome. A slight stimulus may provoke a seizure of severe abnormal sensations.

Suprathalamic Syndrome. Lesions involving thalamocortical sensory fibers also alter somatic afferent sensations contralaterally; however, the loss is not as complete as it is in a thalamic syndrome. In a suprathalamic syndrome (eg, Dejerine's cortical sensory syndrome), there is a severe loss of tactile discrimination, two-point discrimination, passively moved joint-positions, baresthesia, the ability to recognize textures, the ability to recognize numbers drawn on the skin, and stereognosis because cortical function is necessary. However, only a minor or moderate loss occurs of pain, temperature, simple touch, and vibration sensations (Fig. 3.13).

Posterior Fossa Level Lesions

Lesions at the posterior fossa level feature contralateral intersegmental sensory loss below the neck because of interruption of the major ascending tracts and, usually, an ipsilateral sensory loss in the face because of involvement of the trigeminal nucleus (Fig. 3.14). The most common cause of this syndrome is inferior cerebellar artery occlusion (Wallenberg's syndrome).

Spinal Level Lesions

Severe lesions of the spinal cord, proximal to root entry, that interrupt major ascending and descending pathways will produce sen-

Table 3.7. Classic Locations of Segmental Pain

Priority Suspect Nerve(s)	Area of Localized Pain	Priority Suspect Nerve(s)	Area of Localized Pain
Trigeminal	Anterior head and face	*T5—12*	Peritoneum
C1—2, T7—12	Occiput	*T6—10*	Pancreas, spleen
C2—3	Forehead	*T7—9*	Ascending colon
C3, T1—5	Neck	*T8—9*	Gallbladder
C3—4, T1—3	Aortic arch	*T9—10*	Small intestines
C3—4, T1—5	Heart	*T9—11*	Transverse colon
C3—4, T1—8	Head and face	*T10—11*	Umbilical area, ovary, testicle
C3—4, T3—5	Lungs		
C3—4, T6—7	Stomach, cardiac aspect	*T10—12*	Crown of head, scrotum, lower limbs
C3—4, T8—10	Stomach, pyloric aspect		
C3—4, T7—9	Liver	*T10—12, S1—3*	Prostate
C4	Shoulder girdle, temple area	*T10—L1*	Kidney, uterine body
		T11—L1	Urethra, epididymis
C5	Deltoid area	*T11—L2*	Bladder neck, descending colon
C6	Thumb		
C7	First or index finger	*T11—L1*	Suprarenal area
C8	Fourth finger	*T12—L1, S1—4*	Uterine neck
T1	Fifth finger	*T12—L2*	Ureter
T1—4	Thorax	*L1*	Groin
T2	Nipple area	*L1—3, S1—4*	Bladder body, rectum, genital organs
T2—4	Bronchi		
T2—5	Upper limbs	*L3*	Knee, medial aspect
T2—12	Pleura	*L5*	Great toe
T4—5	Mammae bodies	*S1*	Fifth toe
T4—7	Thoracic aorta	*S2*	Thigh, posterior aspect
T5—8	Esophagus (caudal)	*S2—4*	Cervix

Note: Authorities differ somewhat as to exact levels, and variances of a segment above or below are commonly stated by different authorities. The above data are a composite of the findings from several sources (Courtesy of Associated Chiropractic Academic Press).

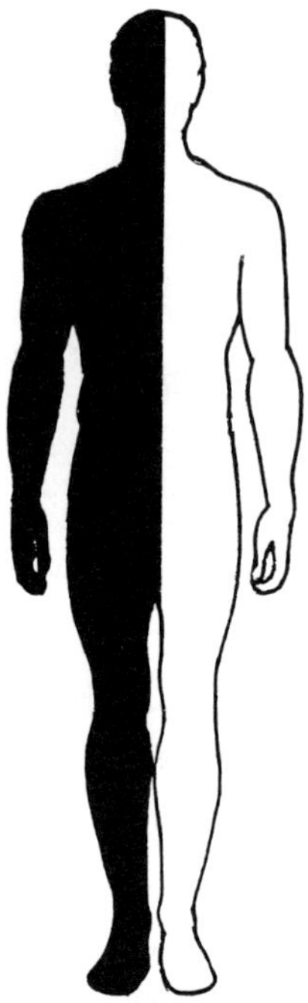

Figure 3.12. Thalamic syndrome, which will exhibit impairment of all sensations contralaterally.

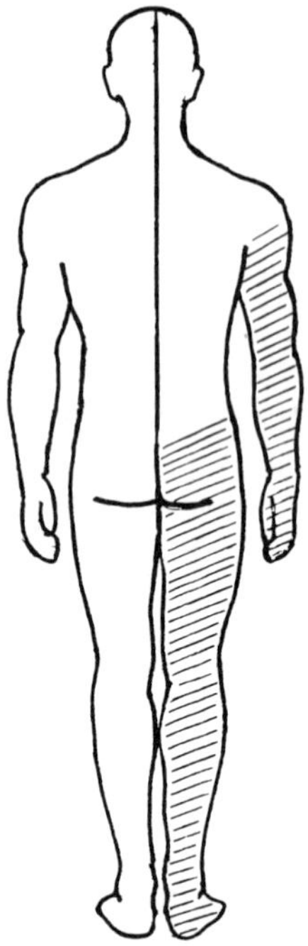

Figure 3.13. Suprathalamic syndrome, which will exhibit severe impairment of sensory discrimative faculties but minor deficits in other sensations.

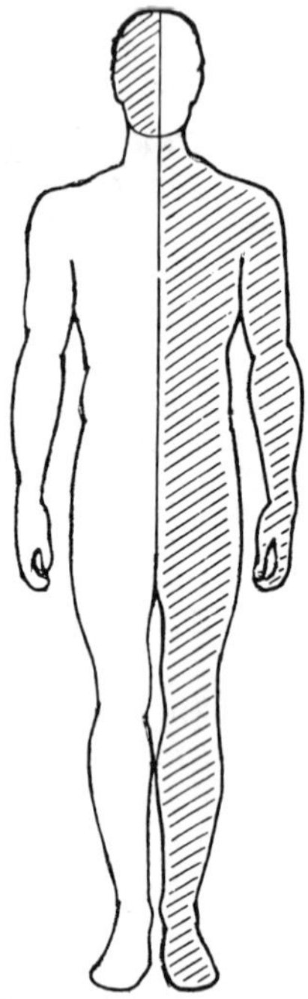

Figure 3.14. Posterior fossa level lesion, which will exhibit impaired pain and temperature sensation on the ipsilateral left face and the right side of the body below the neck.

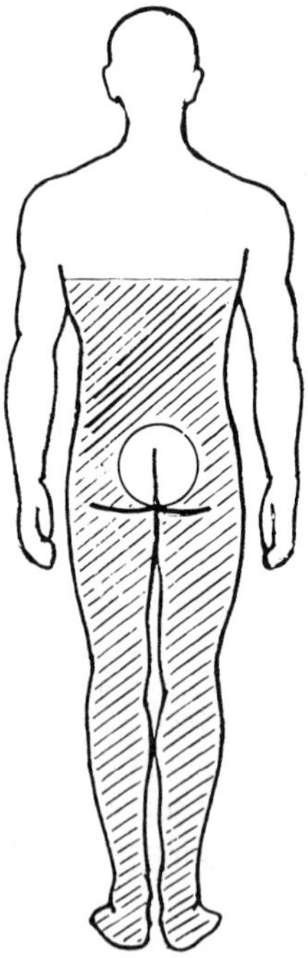

Figure 3.15. Posterior view of a lateral spinothalamic tract syndrome caused by a wide intramedullary lesion, exhibiting bilateral sensory loss with sacral sparing.

sory signs and symptoms at and below the lesion level. Typical examples are paralysis, loss of superficial and deep reflexes, and autonomic disturbances. If sensory tracts are interrupted but reflex motor arcs are not, deep tendon reflexes at and below the level of the lesion will be hyperactive.

Spinothalamic Tract Syndrome. If a lateral spinothalamic tract is interrupted, the patient will exhibit a contralateral loss of pain and temperature sensation from 2—3 segments below the level of the lesion through the lower extremity. Because fibers of the spinothalamic tract run in courses determined by their entry to the CNS (refer to Fig. 3.8), small midspine anterior lesions may spare fibers entering at the sacral area (Fig. 3.15).

Commissural Syndrome. This syndrome is seen when the *central* region of the spinal cord is impaired for several segments. It is characterized by a *bilateral* segmental loss of pain and temperature sensations, because both ipsilateral and decussating fibers are involved. Syringomyelia (cavitation), cord neoplasms, and trauma are the common causes. See Figure 3.16.

Syringomyelia, which produces gliosis around the central canal of the spinal cord, features a severe loss of pain and temperature sensations but retains touch and pressure sensations in the affected parts; ie, *dissociated anesthesia*. See Figure 3.17.

Brown-Séquard's Syndrome. This syndrome is rarely witnessed, but it offers a classic picture of the effects of an unilateral lesion of the spinal cord (Fig. 3.18). The classic picture is described as follows: (1) ipsilateral lower motor neuron paralysis and a zone of anesthesia in the segment of the lesion; (2) ipsilateral hyperesthesia below the zone of anesthesia; (3) ipsilateral upper motor neuron paralysis, loss of proprioception, loss of vibration sense, and loss of two-point discrimination below the level of the lesion; (4) a contralateral zone of hyperesthesia in the segment of the lesion; and (5) a contralateral loss of pain and temperature sensation below the level of the lesion. Common causes include a bullet wound, laceration, hemato-

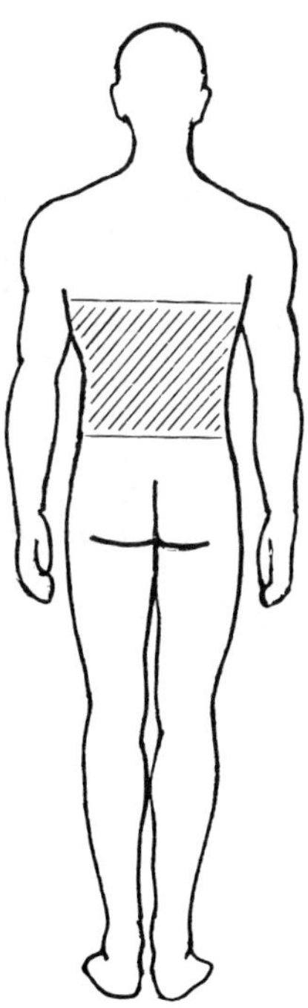

Figure 3.16. Segmental pain and temperature deficit because of midthoracic commissural syndrome.

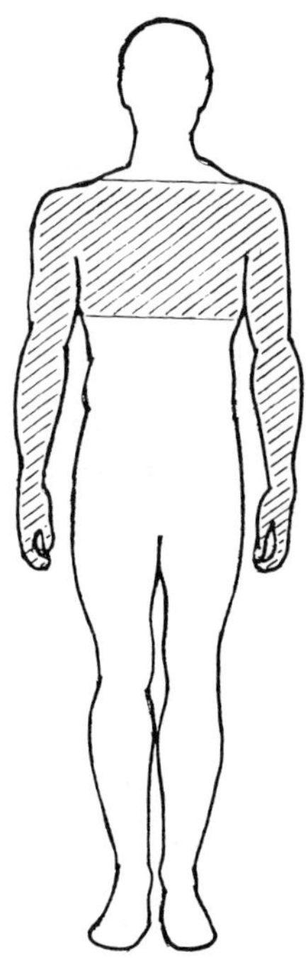

Figure 3.17. Syringomyelia, which will exhibit bilateral segmental loss of pain and temperature sensations.

myelia, cord tumor, and syringomyelia.

Tabes Dorsalis. Because of the interruption of proprioception pathways in the dorsal roots and posterior columns, this syndrome features marked sensory ataxia and a characteristic gait. At times, subjective sensory disturbances (tabetic crises) manifest as severe painful cramps in the larynx, stomach, and other viscera.

Posterolateral Sclerosis. In advanced cases of pernicious anemia, for example, combined degeneration of the posterior and lateral columns of the spinal cord occurs. The syndrome features marked sensory and motor disturbances. An early sign is a diminished vibration sense, with diminished discrimination faculties following (Fig. 3.19).

Multiple Sclerosis. This disorder is caused by disseminated patches of gliosis in the spinal cord and brain. It features early patches of numbness and paresthesias, followed by marked sensory and motor disturbances.

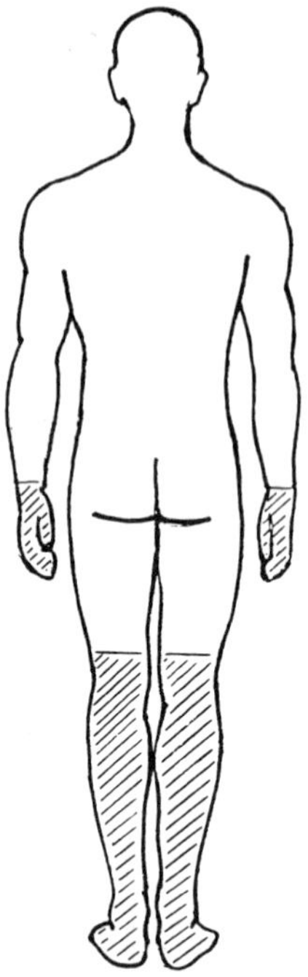

Figure 3.19. Posterolateral sclerosis, which will exhibit diminished vibration, two-point discrimination, and joint-position sensations bilaterally.

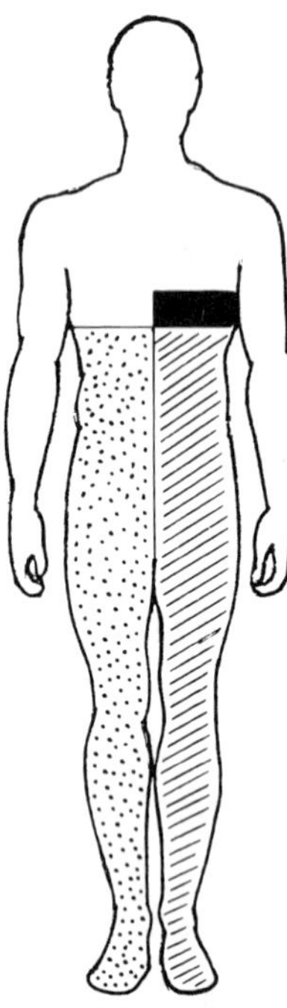

Figure 3.18. Brown-Séquard's syndrome. Loss of all sensations unilaterally at the level of the lesion; loss of proprioception, vibration, two-point discrimination, and joint-position sensation ipsilaterally; motor deficit ipsilaterally; and and impaired pain and temperature sensation contralaterally below the lesion.

Root Lesions. Nerve root syndromes are frequently encountered in chiropractic practice. They may involve neuronal compression, stretching, or inflammation and induce sensory disturbances such as pain, hyperesthesia or hypesthesia, and paresthesias along the anatomical distribution of the affected root. This typically manifests in a dermatomal pattern (Fig. 3.20). The associated pain (usually lancinating) is commonly aggravated by any act that increases intrathecal pressure such as in coughing, sneezing, abdominal straining, or any maneuver that stretches the involved root. Typical causes include acute subluxations, IVD protrusions, spondylitis, cord tumors, vertebral fractures, and meningitis.

In singular lesions, the perception of touch in dorsal root lesions is retained to a large degree because of the segmental overlap to adjacent segments; eg, the segmental distribution of T5 overlaps half of T4 and T6, T6 overlaps half of T5 and T7, etc. As most of the skin is innervated by an overlapping nerve supply from adjacent nerve branches, it is difficult in testing cutaneous sensations to isolate a specific spinal nerve that may be affected. In certain parts of the body, however, there are isolated areas of cutaneous innervation by a specific nerve. These areas are known as *diagnostic sensory areas.* Skully lists the more important areas as follows:

- The *radial* sensory area, located on the back of the hand and the lateral aspect of the thumb.
- The *median* area, occupying more than half of the palm and the posterior tips of the index finger, middle finger, and half of the ring finger.
- The *ulnar* area, limited to the anterior and posterior surfaces occupied by half of the ring finger and the small finger, from fingertip to wrist (Fig. 3.21).
- The *musculocutaneous* area, located on the medial aspect of the forearm.
- The *axillary* area, found over the point of the shoulder.
- The *femoral* area, situated on the anterior medial aspect of the thigh.
- The *femoral lateral cutaneous* area, located over the distal part of the lateral surface of the thigh.
- The *common peroneal* area, exhibited

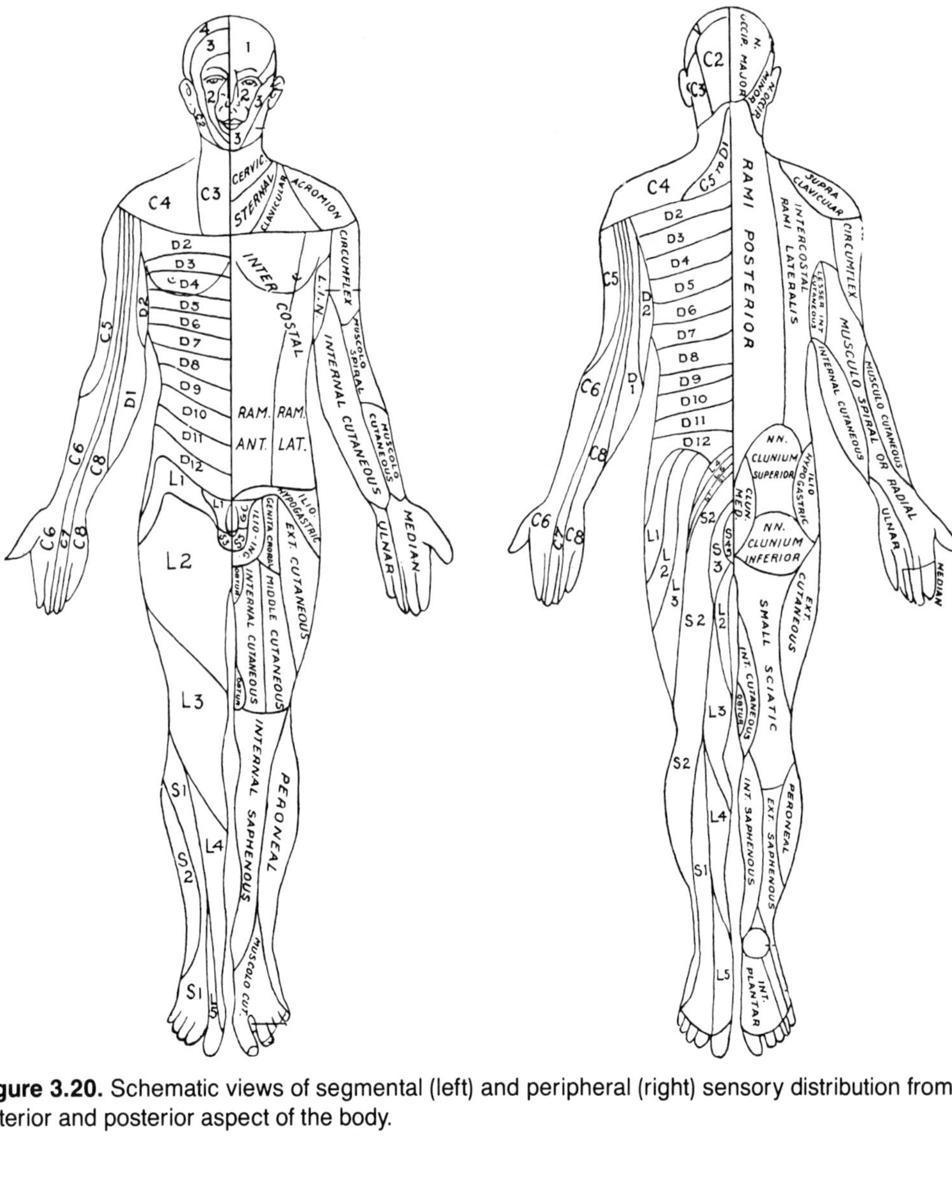

Figure 3.20. Schematic views of segmental (left) and peripheral (right) sensory distribution from the anterior and posterior aspect of the body.

as a vertical strip on the front of the ankle.

• The *sciatic* sensory area, occupying the entire foot and ankle except the medial aspect.

Peripheral Lesions

Nerve course varies little with body type. Some nerves that normally pass over or under a muscle, may pass through it—thus subjecting them to abnormal stress during motion. The sciatic nerve, for example, may pass over, under, of through the piriformis muscle, or it may be divided. Peripheral nerve courses sometimes do not follow the specific descriptions shown in textbooks, which exhibit average paths.

Because a peripheral nerve contains mingled sensory, motor, and autonomic fibers, it is almost impossible that a peripheral nerve injury would result in only a sensory loss. Thus, numbness, absent stretch reflexes, flaccid paralysis, atrophy, and trophic disturbances can be expected if a peripheral nerve is severed. If a peripheral nerve is affected by an irritating lesion that results in hypersensitivity, pain, hyperesthesia, tenderness, paresthesias, possible hyperreflexia, and hypertonicity can be expected. In either situation, the sensory signs will manifest in a segmental manner.

A noxious peripheral stimulus is usually perceived in a well localized area. It is commonly described as a burning or prickling type of pain that is often worse at night and unrelated to position.

Neurogenic pain manifests within the involved nerve's distribution, on the surface or deep, and it usually radiates. There is an excessive response to stimulation. It is difficult for the patient to describe its character as it is unlike any other type of pain and usually is a combination of painful sensations. It is provoked by any peripheral stimulation in the involved zone, and stimulated trigger points cause spontaneous paroxysms. The patient vigilantly guards the involved part and shows great apprehension.

Pain that is accentuated by heat suggests neuritis. In contrast, pain that is relieved by heat usually suggests something producing abnormal myotonia. Pain of intrinsic neurologic origin is generally accompanied by paresthesias and root signs. When throbbing pain is present, vascular congestion, crush syndrome, a vasomotor disturbance, or possibly Paget's disease should be the first suspicions.

Neuralgia. Neuralgia is a general term that refers to any sharp, severe, stabbing, paroxysmal, remittent pain with temporary abatement in severity that travels along the course of one or more nerves. It is usually limited to tissues supplied by the branches of a specific nerve. The sharp pain, often described in terms of "lightning-like" or "like an

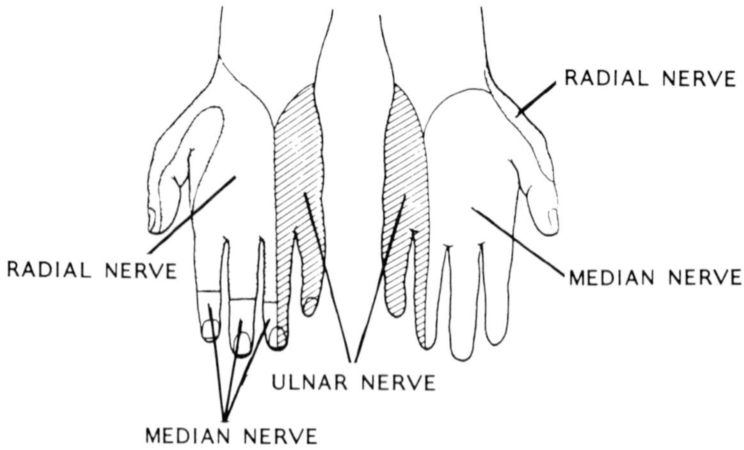

Figure 3.21. The superficial innervation of the hand.

electric shock," is usually associated with tenderness along the course of the nerve and violent episodic spasms in the muscles innervated. Although the term *neuralgia* is nondiagnostic, it is often used in situations where the exact etiology and pathology involved are idiopathic. Neuralgia rarely subsides spontaneously, and it is often so severe that the victim becomes totally incapacitated and frequently addicted to narcotics. Depression is a common associated factor, and suicidal tendencies are not infrequently seen. Morphologic changes cannot usually be detected early in a pure neuralgia or neurodynia. The term *neurodynia* is often used to describe a similar pain that is less severe; ie, a deep ache.

Neuritis. The term *neuritis* technically refers to inflammation of any nerve or nerves, but it is commonly restricted to inflammatory disorders of peripheral nerve disorders. The syndrome may consist of neuralgia in the affected part, hyperesthesia, anesthesia, paresthesia, dysesthesia, muscular atrophy, possible paralysis, and diminished reflexes—depending upon the cause and the scope of degenerative processes involved. During the early stages, pain and tenderness is prominent along the course of the nerve involved. Later, motor and sensory deficits occur and involved normal reflexes are lost or greatly diminished. Causes include (1) *mechanical factors* (eg, trauma, compression, contusion); (2) *infections* (eg, leprosy, malaria, measles, tetanus, tuberculosis); (3) *vascular factors* (eg, peripheral vascular disease); (4) *toxicosis* (eg, heavy metal poisoning, alcohol, carbon tetrachloride); or (5) *metabolic factors* (eg, diabetes, gastrointestinal malfunction, thiamine deficiency, toxemia of pregnancy).

Radiculalgia. Radiculalgia refers to the pain of spinal root disease, which arises primarily from the posterior roots. Inflammation or a grating compression of posterior nerve roots irritates nociceptive fibers and commonly produces pain that is felt along the anatomical distribution of the roots affected. The pain radiates to the periphery, is usually deep seated, and is directly related to paravertebral muscle tension enhanced by any movement that would cause stretch or contraction of the involved muscle(s). The unmyelinated fibers in the posterior roots are responsible for *dull pain*, while the myelinated fibers are responsible for *sharp pain*. In either case, the pain is aggravated by any maneuver (eg, Valsalva's) that increases intraspinal pressure. Thus, coughing, laughing, sneezing, or straining at the stool will aggravate the pain of spinal root disease. Sensory changes such as hyperesthesia and abnormal reflexes may also accompany inflammatory spinal root disease.

Causalgia. Causalgia refers to an agonizing burning pain, usually associated with a history of severe trauma, that is essentially a reflex vasomotor dystrophy. It consists chiefly of sympathetic phenomena involving one or more limbs. It is often followed by organic changes such as bone atrophy and mottling, resulting from persistently recurring nutrient artery spasms as well as skin and muscle dystrophy and atrophy. The vasospasm produces an excruciating, diffuse burning pain that may involve either or both the lower or upper extremities. Joint immobility with or without pain, scleroderma, and contractures may occur. Emotional disturbances are often associated. Any slight tactile, thermal, or even psychic stimulus may produce an explosive attack.

Hyperalgesia. Hyperalgesia literally means an excessive sensitivity to pain. A painful tenderness produced by external pressure frequently results from trigger points, traumatic lesions of sensitive subdermal tissue, the development of a toxic accumulation, or a deep-seated inflammatory irritation. An extremely "ticklish" person is one whose superficial reflexes (skin and tendon) are very lively, thus low pain and temperature thresholds can be anticipated.

Nerve Tracing. There may be a condition that will cause tenderness if pressure is exerted, but no abnormal sensation is felt if there is no pressure. It is upon this fact that *nerve tracing* is based. Nerve tracing is the palpable act of following the course of tenderness over spinal nerves that are irritated or impinged that will usually assist in locating the focus of pain, tenderness, or headache. It is a diagnostic art that is used more in chiropractic than any other healing art. The technique of nerve tracing will be described in a subsequent chapter.

Peripheral vs Central Lesions

By evaluating the sensory bed, it is often possible to determine if a lesion is in the peripheral nerves or whether it is in the central (upper) system such as within the cord or brain.

• Peripheral lesions give a segmental loss picture, and the loss will be on the same side as the lesion (eg, nerve root compressions).

• Central lesions cause a sensory loss from the level of the lesion caudally in the following manner: (a) the loss will be on the side opposite the lesion for exteroceptive sensations; (b) the loss will be on the same side as the lesion for proprioceptive sensations. The reason for this is that exteroceptive fibers transverse the cord while proprioceptive fibers do not.

The Components of Pain

Pain can be defined as any sensation of severe discomfort or distress because of sensory receptor provocation that is difficult to ignore. It is the result of central interpretation arising from an abnormal condition within the body or from an external stimulus that has a detrimental effect upon the body. It is a feature of physical as well as psychologic illness, and its perception may vary from mild discomfort to excruciating, intolerable agony.

In regard to pain, Chatton defines the clinician's concern: "The reaction to pain, a function of the higher centers, is extremely variable and influenced by many factors depending upon the individual patient (the affective component) and the situation (the sensory component). When pain becomes chronic, the multifactorial influences (eg, anxiety, depression, social, cultural, and economic factors; and secondary gain) play an even larger role." Thus, whenever possible, the primary cause, its pathophysiology, and the contributing factors involved must be determined.

The experience of pain contains six sequential components:

1. The reception of homeostatic-threatening stimuli (mechanical, chemical, thermal, psychic) by algesic substances acting on transducer-like pain receptors. The most common algesic substances appear to be accumulations of bradykinins, certain prostaglandins, hydrogen ions, and potassium chloride following cellular damage by pathologic inflammation or trauma. Cailliet and Travell/Rinzler point out that certain functional disorders may also enhance the excitability of pain receptors. For example, the pain receptors located within muscles and tendons are activated or primed by excessive tone such as seen in hypertonic syndromes or the effects of poor biomechanics.

2. The transduction of energy changes from its origin at pain receptors into sequential nerve impulses.

3. The conduction of the pain impulses by intact peripheral, spinal, and higher center nerves.

4. The unconscious modulation and integration of impulses within the central nervous system.

5. The conscious perception (experience) of pain.

6. The voluntary and automatic reactions to pain such as are contained within various physical and psychologic responses.

Thus, pain is a complex "mind-body" experience involving the total person rather than only the mind or the body; ie, the mental and physical experiences of pain are inseparable. See Figure 3.22.

Pain gives information about a patient's biologic status; but, unlike other reported sensations, it does not indicate the nature of the stimuli. With healthy afferent pathways, pain results from tissue damage; but with hypersensitive receptors, normally nonnoxious stimuli may also evoke pain.

Basic Types of Pain

Fast vs Slow Pain. A painful stimulus may cause two sensations: (1) an initial sharp, localized sensation is perceived; (2) a following dull, aching, more diffuse and longer lasting response. Guyton, Daube/Sandok, Chusid, and others frequently refer to these different sensations as *fast* or *first* pain and *slow* or *second* pain, respectively. Various combinations of fast and slow pain determine the character of the pain experienced; eg, local, diffuse, sharp, dull, burning, prickling, gnawing, knifelike, etc. These descriptors and whether the pain is constant or intermittent frequently help to localize the underlying site and character of the distress.

The primary explanation for these two sensations has been that fast pain is mediated centrally by small myelinated A-delta (type III) fibers and transmitted cephally by direct lemniscal pathways, while slow pain is conducted centrally by extremely small and slower conducting C (type IV) unmyelinated fibers and transmitted cephally by multisynaptic nonlemniscal tracts. Guyton states that C fibers constitute over two-thirds of all fibers within the peripheral nervous system. It has also been noted that the farther the initial stimulus is from the brain, the greater the temporal separation of these two painful sensations. Lewis/Pochin feel that much of this temporal separation between the perception of fast pain and slow pain is due to the fact that nerve fibers conveying pain impulses from muscles and those conveying sense of position, or of local tension, are separate. While the difference in conduction rates between type III and IV sensory fibers can explain the timing difference, it does not explain the difference in the quality of pain perceived.

It is generally taught that afferent fibers enter the spinal cord through the posterior roots and efferent fibers leave the cord through the anterior roots. In 1977, however, Coggeshall and Ito showed that some C fiber afferents enter the cord through the *anterior* roots. Whether these are nociceptive fibers or not and how they connect with ascending sensory tracts has not been firmly determined, but this finding has certainly added to the complexity of neuroanatomy and associated clinical concepts.

Superficial vs Deep Pain. Unlike superficial pain, deep pain is poorly localized and often associated with autonomic symptoms such as nausea, sweating, and blood pressure alterations. Reflex contractions of skeletal muscles near the origin of the noxious stimuli are often found, and such contractions will lead to myoischemia, stimulating muscle nociceptors, which will contribute to the painful syndrome. Deep somatic pain and visceral pain are frequently not perceived at the site of the lesion but *referred* to distant somatic tissues. Such pain is usually referred to a structure that developed from the same embryonic dermatome, myotome, or sclerotome.

Pain can also be generally classified into the two general divisions of *objective* pain and *subjective* pain. See Table 3.8. Objective pains are those that arise from some foreign agent or condition which is abnormal to the area in which it is excited. Objective pain can be further divided into *central* objective pain and *peripheral* objective pain. Central pain is that for which no peripheral cause

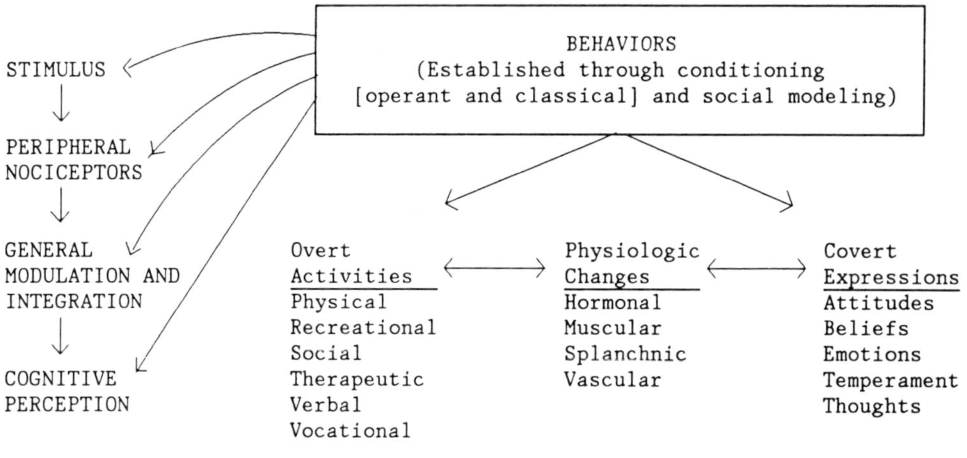

Figure 3.22. Schematic of theoretical nociceptive determinants (modified from Brena/Chapman).

exists at the time the pain is perceived by the patient. Subjective pains are those that have no organic cause; rather, they arise primarily through a mental process.

Central Objective Pain. Central pains are mainly due to lesions in the optic thalamus (eg, thrombosis of a branch of the posterior cerebral artery perfusing the thalamus), which causes transient paralysis, marked loss of position, abnormal vibratory and touch sensations on half of the body, and moderate loss of pin-prick perceptions that are followed by severe painful dysesthesias. A central lesion that can cause extremity pain is secondary to paralysis from either a loss of spinal cord or corticospinal tract function that is always related to immobilization of a joint or spasticity. It is differentiated from thalamic pain in that there is no dysesthesia, and movement of an extremity, especially of the proximal joints, increases the pain.

Causalgias, phantom limb pains, and central pains are sometimes referred to collectively as central pain syndromes even though their etiologies differ. Causalgia from injury to a peripheral nerve is sometimes listed separately from central pain and from lesions within the CNS that affect pain pathways, but the fact remains that causalgia, phantom limb pain, and central pain are all related.

Peripheral Objective Pain. Peripheral objective pain may be either intrinsic or extrinsic:

• *Peripheral pain of intrinsic origin.* In a sprain, for example, the ligaments are overly stretched. There are sensory impressions constantly arising from the injured tissues that reach the brain, are interpreted, and then efferent impulses are directed to the point from which the impression originated. The experience of pain, however, occurs in the brain. Other examples of intrinsic pain include the parenchymatous types that arise from inflammations, masses, colic contractions, or displacements.

• *Peripheral pain of extrinsic origin.* Pain from a bruise, for example, has a protective function to prevent further use of the injured part until it can be properly and naturally repaired. After a scratch, signals are sent to the brain where they are interpreted as pain. Motor impulses are then sent back to the muscles, which causes them to contract to withdraw the part from further injury. Other examples of extrinsic pain are those that register from functional pressure upon nerves or their terminals such as new growths, swollen organs, tensed tendons, stretched ligaments, and spastic muscles.

The mechanisms of pain, its perception, and the various characteristics of reported pain that aid the diagnosis of its cause will be described from additional viewpoints in Chapter 8.

THE MOTOR SYSTEM

In a manner similar to that of the afferent sensory system, the efferent motor system consists of a complex network of pathways and centers at all levels of the neuraxis, which interact with multiple integrating sensory centers that modify and initiate appropriate motor responses.

All body movements (somatic, visceral, or glandular) result from muscle contraction. The integration of sensory and motor impulses is carried out essentially by stereotyped responses to a specific sensory stimuli (reflexes) in which action potentials from sensory neurons activate action potentials of motor neurons, which, in turn, initiate a stri-

Table 3.8. General Categories of Pain

1. Objective pain	2. Subjective (psychic) pain
a. Central objective pain	a. Emotional pain
b. Peripheral objective pain	b. Habitual pain
(1) Intrinsic	c. Hysterical pain
(2) Extrinsic	d. Occupational pain

ated muscle or autonomic motor response.

During the neurologic examination, testing procedures are directed to the functioning of the entire reflex arc, all of its parts, as well as the interrelation between various structures of the nervous system. The most simple reflex is that exhibited by a deep tendon reflex (eg, knee jerk), which occurs strictly on the horizontal level of a spinal cord segment. It consists of a first-order sensory neuron, an internuncial neuron that connects the anterior and posterior horns of the spinal cord, and the final common efferent pathway.

Basic Sensory and Motor Segmental Mechanisms

Sensory impulses initiated from receptors in muscles, joints, skin, or viscera travel to the posterior root ganglia by way of unipolar neurons and then to the spinal cord. Some of these impulses are transmitted to higher control centers where they may or may not reach conscious awareness. The majority of these sensory impulses are instantly relayed via cord interneurons (flexor, extensor, excitatory, inhibitory) to motor neurons located at the same segmental level (ipsilaterally or contralaterally) as the entering posterior root to determine whether muscles will act as prime movers, accessories, antagonists, or synergists. A minority of sensory impulses synapse directly with motor neurons without assistance from interneurons; these allow the *stretch reflex*.

Because most afferent impulses travel a multisynaptic course, each motor neuron at the segmental level is subject to numerous contralateral and ipsilateral influences, communications from superior and inferior adjacent segments, and influences from higher centers transmitted via the descending pathways. The integrating net effect of these influences determines motor neuron potential and the resulting state of effector organ excitability.

Functional Anatomy: An Overview

The primary efferent component is the *motor unit.* A motor unit consists of (1) a single cell body of a lower motor neuron (located in the anterior gray horn of the spinal cord or brain stem), (2) its axon and many branches (extending from the CNS through an anterior root via a peripheral nerve), (3) the motor end plates and neuromuscular junctions, and (4) the particular muscle fibers innervated.

A motor unit is also called a *lower motor neuron* or an *alpha motor neuron.* In addition to alpha neurons, there are also smaller neurons in the anterior horn, the *gamma motor neurons,* which innervate muscle spindles, and the *interneurons,* which provide connections with other neurons. A neuron conveying impulses from the cells of the motor area of the cerebrum, through the internal capsule, to an anterior horn cell in the brain stem or spinal cord is called an *upper motor neuron.*

Gamma motor neurons have a lower firing threshold than do alpha motor neurons. Thus, stimuli sufficient to fire a gamma neuron may be insufficient to fire an alpha neuron and stimuli just strong enough to fire an alpha neuron may exert a pronounced effect on gamma neurons.

Each lower motor neuron is *directly* influenced by input from (1) the sensory system (eg, simple reflexes), (2) the direct activation pathway (pyramidal tract), and (3) the indirect activation pathway (extrapyramidal tract). It is also *indirectly* influenced by the control circuits. See Figure 3.23.

The *direct activation pathway* conveys unsynapting impulses directly from the cerebral cortex to contralateral anterior horn cells to initiate voluntary movements (especially fine, skilled motions). The major pyramidal tract is the corticospinal tract. The shorter, more complex, multisynapsing tracts of the *indirect activation pathway* also convey impulses from the cerebral cortex to the anterior horn cells but they essentially mediate conscious and unconscious gross automatic activities (eg, posture) where the coordination of many muscles is required. The major coordinating tracts are the reticulospinal, vestibulospinal, and rubrospinal tracts.

The motor pathways originating in the cerebral cortex include five basic systems: the corticospinal, corticobulbar, corticotectal, corticorubrospinal, and corticoreticulospinal tracts. In the brain stem, the descending corticospinal tracts are joined by tracts from the midbrain, pons, medulla, and vestibular apparatus. In general, the pathways that pass through the spinal cord to the *anterior* portion of the gray matter generally tend to facilitate extensor activity and inhibit flexor activity. Conversely, the pathways that synapse in the *posterior* portion of the gray matter tend to facilitate flexor and inhibit extensor neurons. This point is helpful during the analysis of paralysis (spastic or flaccid).

The two major components of the *control circuits* are the cerebellum, the basal ganglia, and their connections to components of the motor system. The cerebellum, which coordinates and refines muscle motion, and the basal ganglia, which provides background support of static motor activity and some autonomic activity, receive input from the direct and indirect activation pathways, and, in turn, the cerebellar and basal ganglia systems modulate the activities of the direct and indirect activation pathways.

Some authorities view motor control in a slightly different manner. Skeletal activity is described as the net result of the influences upon alpha and gamma motor neurons of the spinal cord and upon the motor components of the cranial nerve nuclei. Such activity is primarily controlled by several descending motor pathways which directly or indirectly are under the management of the cerebral cortex, certain brain stem nuclei, the basal ganglia, and the cerebellum. These structures are, as a whole, called the *suprasegmental motor system* (Fig. 3.24).

The Final Common Pathway

It has been previously explained that each lower motor neuron is directly influenced by

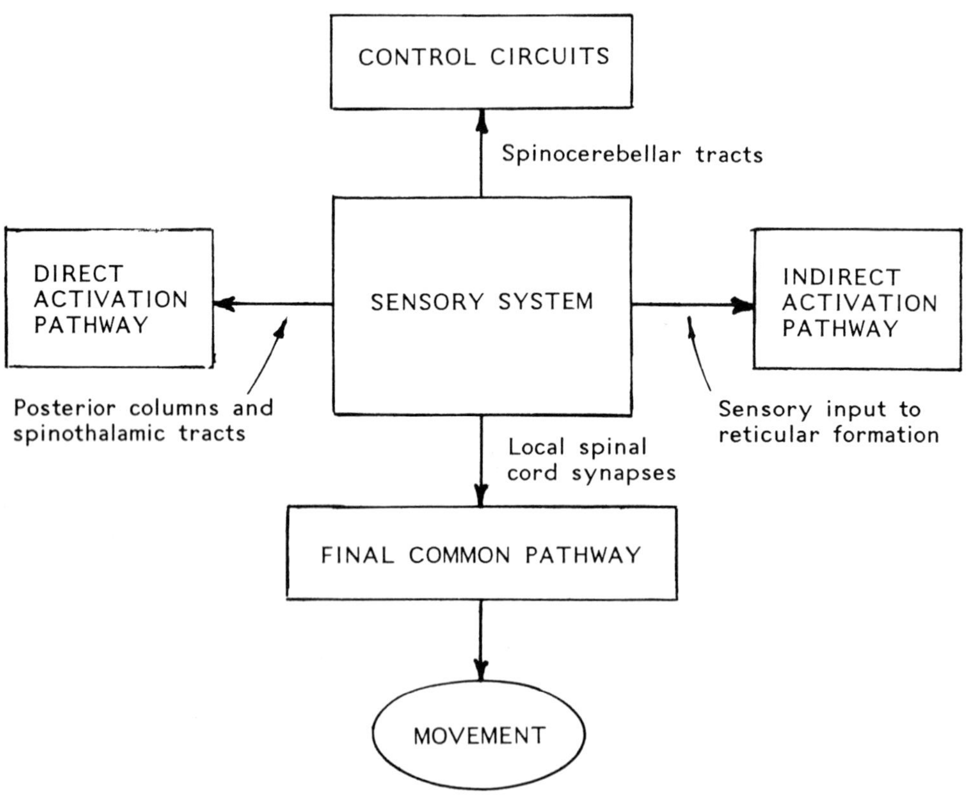

Figure 3.23. General organization of the major divisions of the motor system and the sensory pathways that act upon the motor system.

input from sensory neurons, the direct activation pathway, and the indirect activation pathway, and is indirectly influenced by the control circuits. The neurologic unit through which the motor system finally acts via the lower motor neuron is called the *final common pathway.*

It is well to think of a skeletal muscle as one part of a three-part nerve-muscle-skeleton unit. That is, an intact spinal level and motor nerve is necessary to stimulate muscle contraction, the muscle itself must be able to contract and to relax, and the power of the contraction must be transmitted to a skeletal attachment to produce the desired movement. When any one part of this three-part unit cannot function normally, total function suffers.

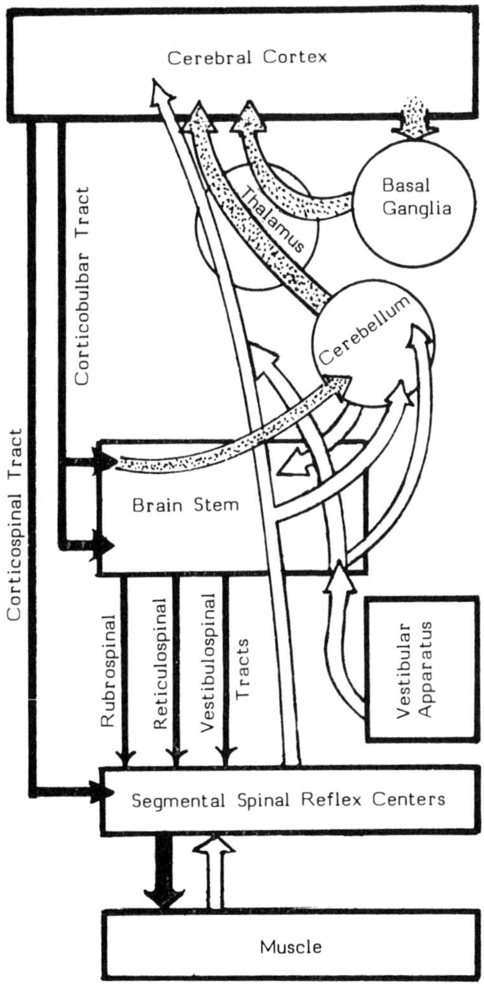

Figure 3.24. Diagram of the relationships between the major components of the suprasegmental motor system and the segmental spinal reflex centers. The main descending efferent tracts are shown in black, the ascending afferents in white, and the interconnectors by stippled areas.

The Spinal Cord and Peripheral Motor Cells

The final common pathway consists of lower motor (alpha) neurons. The bodies of the alpha motor cells in the anterior horn of the spinal cord are compratively large (50—80 μm). About half the myelinated peripheral nerves extending from the anterior root consist of large (6—20 μm diameter) alpha motor neurons that innervate muscle fibers (extrafusal muscle fibers) and about half consist of smaller (6—10 μm diameter) gamma motor neurons that extend to muscle spindles (intrafusal muscle fibers). Alpha fibers bifurcate several times to richly supply numerous muscle fibers. The smaller gamma fibers that supply muscle spindles provide indirect central control via a neural loop.

The relatively large motor cells arranged in columns within the anterior gray horn of the spinal cord and brain stem are influenced by:

1. The activity of the descending (a) corticospinal, (b) rubrospinal (from the contralateral red nucleus), (c) vestibulospinal (from the ipsilateral dorsal vestibular nuclei and contralateral vestibular nuclei), (d) olivospinal (from the ipsilateral olivary nucleus), (e) reticulospinal (from the ipsilateral reticular nuclei), and (f) tectospinal (from the contralateral tectum) tracts. See Figure 3.25.

2. Various intersegmental and intrasegmental reflex neurons such as (a) ipsilateral reflexes of the same segment of the cord, (b) contralateral reflexes of the same segment of the cord, (c) ipsilateral reflexes from other segments of the cord, and (d) contralateral reflexes from other segments of the cord. See Figure 3.26.

3. The convergence from many *afferent* sources. That is, sensory impulses from several segments (involving many types of receptors) may influence the function of the

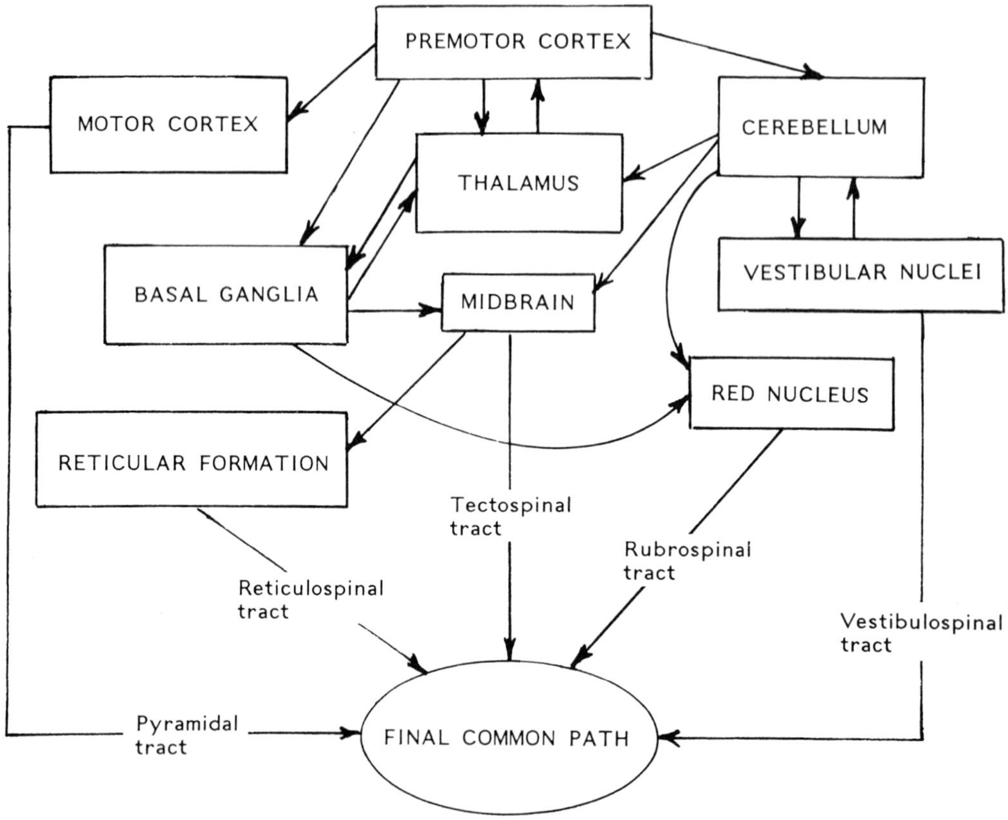

Figure 3.25. Major areas of the brain and descending tracts that influence the final common pathway.

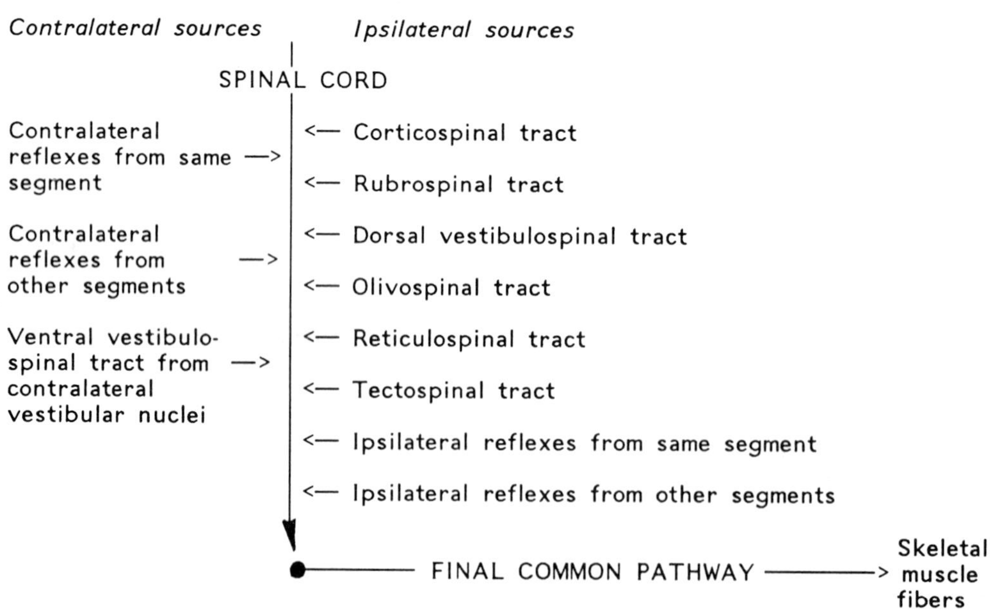

Figure 3.26. Sources of input at the spinal cord level upon the final common pathway.

anterior horn cells. If input from several sources compete for the final common pathway at one time, allied impulses may reinforce each other. If incompatible, those impulses (usually nociceptive) that are protective have priority.

Muscle Fibers

Basic muscle tissue consists of (1) active contractive elements within the muscle fibers and (2) inactive spring-like yielding connective tissue that allows muscle tension to be transmitted smoothly and for elongated fibers to recover. The quantity of noncontractile connective tissue decreases and the length of muscle fibers increases as muscles are located more proximally in a limb. Much of the connective tissue element of muscle tissue is quite elastic. During work, there is no load on or shortening of the active contractile fibers until the load first stretches the inactive elastic connective-tissue components.

Muscle Fiber Blood Supply

Muscle tissue is rich in blood vessels. Arteries and veins course through the epimysium, arterioles and venules travel along the perimysia, and capillaries run longitudinally between muscle fibers in the endomysia. There are many collateral links and tiny reservoirs between many of these vessels to form a rich pool-like network that supplies oxygen and other necessary nutrients during prolonged effort where severe contraction may restrict capillary flow. During rest, many of these pools are closed, but they open when contraction makes it necessary. In this manner, the blood supply to a muscle is normally in accord with the degree of physical activity.

Typical Motor Reflexes

The body's ability to respond to internal and external environments depends on the functional integrity of all parts of simple and complex reflex arcs. If any part of the arc is disturbed, the function of the body with regard to responsiveness to a particular stimulus is disturbed and can be evaluated.

Although motor reflexes will be described in the next and several subsequent chapters, brief mention of their function will be made here so that an overview of their action and association with the longitudinal neurologic systems can be recognized.

The Reflex Arc and Its Components

A reflex arc can be described as that mechanism whereby an internal or external originating stimulus is received, where the nerve impulse so created is sent to central interpretive centers, and where various centers within the CNS are stimulated to cause an impulse to be created to accomplish a specific purposeful function such as to contract a muscle. Thus, the basic parts of the reflex arc are (1) the receiver mechanism or afferent (sensory) limb of the arc, (2) the interpretation center or internuncial limb of the arc, and (3) the activator mechanism or efferent (motor) limb of the arc. See Figure 3.27.

• The sensory limb originates in the receptors of the skin, muscles, joints, ligaments, and viscera. Impulses travel the afferent fibers to parts of the CNS such as the spinal cord, brain stem, cerebral cortex, and/or cerebellum. General sensory fibers have their cells of origin located in the dorsal root ganglia. Somatic afferent fibers carry the exteroceptive and the proprioceptive impulses from the sensory endings in the body wall, tendons, and joints. Visceral afferent fibers

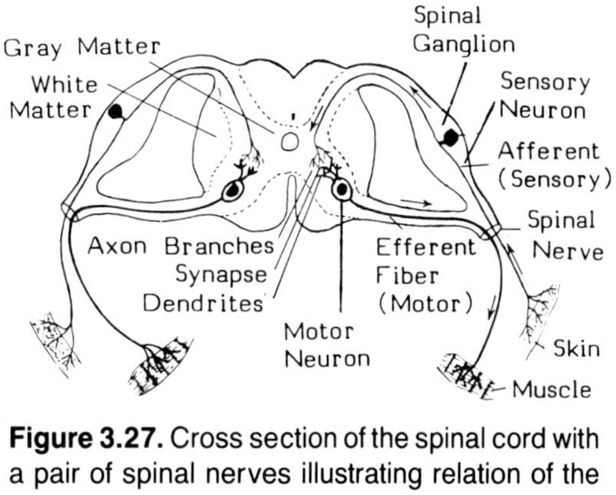

Figure 3.27. Cross section of the spinal cord with a pair of spinal nerves illustrating relation of the neurons and the mechanism of a simple reflex cycle. Arrows indicate the path of a nerve impulse.

carry sensory impulses from the internal organs.

• The internuncial limb carries impulses to an interpretative center and thus connects the stimulating point with a center that will create a responsive impulse.

• After interpretation of the stimulus, a center of the CNS creates an impulse that is sent to an effector organ such as a muscle or gland via the efferent or motor limb of the arc. Somatic motor fibers innervate the striated musculature derived from the myotomes of somites. Visceral (autonomic) motor fibers innervate smooth and cardiac muscle and regulate glandular secretions.

Stretch Reflexes

Some of the proximal fibers conveying unconscious proprioception signals from muscle spindles pass directly through the posterior gray matter to the anterior gray matter. These fibers constitute the afferent limb of *stretch reflexes* such as are induced clinically by testing tendon reflexes with a percussion hammer. The normal result is contraction. This reaction is the effect of a typical *local segmental reflex.*

Lengthening Reflexes

The Golgi organs offer the most important sensory feedback from tendons. As contrasted with stretch receptors, Golgi organ impulses reflexly *inhibit* contraction of the muscle of origin and its synergists. For example, if a spastic muscle is stretched to the threshold of the Golgi tendon organs, the muscle will suddenly give way (clasp-knife reflex). This reflex restraint, a protective mechanism, is called *autogenic inhibition* and has an important therapeutic application in relaxing functionally spastic (splinting) muscles.

Nocifensive Reflexes

A skin receptor that is stimulated by injury (nociceptor) or the anticipation of traumatic stimuli will induce a protective reflex response. For example, a limb will automatically withdraw from a stimulus that is irritating or perceived to be irritating. This usually unilateral and usually contraction response will also involve an opposite reaction in the ipsilateral antagonist and contralateral limb's flexors and extensors.

Reciprocal Innervation

The term *reciprocal innervation* is used to describe the cord level reflex activity that coordinates functionally opposite groups of muscles such as agonist-antagonist coordination of the hip and lower extremity muscles during gait. This mechanism helps to make possible self-regulation of rhythmical movements. Reciprocal innervation is thought to be due to division within the spinal cord of connector neurones for each af-

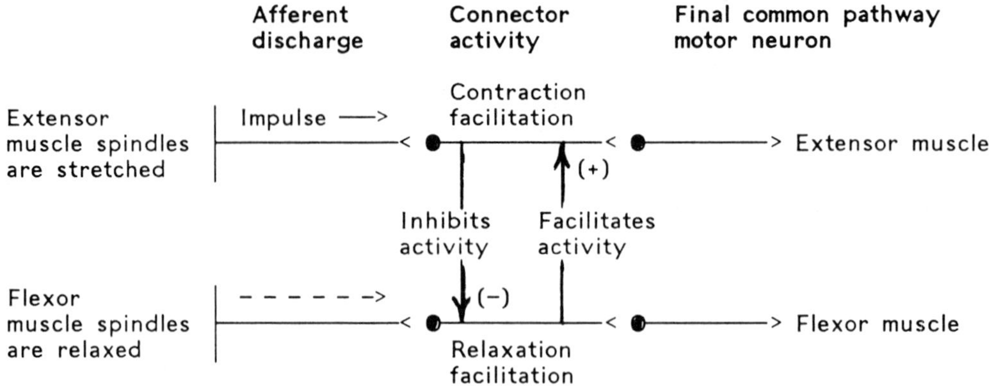

Figure 3.28. Schematic of reciprocal innervation when a limb is flexed.

ferent nerve so that one branch excites extensor motor neurons and the other branch inhibits flexor motor neurons (Figs. 3.28 and 3.29).

The Direct Activation Pathway

The *direct activation pathway* derives its name from the fact that fibers from the cerebral cortex (especially the motor areas of the frontal lobe) course to the anterior horns of the spinal cord *without synapsing* (ie, primarily corticospinal). The major function of this pathway is involved in the planning (based upon past experience) and directing of skilled voluntary motions (Fig. 3.30). In right-handed people, for example, a large part of the facial area of the lower left hemisphere provides motor centers for speech. The same is true of the lower right hemisphere in left-handed individuals.

Course

Because corticospinal fibers mainly arise from the precentral cortex (only a few arise from the postcentral cortex and several other lobes) and pass through the pyramid of the medulla during their course, they are often referred to as the *pyramidal tract*. About 80% of corticospinal fibers decussate in the pyramidal decussation of the brain stem and descend contralaterally in the lateral column via the lateral corticospinal tract (Fig. 3.31). From the lateral corticospinal tract, action potentials from the cerebrum (essentially phasic) synapse directly with lower motor neurons or connect via interneurons. The influence is on all cells of the anterior horn; ie, alpha motor neurons especially but also gamma neurons.

The 20% of uncrossed fibers descend in the much smaller anterior column via the anterior corticospinal tract. Whether or not some of these decussate in their descent is undetermined.

Corticobulbar fibers are also considered part of this pathway because they are grouped with corticospinal fibers in the cerebrum; however, they do not pass through the pyramids. Corticobulbar fibers separate from corticospinal fibers at several levels in

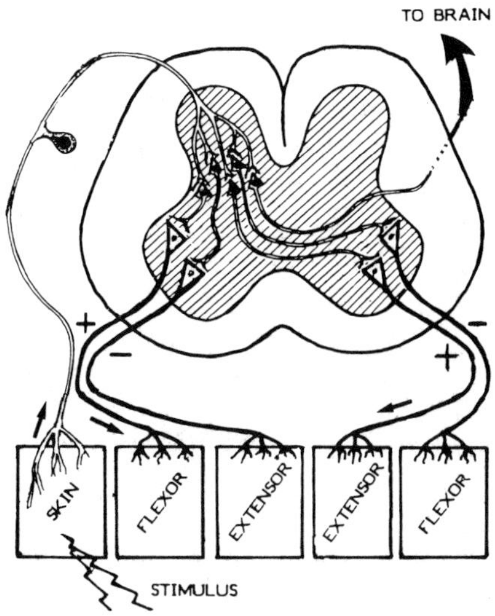

Figure 3.29. Reciprocal innervation mechanism, showing a single interneuron between the afferent and efferent fibers where there normally are many. In this example, a painful stimulus on the skin produces unilateral flexor excitation and extensor inhibition, and contralateral extensor excitation and flexor inhibition, as seen in a typical nocifensive response.

the brain stem, with most decussating, to connect with the motor nuclei of eight of the twelve cranial nerves.

Because 80% of pyramidal fibers decussate, lesions will primarily exhibit themselves on the contralateral side relative to the hemispheric origin of the neurons involved. Thus, understanding this course is important during the diagnosis of many common motor disturbances.

Clinical Significance

Disturbances of the corticospinal tract may be either stimulative (irritative) such as in epileptic seizures or depressive (inhibiting) such as in flaccid paralysis, depending upon the type of lesion present and how it is affecting the transmission of action potentials.

A general rule holds that muscle groups which commonly act in unison in an agonist-antagonist manner (eg, the paraspinal muscles) are usually innervated bilaterally; ie, they receive input from both hemispheres. In

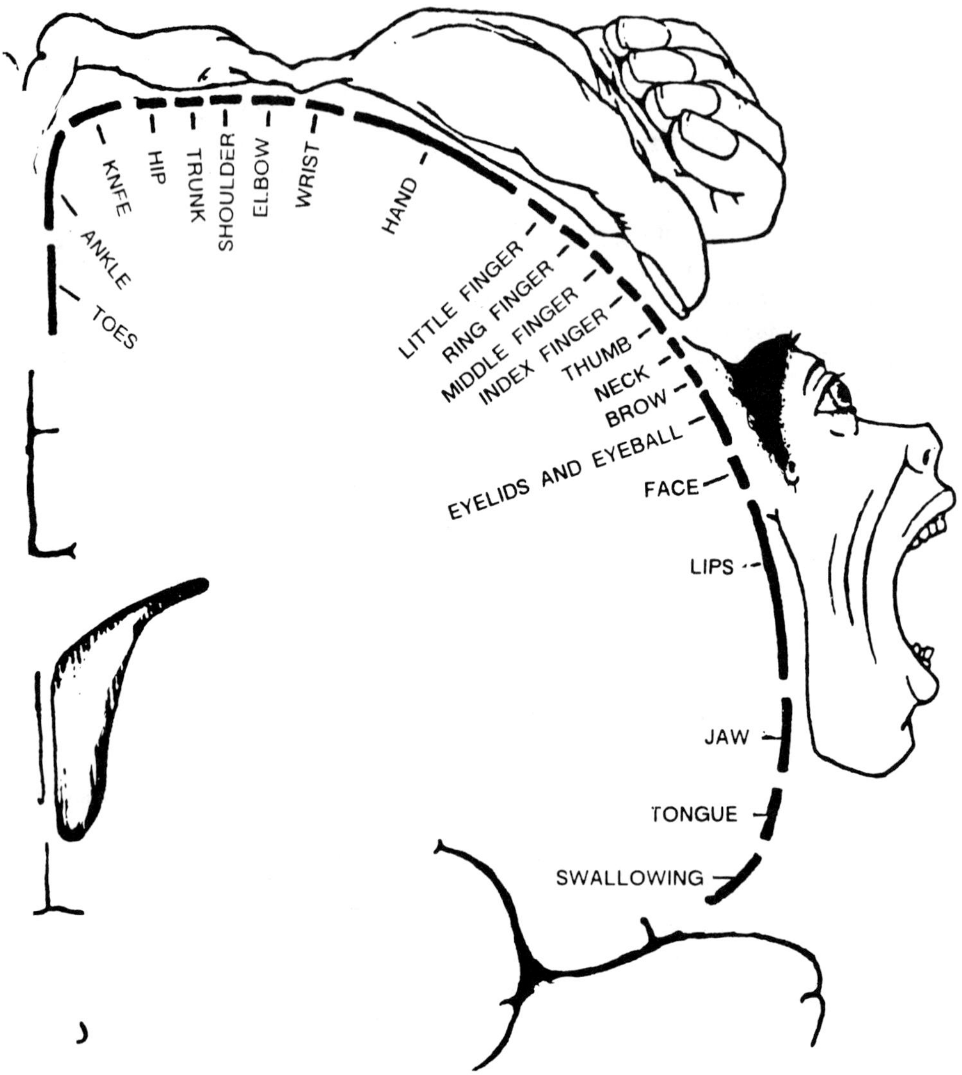

Figure 3.30. Motor representation of the premotor areas of the frontal lobes in the precentral gyrus as portrayed along the cerebral cortex. The fiber arrangement originating from this somatotopic organization persists to a great extent throughout the descending corticospinal pathway. Note the large area for neuron origin for the hands and the muscles involved in speech, enabling the performance of intricate complicated skills necessary for refined actions in manual dexterity and articulation. Redrawn from Penfield/Rasmussen.

contrast, delicate muscles that habitually act in a learned, isolated manner (eg, lower facial muscles and the muscles of the fingers) are primarily activated by impulses originating in the contralateral hemisphere. For this reason, a unilateral cerebral lesion (eg, hemorrhage, tumor) involving motor areas typically manifests as slurred speech and severe contralateral body weakness that spares to a considerable extent the paraspinal muscles and the muscles of the upper face.

Conduction Blocks. Conduction blocks of the pyramidal tracts are especially characterized by impairment of fine voluntary digital movements, hypotonia, a lack of atrophy, and minor, if any, hyporeflexia. There are, however, some exceptions to the hyporeflexia being minor. For example, although tendon reflexes may appear near normal, a unilateral loss of the segmental abdominal and cremasteric reflexes is a cardinal feature because these reflexes depend upon an intact corticospinal tract. Babinski's plantar reflex and the grasp reflex are also prominent because the withdrawal effect expressed in these pathologic reflexes is normally inhibited by corticospinal action potentials.

The extent and location of the somatic peripheral weakness depends upon the scope and site of the lesion. For example:

• Limited cortical lesions manifest on one side of the face or in one limb. Pyramidal medulla lesions exhibit contralaterally below the level of the lesion on one side of the body. The unusual occurrence of a positive Babinski response and flaccid paralysis distally signifies a lesion in the primary motor area of the cerebral cortex.

• Lesions of the anterior aspect of the frontal lobe often spare the primary motor centers. If this occurs, there will be no somatic weakness but delicate volitional control will be severely impaired (viz, motor apraxia).

Irritative Lesions. Stimulating lesions of the direct activation pathway are rarely found below the corona radiata level. One common exception to this is seen in the *early* stages of amyotrophic lateral sclerosis in which the anterior horn cells are highly irritable and produce widespread fasciculations and spasticity. Once the lower motor neurons degenerate, atrophy and flaccid paralysis occur.

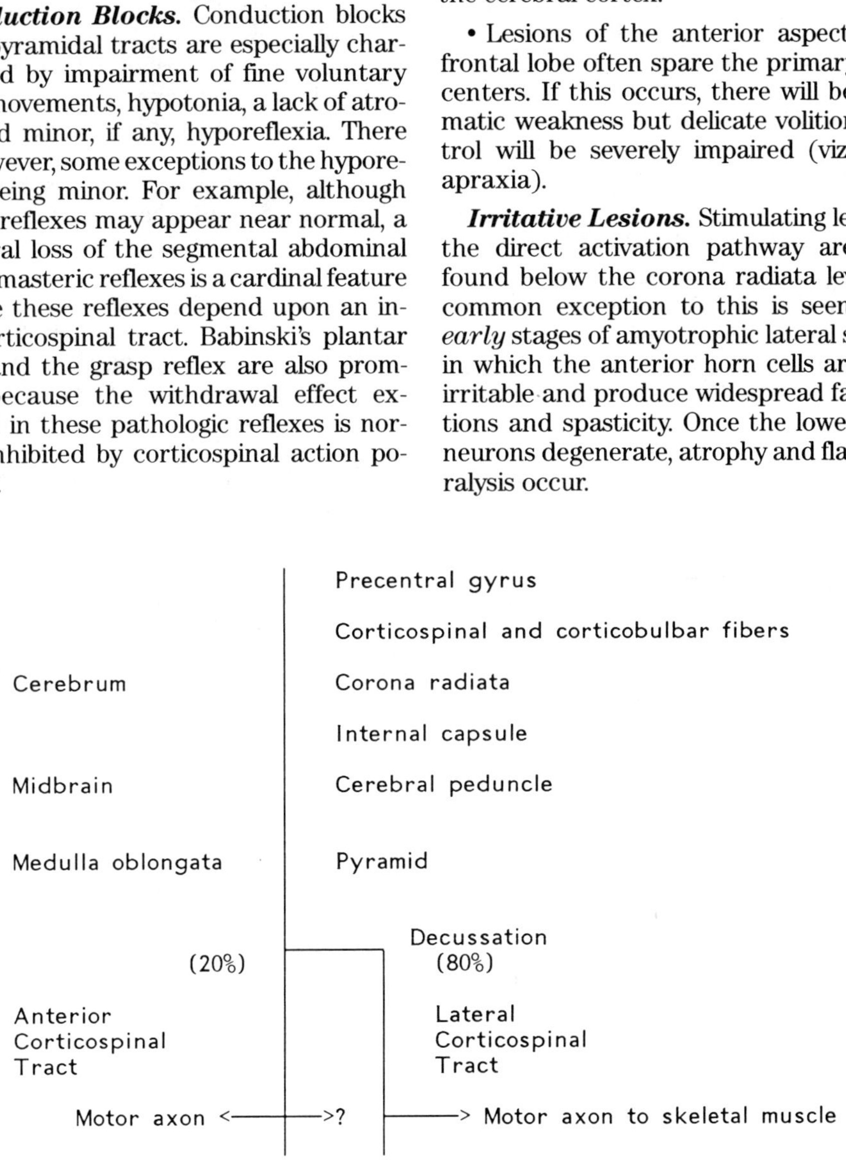

Figure 3.31. The corticospinal tract, shown coursing without synapses from the cerebral hemispheres through the brain stem and spinal cord.

The Indirect Activation Pathway

The *indirect activation pathway* is more complicated than the direct pathway. This extrapyramidal system consists of neurons originating in the cerebral hemispheres that extend to (1) the red nucleus and the rubrospinal tract, (2) the reticular formation and the reticulospinal tract, (3) the vestibular nuclei and the vestibulospinal tract, and (4) the tectospinal tract. The major function of this pathway is involved in the maintenance of *muscle tone* and *gross posture*, thus providing a framework upon which action potentials for skilled volitional skills expressed through the direct activation pathway may manifest.

Influences from the Red Nucleus

The red nucleus receives input from the cerebral cortex, basal ganglia, and cerebellum. The comparatively scarce descending rubrospinal fibers are closely intertwined with those of the corticospinal tract in the spinal cord and their terminations are essentially at the same areas. The effect of rubrospinal impulses is to *activate flexor* muscles and *inhibit extensor* muscles, thus providing muscle coordination. Because few rubrospinal fibers extend past midthoracic levels, their influence is mainly on the muscles of the upper extremity.

Postural Control: Neuronal Reciprocity

The motor neurons controlling posture are directed supraspinally from neurons originating in the pons and medulla. Their basic function is to *activate extensor* activity and *inhibit flexor* activity, and these pontobulbar functions are modulated (±) by impulses from forebrain structures that *activate flexor* and *inhibit extensor* activity. If the counterbalancing impulse conduction from the forebrain structures is suppressed, pontobulbar function is left unchecked and extensor spasticity (or at least hyperexcitability) results. Just which specific extensors will be affected depends upon the level of the lesion.

Influences from the Reticular Formation

The reticular formation is a collection of small nuclei scattered between the large nuclei and tracts of the medulla, pontine tegmentum, and mesencephalic tegmentum. Its purpose is to control the overall degree of CNS activity.

The ascending reticular activating system has its origin in the lower brain stem, extends upward through the mesencephalon and thalamus, and is distributed throughout the cerebral cortex via two paths. One pathway extends through the brain stem portion of the reticular formation and the other smaller pathway extends through subthalamic, hypothalamic, and adjacent structures.

The reticular activating system has two general functions: (1) two areas of the system produce contrasting (excitatory and inhibitory) yet consistent motor effects, and (2) it mediates ascending sensory activity and consciousness (eg, attention, wakefulness, and sleep states). This second general function will be described later in this chapter. The emphasis here concerns the postural motor effects:

- *Posterolateral reticular fiber influences.* Action potentials traveling this course activate the gamma motor neurons in the anterior horn of the spinal cord that serve to *activate extensor* motor neurons and *inhibit flexor* motor neurons in the maintenance of postural tone.
- *Anteromedial reticular fiber influences.* Action potentials traveling this course have mixed effects depending upon various synaptic influences, but their primary function (like rubrospinal impulses) is to *activate flexor* motor neurons and *inhibit extensor* motor neurons in the maintenance of postural tone. Thus, they tend to counterbalance posterolateral reticular influences.

Influences from the Vestibular Nuclei

The vestibular nuclei of the brain stem receive input from the vestibular apparatus and cerebellum, and, in turn, project efferents to (1) the cerebellum, (2) other cells within the brain stem via ascending and descending fibers (medial longitudinal fasciculus) to modulate eye and neck muscle activity, and (3) the spinal cord via descending fibers (lateral vestibular fasciculus) to modulate spinal motor neurons (essentially the activation of motor neurons supplying flexor muscles).

Influences of the Tectospinal Tract

Few facts about this tract are known. It arises from the superior colliculus, decussates in the brain stem, descends near the medial longitudinal fasciculus, and then travels inferiorly via the anterior funiculus to terminate in the anteromedial region of the cervical cord. Fibers are not found below the cervical level. It is generally believed that this tract plays a role in mediating reflex movements of the neck in response to visual and auditory stimuli.

Clinical Significance

Severe brain stem lesions produce effects that are not conducive to sustaining life. Thus, from a clinical standpoint, the common diagnostic concern involves isolated lesions. When vital functions are not impaired, specific muscle weakness and poor reflex reactions will often point to a lesion of the indirect activation pathway. For example:

- Conduction block lesions in the *rubrospinal system* and *anteromedial reticulospinal system* manifest as *flexor* weakness.
- Conduction block lesions in the *posterolateral reticulospinal system* feature *extensor* weakness.
- Conduction block lesions of the *vestibulospinal system* are characterized by a *tendency to fall* after rapid turning movements.
- Conduction block lesions of the *tectospinal tract* result in *delayed postural responses* of the neck and head to potentially harmful visual and auditory stimuli.

The level of a lesion in the indirect activation pathway will determine its effects. Examples are shown in Table 3.9. The major points in differentiating an indirect activation pathway lesion from a direct activation pathway lesion are shown in Table 3.10.

If the descending tracts to alpha and gamma motor neurons of the spinal cord are severed, initially all motor and reflex activity is lost and muscles become flaccid. In time, however, the lower motor neurons will usually recover their excitability so that reflexes become overactive but postural and voluntary motor activity will remain lost.

The Control Circuits

In order for motor activity to be smooth and well coordinated, the integration of a large amount of sensory input is necessary. This input is derived from skin receptors,

Table 3.9. Lesions of the Indirect Activation Pathway

Level	Effects
Above midbrain and red nucleus	Increased flexor tone in arms and increased extensor tone in legs (decorticate posture) because of loss of descending pathway inhibition.
Midbrain below the red nucleus	Weak arm flexors, spastic and hypertonic arm extensors (decerebrate posture). A bilateral lesion will produce extensor spasm in all extremities.
Below medulla	Generalized flaccidity because of loss of descending input.

muscle receptors, joint receptors, the coordination of the activity in the direct and indirect activation pathways just described, and the highly important control circuits of the basal ganglia and cerebellum. To sustain smooth and efficient skeletal muscle activity, these circuits have some influence on the descending tracts but their major function is to integrate and coordinate motor action potentials at the *cerebral cortex* level.

Input from the *cerebellum* integrates, coordinates, and directs especially carefully synchronized agonist-antagonist motor activity. Input from the *basal ganglia* integrates and coordinates motor activity concerned with posture and background static muscle contractions. In addition, circuits exist for intercommunication between the cerebellum and basal ganglia.

Basal Ganglia Influences

The cerebrum exerts its control over lower motor neuron activity either directly through the corticospinal and corticobulbar (pyramidal) tracts or indirectly through the polysynaptic extrapyramidal pathways such as the corticoreticulospinal and corticorubrospinal tracts. The many circuits and feedback loops within and between the structures related to the basal ganglia of the hemispheric subsubstance and rostral part of the brain stem interact with the cerebral cortex and cerebellum to affect indirectly the activity of the lower motor neurons reflex centers via thalamic circuits and midbrain nuclei.

The basal ganglia control circuits provide a braking system, thus:

• *Abnormal activity* in this circuit leads to slowed skeletal muscle activity (hypokinesia), hypertonicity, stiffness, and increased resistance to passive motion (rigidity). Abnormal postures are assumed, and motions are difficult to stop precisely (eg, past-pointing phenomena). The substantia nigra is the most common site for a lesion in the basal ganglia control circuit.

• *Subnormal activity* in this circuit leads to somatic hyperactivity (hyperkinesia), resting tremor, athetosis, chorea, hemiballismus, and dystonia. Parkinsonism and Huntington's chorea are classic examples of subnormal basalganglia control circuit function.

Cerebellar Influences

The cerebellum is the director of somatic synergy throughout the body. It coordinates the activity of muscle groups spatially and times contractions so that motion will be smooth and accurate. In spite of the fact that the cerebellum receives an abundance of afferent fibers, its efferent fibers do not give rise to consciousness of sensation in the cerebellum, nor are these sensations perceived elsewhere in the brain. Cerebellar input is derived primarily from the cerebral cortex, the vestibular apparatus, the vestibular nuclei of the brain stem, muscle spindle stretch receptors, Golgi tendon organs, and joint and periarticular proprioceptive afferents.

Table 3.10. Signs of Activation Pathway Lesions

Indirect Activation Pathway Lesions	Direct Activation Pathway Lesions
Clasp-knife response to passive stretch	Absent abdominal reflexes
Clonus	Babinski plantar reflex positive
Crude exaggerated motions	Distal weakness
Decerebrate or decorticate posture	Grasp reflex positive
Hypertonic arm flexors and leg extensors	Tendon hyporeflexia
Tendon hyperreflexia	Muscle hypotonia
	Loss of fine, skilled, voluntary motions

Cerebellar afferents transmit impulses from the vestibular system, the cerebral cortex (pontine nuclei), the basal ganglia (rubroreticulo-olivocerebellar tract), and/or the spinal cord (posterior spinocerebellar tract). Cerebellar efferents transmit impulses from the flocculonodular lobe to vestibular nuclei, anterior lobe and vermis to the red nucleus and reticular formation, and posterior lobe to the red nucleus, thalamus, and cerebral cortex.

In contrast to the cerebrum, the cerebellar influence on movement is ipsilateral. Voluntary movement and its power, intellectual faculties, and sensory perception can be achieved without cerebellar assistance, but the motions will be awkward and disorganized such as are typified in the inaccuracy and intention tremor of dyssynergia, cerebellar ataxia and hypotonia, dysmetria, and certain speech impairments (ataxic dysarthria) where deficits in rapidity, pitch, rhythm, and volume are heard.

Clinical Considerations

The most common features associated with diseases of the motor system are muscle weakness, spasm, stiffness, paralysis, atrophy and wasting, incoordination, and smooth muscle dysfunction. Less common efferent nerve lesions take the form of tremors, tics, gait disturbances, loss of interest or drive or energy, major or minor convulsions, dysuria, and difficulties in talking, swallowing, or writing.

In evaluating the motor system, the equipment usually required includes a percussion hammer, tongue blades, sterile pads, penlight, ophthalmoscope, laryngoscope, skin pencil, flexible tape, wristwatch, drinking water, and a solid food. Common accessory equipment includes an electric muscle stimulator and/or an electromyograph.

Any lesion producing an interruption of connections between the motor cortex or subcortical levels and the motor axons found in the anterior horn of the spinal cord is considered to be an upper motor neuron lesion. Such a lesion may interrupt direct or indirect activation pathway fibers, or both, because the pyramidal and extrapyramidal systems are so closely associated that lesions involving one will invariably affect both. On the other hand, any lesion damaging motor neurons whose axons reach skeletal muscle fibers produces a lower motor neuron lesion, whether the destruction is in the anterior horn, ventral roots, peripheral nerves, or neuromuscular junction.

Diagnostic Reflexes

While a diagnosis of a neurologic disorder cannot be determined by reflexes alone, they are important aids in establishing the type and location of a lesion. Diagnostic reflexes are divided into *deep reflexes* (eg, tendon, periosteal), *superficial reflexes* (skin, pharyngeal), *visceral reflexes* (eg, pupillary, carotid sinus, bladder), and *pathologic reflexes* (eg, Babinski's). Deep reflexes vary in direct proportion to muscle tone. Superficial reflexes involve any reflex phenomenon that may be induced by a light tactile stimulus (eg, stroking the skin with a wisp of cotton, resulting in horripilation [gooseflesh] or muscle contraction).

It is important to realize that: (1) In upper motor neuron or pyramidal fiber lesions, the deep tendon reflexes are exaggerated but the superficial skin reflexes are decreased or absent. (2) In lesions of a lower motor neuron or the motor fibers from the anterior horn cells of the cord, both the deep and the superficial reflexes are decreased or absent.

Upper Motor Neuron Lesions: Summary Review

Upper motor neurons convey impulses from the motor area of the cerebrum via fibers that pass through the internal capsule, the brain stem, and the spinal cord to synapse in the anterior gray horn cells of the spinal cord. At the synapse, connections are made with lower motor neurons.

Lesions of the upper motor neurons may occur anywhere along their course and may be the result of hemorrhage, thrombosis, inflammation, birth injuries, neoplasms, trauma, or a degenerative process. From a clinical standpoint, any lesion producing an interruption of connections between the motor cortex, especially the cortical area 4 of Broadman, or subcortical levels and the motor axons found in the anterior horn of the spinal cord is considered to be an upper motor neuron lesion. Such a lesion may interrupt corticospinal fibers or extrapyramidal fibers, or both, since the pyramidal and extrapyramidal systems are so closely associated that lesions involving one will invariably encompass both. On the other hand, any lesion damaging motor neurons whose axons reach skeletal muscle fibers produces a lower motor neuron lesion, whether the destruction is in the anterior horn cells of the spinal cord, ventral nerve roots, or the spinal or peripheral nerves. See Table 3.11.

The classical clinical picture of an upper motor neuron lesion is described by Tran and others as follows:

1. Spastic type of paralysis or paresis on the opposite side of the body and below the level of the lesion if the lesion is at or above the medullary pyramidal decussation; eg, in the motor cortex, internal capsule, pes pedunculi, or pons. Weakness is especially pronounced in the musculature of the limbs, and there is great difficulty with movements of the hands. Increased muscle tone will be witnessed as firmness and stiffness, especially in the arm flexors and the leg extensors.

2. Minimal or no atrophy of the muscles involved. However, there will be a later disuse atrophy. After a few days to a few weeks, stretch reflexes return in the involved muscles and usually become more active than usual. Muscle resistance to passive movements is exaggerated. It is often strong at the beginning of movement and then collapses in a peculiar "clasp-knife" method as more force is applied.

3. An increase response of deep reflexes since the normal operation of gravity against the weight of the body may initiate stretch reflexes. The reflex contractions are exaggerated because of a loss of the inhibitory mechanism from the higher central level. The combination of this effect with contractions resulting from continuous discharge of brain stem excitatory mechanisms leads to a hypertonic state. Increased tone is characterized by firmness and stiffness, especially in the flexor muscles of the arm and the extensors of the leg.

4. The superficial reflexes (eg, abdominal, cremasteric) are abolished.

5. The nociceptive flexor reflex and a positive Babinski sign can be observed. The nociceptive reflex evokes withdrawal of a body

Table 3.11. Differentiation of Upper and Lower Motor Neuron Lesions

Consideration	Upper Motor Neuron Lesion	Lower Motor Neuron Lesion
Site	Cerebral cortex or pyramidal tract	Anterior horn or peripheral motor neuron
Distribution	Diffuse or patchy	Segmental (number)
Reflexes		
Superficial	Absent	Absent
Deep	Exaggerated	Absent or hypotonic
Atrophy	Disuse, not prominent	Rapid extension, trophic
Trophic lesions	Minimal	Intense and extensive
Pathologic signs and reflexes	Present	Absent
Fasciculations	Not present	Present
Paralysis		
Type	Spastic and rigid	Flaccid
Location	Contralateral or ipsilateral hemiparesis, depending upon lesion site.	Paresis limited to specific muscles

part by action of flexor muscles at one or several joints, depending on the severity of the stimulus, in response to actual or potential injurious stimuli such as pricking, pinching, or burning. A variation of the flexor reflex is the famous Babinski reflex. In a patient with a pyramidal tract lesion or an infant in whom the tract is not yet functional, the Babinski reflex will be positive. The anatomical basis of the change of response is not totally understood. Hoffmann's sign is usually present, but it is not a reliable sign since it is seen occasionally in normal individuals.

No reaction of degeneration will be present in an upper motor neuron lesion. If the peripheral nerve responds to galvanic or faradic stimulation, it can be assumed that the lesion is in an upper motor neuron.

Lower Motor Neuron Lesions: Summary Review

The lower motor neuron has its cell body in the anterior gray column of the cord and its axon passes via the peripheral nerves to the motor end plates of the muscles associated. This course is known as the final common pathway because the corticospinal, rubrospinal, olivospinal, vestibulospinal, reticulospinal, and tectospinal tracts as well as the intersegmental and intrasegmental reflex neurons travel this route as a final pathway through which efferent impulses reach the muscles.

Lesions of lower motor neurons result from infection, toxins, trauma, fractures, vascular disorders, tumors, congenital malformations, and degenerative processes. Lesions involving spinal nerves or peripheral nerves induce both motor and sensory losses and often reflex changes. The major neurologic signs involved in the cervical and lumbosacral radiculopathies, for example, are shown in Table 3.12.

In a lower motor neuron lesion, neuronal impulses from the upper central level or from the anterior gray horn of the spinal cord cannot reach the appropriate muscle fibers; thus, the characteristic clinical picture will be as follows:

1. A flaccid type of paralysis is seen if there is no regeneration; ie, the muscles involved eventually shrink and possibly are replaced by connective and adipose cells. Muscle tone no longer exists because the peripheral nerve is unable to maintain muscle tone. The involved muscles become soft and limp.
2. Severe muscle atrophy is observed within a few weeks due to a lack of efferent impulses that results in degenerated muscle fibers.
3. Fibrillations and fasciculations are present only in the early stage during which the muscles are undergoing atrophic changes.
4. There is a loss of both superficial and deep reflexes. Stretch and tendon reflexes are abolished, thus producing a hypotonic state, and the classic pathologic reflexes are not exhibited.

Reaction of degeneration is seen 10—14 days after the injury. The nerve is unable to conduct a galvanic or faradic current because of structural alterations.

Control of Locomotion Patterns

Large motor units are required for powerful gross movements where the muscle fasciculi are large and coarse. Fine precise movements require smaller motor units where the fasciculi are small in proportion to adjacent connective tissue. Different motor units respond differently to identical stimulus intensities and manifest different frequency peaks and discharge rhythms.

In repetitive activities such as during gait and exercising, muscle flexor and extensor groups must be fired and depressed at the proper time to afford smooth reciprocal actions, body part coordination, and adjustments to speed and external forces and conditions. During moderate gait, conscious control is only primary when gait is started, stopped, or during fatigue. This requires various sustaining excitatory and inhibitory spinal cord mechanisms acting on ipsilateral and contralateral muscle groups.

A pair of genetically determined *pattern generators* in the cervical spinal cord for the upper extremities and a pair in the lumbosacral cord for the lower extremities are believed to control action by exciting or inhibiting alpha and gamma motor neurons in proper sequence. The activity level of the patterns are thought to be set by the midbrain. The generators receive specific and nonspecific input from the periphery, especially specific prompters from hip and shoulder capsules, and they are also modified by the descending tracts and spinal reflexes to adapt to load and balance changes.

The Development of Motor Skills

Motor skill development is a complex process of adjustment where constant attention must be concentrated on the component spatial movements, the power and extent of movements, and the correlation of visual and proprioceptive input. At this early stage, performance is under the control of the *motor* area of the cerebral cortex. With practice, the proper sequence of movements is "learned" and control is transferred to the *premotor* cerebral area where constant attention is no longer necessary. Concurrently, visual and proprioceptive data have been so correlated that the action can be carried out blindfolded and guided solely by proprioceptive input.

Clinical Reflexes

The human body exhibits an astonishingly complex array of neural circuitry. While the study of reflex communication between tissues under "voluntary" control and tissues under "autonomic" control (and their excitatory and inhibitory effect on one another) is still in its infancy, the answers to why so many visceral disorders mimic musculoskeletal disorders and why so many musculoskeletal disorders mimic visceral disorders appear to be on the horizon. Hypotheses are also being presented that help to explain the progressive reaction spread of some dis-

Table 3.12. Neurologic Signs in the Cervical and Lumbosacral Radiculopathies

Nerve Root Affected	Major Sensory Disorder (Hypalgesia)	Major Motor Disorder (Weakness)	Reflex Changes (Reflexes)
C5—C6	Lateral arm	Biceps, supraspinatus, infraspinatus, infraspinatus, deltoid	Biceps
C6—C7	Middle finger	Triceps	Triceps
C7—T1	Lateral forearm and thumb	Brachioradialis	Brachioradialis
C8	Little finger	Wrist and finger flexors	None
T1	Medial forearm	Intrinsic hand muscles	Finger flexors
L2—L4	Medial calf	Quadriceps, iliopsoas; sometimes thigh adductors	Knee jerk
L5	Lateral calf, dorsomedial foot and great toe	Toe/ankle extensors	Usually none, possibly ankle jerk
L5—S2	Posterior calf; sometimes lateral aspect of the foot	Possible weakness of toe extensors	Ankle jerk

orders that fail to respond to conventional therapies. These basic types of clinical reflexes have numerous diagnostic and therapeutic significances that will become obvious in subsequent chapters.

These reflexes can be classified into four broad categories; ie, those communicating from:

1. A site on the body wall, cranium, or limb to another site on the body wall, cranium, or a limb *(somatosomatic reflexes);* ie, a somatosomatic reflex develops when a sensory receptor in the skin, subcutaneous tissues, fascia, striated muscle, a tendon, a ligament, or a joint is stimulated to trigger a volley of action potentials to another anatomical location of this type via efferent somatic or autonomic fibers.

2. A site (cutaneous, subcutaneous, musculoskeletal) in the body wall, cranium, or a limb to an internal organ or gland *(somatovisceral reflexes);* ie, a somatovisceral reflex is initiated when a sensory receptor in the skin, subcutaneous tissue, fascia, striated muscle, a tendon, a ligament, or a joint is stimulated to trigger a volley of reflex efferent impulses to viscera or glands.

3. An internal organ or gland to a site on the body wall, cranium, or a limb *(viscerosomatic reflexes);* ie, a viscerosomatic reflex develops when a sensory receptor in an internal organ, a gland, or a vessel is stimulated to trigger a volley of reflex efferent impulses to the skin, subcutaneous tissues, fascia, a striated muscle, a tendon, a ligament, or a joint.

4. An internal organ or gland to another internal organ or gland *(viscerovisceral reflexes);* ie, a viscerovisceral reflex develops when a sensory receptor in an internal organ, a gland, or a vessel is stimulated to trigger a volley of reflex impulses to another anatomical location of this type via efferents of the autonomic nervous system.

It must also be considered that these reflexes usually have segmental, propriospinal, and/or suprasegmental implications.

Evaluation of the Motor System

Although the basic points involved in the clinical evaluation of the motor system have been described in this chapter, this subject will be described in greater depth in Chapter 9.

THE RETICULAR ACTIVATING SYSTEM

The reticular activating system (RAS) plays dual roles: it is both an afferent and an efferent system. It receives direct or indirect signals from the spinoreticular, spinotectal, spinothalamic, auditory, and visual tracts, as well as others. It also transmits signals superiorly to the cerebrum and inferiorly to the spinal cord (as previously described). In fact, many RAS neurons divide so that one branch is sent upward while another is sent downward.

Functional Anatomy: An Overview

It has been previously described that the ascending reticular activating system extends from the lower brain stem upward through the mesencephalon and thalamus and is distributed throughout the cerebral cortex via one pathway that passes through the brain stem portion of the reticular formation and another smaller pathway that passes through the thalamic area.

The mesencephalic portion of the RAS is basically responsible for maintaining the degree of wakefullness of the brain. The thalamic portion has two basic functions: (1) it transmits general facilitatory signals from the mesencephalon to all parts of the cerebral cortex to activate consciousness. (2) it transmits specific facilitatory signals to selected areas of the cerebral cortex. This latter role is thought to be involved in the direction of attention to specific mental activities (eg, imagination, conceptual development).

The reticular activating system merges into that part of the brain called the *limbic system.* The main structure of the limbic system is the U-shaped hippocampus, which processes messages from short- and long-term memory so vital for learning. Lateral to the hippocampus is the amygdala and above is the hypothalamus, which together generate sex drives, thirst, hunger, heightened emotions, and many altered states of consciousness. The hypothalamus is responsible for both the sympathetic "fight-or-flight" response and the parasympathetic relaxation response.

Arousal and Sleep States

Our ability to think, to concentrate, to perceive, and to respond to a stimulus with anything beyond a simple reflex is due to the cerebral cortex complex. But the cortex cannot function adequately unless it is aroused or awake, and the cortex cannot awaken itself from the sleep state. The RAS, at the superior level of the brain stem, is extremely important in arousing the awareness level of the cerebral cortex. Without it, consciousness is impossible. Without it, we cannot be *aware*.

During the sleep state, the RAS is depressed but almost any sensory input (proprioceptive, nociceptive, visual, auditory, visceral) can reactivate the system. Guyton states that pain and somatic proprioception impulses appear to be the most potent arousal stimuli. Motor activity also has the effect of arousing and maintaining wakefulness.

In addition to arousing the cortex from a sleep state, the RAS monitors and regulates all muscular activity and sensory perceptions, switches on the cortex during sleep to produce vivid dreams, and inhibits the whole spinal cord to prevent sleepwalking. Stimulating some areas of the RAS with an electric current causes all muscular efforts and sensory perceptions to become exaggerated, as if the impulses themselves were stronger. Stimulating other areas of the RAS causes muscles and sensory perceptions to become weaker.

Attention

During normal wakefulness, a normal individual has the ability to focus attention on certain mental activities or aspects of the external environment to the exclusion of others. How this occurs from an anatomical-physiological standpoint is not known—although the faculty has been explored from diverse applied viewpoints in neurology, psychology, religion, and metaphysics.

Recent studies, however, have revealed three clues. First, the degree of overall attentiveness seems to be controlled by the pons and mesencephalon, probably in the same manner that wakefullness is controlled. Second, mild stimuli in the thalamic portion of the RAS activate only a small area in the cerebral cortex. Third, the pathways from all sensory areas of the brain extend centrifugally towards the lower centers so that the intensity of input at the cortex can be either facilitated or inhibited at the cortical level. For example, the auditory, visual, and somesthetic areas of the cortex can either enhance or dampen signals from the cochlea, retina, and musculoskeletal tissues.

Clinical Observations

The cortex and reticular system operate in a feedback mode in an attempt to maintain an optimum level of stimulation. Impulses reaching the cerebral cortex are fed back to the RAS. If the activity level becomes too high, the RAS sends inhibitory signals to the cortex to reduce the level of excitation, or vice versa if need be. It can thus be postulated that many spastic/anxiety disorders or subtonic states can be attributed to a failure of the inhibitory or excitatory function of the RAS to maintain control within optimum levels.

When faced with stress (functional, physical, or emotional), it appears that the dominant hemisphere delegates, via the RAS, automatic chores to the less dominant and less competent side for temporary control. When the stress level is reduced, control is "switched back" to the finely organized dominant side. For some reason, this "switch back" may fail, and the result may be abnormal neuromuscular effects. Frequently reversing requested directions, mirror writing, and other "switched" reactions are said to be associated overt signs.

According to the empiric studies of applied kinesiologists, unilateral neuromuscular disorders (eg, torticollis or low back pain) are frequently related to contralateral cerebral hemisphere dominance. Examination will typically reveal specific muscle hypotonicity with contralateral hypertonicity. In such disorders, Walther and Stoner (in reference to Goodheart's studies in applied kinesiology) note that if the head of a supine patient is turned contralaterally toward the side of hypotonicity and the patient goes through the active motions of cross-crawling 10—12 times, a reduction in the tone of the spastic muscles will result. This effect can apparently be reversed by having the patient move the arm and leg in unison on the side of hypertonicity, with the head again turned towards the weak muscle.

THE VISCERAL SYSTEM

The visceral nervous system (the magnificent servant) attends to the voluminous neural activities that must be conducted each second to maintain homeostasis. Because of this, and unlike the somatic system, the vegetative system is continually active. The regulation of heart and pulmonary rate, body temperature, perspiration, endocrine activity, and digestive and elimination processes are just a few examples of the complex functions that must be coordinated and regulated. The vast majority of these functions is conducted subconsciously. Conscious awareness of visceral function is minimal except in disease states, and, even then, conscious control is normally meager.

Almost all organs are innervated through the generally antagonistic *sympathetic* and *parasympathetic* divisions of the autonomic nervous system. The sympathetics are widespread in their distribution. Through their innervation of blood vessels, sympathetic fibers reach every tissue of the body. They control blood vessel constriction, subdermal structures, heart muscle, sphincter system of the gut and urinary apparatus, parts of the bladder and genitalia and reproductive organs, inhibit many structures in the head and chest, and reach the enteral system's muscles and glands. The sympathetics are concerned with the expenditure of energy, protection of the organism, and influencing environmental relationships. Thus, the sympathetics are referred to as the *catabolic* system.

The parasympathetics activate the intrinsic eye muscles, glands of the peripheral head, bronchi muscles and glands, the entire enteral system, body of the bladder, and inhibit the heart and provide vasodilation in many structures (especially of the head and penis). The major functions of the parasympathetics are the digestion of food, storing of energy, and maintaining of function holistically. Thus, the parasympathetics are referred to as the *anabolic* system.

Disturbed activity balance of these two divisions invariably results in some degree of visceral dysfunction. In health, the divisions are tonically stimulated to maintain a reciprocal physiologic balance, even though most organs appear dominantly controlled by one system or the other. For various reasons, this harmony may be shifted in favor of one or the other division and create visceral dysfunction and maladjustments.

Functional Anatomy: An Overview

There are both intrinsic and extrinsic factors responsible for physiologic function. The three major intrinsic systems are the electrolytes, the endocrine glands, and the visceral organs—together forming the activating, correlating, and integrating systems that preside over vegetative structures.

The vegetative effector system comprises the muscle of the heart, the smooth muscle system, and all glandular structures of the body. All life-essential functions such as respiration, circulation, digestion, reproduction, and all other parts essential to maintain a person as an individual and to perpertuate the species are parts of the vegetative system. Embryologically, the somatic structures appear late in development as compared to the vegetative nervous system, which serves as the chief integrating and correlating system of all visceral and glandular structures.

General Organization

The vegetative nervous system is a peripheral system whose ganglia contain cells from which fibers arise and are located without the CNS. These ganglia are arranged either

(1) along the spinal column as the gangliated cord or more peripherally at convenient sites for sending out nerve fibers to supply the various viscera, or (2) they may lie in the walls of the viscera themselves (eg, plexuses of Auerbach and Meisner). See Figure 3.32. The ganglia are connected to the CNS by connector nerves arising from cells within the gray matter of certain segments of the spinal cord and similarly in the medulla and midbrain. Also, certain ganglia are located in the brain and cord that serve as control stations for receiving and distributing impulses which result in the correlation and integration of complicated acts involving several widely separated structures. These stations distribute impulses to visceral, glandular, and skeletal structures, thus bringing the total body habitus into a unity of and for action.

Preganglionic Fibers. Preganglionic *sympathetic* neurons are found with thoracic nerves T1—T12 and lumbar nerves L1—L2. Their cell bodies lie in the intermediolateral horn of the spinal cord. Their fibers pass through the anterior root, enter and course with spinal nerves until they exit their IVFs, then separate and pass through *white rami* into the ganglia of the paravertebral sympathetic chain. From here, these fibers can take one of three courses:

- Synapse with postganglionic neurons in the ganglion entered at that level.
- Ascend or descend longitudinally in the chain to synapse with postganglionic neurons at higher or lower horizontal levels.
- Ascend or descend longitudinally in the chain and then project horizontally to synapse in a peripheral ganglion.

Preganglionic *parasympathetic* neurons are found with cranial nerves I, III, VII, IX, and X, which have their cell bodies in the gray matter of the brain stem and with sacral nerves S2—S4, which have their cell bodies in the middle three segments of the sacral cord. Except for a few cranial parasympathetic fibers and those sacral axons that supply the plexuses of Meissner and Auerbach in the intestinal tract, parasympathetic neurons are preganglionic; ie, they pass without synapsing directly to their peripheral synapses with short postganglionic fibers in the wall of the organ or gland innervated.

Postganglionic Fibers. Postganglionic *sympathetic* neurons originate in either a ganglion of the paravertebral sympathetic chain or in one of the prevertebral ganglia. From either source, the fibers then extend to their destination (ie, visceral tissue or other ganglia). Many postganglionic sympathetic fibers pass back from the paravertebral chain at all levels via the *gray rami* and travel along with spinal nerves (Fig. 3.33). Guyton states that about 8% of a typical spinal nerve consists of these type C sympathetic fibers.

Postganglionic fibers outnumber preganglionic fibers by a ratio of 32:1. Because of this design, a single preganglionic axon serves to discharge a large number of ganglionic cells. It is in this manner that a few CNS connections can transmit impulses to a large number of effectors.

As mentioned above, most postganglionic *parasympathetic* neurons are extremely short because their cell bodies are located in or near the tissues innervated. Thus, their length is quite different from that of the majority of postganglionic sympathetic fibers, which have their cell bodies in the paravertebral or prevertebral ganglia.

Activation and Inhibition Mechanisms

Stimuli that act upon muscle or secreting cells exhibit either an activating or inhibiting effect. As noted in the study of skeletal muscle, a nerve activating a flexor is associated with a stimulus that also inhibits the opposing extensor, and vice versa. This action and inhibition produced by opposing musculature is the result of innervation by different nerves of the voluntary system. However, in the vegetative system, the divisions themselves either are (1) activating or inhibiting to a given smooth muscle or secreting cell or (2) nerves of the same system produce opposing action by different chemical substances through which they transmit their effects to motor cells; ie, cholinergic or adrenergic functions. Thus, vegetative nerves often consist of two systems that are reciprocally antagonistic for the most part. In addition, each system contains neurons that often

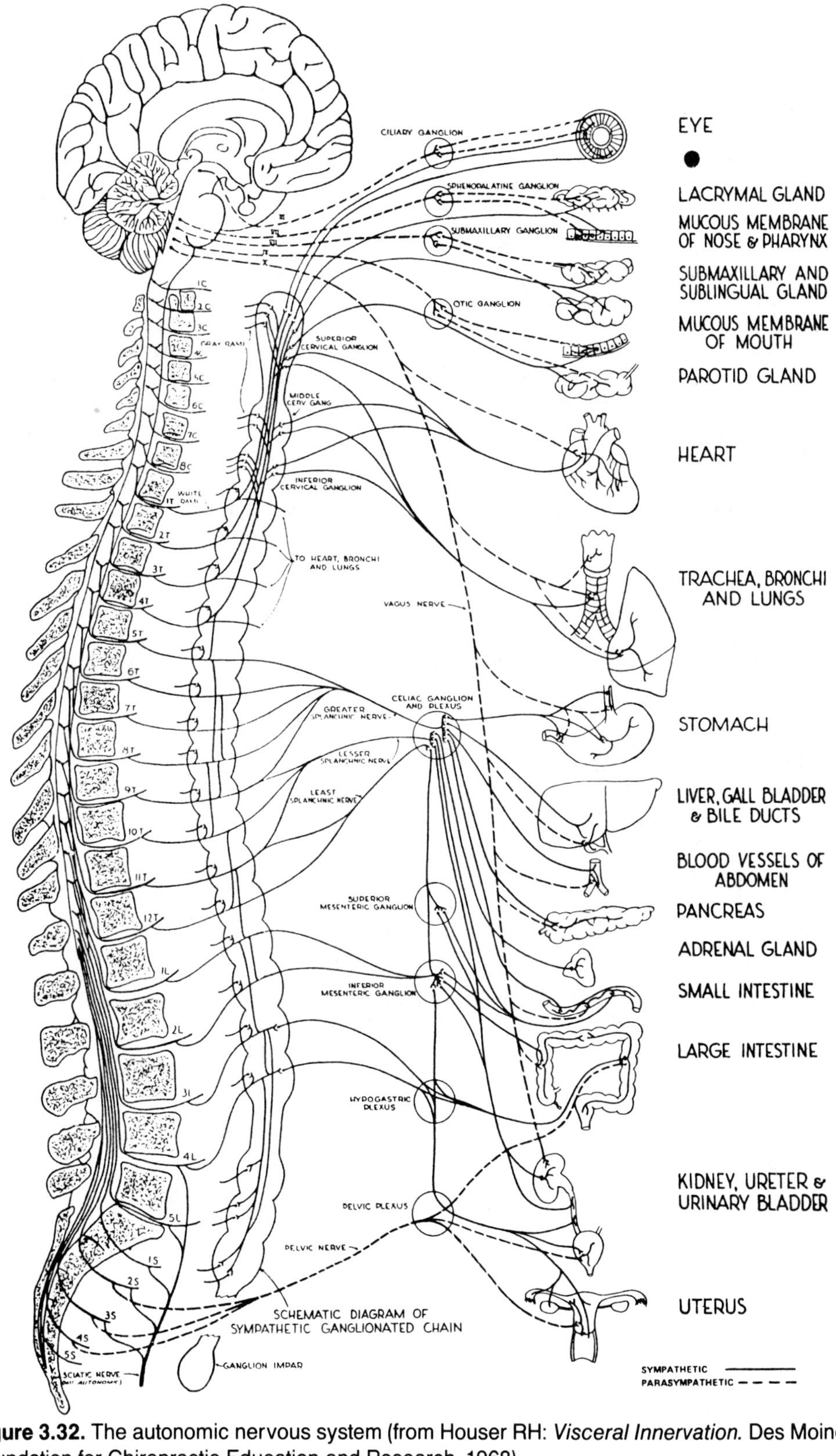

Figure 3.32. The autonomic nervous system (from Houser RH: *Visceral Innervation.* Des Moines, IA, Foundation for Chiropractic Education and Research, 1968).

produce effects opposite to those which are common to that system, and sometimes the function of one system in a dual innervated organ has not be determined. This challenges the common idea that the two systems are *always* antagonistic.

The sympathetics arising from the thoracic and lumbar cord are reciprocal opponents of the parasympathetics arising from the midbrain, medulla, and sacral cord segments when they supply the same viscera, but this is true only when the transmitting substance (which results from stimulating the nerves) is that which is usual to that system. A few structures are supplied by one system only, but most are supplied by both systems. See Figure 3.34. For example, a situation that causes one system to activate an organ simultaneously produces an inhibition of the opposing system. See Table 3.13.

In addition to the specific effects of sympathetic and parasympathetic stimulation shown in Table 3.13, there are also various systemic effects. Those effects that are thought today to be under the sole control of the sympathetic division are shown in Table 3.14.

Visceral nerve action varies according to (1) the state of activity of the organ when it receives the stimulus and (2) the transmitter substances that are liberated at the site of action. For the most part, parasympathetic effects in the visceral tissues are cholinergic and the sympathetic effects are adrenergic. But this is not exclusively true because there are some cholinergic sympathetic fibers and adrenergic parasympathetic fibers.

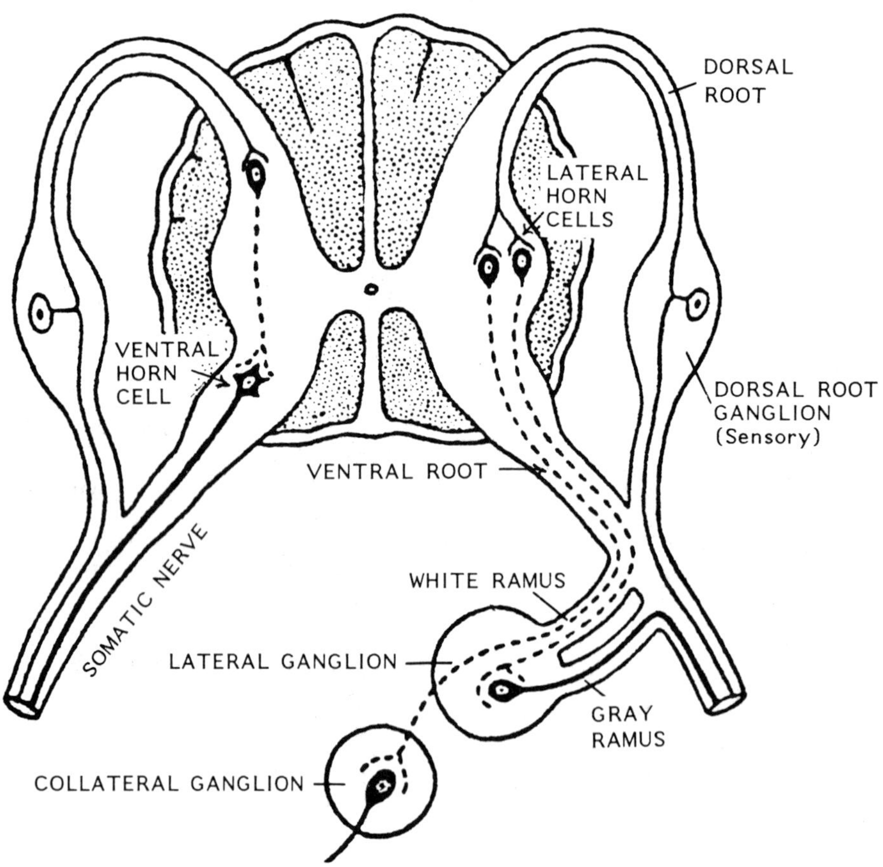

Figure 3.33. Autonomic afferent and efferent pathways in and near the spinal cord.

Viscerosensory Pathways

In the vegetative system, the afferent sensory component is much larger than the efferent motor component. For example, the vagus nerve is one of the largest nerves of the body, second only to the sciatic nerve, and consists of 80% viscerosensory fibers. In spite of this large number of sensory fibers, the vagus does not transmit pain impulses.

Viscerosensory Receptors

Peripheral Visceral Receptors. There are three types of peripheral visceral receptors, and they are widely distributed throughout the body: (1) *slowly adapting mechanoreceptors* that respond to tension (stretch); (2) *rapidly adapting mechanoreceptors* that react to pressure and motion stimuli; and (3) *chemoreceptors* that respond to chemical changes (eg, gastric pH, intestinal osmotic pressure, plasma O_2 level, etc). Keep in mind that there are also somatic *nociceptors* present in visceral surfaces and blood vessels that respond to noxious stimuli. Impulses from any receptor, however, if stimulated intensely and long enough, can be interpreted in the CNS as pain if they reach consciousness. This is true for both the somatic and the visceral systems.

The specialized receptors for taste and smell closely resemble visceral chemoreceptors. Mechanoreceptors are also found in the somatic system, but chemoreceptors are not (according to current belief).

Impulses from visceroreceptors are con-

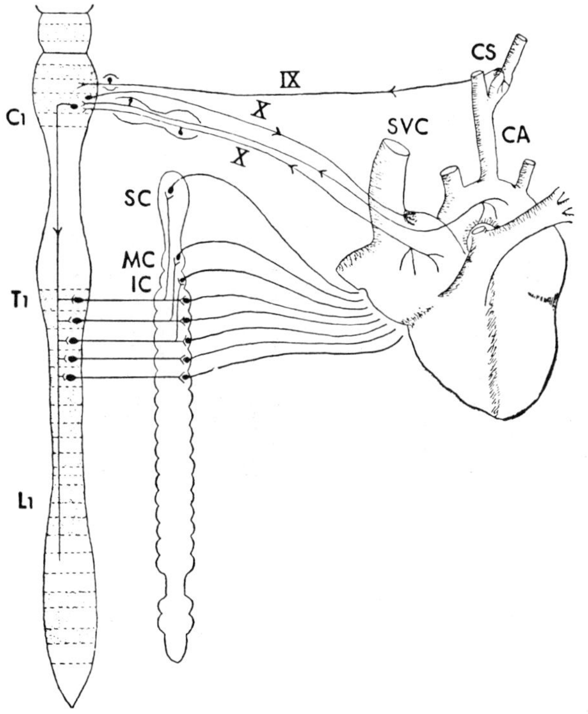

Figure 3.34. Nerve supply of the heart: *IX,* glossopharyngeal nerve; *CS,* carotid sinus; *X,* vagus nerve; *SVC,* superior vena cava; *CA,* carotid artery; *C1,* first cervical segment; *SC,* superior cervical ganglion; *MC,* middle cervical ganglion; *IC,* inferior cervical ganglion; *T1,* first thoracic segment; *L1,* first lumbar segment. Stimulation of the sympathetics to the heart (T1—5) increases the rate and force of contraction and dilates the coronary arteries. Stimulation of the counterbalancing parasympathetics to the heart (vagus) decreases the rate and force of contraction and constricts the coronary arteries.

Table 3.13. Sympathetic and Parasympathetic Activation

Structure	Sympathetic Division		Parasympathetic Division	
	Supply	Effect of Stimulation	Supply	Effect of Stimulation
Thyroid	T1	Increases secretion	X	Decreases secretion
Mucous membranes of head	T1—2	Vasoconstriction	VII	Vasodilation
Salivary glands	T1—2	Increases organic substances	IX	Increases watery substances
Pupils	T1—2	Dilation	III	Constriction
Lacrimal glands	T1—3	Vasoconstriction	VII	Secretion
Heart	T1—5	Increases rate and force of contraction, dilates coronary arteries	X	Decreases rate and force of contraction, constricts coronary arteries
Upper limbs	T1—6	Vasoconstriction, sweating, piloerection		
Bronchi and lungs	T1—7	Dilation, vasoconstriction	X	Constriction, vasodilation
Sphincter of Oddi	T4—8	Constricts	X	Relaxes
Gallbladder	T4—8	Relaxes muscle, constricts sphincter	X	Constricts muscle, relaxes sphincter
Stomach	T5—9	Decreases secretion and motility	X	Increases secretion and motility
Spleen	T6—8	Contracts smooth muscle	X	Relaxes smooth muscle
Pancreas	T6—9	Decreases secretion	X	Increases secretion
Liver	T8—10	Increases glycogen to glucose, increases protein metabolism, vasoconstriction	X	Opposite
Pyloric sphincter	T9	Increased tone, contraction	X	Relaxation
Adrenals	T9—10	Increases secretion	X	? (unknown)
Small intestine	T9—L1	Slightly decreases peristalsis and secretions, vasoconstriction	X	Increases peristalsis and secretions, relaxes sphincters
Kidneys	T10—L1	Vasoconstriction, inhibits	X	? (unknown)
Prostate	T10—L1	Contracts muscle and spermatic vein	S2—4	Increases secretion
Fallopian tubes	T10—L1	Contracts muscle		? (unknown)
Urinary bladder	T12—L2	Constricts sphincter, relaxes wall	S2—4	Relaxes sphincter, constricts wall
Lower limbs	T12—L2	Vasoconstriction, sweating, piloerection		
Uterus	L1	Contracts body	S2—4	Relaxes body, contracts cervix
Ileocecal valve	L1	Contracts	S2—4	Relaxes
Penis, clitoris	L1—2	Duct contraction, ejaculation	S2—4	Erection
Colon and rectum	L1—3	Decreased peristalsis	S3—5	Increased peristalsis
Anal sphincter	L3	Contracts	S3—5	Relaxes

veyed via plexuses to autonomic ganglia located in or near their associated organ, and from there they may either synapse to initiate a local peripheral reflex or be transmitted to the CNS. Visceral afferents from thoracic, abdominal, and pelvic organs enter the cord via the pelvic, hypogastric, and splanchnic nerves. The response is usually a diffuse reaction (including pain). Visceral afferents in the cranial nerves go directly to the brain stem, but the response is far more discrete and localized.

Central Visceral Receptors. In addition to the peripheral visceral receptors described above, there are also mechanoreceptors and chemoreceptors in the CNS that respond to circulating hormones, toxins, and changes in blood pressure, pH, O_2 and CO_2 levels.

Distal Viscerosensory Fibers

Peripheral visceroafferents are small, slow conducting fibers, some of which are unmyelinated. Axons involved in a local peripheral reflex (ie, synapse with a visceroefferent within the organ) or that connect with a peripheral ganglion have their cell bodies in or near the organ innervated. Some authorities believe that these circuits provide a degree of control that is independent of the CNS system. Axons entering the CNS have their cell bodies in posterior root ganglia or cranial nerve nuclei.

Threshold Factors. Full activation of a somatic nerve is in the range of 75—200 impulses per second (ips). The threshold for an autonomic nerve is far lower and an important consideration in electrotherapy. An autonomic nerve, sympathetic or parasympathetic, will generally produce a response sufficient to maintain minimal effect with 1 ips and reach full activation with a 10—20 ips discharge.

Proximal Viscerosensory Fibers

Visceral afferents entering the spinal cord have their cell bodies in the posterior root ganglia, as do those of the somatic sensory system. Fibers from viscera either (1) follow along with splanchnic, hypogastric, or pelvic nerves to join the paravertebral sympathetic chain of ganglia or (2) join with mesentery nerves that travel directly to a posterior root. Fibers from the extremities either (1) follow the blood vessels centrally to join the sympathetic chain and then pass to the spinal nerve and posterior root via the rami communicates or (2) join with somatic nerves that travel directly to a posterior root.

Spinal Cord Level Entry. Viscerosensory fibers entering the spinal cord make many connections. The two major connections for

Table 3.14. Systemic Effects of Autonomic Stimulation

Structure/Process	Effect of Sympathetic Stimulation	Effect of Parasympathetic Stimulation
Adrenals	Secretion increased	Unknown
Apocrine glands	Thick, odoriferous secretion	Unknown
Basal metabolism	Increased (—>100%)	Unknown
Blood coagulation	Increased	Unknown
Blood glucose	Increased	Unknown
Blood vessels	Vasoconstriction	Unknown
Kidney function	Decreased output	Unknown
Mental activity	Increased	Unknown
Piloerector muscles	Excited	Unknown
Skeletal muscle	Increased glycogenolysis and strength	Unknown
Sweat glands	Hyperhidrosis	Unknown

horizontal activity are (1) with somatomotor axons to produce related somatic activity (eg, parietal spasm) or (2) with visceromotor axons for simple viscerovisceral reflex activity. For longitudinal correspondence upward, two routes are also taken: (1) Synapses are made with ascending fibers in the lateral spinothalamic tract and posterior columns to the hypothalamus, thalamus, and reticular formation. (2) Synapses are made with sensory neurons in the posterior horns that also receive peripheral somatosensory input. This convergence of viscerosensory and somatosensory impulses is the basis for the overlying segmental hyperesthesia (superficial referral) so often seen with irritating visceral disorders.

Posterior Fossa Level Entry. At this level, viscerosensory impulses through various cranial nerves reach the CNS via the midbrain (III), pons (VII), and medulla (IX and X). Impulse connections are made in the brain stem that are transmitted to the hypothalamus, thalamus, and reticular formation, with a few extending to the cerebral cortex.

Supratentorial Level Input. Some fibers within the olfactory nerve transmit impulses to the rhinencephalon. These fibers terminate in the amygdala, temporal lobe, and cerebral cortex (medial and frontal lobes). A few fibers from other viscerosensory nerves communicate with the cerebral cortex and most of these arise from the hypothalamus.

Central Visceral Control

Central control of the autonomic nervous system is conducted in the reticular formation in the brain stem and in the hypothalamus and cerebral cortex at the supratentorial level. Impulses from the rhinocephalic cortex participate in bladder and bowel control.

Because we know that the vegetative nervous system is abundant in afferents and only a few reach the conscious level, it can be logically deduced that much afferent activity is involved in reflex activity that is mediated in the spinal cord and brain stem. The spinal cord's cervical segments and the lower lumbar and upper sacral segments are not connected with the vegetative ganglia by efferent connective fibers; rather, they are left to innervate the arms and legs, as far as their nervous outflow is concerned.

Cortical Control

Healthy individuals are rarely aware of visceral sensations except for those of sweating and a distended stomach, bladder, or rectum. During illness, however, visceral-related pain or nausea may be severe. Unfortunately or fortunately, depending upon the circumstances involved, the conscious awareness of visceral dysfunction is minimal.

Human will, at least for normal consciousness, has limited power to direct visceral effects as one would direct a skeletal muscle because vegetative functions must be conducted whether one is awake or asleep. In certain acts, however, voluntary and vegetative nerves supplement one another such as in swallowing, breathing, defecation, and urination. Thus, the voluntary and vegetative nervous systems are intimately connected and brought into reflex connection so that visceral stimulation has somatic expression and skeletal muscle messages are expressed in visceral tissues. The body is a whole in neural integration.

Although the number of viscerosensory fibers in the body far exceeds that of somatosensory fibers, the number of visceral sensations that can be interpreted consciously is quite limited and these are frequently misinterpreted. For example, the perception of a burning sensation arising from visceral tension, compression, or ischemia resembles the feeling perceived when superficial thermal receptors are stimulated. To further complicate clinical discrimination, a sensation arising from one site may be perceived by the patient to be located in an entirely different area. Nowhere else within the study of clinical neurology is the differentiation of referred symptoms more difficult or more frustrating.

Role of the Limbic System and Hypothalamus

Autonomic and somatic afferent and efferent activity is integrated and coordinated at the supratentorial level by the *limbic system*. The limbic system consists of an array of cortical and subcortical structures (especially the hippocampus, amygdala, and gyrus formation), which are located at or near the edge (limbus) of the medial wall of the cerebral hemispheres. Connections are made with the septal area, hypothalamus, and medial zone of mesencephalic tegmentum. Via the latter connection fibers, the limbic system exerts an important influence upon the autonomic nervous system—especially those that affect mood and motivation and direct other affective and emotional states.

The hypothalamus, the center of homeostatic activity, forms the floor and a part of the anterolateral walls of the third ventricle. It contains the optic chiasm, the stalk of the pituitary, the mammillary bodies, and an abundance of hypothalamic nuclei. Fiber connections are numerous and complex, with connections with the cerebrum, brain stem, spinal cord, and intrahypothalamic fibers.

The hypothalamus mediates the major reflex activity for the vegetative system (via fast, specific, short duration stimuli over neural pathways to the brain stem and spinal cord) and endocrine system (via slower, more generalized, longer lasting stimuli over hormonal pathways).

A lesion in the rostral (supraoptic) region or caudal portion results in sympathetic dominance. Other effects of a hypothalamic lesion are diabetes insipidus, appetite abnormalities, Fröhlich's syndrome, neurogenic fever, and antisocial behavior.

Reticular Formation Control Centers

The reticular formation is a group of nonspecific neural centers that surround the central core of the brain stem from the medulla to the pons. It receives viscerosensory impulses from the hypothalamus and the periphery.

At the medulla level, centers controlling vomiting, respiration, and cardiovascular activity are located. It also has specialized receptors at the medulla level that are sensitive to various alterations in the blood (eg, hormones, metabolic debris, pH, CO_2 levels) and blood pressure (pressor and depressor centers). There is also a respiratory center located at the pons level.

Visceromotor Pathways

Unlike the somatic motor system, in which the spinal pathway from the cord to a skeletal muscle consists of a single fiber, there is no final common pathway in the autonomic system. This is because of the dual paths in the sympathetic system, consisting of two fibers (preganglionic and postganglionic). In addition, some activities are controlled entirely in the periphery.

Tracts: Summary Review

Sympathetic impulses from the hypothalamus and reticular formation are conveyed through the spinal cord via the lateral funiculus to thoracic and upper lumbar neurons that mediate the visceral activities of the thorax, abdomen, and pelvis. Impulses are then transmitted over short preganglionic fibers, which primarily terminate in the nearby paravertebral ganglia and act upon long postgangionic axons that extend to visceral receptors.

Parasympathetic impulses are transmitted to the nuclei and axons of several cranial nerves (III, VII, IX, and X) and down the lateral funiculus of the spinal cord to connect with sacral autonomic efferents. Impulses are then conveyed over long preganglionic axons, which ultimately synapse in peripheral ganglia with the shorter postganglionic fibers that innervate the visceral effectors.

Visceral Ganglia and Plexuses

A ganglion is a group of nerve cell bodies and associated fibers, lying outside the CNS, that is contained within a connective tissue capsule. Some visceral neurons are found in the paravertebral ganglia or in peripheral ganglia near the organs they innervate, and others are found in the posterior root ganglia.

A nerve plexus is a complex network of axons that extend from one area to another.

There are 41 differentiated nerve plexuses associated with the peripheral autonomic nervous system. The large plexuses contain mingled direct viscerosensory axons, preganglionic parasympathetic axons, and postganglionic sympathetic axons.

Hormonal Mechanisms

The hormonal pathway is a nonneural pathway. It consists of the hypophyseal portal system and various releasing factors secreted by the hypothalamus that modulate secretions of the anterior pituitary gland such as somatostatin, the thyrotropin-releasing factor, and the luteotropin-releasing factor. See Figure 3.35.

Visceral Effector Organs

Most end organs of autonomic efferents act upon smooth muscle fibers of the viscera, glands, blood vessels, skin, eyes, and genitals. Although smooth muscle has the same characteristics of excitability and contractability as striated muscle, it also has three unique properties:

1. *Adaptation.* Smooth muscle contains an inherent ability to adapt (alter) the strength and rhythm of contractions that is unrelated to mechanical influences (eg, distension stretch). Smooth muscle also readily adapts to humoral and chemical influences.

2. *Automatism.* The term *automatism* refers to the ability of smooth muscle that has been isolated from any innervation to continue to spontaneously contract in a rhythmic manner in response to *local* stimuli. The stimuli for this effect arise from functional *pacemakers* whose impulses spread from one area of tissue to another. These are *functional* areas, not structural entities, as they may shift from one area to another as the result of changing needs. In

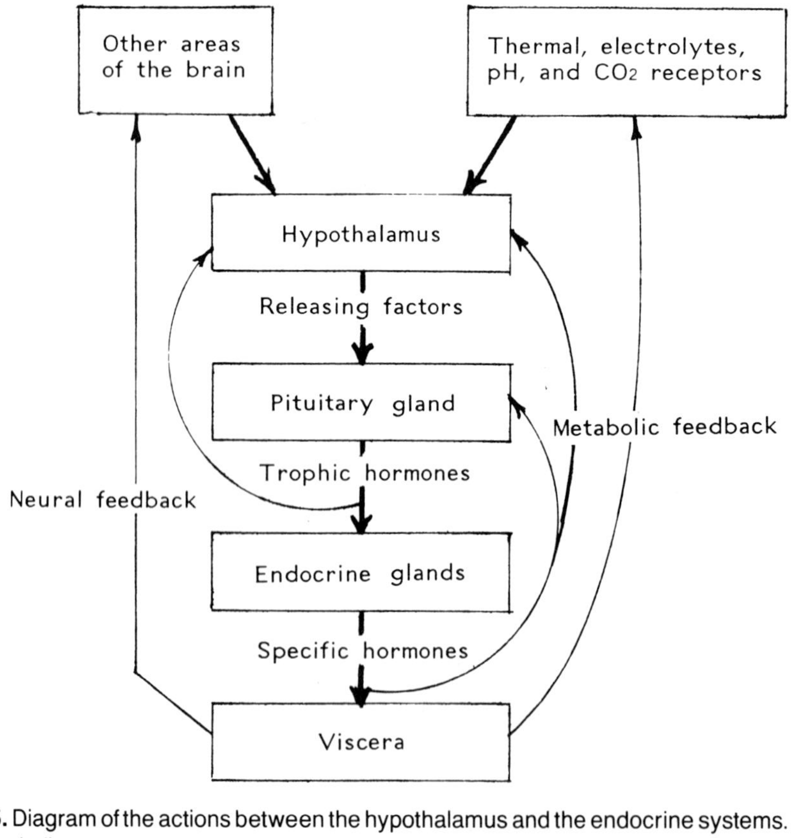

Figure 3.35. Diagram of the actions between the hypothalamus and the endocrine systems. The heavy direct arrows indicate control; lighter loops depict feedback pathways.

this manner, smooth muscle and many glands may continue to function in the absence of an outside source of action potentials. It is for this reason that autonomic neural disorders express clinically in a far less overt manner in their early stages than do somatic neural disorders.

3. *Intramural conduction.* If a local area of a vegetative organ (eg, intestine) is stimulated, local contraction occurs that slowly travels along the length of the organ. This spread is made possible by *intramural connections.*

Types of Autonomic Neurotransmitters

An autonomic nerve that stimulates the release of epinephrine or an epinephrine-like substance is said to be functionally *adrenergic* (a term derived from *adrenaline,* the British word for epinephrine). An autonomic nerve that stimulates the release of acetylcholine is called *cholinergic.*

Preganglionic Autonomic Axons. All preganglionic autonomic neurons, sympathetic and parasympathetic, stimulate the release of acetylcholine. From this, it can be deduced that a preganglionic sympathetic fiber will excite both postganglionic parasympathetic and sympathetic fibers, and vice versa. Some preganglionic sympathetic axons extend to the medullae of the adrenal glands and terminate on special cells where they stimulate the release of epinephrine and norepinephrine directly into the blood stream to produce widespread sympathetic effects.

Postganglionic Autonomic Axons. All parasympathetic postganglionic axons are cholinergic. Most postganglionic sympathetic axons are adrenergic, but postganglionic sympathetic fibers to the sweat glands and a few blood vessels are cholinergic.

Autonomic Neurotransmitter Actions

Adrenergic and cholinergic neurotransmitter substances have a different effect on different areas of cell membrane according to the type of receptor present. For example, acetylcholine activates nicotinic and muscarinic receptors. These receptors are so named because these poisons, nicotine and muscarine, activate only these receptors.

Muscarinic receptors are activated by postganglionic parasympathetic neurons

Table 3.15. Transmitter-Receptor Effect in the Vegetative System

Usual Transmitter	Typical Receptor	Action Location	Effect
Acetylcholine	Muscarinic	Smooth and cardiac muscle	Temporary depolarization
Acetylcholine	Nicotinic	Smooth muscle, ganglia, and striated muscle	Prolonged depolarization
Norepinephrine	Alpha-adrenergic	Smooth muscle	Depolarization, contraction
Epinephrine	Alpha-adrenergic	Smooth muscle	Depolarization, contraction
	Beta-adrenergic	Smooth muscle	Hyperpolarization, relaxation

and postganglionic sympathetic cholinergic neurons. Nicotinic receptors are found at the synapses of both preganglionic sympathetic and parasympathetic neurons and at the terminal connections of both sympathetic and parasympathetic neurons. See Table 3.15.

There are two different types of adrenergic receptors: alpha and beta (ß1 and ß2). Norepinephrine activates alpha-adrenergic receptors, with a minimal effect on beta-adrenergic receptors. Epinephrine activates both alpha-adrenergic and beta-adrenergic receptors to an equal degree.

Either type of adrenergic receptor (alpha or beta) can be either excitatory or inhibitory, depending upon the affinity of the hormone for the receptors in a particular effector organ. Table 3.16 shows the reaction of these receptors to activating stimuli in some organs and systems under the dominance of the sympathetics, according to Guyton.

It is well to keep in mind when treating patients who are on drugs which affect the autonomic nervous system that synthetic drugs may or may not act upon receptors in the same manner that these natural substances do. For example, synthetic isopropyl norepinephrine activates a strong reaction in beta receptors but has no effect on alpha receptors.

The Adrenal Medullae

Activation of the entire sympathetic system is the typical effect when a significant portion of it is stimulated. Thus, epinephrine and norepinephrine are invariably released by the adrenal medullae into systemic circulation simultaneously whenever local sympathetic stimulation occurs. In this manner, vegetative tissues are acted upon by two supporting influences: neural and hormonal. Because hormones are removed from the circulation slowly, the effects of adrenal medulla secretion last about 10 times longer than direct sympathetic stimulation.

Because of the dual action of sympathetic innervation and the adrenal medulla hormones, complete loss of local innervation will be supported by the adrenals or bilateral loss of the adrenals will be supported by local innervation. In most cases, these compensating events will completely hide deficits from the clinical picture.

Epinephrine and norepinephrine react on tissues in a similar manner, but there are some differences. In comparison to norepinephrine, epinephrine has a greater effect on heart muscle and output; has a far greater effect on basal metabolic rate, liver and muscle glycogenolysis, and glucose release into the blood; but causes weaker vasoconstriction in skeletal muscle.

Adrenal medullae hormones also stimulate processes that are not directly innervated by sympathetic fibers. For example, although a small percentage of body cells receive direct sympathetic innervation, epinephrine and norepinephrine increase the metabolic rate of every cell in the body.

Clinical Considerations

For most of the history of chiropractic, most chiropractic practices were family oriented; ie, almost any type of case was accepted that was within the scope of a particular

Table 3.16. Functions of Adrenergic Receptors

Alpha Receptors	1 Receptors	2 Receptors
Intestinal relaxation	Cardiac acceleration	Bronchodilation
Intestinal sphincter contraction	Increased heart strength	Calorigenesis
Pilomotor contraction	Lipolysis	Glycogenesis
Pupil dilation		Intestinal relaxation
Urinary bladder sphincter contraction		Urinary bladder relaxation
Vasoconstriction		Uterine relaxation
		Vasodilation

state's practice act except those that required surgical, pharmaceutical, or psychiatric attention. About 75%—80% of entering complaints reported could be classified under the broad category of visceral dysfunction and minor infections (eg, colds, influenza, childhood diseases), with the remaining 20%—25% classified under musculoskeletal disorders. During the 1970s, these percentages became almost reversed—parallel with the inclusion of chiropractic within Medicare, Medicaid, and the passing of insurance equality laws. While it is fortunate that this turn in events has increased our knowledge and improved our efficiency in the treatment of biomechanical disorders, it is unfortunate that recent years have seen a neglect of the role of chiropractic in treating visceral disorders.

Wiles/Diakow reported in 1982 that bronchial asthma, idiopathic dysmenorrhea, and essential hypertension are three of many visceral disorders frequently treated in a chiropractic office. Structural adjustments, nutritional therapy, and a variety of therapeutic modalities are commonly used.

Imbalance Manifestations

The contributions of Pottenger cannot be overlooked in proving that imbalance in the vegetative nerves is capable of producing a wide variety of symptoms. Clinically, a recognizable imbalance is produced in all visceral diseases that reach a sufficient magnitude to be recognized by the patient.

Autonomic imbalance implies visceral instability wherein the normal physiologic control of visceral activity throughout the body, or in some organ or system, is so unstable that a comparatively mild stimulus, when applied to the system of unstable cells, is sufficient to produce a marked effect. This effect often overcomes all antagonistic forces and produces a pathologic state. Patients having such an imbalance show reactions beyond what is natural for the stimulus applied. For instance, such factors as subluxations, emotions, fatigue, weather changes, and toxemia produce changes in such individuals that are far greater than would normally be expected.

Skin Reactions

The piloerector muscles, sweat glands, and blood vessels of the skin are innervated by cholinergic sympathetic fibers arising from T1—T6 for the upper limbs and T12—L2 for the lower limbs. These sympathetics also supply the apocrine glands, but the fibers are adrenergic. It is on this rationale of sympathetic dominance of the skin that instruments which measure skin resistance or surface temperature are often used in chiropractic to gather data as to the efficiency of local sympathetic innervation. The function of parasympathetic fibers in the extremities has not been determined.

A point of interest made by Guyton is that the sympathetic fibers supplying most of the structures of the skin are activated primarily by hypothalamic centers that are usually considered to be parasympathetic centers. Fibers supplying the apocrine glands are controlled by CNS sympathetic centers rather than parasympathetic centers.

During general sympathetic overactivity (eg, anxiety, fear), the blood vessels constrict, the sweat glands secrete, "goose pimples" arise, and hairs sometimes erect. The result is a cool, clammy, unsmooth skin. During sympathetic underactivity (eg, Horner's syndrome), the blood vessels dilate, the sweat glands are inhibited, and the piloerectors relax. The result is a warm, dry, smooth skin.

Circulatory Reactions

Besides the influence upon smooth muscle, much of visceral function is regulated by blood vessel size and heart output. Vessel lumen diameter is under the control of the sympathetic system, heart rate and contraction strength are the product of both sympathetic and parasympathetic influences, and both vascular size and heart efficiency receive specific and nonspecific sensory input from receptors within the blood vessels, heart, and CNS. If lesions affect these receptors, functional blood pressure abnormalities and cardiac disorders arise, which are often the result of poor adaptation to normal stress.

During undemanding activity, sympathetic stimulation to blood vessels keeps the vessels of the body constantly constricted to about 50% of their maximum. This is the basis of peripheral vasculature *tone*. If it were not for this fact, inhibited sympathetic control could not produce vasodilation.

Inasmuch as activated sympathetics increase heart strength and constrict blood flow within peripheral circulation, the role of sympathetic overactivity is an important factor to be considered in managing cases of vasotonic high blood pressure.

Studies conducted so far indicate that stimulation of the parasympathetics does not appear to have any effect on arterial diameter; ie, it does not induce vascular relaxation. One exception to this is facial blushing. As sympathetic stimulation induces vascular contraction and sympathetic inhibition induces vascular relaxation, the peripheral vascular system is currently considered under the essential control of the sympathetics. The same appears to be true for the sweat glands, pilomotor muscles, apocrine glands, kidneys, skeletal muscle, adrenal cortex, basal metabolism, and mental activity. However, it would be a narrow belief that the parasympathetic system has no role on these structures or processes even if that purpose has not yet been determined.

Pupil Reactions

The size of the pupils is under the control of the autonomic nervous system, and size changes are responses to both external (light) and emotional stimuli. Pupil constrictors and the degree of lens convexity are controlled by parasympathetic fibers traveling in the oculomotor nerve. Pupil dilators are regulated by sympathetic fibers originating from spinal segments T1 and T2 via the sympathetic chain. Thus, a pupil that does not respond to light during examination likely indicates either sympathetic underactivity or parasympathetic overactivity.

Duct Glands and Gut Reactions

The lacrimal, nasal, salivary, upper gastrointestinal glands (mouth to stomach), and pancreas are under the dominance of the parasympathetics. The glands of the enteric system are controlled for the most part by local factors rather than autonomic innervation from the spinal cord.

Although the autonomics play a minimal role in intestinal glandular activity, they serve a primary role in intestinal tone and motility. Sympathetic stimulation (T9—L1) decreases peristalsis. Parasympathetic stimulation (Cranial X) increases peristalsis and plays an essential role in maintaining the sustained tone of intestinal smooth muscles.

Endocrine Reactions

Sympathetic activation increases the secretion of the adrenal medulla, pancreatic islets, pineal gland, and thyroid. The parasympathetics have a reverse or unknown effect.

Micturition

The urinary bladder is innervated by sympathetic, parasympathetic, and some somatic fibers (external sphincter), and they all arise from the lower segments of the spinal cord. Sympathetic afferents are believed to originate in detrusor muscles of the body of the bladder, and efferents are provided by the T12—L2 segments of the spinal cord. Parasympathetic afferents pass via the pudendal nerve to the S2—S4 segments of the cord, and efferents extend from these segments to the bladder via the hypogastric plexus.

The voluntary initiation and stopping of micturition arises primarily from impulses in the paracentral lobule of the cerebral cortex. Sympathetic stimulation relaxes the muscular wall and constricts the sphincter; parasympathetic stimulation has the opposite effect. Dysfunction in micturition may be the result of inadequate sensory input, poor motor output, a lesion involving reflex interneurons in the spinal cord, or a lesion disrupting longitudinal ascending or descending impulses.

Defecation

The rectum, as the urinary bladder, is innervated by sympathetic, parasympathetic, and somatic fibers (abdomen, external anal sphincter). Sympathetic innervation is provided from L1—L3 segments, and the parasympathetic supply is from the S3—S5 segments of the spinal cord. Sympathetic stimulation contracts the internal anal sphincter and decreases peristalsis. Parasympathetic activation has the reverse effect. Voluntary assistance by the abdominal muscles is provided by somatic motor nerves T6—T12.

Sexual Function

Sexual function is a product of both sympathetic and parasympathetic influences. In the female, sympathetic stimulation contracts the fallopian tubes (T10—L1), contracts the body of the uterus (L1), inhibits vaginal secretion, and relaxes the clitoris. Generally, parasympathetic stimulation (S2—S4) has the opposite effect.

In the male, sympathetic stimulation (T10—L1) contracts the prostate muscle, spermatic vein, and genital ducts, and initiates ejaculation. Parasympathetic stimulation (S2—S4), produces vasodilation for penile erection, relaxes the genital ducts, and increases prostate secretion.

Factors Involved in Vegetative Imbalance

Vegetative functional activity and control are complex affairs conducted by the cells, the electrolytes, chemicals of the various hormones, and the sympathetic and parasympathetic nerves. The action of these systems is interdependent and can be understood only when considered together because imbalance in one may mean imbalance in all. Imbalance may have as its chief cause a disturbance in any one or more of these factors. The cells may be at fault, the electrolytes that have an important part to play in cellular activity may be abnormal in their proportions, or the chemical or nervous regulators may create too little or too much activity. Usually, the cells will do their job if the environment is right. This puts the onus on nerve supply, electrolytes, lymph circulation, and nutrition. Regardless, deviations from the norm result in abnormal or subnormal function.

Normal vegetative function can be maintained if proper nutrition is supplied the cells and their colloidal phases are usual for the structure under consideration provided (1) the necessary electrolytes are supplied in the right proportions, (2) the hormones from the various endocrine glands and vitamins are supplied in normal amounts, and (3) the activating and inhibiting impulses that are carried to the cells by nerves balance each other or at least fail to overbalance each other. If these factors are not provided, deviations from the normal will lead to vegetative imbalance.

Trophic Reactions. Trophic lesions of the joints, muscles (atrophy), skin, and nails are common. They blend and are somewhat explained as the result of vascular changes (vasomotor). Herpes labialis (cold sores) and herpes zoster (shingles) appear to give evidence of being due to nutritive disorders in the ganglia, not to vascular changes, predisposing to virus infection. In brain lesions, trophic and vasomotor changes are much less common than in diseases of the cord and peripheral nerves. The acute bedsores that form in myelitis, the angioneurotic local swellings that appear here and there in certain people, and the local syncope or asphyxia that sometimes lead to Raynaud's form of gangrene seem to require both nerve and vascular changes to explain them.

The Character of Visceral Pain. The character of visceral pain reaching consciousness that is associated with a visceral dysfunction is sometimes helpful during diagnosis. Visceral pain entering directly with peripheral nerves is sharp and quite localized, while pain entering directly from pelvic nerves is perceived as various degrees of fullness. Visceral pain impulses entering through the sympathetic trunk is usually perceived as being diffuse, dull, and aching, regardless of cause (tension, compression, or ischemia).

Associated Factors in Visceral-Related Pain. In the context of pain-related visceral dysfunction, Pottenger pointed out that hyperalgesia of soft tissues is not uncommon in the areas that have been the seat of reflex sensory pain. For example, subcutaneous soreness within the shoulder and upper arm muscles is often associated with inflammatory diseases of the lungs. He also reported that cutaneous hyperalgesia is a common finding in visceral disease. Hyperalgesic skin frequently overlies an area of pleurisy, a tubercular cavity, a peptic ulcer, or an inflamed ovary. Zones of hyperalgesia (often associated with cutaneous vasoconstriction and hypermyotonia) are more commonly associated with acute and subacute visceral disease rather than chronic disorders. See Figure 3.36. The afferent fibers occupying the pre- and post-ganglionic pathways of the autonomic system from soma and viscera have a segmental arrangement when pain is a factor (refer to Table 3.7).

Head's Law. During the differentiation of visceral pain with hyperalgesia, it is well to keep in mind that visceral distress is manifested in two ways: (1) an uneasy dull discomfort in the viscera itself and (2) a truly painful sensation on the overlying surface of the body. Head's law states:

When a painful stimulus is applied to a part of low sensibility (eg, a viscus) in close central connection with a part of much greater sensibility (eg, the skin), the pain produced is felt in the part of higher sensibility to a far greater extent than is perceived in the part of lower sensibility to which the stimulus was applied.

Sympathicotonia and Vagotonia: Basic Considerations

The parasympathetic system tends to express itself in a local, specific manner (eg, anabolic activity); while the sympathetic system expresses in a diffuse, less specific manner (eg, preparatory "flight or fight" responses).

Any deviation from normal vegetative functional activity is called a vegetative imbalance. The two common deviations are called sympathicotonia and parasympathicotonia (vagotonia). Vagotonia is a condition indicating excessive action in cranial X expressing itself in the tissues of the body. The opposite is sympathicotonia. These disorders

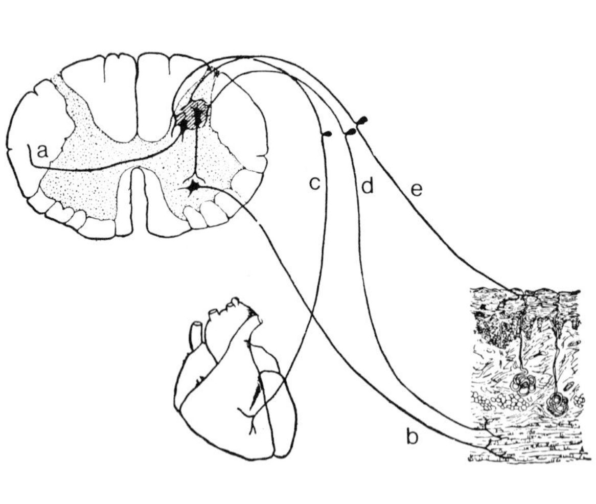

Figure 3.36. Diagram showing possible neural path for referred pain of cardiac origin. Nerve impulses *(c)* from a disturbed heart bring about an "irritable" area in the gray matter of the anterior horn. Nerve fibers from the overlying skin and muscle *(d and e)* enter the same area. Nerve fibers from this region transverse the cord *(a)* to join with fibers of the spinothalamic tract whose impulses are carried to the cerebral cortex and over another path *(b)*, via interneurons to the ipsilateral anterior horn, which synapse with efferent neurons to the chest muscles that contract in an exaggerated manner.

may be general or limited to certain systems or organs.

Although vegetative disorders are expressed in terms of sympathetic and parasympathetic action, this does not mean that the nervous system is primarily at fault: remembering that the fault may lie with the cells, electrolytes, hormones, vitamins, or the autonomic nerves. Regardless of cause, there are large numbers of people who have a marked tendency to respond to stimuli that act on one or the other part of the vegetative system to such a degree that it amounts to disease.

Pottenger stated that sympathicotonics react more markedly than normal to cold, toxins, and emotions in an epinephrine-like manner. They readily produce reflexes wherein the sympathetics are involved. Contrarywise, parasympathicotonics are particularly susceptible to allergic excitants and respond in an atropine-like manner.

These syndromes may be produced by stimuli that act either centrally or peripherally. Toxins, for example, act centrally and result in widespread sympathetic effects. Inflammation in an organ, on the other hand, may act upon the nerve endings therein and create reflex sympathetic or parasympathetic effects only in the specific organs or tissues whose nerves receive the reflex stimulation.

A patient need not be sympathicotonic or vagotonic throughout the vegetative structures. He may have a sympathicotonic heart while the rest of the structures are normal, or he may express symptoms of vagotonia elsewhere such as hyperchlorhydria or spastic colon. The important thing during diagnosis is to assign these phenomena when they arise to the components of the vegetative nervous system to which they belong. Exophthalmic goiter is a good example where sympathetic imbalance can be found in one organ and parasympathetic imbalance in another.

Psychic Influences. Stimuli to the sympathetic-accelerator side of the autonomic nervous system are initiated frequently by emotions as well as by related exercise. Within a reasonable time, the symptoms created by the stimuli should return to normal. However, if these stimuli are too prolonged or pronounced, then the balancing parasympathetics (eg, the vagus nerve) should be investigated to see why it is not exerting its proper opposition force or why it is underactive.

Activation of the parasympathetic-brake side of the autonomic system is often initiated by bad news, fright, or shock. Again, within a reasonable time, the patient should recover from the effects of these stimuli and the emotions returned to normal. If these stimuli are too prolonged or pronounced, then the balancing sympathetics should be investigated to see why they are not exerting their proper opposition forces or why they are underactive.

The clinical evaluation of the autonomic nervous system and interpretation of findings are described in Chapter 10.

THE VASCULAR SYSTEM

In the longitudinal systems described previously, the signs of dysfunction were the result of direct neural damage. This is not true for the vascular system. Being a supporting system, defects in the vascular system supplying the nervous system generally manifest as secondary neurologic deficits.

Functional Anatomy: An Overview

Lassen and associates found that even at rest the blood flow to the brain is not uniform. They found that engaging the senses increased cortical blood flow and brought into action cerebral regions in a special pattern.

The major blood supply of the brain has been described in Chapter 2. See Figure 3.37.

Circulation of the Spinal Cord

Arterial Supply. Each cervical vertebral artery offers a branch at the brain stem to form a single anterior spinal artery that runs the length of the spinal cord, lying over the median fissure. It tapers as it courses downward in the thoracic cord and gives off central branches at intervals of about 2 mm which, in turn, branch both peripherally and centrally. The anterior spinal artery supplies all the cord with the exception of the posterior columns and horns.

The vertebral arteries also contribute a branch to unilateral posterior spinal arteries that form longitudinal plexiform channels as they progress caudad to supply the posterior columns and horns. The anterior spinal artery appears to be the main source of blood supply to the posterior arteries below the upper thoracic level.

Radicular Support. The arterial system of the cord does not have extensive collateral circulation. It relies heavily on extraspinal *radicular artery* sources. Any interruption of these (eg, IVF encroachment) can produce serious neurologic damage. The superior portion of the anterior spinal artery is assisted by radicular arteries that enter through the IVFs of the midcervical, lower cervical, and upper thoracic levels. A large radicular artery *(great spinal)* enters between the T9 and L3 levels and is believed to be responsible for ¼—½ the blood supply of the cord below this level. A severe drop in blood pressure for 3—5 minutes can so compromise radicular circulation that necrosis of the thoracic neurons occurs.

Venous Supply. The abundant veins of the spinal cord drain into the intervertebral veins that communicate with other plexuses. The immediate part of the system involves the (1) *internal plexuses*, whose pia branches drain the contents of the vertebral canal, vertebral arch, and posterior vertebral body and leave via the IVF and (2) the *external plexuses*, which drain the anterior and lateral aspects of the vertebral body and its associated tissues (Fig. 3.38). If the prostate is cancerous, pelvic blood returning to the heart via the vertebral plexuses rather than the inferior vena cava may initiate spinal metastasis.

Circulation of the Spine

The Arterial System. An *anterior artery*, descending in the ventral median sulcus, and two *posterior arteries*, descending along the posterolateral sulcus, supply the spine (Fig. 3.39). The latter arise from either the vertebral arteries or the posteroinferior cerebellar arteries. These anterior and posterior axial conduits are often small, irregular, and must be reinforced at intervals by radicular arteries that branch from nearby spinal arteries arising outside the vertebral column.

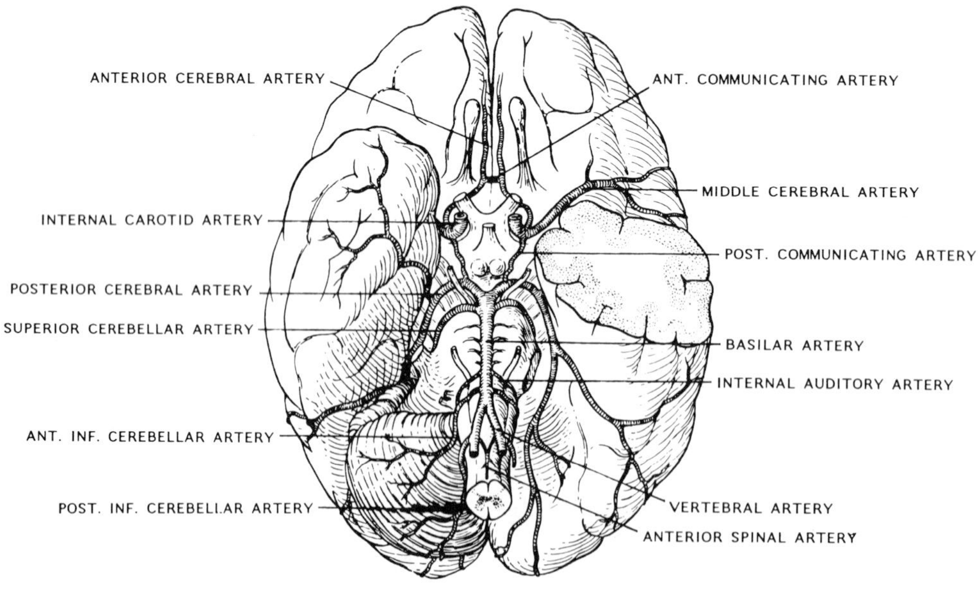

Figure 3.37. The arterial supply of the brain as viewed from its base.

In the cervical area, the vertebral artery runs in the foramen transversarium of the transverse processes of C2—C6 and offers branches to each segment. Similar arteries arise from the intercostal and lumbar arteries branching from the aorta. The lateral sacral arteries give branches to the sacral segments. In each instance, the segmental artery offers several anterior twigs to the front and sides of the vertebral body and posterior divisions to the spinal muscles and IVFs. After a posterior division passes through the IVF, it enters the vertebral canal and divides into three branches: (1) an *anterior branch*, which (a) supplies the posterior aspect of the vertebral body to anastomose with the lateral and anterior twigs of that part of the artery that did not enter the IVF, and (b) ascending and descending twigs; (2) an *intermediate branch*, which supplies the nerve root and spinal dura; and (3) a *posterior branch*, which supplies the vertebral arch, extradural contents, and dura.

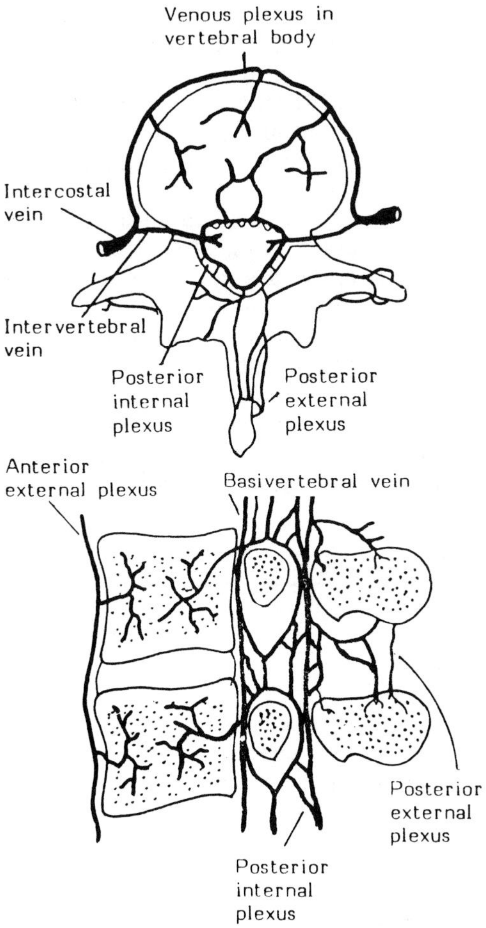

Figure 3.38. *Top,* schematic of the venous supply of the vertebral area, as viewed from above. *Bottom,* a lateral midsagittal section of the area, showing the relationship of the major veins to the osseous structures and soft-tissue areas.

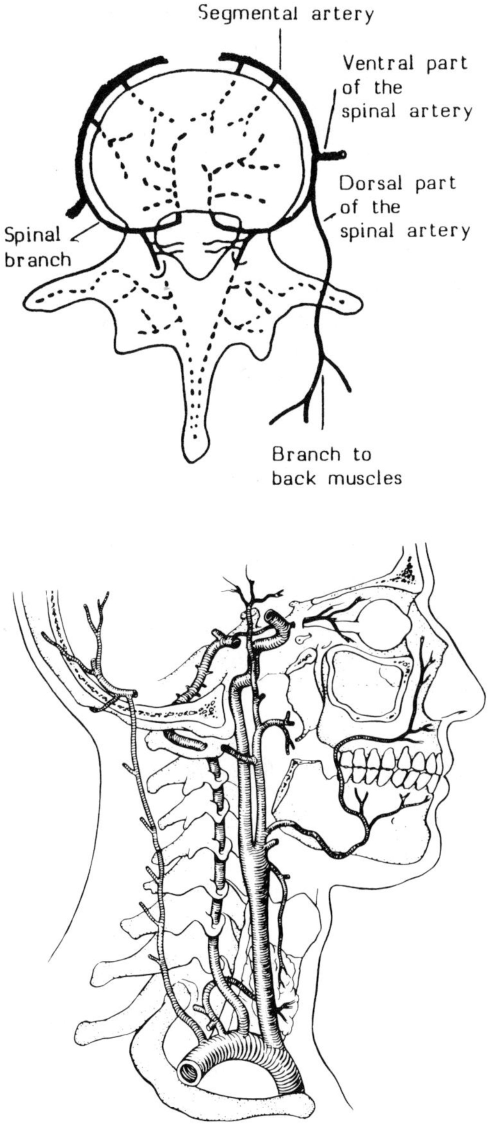

Figure 3.39. *Top,* schematic of the arterial supply of the vertebral area, as viewed from above. *Bottom,* course of the major arteries of the neck. Note the route of the vertebral artery through the transverse foramina of the cervical vertebrae.

The Venous System. The venous system of the spine *(Batson's plexus)* is a valveless plexus separate from that of the thoracoabdominal cavities. It is derived from the veins of the extremities, body wall, neck, and head. Any increase in intrathoracic or intra-abdominal pressure (eg, Valsalva maneuver) shunts venous blood to the vertebral system. The resulting engorgement contributes to the spinal pain of many patients with spinal faults. The close tie between spinous venous pressure and neurologic integrity is clearly exhibited when the *jugular compression test* elicits paresthesia in the lower extremities.

Clinical Considerations

Space-occupying lesions within the cranium commonly result from hemorrhage, an aneurysm, or a tumor. The primary characteristics of such lesions are shown in Table 3.17.

Extradural Hematoma

The dura mater in the adult does not adhere to the entire skull. Thus, it is possible for fluid to be forced between the cranium and the dura, and the increased pressure tends to dislodge attached dura from its points of skull connection. As branches of the middle meningeal artery nourish both the dura and the surrounding bone of the skull, bleeding from torn vessels forms between the skull and the dura and produces an extradural hematoma. It is controversial whether this condition is commonly associated with concussion: opinions vary from frequently to rarely.

Extradural hematoma can result when a fracture tears the middle meningeal artery. A characteristic feature is the appearance of paralysis of the arm, leg, and face on the contralateral side of the lesion. The semiconscious patient will not respond to supraorbital pressure on the affected side. When hemiplegia is suspected, corroborating signs must be sought such as increased deep reflexes, absent abdominal reflexes, and a positive Babinski response. In early cases, the arm is more affected than the leg. Other features include early but brief unconsciousness, followed by drowsiness, headache, and vomiting.

The probability of extradural hematoma should always be suspected when hematoma of the temporalis muscle, gradual onset of hemiplegia, deepening coma, Hutchinson's pupils, and the lucid interval are exhibited. The differential diagnosis should first exclude a depressed skull fracture, intracerebral hematoma, and subdural hematoma.

In addition to the general characteristics of increased intracranial pressure, the typi-

Table 3.17. Primary Features of CNS Space-Occupying Lesions

Above the Foramen Magnum	
Cranial nerve palsies, unilateral	Papilledema
Headache, persistent	Perceptive deafness, unilateral
Hemiplegia, slowly progressing	Personality changes
History of seizures	Progressive onset of symptoms
Increased intracranial pressure	Visual field cuts
Below the Foramen Magnum	
Bladder disturbances	Paralysis, slowly progressing
Cutaneous electrical resistance changes	Progressive onset of symptoms
Muscle weakness and atrophy, unilateral or bilateral	Radicular pain
	Rectal sphincter disturbances
	Trophic changes

cal clinical picture exhibits an abrupt onset, hemispheric or brain stem compression signs, and rapidly evolving coma. X-ray films will likely show a possible fracture across the middle meningeal artery, and a pineal shift is probable. There is a positive brain scan, and EEG depression over site.

The many characteristics of neurovascular injury following severe head injury are listed in Table 3.18.

Subdural Hematoma

Subdural hemorrhages are caused by rupture of bridging veins crossing the space between the dura and the arachnoid. They are characterized by headaches, drowsiness, poor concentration, mild confusion, progressively decreasing levels of consciousness, and motor deficits (eg, hemiparesis). These symptoms may be immediate or delayed for weeks or months after injury. Although larger in size than an extradural hemorrhage, a subdural hemorrhage is confined unilaterally because the dura is firmly fixed to the falx between the hemispheres.

Acute Subdural Hematoma. This is the most frequent cause of death in falls and sports injuries. It is much more common than extradural hematoma and shows no lucid interval. Lateralizing signs, however, are similar. Inequality of pupils (anisocoria) is of considerable localizing value. Hutchinson's pupil from compression of the 3rd cranial nerve against the free edge of the tentorium is often seen. Widely dilated and fixed pupils bilaterally indicate that death is approaching. Severe acute subdural hemorrhage is usually associated with cerebral laceration.

Table 3.18. Neurovascular Features of Severe Head Injury

Abnormal auscultated vascular sounds in skull	Hemianopsia
Abnormal auscultated vocal sounds in the skull	Hyperglycemia
Abnormal lip and/or mouth color	Impaired sensory interpretation
Abnormal movement of head or face	Irritability
Amnesia	Lucid interval
Anxiety	Mouth breathing
Aphasia	Nausea
Autonomic dysfunction	Nuchal rigidity
Battle sign	Palpable abnormal elevations or depressions
Behavioral changes	Palsy or paralysis
Bloody or nonbloody otorrhea	Papilledema (late usually)
Bloody or nonbloody rhinorrhea	Postnasal bleeding
Bloody spinal fluid	Progressing fever
Consciousness disturbances	Pulsating exophthalmos
"Cracked-pot" sound on skull percussion	Raccoon sign
Cranial nerve malfunction	Respiratory rhythm changes
Cyanosis	Restlessness (severe)
Decerebrate rigidity	Roentgenographic findings
Diplopia	Scalp laceration (possibly)
Disorientation	Shock
Dizziness/vertigo	Speech impairment
Ecchymosis	Stertorous breathing with cheek puffing
Eyelid edema and/or malfunction	Strabismus
Facial swelling	Tongue protrusion deviation
Headache	Unequal pupils
	Unilateral facial palsy
	Vomiting

Bleeding from the brain itself seeps into the subdural space, adding to probable dura, pia, and arachnoid bleeding. In the late stage, signs of herniation and oculomotor paralysis appear. The incidence is high in the elderly because cortical atrophy increases the space in which the veins must traverse. The incidence is also high in boxers, other contact-sport athletes, and alcoholics because of increased head trauma.

Features include pronounced and progressive headache, drowsiness, stupor, epileptic attacks, temperature increase, reduced pulse and respiratory rates, increased pulse pressure, progressive contralateral paralysis, sphincter relaxation, severe shock, and coma. Besides the general characteristics of increased intracranial pressure, other major signs are: skull fracture (probably), possible pineal shift shown on x-ray films, positive brain scan, EEG depression over site, inhibited mental functions, lateralizing signs (if unilateral), and progressive obtundation. The localizing features following intracranial trauma are shown in Table 3.19.

Chronic Subdural Hemorrhage. Chronic subdural hemorrhage presents with symptoms of anorexia, vomiting, blurred vision, drowsiness, personality changes, and gait disturbances. These not infrequent sequel of head injury are often related to a mild initial cranial trauma, insufficient to cause loss of consciousness. The accident is often forgotten by the patient. Headache, mental changes, and drowsiness develop some months later. This is caused by the clot attracting nonprotein fluids that cause gradual enlargement of the mass; ie, the osmotic tendency of any fluid of lighter density to pass through a semipermeable membrane to join fluid of greater density. Symptoms are often marked at times, disappear, and return later with greater severity. Albuminuria is a striking concomitant finding, and xanthochromic spinal fluid is a common finding. Motor involvements, emotional disturbances, and greatly altered deep reflexes are usually present. Less frequently, cranial nerve involvement, Jacksonian convulsions, aphasia, vomiting, slow pulse, and choked disc are exhibited. The differential diagnosis should exclude bromide intoxication, general paresis, and subdural hygroma and other space-occupying cerebral lesions.

Apoplexy

The most dangerous effect of high blood pressure is hemorrhage. This commonly

Table 3.19. Localizing Features Following Intracranial Trauma

Feature	Location
Impaired recognition of ordinary sensations	Postcentral gyrus
Irregular explosive speech	Cerebellar involvement
Movement difficulties with spastic paralysis and/or hypertonicity and rigidity of contralateral side	Precentral gyrus and adjacent frontal gyri
Lucid interval	Middle meningeal (extradural) artery hemorrhage, usually
Nasal speech	Palatal paralysis
Olfactory hallucinations	Temporal lobe
Personality changes	Prefrontal area of cerebrum
Recent-event amnesia, poor recognition of sounds and their significance	Temporal lobe
Severe, intractable, poorly localized pain	Thalamic lesion
Slurred speech	Upper or lower motor lesion
Vasomotor and autonomic disturbances	Hypothalamic lesion
Visual disturbances of recognition	Occipital lobe

occurs into the cerebrum from a terminal branch of the middle cerebral artery. Hemorrhages into the ventricles of the brain or meninges may also be found. Intracranial hemorrhages may be small and localized or massive and diffuse. They may be suddenly fatal or cause a paralysis that corresponds to the portion of the brain damaged. Nosebleed is a common warning sign. Intracerebral hemorrhage can be associated with either extradural or subdural hematoma, or it may be the sole lesion. Lateralizing signs are usually absent. Hemorrhages less frequently occur into the spinal cord.

The most common sites and causes of cerebral hemorrhage are shown in Table 3.20. The onset may be slow or spontaneous (stroke), and symptoms will vary depending upon the severity and site of the hemorrhage; eg, abrupt headache (usually suboccipital), torticollis, vomiting, mental confusion, weakness, possible sensory loss, visual field defects, possible skull bruit, possible aphasia, unconsciousness, xanthochromia, late upper motor lesion signs, hemiparesis, and coma.

In cases of intracranial hemorrhage, Babinski's sign is most significant and the one most frequently present. It usually denotes a hematoma on the opposite side of the brain. Aphasia may be the first lateralizing sign in a left side lesion in a right-handed person. Broca's area is usually on the left side.

Infarction from either embolism or thrombosis often mimics hemorrhage. Hemorrhage gives little warning, infarction usually does. Cortical defects are rare with hemorrhage but common to infarction. Stiff neck, papilledema, and a shifted pineal gland are typical signs of hemorrhage but rare with thrombosis. However, inasmuch as both are medical emergencies, the need for differentiation in a chiropractic office is rare. When suspicions arise, immediate neurologic consultation is recommended.

Vertebrobasilar Insufficiency

The posterior vertebral arteries pass through the transverse foramina of the cervical vertebrae and the foramen magnum before forming the posterior portion of the circle of Willis. As Zeoli points out, cervical subluxation syndromes, muscular spasms, scolioses, and the size and position of the foramen magnum may adversely affect cranial blood supply. These syndromes will be described in subsequent chapters. Major features such as headache, nausea, vertigo, lip and tongue tingling, dysarthria, diplopia or blindness, ataxia, increased cranial pressure, and hemiparesis or tetraparesis may result.

Other Common Considerations

A large number of intracranial lesions produce increased intracranial pressure. The general features of pressure build-up, which are common to most all etiologies, include:

- Blurred vision
- Decreased alertness
- Diplopia
- Dizziness
- Fever (possibly)
- Frequent yawning
- Headache

Table 3.20. Common Sites and Causes of Cerebral Hemorrhage

Site	Cause	
Intracerebral hemorrhage	Aneurysm Arteriovenous malformation Bleeding disorders	Hypertension Trauma
Subarachnoid hemorrhage	Aneurysm Arteriovenous malformation	Bleeding disorders Trauma

- Hiccuping
- Nausea
- Papilledema (usually late)
- Projectile vomiting
- Tinnitus

Specific disorders causing increased intracranial pressure are listed in Table 3.21. Some other cerebrovascular disorders not previously mentioned are briefly described below.

Cerebral Aneurysm. The most common cause of a cerebral aneurysm is an atheroma of the internal carotid. The primary symptoms vary, depending upon the exact site of the lesion; eg: (1) frontal headache and isolated oculomotor paralysis (origin of posterior communicating artery); (2) ophthalmoplegia, possible ocular bruit, and trigeminal sensory loss (carvernous sinus); or (3) optic atrophy and visual loss (suprasellar region).

Cerebral Angioma. This is a congenital arteriovenous defect that usually exhibits in early to middle adulthood. Major symptoms include focal epilepsy, a cranial bruit, and constant migraine-like headaches.

Cranial Arteritis (Cerebral Vasculitis). This inflammatory disorder leads to a clinical picture of peripheral symmetric or mononeuropathy multiplex. In addition to the general characteristics of intracranial pressure, the onset is sudden, and the signs are similar to those of hypertensive encephalopathy. Skull x-ray films are negative, brain scan positive (usually), and EEG shows focal-to-diffuse abnormalities.

Diffuse Cerebral Atherosclerosis. As a result of a series of minor strokes, progressively deepening symptoms of intellectual impairment, personality changes, dysarthria, dysphagia, bladder disturbances, shuffling gait, parkinsonism, and signs of progressive pseudobulbar palsy are typical.

Internal Carotid Disease. Brief, frequent episodes of confusion, transient ipsilateral monocular blindness, possible contralateral hemiplegia and sensory loss, dysphagia (dominant hemisphere), and Horner's syndrome are characteristic.

Migraine. The cardinal symptom is paroxysmal headache that is usually unilateral and of long duration (from several hours to days). Early prodromal aura and facial or arm paresthesia are often associated. Depending upon severity, photosensitivity, hyperlacrimation, nasal congestion, unilateral ptosis and contracted pupil, anorexia, and vomiting may be associated.

Posterior Cerebral Artery Syndrome. The major feature of this disorder specifically depends on the site of the lesion. For example:

- Medial temporal lobes (bilateral) - global amnesia
- Medial temporal lobe (unilateral) - specific memory defect(s)
- Occipital lobe - visual field defect
- Subthalamus - hemiballismus
- Thalamus - loss of tactile sensation and pain contralaterally.

Sagittal Sinus Thrombosis. Possible skull fracture should be ruled out. In addi-

Table 3.21. Disorders That Produce Increased Intracranial Pressure

Cardiopulmonary disease	Heavy metal poisoning	Paget's disease
Cerebral edema	Hydrocephalus	Parasitic infestation of brain
Cerebral vasculitis	Hypertensive encephalopathy leading to apoplexy	Polyneuropathy
Cerebral venous thrombosis	Intracranial abscess	Poststatus epilepticus
Demyelinating diseases	Leptomeningeal cyst	Primary neoplasm
Diabetes mellitus	Mediastinal disease	Reye's syndrome
Empyema, epidural or subdural	Meningeal neoplasm	Sagittal sinus thromb.
Epidural hematoma	Meningismus	Spinal cord tumor
Fluid/electrolyte imbalances	Meningitis	Subarachnoid bleeding
Granulomatous diseases	Metastatic neoplasm	Subdural hematoma
	Mycotic aneurysm	Viral encephalitis

tion to the general characteristics of intracranial pressure, seizures are common that slowly progress in severity. There are neurologic focal signs, a negative brain scan, and EEG findings are normal or show diffuse slowing.

Venous Sinus Thrombosis. Whether or not the cause is trauma or an infection, this disorder has three major forms; ie, (1) *lateral sinus thrombosis* from mastoid disease exhibits headache, papilledema, fever, and vomiting; (2) *cavernous sinus thrombosis* from facial or nasal sinus disease is associated with ocular proptosis, severe eye pain, chemosis, and possible papilledema and ophthalmoplegia; and (3) *superior sagittal sinus thrombosis* from facial or nasal sinus disease manifests as focal neurologic and epileptic signs. In addition to the general characteristics of any cause of increased intracranial pressure, the syndrome features include a sudden onset, focal neurologic signs, and seizures. Skull x-ray films are negative, brain scan is possibly positive, and EEG shows focal-to-diffuse abnormalities.

THE CONSCIOUSNESS SYSTEM

The term *consciousness* refers to the mental state of perception and responsiveness to environmental stimuli. *Perception* is the process of being aware; the receiving, elaboration, and usually the localization of a sensory impressions; the mental linking of cause and effect. *Apperception* refers to full comprehension such as the recognition or identification of the source of a stimulus, and this depends greatly on association with past experiences. These faculties of *awareness* are primarily integrated, modulated, and coordinated by the cerebral cortex (Fig. 3.40).

Central Neural Control Mechanisms

Whether a person is awake or asleep, the brain is constantly bombarded by input from all skin and internal receptors. This barrage of incoming messages is examined, valued, and translated relative to a framework composed of instincts, experiences, and mental conditioning. In some as yet undiscovered manner, an appropriate decision is arrived at that is transmitted to all muscles necessary for the response desired. By means of varying synaptic facilitation and restraints within the appropriate circuits, an almost limitless variety of neural integration and signal transmission is possible. For review, a diagram of a typical motor and sensory circuit is shown in Figure 3.41.

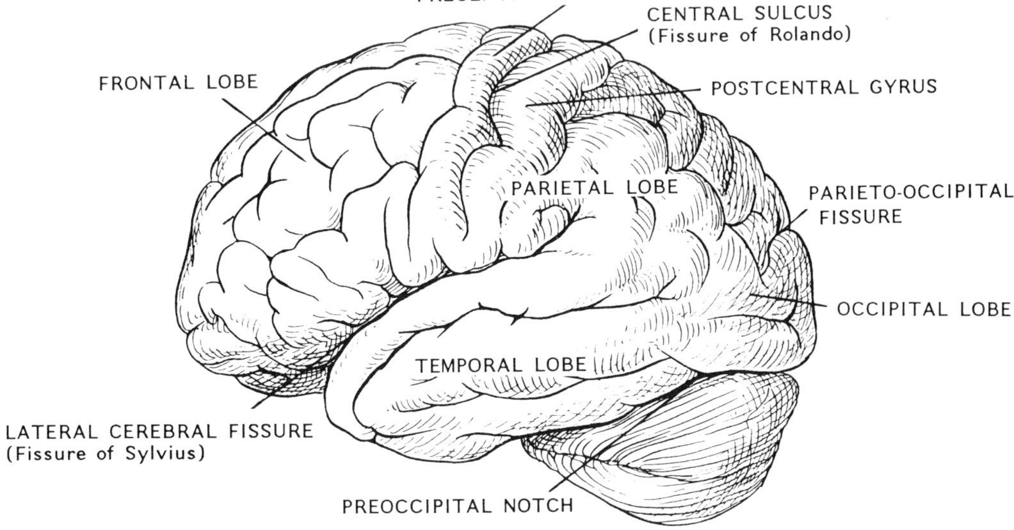

Figure 3.40. Superior and lateral views of the cerebral hemispheres.

In terms of motor function, the cerebral cortex can be discussed as three distinct regions that control specific muscle groups associated with specific joints. The *primary motor region* of the cerebral cortex is primarily concerned with delicate *voluntary movements*, particularly of the facial and distal flexor muscles of the extremities. Its left aspect controls the right side of the body, and its right aspect controls the left side. The *supplementary motor area* is concerned primarily with bilateral synergistic movements. The *premotor area*, the cortical *extrapyramidal* center, is involved in the development of motor skills, and its fibers are linked to the cerebellum via thalamic nuclei.

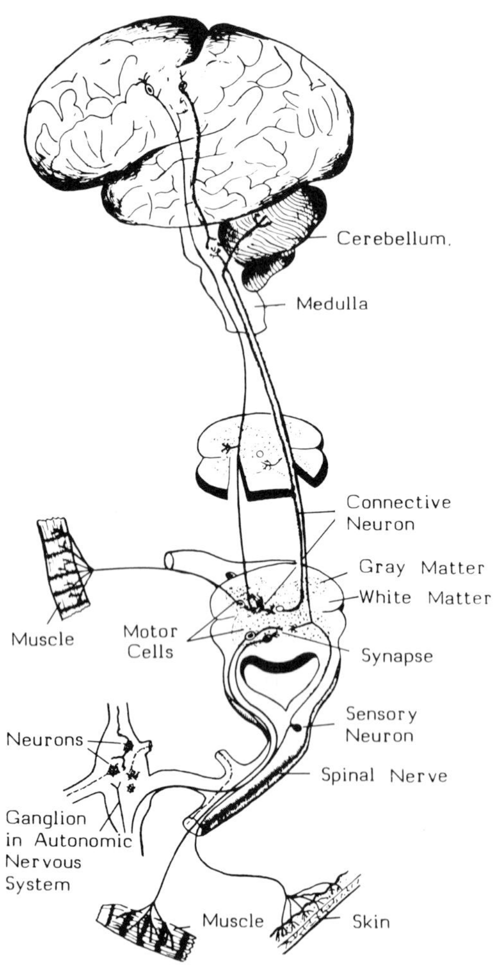

Figure 3.41. Schematic showing sensory and motor circuits of the brain and spinal cord.

Memory

The vast majority of activity of the nervous system is initiated by stimuli acting on one or more types of receptor end organs that are transmitted into the CNS via spinal and cranial nerves. This sensory experience may or may not initiate a motor response (eg, muscular or glandular activity). Because of the vast number of sensory receptors of the body and because of the multitude of stimuli to which it is exposed to each second, Guyton states that more than 99% of all sensory information entering the CNS is discarded by the brain as being irrelevant and unimportant. Much of this selective filtering process is conducted at the synapses.

Whether a motor response to sensory impulses is initiated or not, the memory of the experience may be stored (from seconds to years) within the nervous system (primarily by facilitation at the supratentorial level) and be used to modify (±) similar experiences that might occur in the future. Without such sensory input and its memory, the conscious being would have no communication with or knowledge of its environment, have no capacity to learn and adapt, or be unable to draw attention to or away from specific impressions.

Just as there are certain tensions, mechanical vibrations (sounds, pressure waves), electromagnetic wavelengths, smells, and tastes that are above and below conscious perception, it can be postulated that many events occur within the external and internal environment to which the brain at either conscious or unconscious levels is unaware because there are no receptors that are sensitive to the type or level of stimuli produced.

Cortical Hemispheric Dominance

It can be said that the brain has three levels corresponding to its evolutionary ancestry: (1) the brain stem from the reptilian period, (2) the limbic system from the mammalian level plus the cerebellum added to the brain stem, and (3) the higher cortex. The later levels are further divided into right and left hemispheres, and the whole brain has certain preferred communication paths. The brain stem is linked through the limbic levels to the cortex, and there are massive communication links between the two halves of the cortex.

The structurally ideal biped would be ambidextrous, but most people present with a hemispheric dominance as expressed, for example, in right- or left-handedness, as well as in a dominant eye, ear, and foot. About 90% of the population has a genetically dominant right side that becomes firmly established about the age of 8 years. Attempts in maturity to acquire balanced bilateral motor activity interferes with one's normal speed, rhythm, and endurance.

Primary consciousness resides in the dominant hemisphere, and this side is responsible for such operations as logical thought, time-sequential analysis, categorizing, and speech. The nondominant side is responsible for such abilities as recognizing familiar people, places, and things; understanding maps and other abstractions; appreciating art and music; and perceiving holistic concepts.

Cerebral Asymmetry

While accepting the fact of hemispheric dominance, most people think of the hemispheres of the brain as being symmetrical. They are not. Asymmetries in the occipital lobes and lateral ventricles are correlated with hand preference. Asymmetries in the auditory region and in the Sylvian fissure are present even in the fetus, and it is possible that these differences relate to right-left differences in function and to language lateralization. The studies of Galaburda and associates have led them to believe that anatomical asymmetries help to explain the range of human talents, the recovery from acquired disorders of language function, certain childhood learning disabilities, and some dementing illnesses of middle life.

Brain Waves

The brain constantly emits varying waves of electrical activity. These patterns can be recorded from the outer surface of the head or from the surface of the brain during surgery. The recording process is called *electroencephalography* (EEG). The undulating patterns of brain activity vary in intensity and frequency during various levels of excitation during consciousness and sleep, and certain brain disorders offer characteristic patterns (eg, epilepsy, hypertensive encephalopathy, cerebral embolism or thrombosis, brain tumors or abscesses, etc).

The higher the degree of cerebral activity, the higher the frequency of the wave pattern. For example, during general anesthesia the frequency may be 1 ips, while during a seizure it may be 100 ips or more.

For teaching purposes, certain distinct brain wave patterns have been classified into four transient *levels of consciousness:* alpha, beta, theta, and delta.

Beta Waves

This is the normal level of consciousness in which a person conducts everyday affairs. Typical beta waves have a fast frequency of 14—30 Hz and their greatest intensity is found over the frontal and parietal lobes.

Beta waves are divided into two types: beta I and beta II. Beta I waves disappear during mental activity, thus are inhibited by cortical activity. Beta II waves appear during typical mental activity (eg, tension), thus are excited by cortical activity. During normal daily activities, the patterns constantly shift from beta I to beta II waves as attention to sensory stimuli rises and falls.

Alpha Waves

Alpha waves have a typical frequency of 8—13 Hz. They usually have their greatest intensity in the occipital area, but sometimes they are located over the parietal or frontal lobes. These waves are found in healthy conscious individuals during deep relaxation with the eyes closed but are quickly replaced with low-voltage patterns when the eyes are opened. They are not found during sleep or during conscious sensory impression from the environment (eg, visual, auditory, etc). They are prominent just before entering sleep and before full awakening occurs after sleep.

The alpha level has a typical voltage of 50 μv, but this voltage drops immediately when mental activity is aroused. Alpha waves do not occur in the cortex unless thalamic connections are intact, thus it is thought that they originate from a generalized activity of the thalamocortical system.

The alpha level of consciousness has also been associated with yoga and other forms of prolonged meditation, in which thought processes are stilled and the autonomic nervous system is quieted. It is thought by many that this level, when prolonged, affords the optimal level for creativity, inspiration, intuitive perceptions, and unusual psychic phenomena.

Theta Waves

Theta waves have a frequency of 4—7 Hz and usually have their greatest intensity in the parietal and temporal lobes in children. These levels are recorded in adults during periods of emotional stress (eg, frustration, disappointment) and during certain brain disorders. Theta waves are sometimes found in the parietal and temporal lobes of healthy children and drowsy adults.

Delta Waves

Delta waves, the slowest of brain waves, have a frequency of 3.5—0.33 Hz. They appear to originate from the thalamus and occur during normal deep sleep states, stupor, and general anesthesia; ie, when the cerebral cortex is not being influenced by the reticular activity system. They are also frequently recorded from healthy infants and in severe organic brain disease.

Disorders of Consciousness

Consciousness is the ability of the mind to cognize sensory impulses that are capable of producing physical or mental sensations. It is a function of the combined activity of the cerebral cortex and the ascending reticular activating system (ARAS), thus a product of both supratentorial and posterior fossa activity. If the function of either the cortex or the ARAS become impaired, temporary or permanent consciousness alterations can be expected. Signs may vary from mild sleepiness to deep coma depending upon the site and scope of the lesion.

The *conscious* patient is awake, alert, and oriented in time and space. A *semiconscious* patient responds to painful stimuli but makes no spontaneous movements. An *unconscious* patient is in a condition in which there is no cerebral appreciation of environmental stimuli.

Loss of consciousness may occur gradually or suddenly and may have varying degrees of completeness such as in somnolence, stupor, coma, delirium, and delusion. A patient may also appear dazed, stunned, irritable, irrational, etc. Several disorders of consciousness are briefly described below.

Coma. Coma is an abnormally deep and prolonged state of unconsciousness from which the patient cannot be aroused by even painful stimulation. It is the most severe form of unconsciousness. The patient exhibits absent or depressed pupillary, stretch, and plantar reflexes; a periodic respiratory rhythm and slowed pulse, especially if the lesion is in the brain stem; and little or no spontaneous movement. *Coma vigil* is a severe and grave form of coma in which the patient lies with the eyes open but is entirely unconscious of surroundings. It may be accompanied by a low muttering delirium that is similar to that of a person talking during deep sleep. *Semicoma* is a light state of coma in which the patient is restless (often exhibiting tremors and twitches) and reacts somewhat to painful stimuli.

Concussion. A sudden blow to the head often results in a brief loss of consciousness that is followed by a variable duration of partial amnesia. This loss of consciousness is usually attributed to mechanically altered neuronal function (from stretching or pressure) of neurons critical for consciousness, cerebral ischemia, and/or neuronal hyperpolization or depolarization.

Confusion. A mentally confused individual is often irritable, impatient, angry, and may refuse to talk or cooperate. The ability to think clearly and respond quickly is impaired. The patient is alert but disoriented and excited, presenting some coherent conversation. The disorientation to environment and resulting excitement, which are not in keeping with the total situation, may be temporary and have a psychologic basis in addition to or rather than organic injury.

Convulsions. A convulsion is a series of transient involuntary muscle contractions and relaxations involving the voluntary muscles of a major portion of the body. Convulsive seizures are sudden and violent, and they may vary in intensity from a momentary lapse in consciousness (petit mal) to prolonged violent convulsions (grand mal). Generalized seizures are commonly associated with a loss of consciousness; focal seizures are usually not. Several authorities place some abnormal sensations (eg, paresthesias, hallucinations, and overt behavioral disturbances) under the category of "seizures."

Delirium. Delirium is a state of mental unrest, usually of short duration, which often follows unconsciousness. It often features incoherent speech, delusions, illusions, hallucinations, restlessness, excitement, and sensory perversions—a profound agitated state of confusion.

Delusions, Illusions, and Hallucinations. These states should be differentiated. A *delusion* is an absurd and unfounded belief. An *illusion* is a false interpretation of sensory impressions received from objects that really exist. An *hallucination* is a sense perception without a physical basis. Any or all of these disturbances of consciousness may be found in the insanities, profound neuroses, or typhoid states.

Dizziness. Dizziness, a disturbed subjective relationship with space, is a sensation of whirling, unsteadiness, or being subjected to a tendency to fall. Sometimes a feeling of movement within the head is experienced. It may be a mild form of vertigo or a state of impending syncope, from which it should be differentiated. Dizziness is sometimes caused by simple anxious overbreathing that reduces blood CO_2, which in turn inhibits the metabolism of the balancing center.

Faintness. Faintness, a mild form of syncope, is a sensation of weakness and impending loss of consciousness.

Irrationality. This state, which usually precedes delirium, is characterized by loquaciousness and belligerence. Blunt forehead trauma may be sufficient to injure the frontal lobes of the brain and cause marked behavioral changes, irritability, and seizures (rare).

Stupor. Stupor is a decided loss of consciousness into which the patient may pass and from which he can be aroused only by extraordinary means. It is a borderline state from which a patient may sink into coma or enter when recovering from coma. In stupor, few sensible answers are obtained but the patient might respond to simple forceful commands.

Syncope. Syncope is a brief faint, a transient loss of consciousness. It is usually the result of a generalized cerebral ischemia, for whatever reason. Typical causes include factors producing a reduced pulse, a reduced cardiac output, or pooling of the blood in the periphery. Syncope is usually preceded by *faintness,* which is characterized by a sensation of weakness, giddiness, light-headedness, blurred vision, and impending loss of consciousness. Pallor, a weak pulse, hypotension, and cool perspiration are generally associated.

Transient Ischemic Attacks (TIAs). Transient disorientation, weakness, dysarthria, and numbness result from insufficiency of the carotid artery or one of its branches. These attacks usually precede a major cerebrovascular accident.

Vertigo. Vertigo is not a synonym of dizziness (spatial disorientation), but it is closely related. Vertigo is a hallucination sensation of turning or rotating either of the self (subjective) or the surroundings (objective). The cause of vertigo is usually a disturbance in the equilibratory apparatus—anywhere from the middle ear (semicircular canals, labyrinthitis) to the brain stem through cranial nerve VIII.

THE CEREBROSPINAL FLUID SYSTEM

Functional Anatomy: An Overview

The brain and spinal cord are suspended in cerebrospinal fluid (CSF) that fills the surrounding subarachnoid space. The four ventricles are also filled with this clear watery liquid. The system is constantly being renewed by production and reabsorption equalling a total replacement every 8 hours. Most of the fluid originates from the choroid plexuses of the ventricle walls (Fig. 3.42).

In its superior aspect, there is movement of fluid from the ventricles into the subarachnoid spaces where it is absorbed by cerebral veins. In its inferior aspect, spinal fluid fills the sleeve-like tubular extension of the subarachnoid space around the spinal cord to about S2, far below the end of the spinal cord. Although this sleeve ends as a blind pocket, the exchange of spinal fluid is enhanced by a slow mixing process induced by postural changes. Some authorities believe that this is important from a clinical viewpoint because biomechanical spinal and cranial disorders may interfere with normal spinal dynamics that can result in CSF stagnancy.

Clinical Considerations

Effects of Flow Impairment

Impairment to normal cerebrospinal fluid (CSF) circulation results in ventricular backup, leading to an increase in intracranial pressure. Severe facial or skull trauma, edema, meningitis, brain mass, or anything that will cause blockage along the passageways will produce fluid accumulation in the system resulting in a degree of hydrocephalus. In a few days or weeks, increased pressure inside the sleeve of the dura surrounding the optic nerve may cause the retinal veins to dilate and the pale pink optic nerve head to exhibit papilledema and a choked disc.

Brain tumor compressing part of the ventricular system is the most common cause of papilledema, associated commonly with headaches (dura mater stretching) and vomiting (a parasympathetic center reflex).

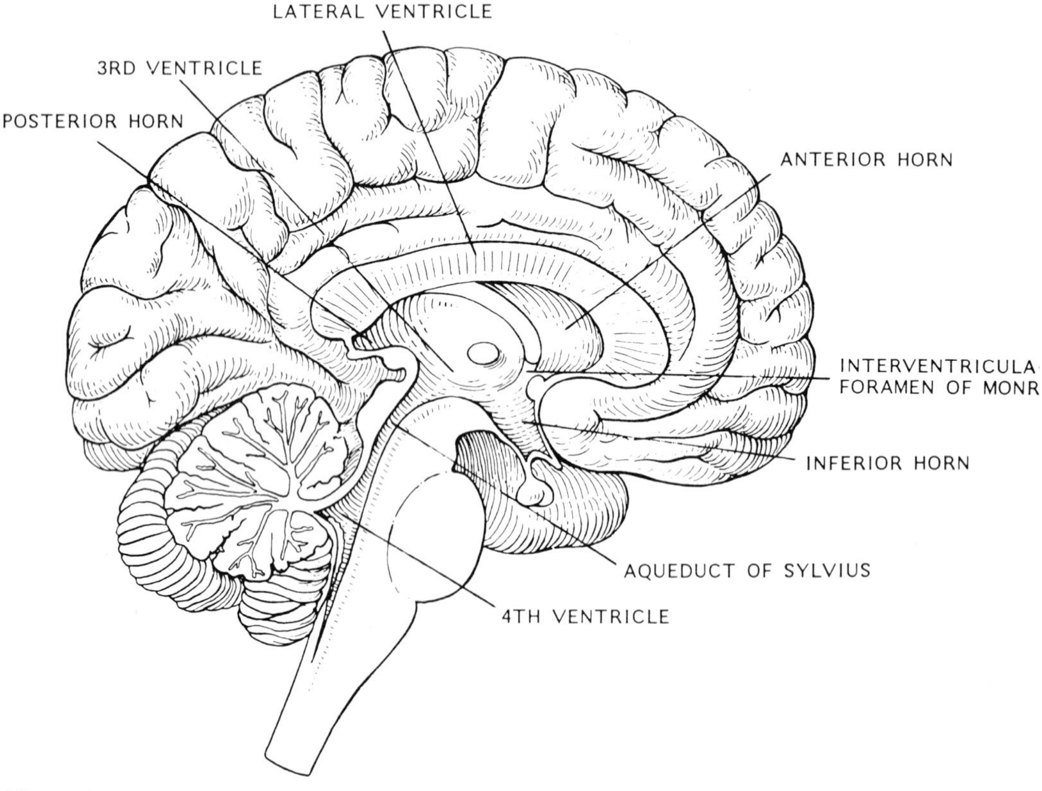

Figure 3.42. Major parts of the cranial ventricular system.

Meningitis, trauma, or anything that will cause blockage along the passageways will produce fluid accumulation in the system resulting in some degree of hydrocephalus. The features of increased intracranial pressure have been previously described in this chapter relative to vascular system disorders.

The Dynamic Craniosacral System

Although cranial sutures are immovable in cadavers and dried skulls, they are minutely movable in the living body, although it is often taught that they are not. The uniting and intervening layers between the edges of adjacent bones in the skull offer a strong bond of union yet one that permits definite but limited movement. It is thought by many that this movement is necessary for tissue respiration of the brain and spinal cord. It is controlled by the following structures and motions: (1) the inherent motility of the brain and spinal cord, (2) the fluctuations of the cerebrospinal fluid, (3) the mobility of the intracranial and intraspinal membranes, (4) the articular mobility of the cranial bones, and (5) the involuntary mobility of the sacrum between the ilia.

Involuntary Cranial Motion. Upledger and other osteopathic researchers have conducted numerous studies of craniosacral motion, its causes, and the results of impairment in the system. They explain that every organ in the body exhibits a pulsation or inherent rhythmic action that features a slow, worm-like movement. The brain and spinal cord are no exception to this: manifesting a slow, rhythmic coiling and uncoiling of the hemispheres and a longitudinal movement of the spinal cord within the spinal dura. This combined motility of the central nervous system and movement of CSF manifest as a hydrodynamic "pump" and a bioelectric interchange. Upon light palpation of the cranium, this pulsation can be felt to have a rate of about 10—14 cycles/min. It is the result of the pull of the dural membranes, the fluctuating CSF, and the inherent motility of the CNS. The sphenobasilar symphysis appears to be the key cranial articulation. Prior to 25 years of age, it has a cartilaginous union; after 25, it has the resiliency of cancellous bone.

Flexion of both the sphenoid and occiput increases the dorsal convexity of the skull and results in elevation of the sphenobasilar symphysis towards the vertex. Extension does the reverse. In other words, flexion of the midline bones appears as a slight increase in convexity; extension, a slight decrease in convexity; ie, the occiput, sphenoid, ethmoid, and vomer. The paired temporals, parietals, and maxillae move in synchronized internal and external rotation with the midline bones. Fixation resulting in impaired reciprocal motion of these bones is the basic hypothesis of cranial therapy in osteopathy and chiropractic.

Associated Involuntary Extracranial Motion. In addition to normal voluntary and postural motions of the sacral between the ilia, the sacrum responds to the inherent motility of the central nervous system, fluctuation of the CSF, and pull of the intracranial and intraspinal membranes in a similar fashion as do the cranial bones. Upon light palpation, it is felt as a slight rocking synchronized with cranial motion. Since all voluntary and involuntary systems are encased in fascial envelopes connected directly or indirectly to the base of the skull through the cervical, thoracic, abdominal, pelvic, and appendicular fascial connections, all organs are subjected to this rhythm in addition to the rhythms of their particular voluntary or involuntary activity throughout life.

Several authorities state that dysfunction of inherent craniospinal motion is noted in almost every case of temporomandibular joint (TMJ) pain and dysfunction, thus the wide range of effects from this disturbance—from cranial nerve impairments to lower extremity disorders. Likewise, the spine, pelvis, and extremities also affect the head and TMJ via the temporals because of the dural strap connecting the sacrum to the cervical spine and occiput.

Bibliography

Adrian ED: Sensory mechanisms: Introduction. In Field J, Magoun HW (eds): *Handbook of Physiology*. Washington, DC, American Physiological Society, vol 1, 1959.

Anderson KV: Endogenous opioid peptides and the control of pain. In Brena SF, Chapman SL (eds): *Management of Patients with Chronic Pain.* New York, Spectrum, 1983, pp 33-46.

Arbuckle BE: Reflexes. *Journal of the American Osteopathic Association*, 46(7), July 12, 1946.

Balduc HA: Overview of contemporary chiropractic science for the Chiropractic Association of Oklahoma. Northwestern College of Chiropractic, Convention notes, April 24, 1983.

Beck JW (ed): *The Management of Pain.* Amsterdam, Elsevier, 1979, pp 306-316.

Berthold CH: Morphology of normal peripheral axons. In Waxman SG (ed): *Physiology and Pathobiology of Axons.* New York, Raven Press, 1978.

Bishop B: Pain: Its physiology and rationale for management. Part I, neuroanatomical substrate of pain. *Physical Therapy*, 60:13-23, 1980; Part II, analgesia systems of the CNS, 60:21-23, 1980.

Black RG: The chronic pain syndrome. *Surgical Clinics of North America*, 55:999-1011, 1975.

Blacker HM: Evaluating sensory and motor systems. *Patient Care*, 17(16):121-136, 1983.

Bonica JJ: Neurophysiologic and pathologic aspects of acute and chronic pain. *Archives of Surgery*, 112: 750-761, 1977.

Brazier MAB: *Electrical Activity of the Nervous System*, ed 4. Baltimore, Williams & Wilkins, 1977, pp 1-12.

Brena SF, Chapman SL: Chronic pain: Physiology, diagnosis, management. In Leek JC, Gershwin ME, Fowler WM Jr: *Principles of Physical Medicine and Rehabilitation in the Musculoskeletal Diseases.* Orlando, FL, Grune & Stratton, 1986, pp 189-216.

Bullock TH: The neuron doctrine and electrophysiology. *Science*, 129:17, 1959.

Burke DC, Murray DD: *Handbook of Spinal Cord Medicine.* Toronto, MacMillan of Canada, 1975, pp 65-70.

Cailliet R: Disuse syndrome: fibrositic and degenerative changes. In Brena SF, Chapman SL (eds): *Management of Patients with Chronic Pain.* New York, Spectrum Publications, 1983, pp 63-71.

Calbe DB, Eisler T: The pathogenesis and medical treatment of extrapyramidal disease. *Medical Clinics of North America*, 63:715-727, 1979.

Cervero F: Deep and visceral pain. In Kosterlitz HW, Terenius LY (eds): *Pain and Society.* Weinheim, Verlag Chemic, 1980, pp 263-282.

Chusid JG: *Correlative Neuroanatomy & Functional Neurology*, ed 19. Los Altos, CA, Lange Medical, 1985, pp 19-37, 66-80, 162-243, 254-257, 269-278, 338-352, 448-470.

Clark WC, Hunt HF: Pain. In Downey J, Darling R (eds): *Physiological Basis of Rehabilitation Medicine.* Philadelphia, W.B. Saunders, 1971, pp 373-401.

Coggeshall RE, Ito H: Sensory fibers in ventral roots L7 and S1 in the cat. *Journal of Physiology*, 267:215, 1977.

Conforti MF: The mind as in a computer. *Occupational Nursing*, 18(12), December 1970.

Coote JH, et al: Reflex discharges into thoracic white rami elicited by somatic and visceral afferent excitation. *Journal of Physiology*, 202:141-159, 1969.

Crue BB, et al: Neurophysiology of pain—peripheral aspects. *Bulletin of the Los Angeles Neurological Society*, 41(1):13-42, 1976.

Curtis DR, Eccles JC: Synaptic action during and after repetitive stimulation. *Journal of Physiology* (British), 150:374, 1960.

Daube JR, Sandok BA: *Medical Neurosciences.* Boston, Little, Brown, 1978, pp 92-111, 114-133, 138-153, 156-191, 194-227, 230-257.

Davis NJ, Kovac MP: The command neuron and the organization of movement. *TINS*, 4(3):73-76, 1981.

DeBacher G: Biofeedback in spasticity. In Basmajian JV (ed): *Biofeedback: Principles and Practice for Clinicians.* Baltimore, Williams & Wilkins, 1979, p 61.

Ditmar E: Cutaneo-visceral neural pathways. *Journal of Physical Medicine* (British), 15:208, 1952.

Eisen A, Hoirch M: The electrodiagnosis evaluation of spinal root lesions. *Spine*, 8(1):98-106, 1983.

Fitz-Ritson D: The anatomy and physiology of the muscle spindle, and its role in posture and movement. *Journal of the Canadian Chiropractic Association*, 26(4): 144-150, 1982.

Fowler WM Jr, Taylor RG: Differential diagnosis of muscle disease. In D'Ambrosia RD: *Musculoskeletal Disorders: Regional Examination and Differential Diagnosis.* Philadelphia, J.B. Lippincott, 1977, pp 93-95.

Freedman BG: The biodynamical aspect of cerebrospinal fluid in disease and health. *Journal of Manipulative and Physiological Therapeutics*, 2:79-84, 1979.

Galaburda AM, LeMay M, Kemper TL, Geschwind N: Right—left asymmetries in the brain. *Science*, 199: 852-856, 1978.

Gandhavadi B, et al: Autonomic pain: Features and methods of assessment. *Postgraduate Medicine*, 7(1):85-90, 1982.

Goodman CE: Pathophysiology of pain. *Archives of Internal Medicine*, 143:527, 1983.

Guyton AC: *Medical Physiology*, ed 4. Philadelphia, W.B. Saunders, 1971, p 557.

Guyton AC: *Textbook of Medical Physiology*, ed 6. Philadelphia, W.B. Saunders, 1981, pp 560-564, 671-677, 679-682, 684-698, 710-718.

Haldeman S: The electrodiagnostic evaluation of nerve root function. *Spine*, 9(1):42-48, 1984.

Haldeman S: Interactions between the somatic and visceral nervous systems. *ACA Journal of Chiropractic*, V:57-64, August 1971.

Haldeman S: Neurophysiological concept of importance to chiropractors. *Journal of the Canadian Chiropractic Association*, 18(3):6, 1974.

Hart FD (ed): *The Treatment of Chronic Pain.* Philadelphia, F.A. Davis, 1974, pp 1, 4, 8, 15, 64, 113.

Hibbard D: Effects of manipulation on gait muscle activity: Preliminary EMG research. *ACA Journal of Chiropractic*, 20(10):49-52, 1983.

Hirschy LD: Utilization of TENS in conjunction with chiropractic methodology in the treatment of acute and chronic pain. *Ortho-Briefs*, ACA Council on Orthopedics, pp 23-29, April 1984.

Howard IP, Anstis T: Muscular and joint-receptor components in postural persistence. *Journal of Experimental Psychology*, 103(1):167-170, 1974.

Huskisson EC: Measurement of pain. *Journal of Rheumatology*, 9(5):768-769, 1982.

Igneizi RJ, et al: Pain and its modulation. *Neurosurgery,* 6(5):577-590, 1980.

Inman VT, Saunders JB: Referred pain from skeletal structures. *Journal of Nervous and Mental Disease,* 99:660-667, 1944.

Janda V: Muscle and joint correlations. In Lewis K, Gutmann G (ed): *Rehabilitácia, Proceedings of the IVth Congress Prague International Federation of Manual Medicine,* Supplement 10-11:154-157, 1975.

Janse J: A concept: The neurological element as it relates to clinical chiropractic. *The Chirogram,* December 1975.

Janse J: The integrative purpose and function of the nervous system: A review of classical literature. *Journal of Manipulative and Physiological Therapeutics,* 1(3), September 1978.

Janse J: *Principles and Practice of Chiropractic.* Lombard, IL, National College of Chiropractic, 1976, pp 243-250.

Jaskoviak PA, Schafer RC: *Applied Physiotherapy: Practical Applications Within Clinical Chiropractic.* Arlington, VA, American Chiropractic Association, 1986, pp 15-44.

Jewett DL, Rayner MD: *Basic Concepts of Neuronal Function.* Boston, Little, Brown, 1983.

Kandel ER: Small systems of neurons. *Scientific American,* 24(3):66, 1979.

Karvinen E, Komi PV: Neuromuscular performance. In Larson LA (ed): *Fitness, Health, and Work Capacity.* New York, MacMillan, 1974, pp 73-78, 81-86.

Keegan JJ, Garrett FD: The segmental distribution of the cutaneous nerves in the limbs of man. *Anatomical Record,* 102:409-439, 1948.

Kellgren JH: Observations on referred pain arising from muscle. *Clinical Science,* 3:175, 1938.

Kellgren JH: On the distribution of pain arising from deep somatic structures with charts of segmental pain areas. *Clinical Science,* 4:35-46, 1939.

Kellgren JH, Samuel EP: The sensitivity and innervation of the articular capsule. *Journal of Bone & Joint Surgery,* 32(B):84-92, 1950.

Kessler RM, Hertling D (eds): *Management of Common Musculoskeletal Disorders.* Philadelphia, Harper & Row, 1983, pp 27-30, 91-98.

Kimber DC, Gray CE, Stackpole CE: *Textbook of Anatomy and Physiology,* ed 11. New York, MacMillan, pp 194-197, 250-260.

Korr IM: The spinal cord as organizer of disease processes: Some preliminary perspectives. *Journal of the American Osteopathic Association,* September 1976.

Krupp MA, Tierney LM Jr, Jawetz E, Roe RL, Camargo CA: *Physician's Handbook,* ed 21. Los Altos, CA, Lange Medical, 1985, pp 34-53.

Kuntz A: Anatomic and physiologic properties of cutaneo-visceral vasomotor reflex arcs. *Journal of Neurophysiology,* 8:421-429, 1943.

Lamb DW: The neurology of spinal pain. *Physical Therapy,* 59:971-973, 1979.

Laporte Y, Emonet-Denand F, Jami L: The skeletal-fusimotor or beta-innervation of mammalian muscle spindles. *TINS,* 4(4):97-99, 1981.

Lassen NA, Ingvar DH, Skinhoj E: Brain function and blood flow. *Scientific American,* 239(4):62-71, 1978.

Laufenberg PC: New dimensions in neurologic evaluation. *The Digest of Chiropractic Economics,* pp 10-12, 105-106, May/June 1979.

Leavitt F, Garron DC, Whisler WW, Sheinkop MB: Affective and sensory dimensions of back pain. *Pain,* 4:273-281, 1978.

Lewis T, Pochin EE: Effects of asphyxia and pressure on sensory nerves of man. *Clinical Science,* 3:141-155, 1938.

Lewis T: Suggestions relating to the study of somatic pain. *British Medical Journal,* 1:321-327, 1938.

Lynch MK, Kessler RM: Pain. In Kessler RM, Hertling D (eds): *Management of Common Musculoskeletal Disorders.* Philadelphia, Harper & Row, 1983, pp 51-72.

MacDonald ML, Stanish WD: Neuromuscular system. In Scott WN, Nisonson B, Nicholas JA: *Principles of Sports Medicine.* Baltimore, Williams & Wilkins, 1984, pp 15-24.

McKenzie RA: *The Lumbar Spine.* Upper Hutt, New Zealand, Spinal Publications Ltd, 1981, pp 9-14.

McNaught AB, Callander R: *Illustrated Physiology,* ed 4. New York, Churchill Livingstone, 1983, pp 220, 246-256, 260, 264-265, 268-270.

Melzack R, et al: Neurophysiological foundations of pain. In Sternbach RA (ed): *The Psychology of Pain.* New York, Raven Press, 1978, pp 1-26.

Melzack R, Wall PD: On the nature of cutaneous sensory mechanisms. *Brain,* 85:331-356, 1962.

Merskey H, et al: The lateralization of pain. *Pain,* 7:271-280, 1979.

Newton RA: Joint receptor contributions to reflexive and kinesthetic responses. *Physical Therapy,* 62(1):22-29, 1982.

Nouwen A, Bush C: The relationship between paraspinal EMG and chronic low back pain. *Pain,* 20(2): 109-123.

Olson WH, Brumback RA, Gascon G, Christoferson LA: *Practical Neurology for the Primary Care Physician.* Springfield, IL, Charles C Thomas, 1981, pp 1-32.

Pastan RS: Diffuse musculoskeletal pain. *Diagnosis,* 5(3):42-46, 1983.

Penfield W, Rasmussen T: The Cerebral Cortex of Man: *A Clinical Study of Localisation of Function.* New York, MacMillan, 1950.

Perl ER: Mode of action of nociceptors. In Hirsch C, et al (eds): *Cervical Pain.* Oxford, England, Pergamon, 1972, pp 157-163.

Phillips RB: The irritable reflex mechanism. *ACA Journal of Chiropractic,* January 1974.

Pinkenburg C: A basis for the theory of manipulative medicine. *Journal of Manipulative and Physiological Therapeutics,* 3(2):81-85, June 1980.

Pomeranz B, Wall PD, Weber WV: Cord cells responding to fine myelinated afferents from viscera, muscle, and skin. *Journal of Physiology* (British), 199:511-532, 1968

Poole PB: Considerations of neurogenic pain. *OrthoBriefs,* Council on Chiropractic Orthopedics of the American Chiropractic Association, Fall 1982.

Pottenger FM: *Symptoms of Visceral Disease,* ed 6. St.

Louis, C.V. Mosby, 1944, pp 183, 187, 189, 266.

Prichard JW: Nerve. In Albright JA, Brand RA (eds): *The Scientific Basis of Orthopaedics.* New York, Appleton-Century-Crofts, 1979, pp 399-405, 408-412.

Rosse C: Muscle action and its control. In Rosse C, Clawson DK (eds): *The Musculoskeletal System in Health & Disease.* Hagerstown, PA, Harper & Row, 1980, pp 64-65, 70-75.

Rossi F: The fine innervation of the articular capsule. *Acta Anatomy,* 10:161-232, 1950.

Rozeiu AM: Clinical decisions: A normative approach. *Journal of the Canadian Chiropractic Association,* 26:102-106, 1982.

Sato A, Kaufman A, Koizumi K, Brooks C: Afferent nerve groups and sympathetic reflex pathways. *Brain Research,* 14:575-587, 1969.

Schafer RC: *Clinical Biomechanics: Musculoskeletal Actions and Reactions.* Baltimore, Williams & Wilkins, 1983, pp 137, 154-156, 221-223, 233, 240-243, 247-249, 397-401, 405-408, 427-428.

Schafer RC: *Physical Diagnosis: Procedures and Methodology in Chiropractic Practice.* Prepublication manuscript, chapters 4 (Clinical interpretation of pain) and 7 (Basic neurologic considerations). Arlington, VA, American Chiropractic Association, 1988.

Schafer RC: *Symptomatology and Differential Diagnosis.* Arlington, VA, American Chiropractic Association, 1986, pp 8-9, 203-219.

Searles RP, Maldinich EK, Messner RP: Isolated trigeminal sensory neuropathy: early manipulation of mixed connective tissue disease. *Neurology,* 28: 1286-1289, 1978.

Shepherd GM: Microcircuits in the nervous system. *Scientific American,* 238(2): 92, 1978.

Sinclair DC, Weddell G, Feindel WH: Referred pain and associated phenomena. *Brain,* 7:184-211, 1948.

Skully RL: The nervous system and its disorders. *The Texas Chiropractor,* March 1975.

Stoner F: *The Eclectic Approach in Chiropractic.* Las Vegas, FLS Publishing, 1975, pp 341-342.

Sutton DC, Lueth HC: Pain. *AMA Archives of Internal Medicine,* 45:827, 1930.

Terrett ACJ, Vernon H: Manipulation and pain tolerance: A controlled study of the effect of spinal manipulation on paraspinal cutaneous pain tolerance levels. *American Journal of Physical Medicine,* 63(5):217-224.

Thomas AH: The anatomy, physiology, and psychology of pain. *Journal of Occupational Medicine,* 7:526-534, 1965.

Tran TA: Clinical correlations of the pyramidal system. *The Chirogram,* November 1976.

Tran TA: Essentials of the neurological examination: Tests for cerebral function. *The Chirogram,* July 1975.

Tran TA: The motor system: A general look at its components and their clinical correlations. *The Chirogram,* October 1976.

Travell JG, Simons DG: *Myofascial Pain and Dysfunction: The Trigger Point Manual.* Baltimore, Williams & Wilkins, 1983, p 663.

Ufberg SH: Muscular nociception. *ACA Journal of Chiropractic,* 14:93-96, September 1980.

Upledger JE: The relationship of craniosacral examination findings in grade school children with developmental problems. *Journal of the American Osteopathic Association,* 77(9):760-776, 1978.

Upledger JE, Vredevoogd JD: *Craniosacral Therapy,* Seattle, Eastland Press, 1983.

Wall PD: Gate control theory of pain mechanisms: a re-examination and re-statement. *Brain,* 101:1-18, 1978.

Walther DS: *Applied Kinesiology.* Pueblo, CO, Systems DC, 1981, vol 1, pp 121-129.

Wayne KM: Disturbances of the nervous system as related to chiropractic. *Journal of the Canadian Chiropractic Association,* 13(2):20-23, 1969.

Werner JK: Trophic influence of nerves on the development and maintenance of sensory receptors. *American Journal of Physical Medicine,* 53(3):127-142, 1974.

Weiss S, Davis D: The significance of the afferent impulses from the skin in the mechanisms of visceral pain: skin infiltration as a useful therapeutic measure. *American Journal of Medical Science,* 176: 517-536, 1928.

Wiles MR, Diakow P: Chiropractic and visceral disease: A brief survey. *Journal of the Canadian Chiropractic Association,* 26:65-68, 1982.

Williams HG: An anatomical-functional review of selected CNS motor control structures. *The Texas Chiropractor,* April 1977.

Wood KW: Myospasm, myosprain and myalgia. *The Digest of Chiropractic Economics,* pp 126-127, May/June 1985.

Wyke B: Articular neurology and manipulative therapy. In *Aspects of Manipulative Therapy.* Proceedings of Multidisciplinary International Conference on Manipulative Therapy. Melbourne, Lincoln Institute of Health Sciences, Carlton, Victoria, Australia, August 1979, pp 67-72.

Wyke B: Articular neurology: A review. *Physiotherapy,* 38(3):94-99, 1972.

Wyke B: Neurological mechanisms in the experience of pain. *Acupuncture and Electro-Therapeutical Research International Journal,* 4:27-35, 1979.

Zeoli NJ: Anatomical and pathological consideration of the circle of Willis. *Digest of Chiropractic Economics,* 14(3):44-45, 1971.

Chapter 4

The Horizontal Neurologic Levels and Related Clinical Concerns

This chapter describes the basic functional anatomy and clinical considerations of the horizontal aspects of the supratentorial, posterior fossa, spinal, and peripheral levels of the nervous system.

OVERVIEW

The reader should keep in mind that the various aspects of the nervous system as described in this manual (eg, longitudinal and horizontal systems) are only reference guides that are visualizations of a patient's nervous system in the upright position. They can be likened to the lines of longitude and latitude on a globe of the earth. Such systems do not exist physically, but they do serve as excellent mental grid-like tools (viewpoints) during localization and areas in which and from which relationships can be described. For example, although the longitudinal systems take a general vertical course within the spinal column there are numerous alterations and they actually become horizontal when decussating. While the horizontal levels are spatially placed in and extend from the CNS in a general segmental manner, they soon take a widely diffuse course as they project toward their destinations. Thus, references to longitudinal and horizontal levels are just general viewpoints.

It is helpful for study purposes to isolate the body into certain systems, as described above, organize systems into organs, organs into tissues, tissues into cells, and cells into their components. However, we should keep in mind that, physically and functionally, there is only one integrated body—and it is more than the sum of its parts. And even the body cannot be thought of as truly separate from its external environment. Although we may do this for study purposes, it is a limited viewpoint.

The human body is the most intricate and efficient electric instrument in the universe. In a state of perfect health, every organ, tissue, and cell functions in perfect unison, one with another. The primary regulator of such activity lies within the CNS. Its higher component, the brain, is much more than a conglomerate of relay stations. It is a highly evolved data gatherer, data processor (selector and organizer), labeler (identifier), *transformer*, and *transmitter* of energy.

We do not actually "see" with our eyes, "hear" with our ears, "taste" with our tongue, "smell" with our nose, or "feel" with our fingertips. Our specialized receptor organs are only peripheral sensors for visual, sound, liquid, gas, and pressure stimuli by which impulses are sent centrally so that we can be aware of our external environment.

It is primarily within the brain where all types of nerve impulse frequencies are transformed from input frequencies and amplitudes to selected (consciously or unconsciously) output frequencies and amplitudes. It is within the brain where sensations are transformed into musculoskeletal dynamics and where the stimuli from light, sound, heat, touch, thought, and other action potentials are each in their turn transformed into other frequencies, each influencing body function (specifically and holistically) in either a beneficial or destructive manner.

TONE

From a basic perspective, it has been previously described that a nerve is a medium in which energy is expressed in various frequencies and amplitudes and directed by various external, internal, and coordinated cause-and-effect processes. The sum of frequencies and amplitudes of a nerve can be stated in terms of nerve "tone." There are ranges of normal tone, and if these ranges are consistently subnormal or abnormal, the nerve can be said to be acting in an unhealthy manner for the situation at hand; ie, inhibited (blocked, suppressed, raised-threshold) or irritated (overactive, hypersensitive, lowered-threshold).

When nerve tone reflects itself upon an effector organ (eg, muscle, gland, vessel), a subservient body part is said to be expressing a certain tone. Such descriptors as spasticity and flaccidness in reference to muscles, parasympathicotonia and sympathicotonia in reference to the autonomic nervous system, or anxiety and depression in reference to psychologic states are just a few selected labels to describe particular states of overall voluntary muscle, autonomic, and psychic tone. Thus, in this context, the sum tone of the individual can be considered to represent the general health status of the individual.

In capitalized letters on the title page of what is generally believed to be his first book, *Text-Book of the Science, Art and Philosophy of Chiropractic*, D. D. Palmer, the father of the science of chiropractic, stated, "FOUNDED ON TONE." On page 7, he continues, "Life is the expression of tone. In that sentence is the basic principle of chiropractic." He went on to state that "Tone is the normal degree of nerve tension. Tone is expressed in functions by normal elasticity, activity, strength and excitability of the various organs, as observed in a state of health. Consequently, the cause of disease is any variation of tone..."

THE SUPRATENTORIAL LEVEL

The neural structures located above the tentorium cerebelli are those of the supratentorial level (Fig. 4.1), all which are derivatives of the primitive telencephalon and diencephalon. The major systems at this level are the cerebral hemispheres, the diencephalon, the telencephalon, the limbic system, and central portions of the optic and olfactory nerves.

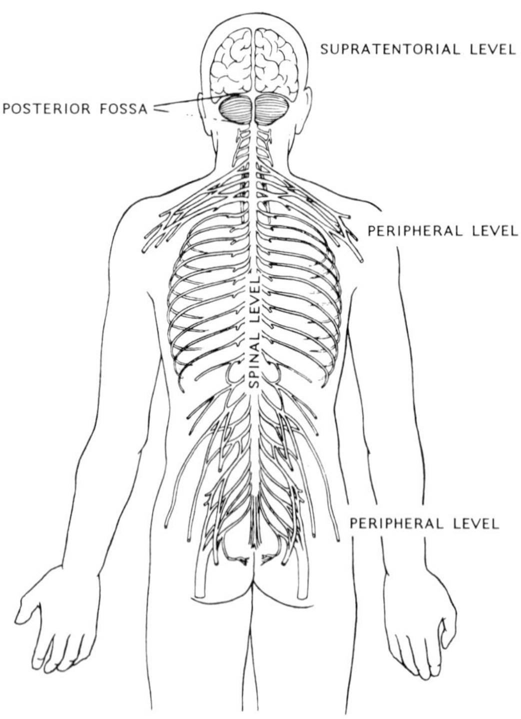

Figure 4.1. The supratentorial and posterior fossa levels of the neuraxis.

The Diencephalon

The structures of the diencephalon, all of which are located between the cerebral hemispheres and the midbrain, surround the 3rd ventricle. The major structures of the diencephalon are the thalamus, hypothalamus, and epithalamus.

The Thalamic Body

The thalamus of each hemisphere is the largest structure in the diencephalon. Its prominent medial portion is called the *pulvinar;* its lateral oval swelling is called the *lateral geniculate body.* The centroposterior aspect of the thalamus is the main body of the thalamus. Its nuclei, arranged in anterior and posterior tiers adjacent to the lateral wall of the 3rd ventricle, serve as relay stations for the several ascending and descending tracts that were described in Chapter 3.

The Anterior Thalamus

That portion of the thalamus which lies between the thalamic body and midbrain is the anterior thalamus. It contains nuclei and passing tracts associated with the control circuits of the basal ganglia and the motor system. The subthalamic nucleus is the major nucleus of the anterior thalamus, and a lesion here produces *hemiballismus.*

The Hypothalamus

The hypothalamus is considered by many to be the central homeostatic core of the autonomic nervous system. It serves as an integrater and regulator of consciousness, defensive emotions (eg, fear, rage), appetitive behavior (eg, hunger, thirst, sex drive), water metabolism, sleep, body temperature, endocrine and cardiovascular functions, and blood osmolality.

The hypothalamus is below and forward to the anterior thalamus and separated from the thalamus by the hypothalamic sulcus. Its major structures are the hypothalamic nuclei in the walls of the 3rd ventricle, tuber cinereum, and mamillary bodies. The hypothalamic nuclei and several tracts are part of the limbic system. Connections are made with all areas of the brain stem and cerebral hemispheres. Although the pituitary gland is not considered part of the hypothalamus, its stalk (infundibulum) attaches to the tuber cinereum. Some authorities consider the optic chiasm as a part of the hypothalamus.

The Epithalamus

The epithalamus lies behind the thalamic body, above the anterior thalamus in the posterior wall of the 3rd ventricle, forming part of the roof of the diencephalon. It contains the posterior commissure and pineal gland. The latter secretes melatonin and endorphin containing hormones. The pineal gland begins to calcify after the age of 20 years. It then can serve as a central landmark, during roentgenography, that may be shifted by a space-occupying lesion.

The Telencephalon

The telencephalon is derived from lateral evagination of the rostral part of the embryonic neural tube. The major structures of the telencephalon are the basal ganglia, the subcortical white matter, and the cerebral cortex. These structures fill the entire cranial vault above the tentorium cerebelli and are separated by the falx cerebri.

The Basal Ganglia

The basal ganglia, which surround the ventricles, are three large masses of gray matter (caudate nucleus, putamen, and globus pallidus) located deep within the cerebral hemispheres, anterolateral to the thalamus (Fig. 4.2). The synaptic complexes of the basal ganglia have important function as a control circuit in regulating muscle tone and motor behavior.

It is within the basal ganglia that many lesions of the extrapyramidal tract occur. Parkinsonism and involuntary movements (eg, athetosis, chorea) are typical examples.

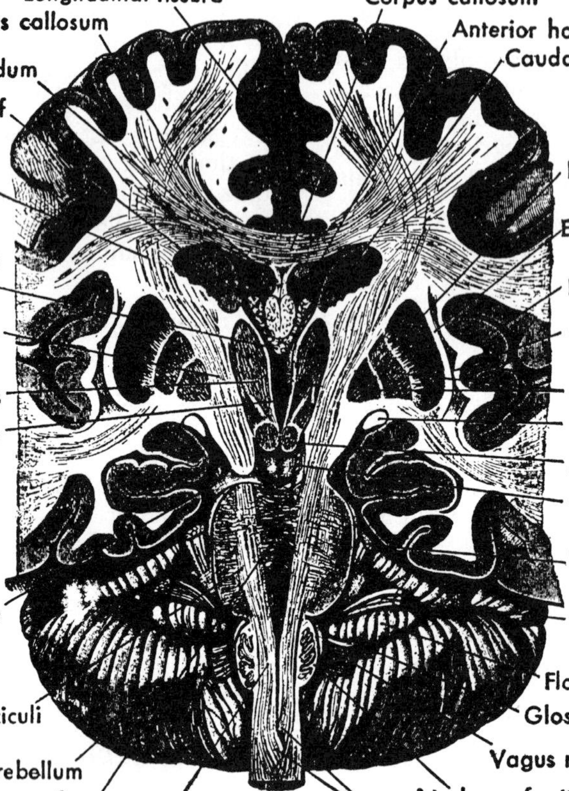

Figure 4.2. Section of the brain showing the basal ganglia, internal capsule, pons, and medulla.

If the internal capsule becomes involved (eg, hemorrhage), contralateral spastic hemiplegia results.

The Subcortical White Matter

The large mass of white matter beneath the cerebral cortex that surrounds the basal ganglia, contains an array of neuroglia and dense unsynapsing myelinated tracts of afferent (corticipetal) and efferent (corticifugal) *projectional neurons* that interplay with cortical neurons and such subcortical structures as the basal ganglia, thalamus, hypothalamus, red nucleus, brain-stem reticular formation, cerebellum, and spinal cord (eg, direct activation pathway). This white matter also contains long and short *association neurons*, which connect ipsilateral hemispheric areas. Short association fibers (eg, subcortical) connect adjacent gyri, while the long fibers connect widely separated areas (eg, the cingulum, fornix, and fasciculi uncinate, arcuate, superior longitudinal, inferior longitudinal, and occipitofrontal).

Numerous transverse *commissural neurons* are also found in the subcortical white matter. They connect homologous areas of the two hemispheres. The largest commissural mass is the broad corpus callosum, which forms the roof of the lateral and 3rd ventricles.

The Cerebral Cortex

The outer neural surface of the five lobes of the brain consists of a relatively thin mantle of gray matter surrounding the subcortical white matter. It has millions of pyramidal and stellate (granule) cell bodies, organized into approximately six laminated layers, and associated vertically and horizontally running axons, dendrites, and blood vessels. Specific functions are shown in Table 4.1. As Guyton points out, we know less about the mechanisms of the cerebral cortex than we do almost all other parts of the brain, though it is by far the largest portion of the nervous system.

The Limbic System

The functionally diverse limbic system includes the limbic lobe of the cerebral cortex, thalamic and hypothalamic areas, and olfactory areas. These structures, arranged in a ring and located deep on the medial surface of the brain, serve to integrate and/or mediate olfaction, behavioral, emotional, memory, and visceral activities. Areas within the frontal lobe (orbital and anterior), medial temporal lobe, and medial parietal lobe are part of the limbic system.

The limbic system as a whole is sometimes referred to as the *visceral brain.* Specific areas within the limbic system have been isolated that play an important role in eating, sleeping, wakefulness states, gastrointestinal and anterior pituitary function, body water regulation, and sexual activities. The limbic system has also been shown to play a role in behavioral modification (reward-punishment reactions) and some modification of pain. However, limbic lesions usually manifest clinically as olfactory, memory, and/or behavioral alterations.

Table 4.1. General Cortical Function of the Lobes of the Brain

Lobe	Primary Function	Lesion Effect
Frontal	Primary motor	Flaccid hyporeflexic paralysis
	Premotor	Spastic hyperreflexic paralysis
	Supplementary motor	Motor seizures (arm elevation with ipsilateral deviation of eyes and head
	Voluntary eye movements	Conjugate deviation of eyes; to opposite side in irritations, ipsilaterally in destructive lesions
	Speech articulation	Speech apraxia
	Prefrontal	Defects in intelligence, memory, emotional control, and motor direction
	Orbital frontal	Visceral and emotional dysfunctions
Limbic	Emotional activity	Personality changes
	Visceral function	Vague vegetative malfunction
Occipital	Vision	Visual impairment
	Visual association	Visual impairment
Parietal	Primary sensory	Sensory deficits
	Sensory association	Graphesthesia, stereognosis, barognosis impairment
Temporal	Auditory	Poor sound localization, discrimination
	Vestibular	Variable equilibrium disturbances
	Language	Variable language defects
	Memory	Variable recall faults

The Olfactory Apparatus

The olfactory nerve is one of two systems solely contained at the cranial peripheral and supratentorial levels. The other is the optic nerve. Both these systems are structured so that they transfer only one type of stimuli. The nose cleans, warms, and humidifies over 500 cubic feet of air every day.

The sensory receptors of cranial nerve I are embedded in the superior nasal mucosa. They are sensitive to gaseous stimuli that are perceived as the sensations of smell. Impulses are conveyed by many small fibers through the cribriform plate to cell bodies in the olfactory bulb, which lies at the anterior aspect of the olfactory sulcus on the orbital surface of the frontal lobe (Fig. 4.3). Upon reaching the bulb, the fibers divide. A medial tract extends to the medial basal portion of the frontal lobe. A lateral tract is projected to the medial portion (piriform) of the temporal lobe, terminating in the uncus (chief olfactory area) and amygdala. From these structures, a network of small links is made with other structures of the limbic system. One example of the complex reflex connections is that it is impossible to sneeze and keep one's eyes open at the same time.

Memory

Memory is a complicated process of labeling, organizing, classifying, storing, retrieving, and transfering acquired and genetic sensory impressions. These sensory impressions may originate extrinsically from the environment or intrinsically by the formulation of images, concepts, and patterns. Although memory is the prerequisite for learning, it is separate from the "thinking" process. This is decidedly demonstrated in various forms of amnesia and agnosia exhibited by otherwise intelligent individuals.

Memory can be divided into several groups such as *visual* memory (descrip-

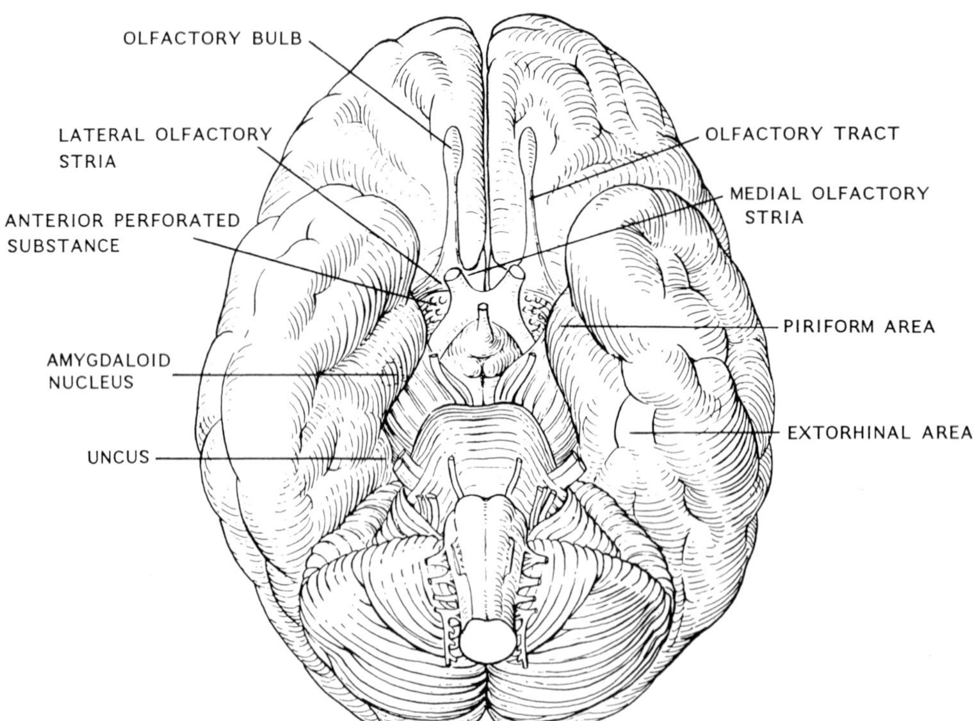

Figure 4.3. The olfactory apparatus.

tions of things out of sight), *gustatory* memory (descriptions of foods not present), *olfactory* memory (descriptions of odors not present), *verbal* memory (description of thoughts spoken previously), and *motor* memory (the repetition of a physical act accomplished previously). Typical examples of inherited memories are instinctive behaviors and the basic urges.

Although some structures are more important for memory than others, there is no isolated area of the brain that regulates the recall of past impressions. Memory stations appear to be dispersed throughout each hemisphere, and data are readily transferred from one hemisphere to the other. Some studies have indicated that areas of the prefrontal cortex store short-term memories and the hippocampus of the temporal lobe stores both complex short-term and long-range memories.

Amnesia

The word *amnesia* refers to the pathologic or physiologic loss of memory. It may be transient or permanent. The two major types are: (1) *Anterograde amnesia*, for events occurring subsequent to the precipitating factor. Some subdivisions are often made; eg, (a) *lacunar amnesia*, a patchy loss of memory for isolated events; and (b) *retroanterograde amnesia*, a situation where past events are referred to the present and vice versa. (2) *Retrograde amnesia*, for events occurring prior to the precipitating factor. Agnosia, astereognosis (tactile memory loss), and certain forms of alexia, agraphia, auditory aphasia (word deafness), and visual aphasia (word blindness), can be considered specific types of amnesia.

Most memory disorders arise within the frontal and temporal lobes. The cause may be gross tissue destruction, a lesion in the association cortex, local cellular changes in the reticular-activating or limbic systems, neurochemical in origin, a RNA synthesis defect, in the neurotransmitters, or in the protein molecules. Infrequently, an obscure low-pressure hydrocephalic condition is involved. It may be subclinical in expression. In overt acute states, fever, headache, nausea, vomiting, and focal signs may be associated.

Orientation

Orientation serves as the foundation for most memory and intellectual processes. Inaccurate knowledge of one's specific orientation with time, place, person, or situation is often reflected in a patient's answers during an interview. It may be exhibited in altered history facts on return visits, the inability to follow simple instructions, the inability to sketch the route taken to the office, the inability to judge the approximate time necessary to conduct a simple task, the inability to judge distances to objects in the environment, etc.

Disorders of the Limbic System

Olfactory Disorders. The patient's sense of smell can be tested with various unlabeled solutions or oils such as cinnamon, peppermint, clove, menthol, vanilla, wintergreen, etc. See Chapter 8.

Memory Alterations. If the patient's level of consciousness and intelligence has been judged adequate, memory can be evaluated for (1) remote events such as childhood residence, employment history, names of siblings, etc; (2) recent events such as current address, telephone number, spouse's age, etc; and (3) immediate recall such as counting seven numbers forward from 57 and counting 5 numbers backward. Memory deficits can occur in any of these three areas. They are most prominent in Alzheimer's dementia, amnesia, encephalitis, lesions of the hippocampus-fornix-mamillary body area, temporal lobe lesions, and the Wernicke-Korsakoff syndrome.

Behavioral Disorders. In every culture, evidence of mental illness has been found in the earliest of civilizations. *Neuroses* are emotional maladaptation problems, characterized by anxiety resulting from some unresolved unconscious conflict(s). They also feature phobic reactions and/or depression. The general term *psychoses* refers to major mental disorders that grossly impair a patient's capability to meet daily demands. They are characterized by regressive behavior, diminished impulse control, delusions and hallucinations, inappropriate moods, schizophrenia, and often violent antisocial behavior. These often complex disorders are the subject of psychologic and psychiatric studies, thus they will only be referred to in this text in passing.

The Visual System

The eyes are remarkable organs. They can perceive more than 1 million simultaneous visual impressions and can discriminate among nearly 8 million graduations of color. Vision accounts for 90% or more of all sensory impressions.

The neural circuits for all direct optic impulses are restricted to the peripheral and supratentorial levels (diencephalon and telencephalon). The ocular muscles are derived from mesoderm; the other nonneural portions of the eye (cornea, sclera, iris, lens, and humors) are derivatives of embryonic ectoderm.

The Peripheral Neural System

The sensory organs of the retina (photoreceptor rods and cones) are the peripheral receptors of the visual system. These receptors are activated by a narrow band of electromagnetic spectrum that is between infrared and ultraviolet wavelengths. The 100-million low-threshold, poorly discriminative, monochromatic rods in each eye are responsible for low-intensity (scotopic) night vision and are found in greatest numbers in the peripheral retina. Rods are absent in the fovea. The higher-threshold, more discriminative, trichromatic cones serve in high-intensity (phototopic) daylight vision, visual discrimination, and color vision. They are found in greatest numbers at the macula.

Central images are projected upon the posterior poles of each eye. Images of the left field of vision are projected on the left nasal and right temporal halves of the two retinas, and vice versa. In addition, the visual image striking the retina is inverted so that the upper portion of the visual field strikes the lower portion of the retina and the lower portion of the visual field is impressed upon the upper aspect of the retina.

A constant image projected upon a specific area of the retina would rapidly lead to receptor adaptation due to the sustained stimulation. Thus, the eyes normally make rapid minute continuous movements (microsaccades) that mistakenly appear as a fixed gaze.

When light rays strike the rods and cones, a breakdown of visual pigments occurs that leads to the set up of receptor potentials. Dendrite impulses are conveyed to peripheral first-order axons (bipolar cells) that synapse with more distal intermediate neurons and then to further distal third-order neurons (ganglion cells). The latter neurons provide the surface of the retina and come into contact with the vitreous humor. The ganglion cells send unmyelinated axons from the peripheral retina to the cup-like optic disc, the axons become myelinated at the disc and then exit the eye as the optic nerve (Fig. 4.4). Ophthalmoscopy will reveal lesions

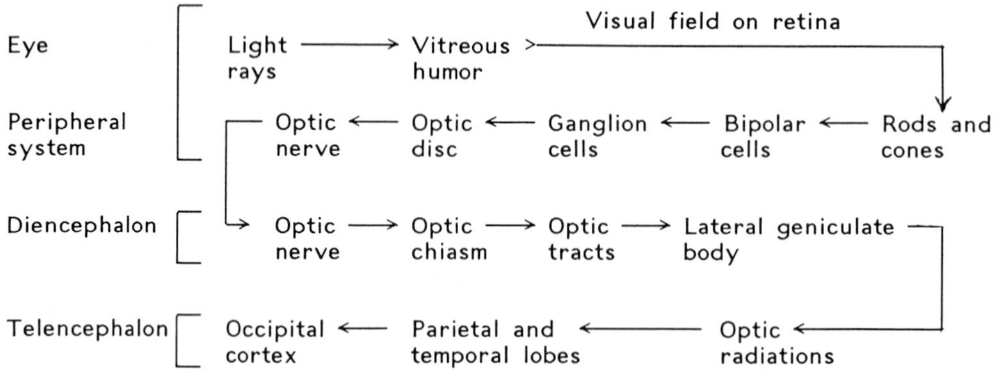

Figure 4.4. Primary course of light stimuli through the optic system.

of the distal optic nerve such as atrophy, neuritis, and papilledema.

The Central Neural System

Proximal to the eye, the major visual structures are located in the diencephalon and telencephalon. The diencephalic structures of the eye include:

1. *Optic nerves.* These tracts of axons extend from each retina, exit through the optic foramen, and unite to form the optic chiasm.

2. *The optic chiasm.* The two optic nerves join at the optic chiasm. The fibers decussate within the chiasm in such an arrangement that the nasal portion from each retina crosses to the opposite side and the temporal portion from each retina remains uncrossed. Thus, lesions in the central chiasm express as binasal hemianopsia; lesions in the lateral portions of the chiasm (rare), manifest as bitemporal hemianopsia.

3. *Optic tracts.* Because of the decussation that occurs in the optic chiasm, fibers from the nasal retina of the left eye join with fibers from right temporal retina to form the right optic tract. Fibers from the nasal retina of the right eye join with fibers from left temporal retina to form the left optic tract (Fig. 4.5). Each optic tract courses posterolaterally and terminates in the respective lateral geniculate body. A few fibers, however, leave the tract before this and are projected to the pretectal area of the brain to form the afferent limb of the *light reflex.*

4. *Lateral geniculate bodies.* Each lateral geniculate body receives the fibers of the optic tract and projects them, following synapse, via the geniculocalcarine tract. In this manner, the entire left visual field is projected to the right hemisphere, and the right visual field is projected to the left hemisphere.

Unilateral lesions of the optic tract, lateral geniculate bodies, or optic radiations mani-

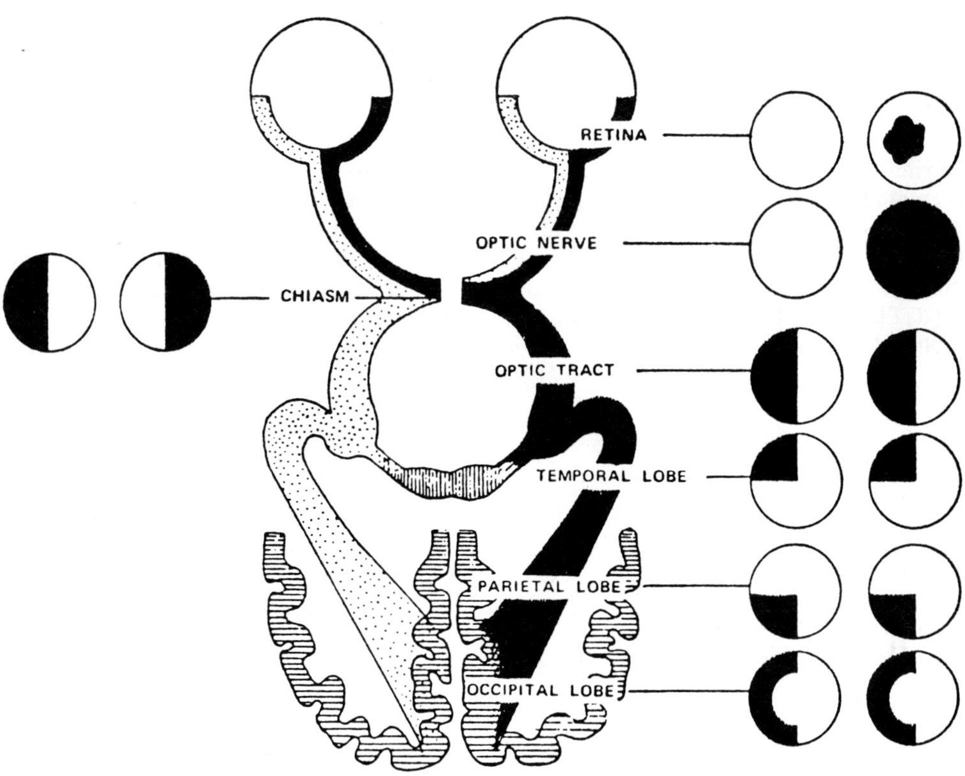

Figure 4.5. Visual field defects produced by lesions at various points along the optic system. Defects in the patient's vision are shown in the circles, representing the perceived visual fields.

fest as homonymous defects in the field of vision of one or both eyes, depending on whether the lesion is partial or complete. Lesions of the optic tract anterior to the optic chiasm produce a defect of vision in only one eye.

The telencephalic structures of the eye include:

1. *Optic radiations.* The fibers of the diencephalic geniculocalcarine tract extend through the retrolenticular aspect of the internal capsule as optic radiations. The posterosuperior fibers of the radiation course the parietal lobe and terminate in the superior calcarine cortex of the occipital lobe. Unilateral parietal lobe lesions produce a contralateral *inferior* quadrant defect. The anteroinferior fibers of the radiation extend around and through the temporal lobe and terminate in the inferior calcarine cortex of the occipital lobe. Unilateral temporal lobe lesions produce a contralateral *superior* quadrant defect.

2. *The occipital cortex.* The inverted image of the visual field on the retina is reproduced in a similar topographic fashion in the calcarine cortex of the contralateral occipital lobe; ie, (a) fibers conducting the lower part of the image terminate in the superior calcarine cortex; (b) fibers conducting central (macular) vision terminate in the posterior aspect of the occipital pole; (c) fibers conducting the upper part of the image terminate in the inferior calcarine cortex; and (d) fibers conducting impulses from the peripheral aspects of the retina terminate in the more anterior portion of the calcarine cortex. It is within the cortex of the occipital lobe that the dual images are integrated into one image.

Fibers originating from the macula are widely distributed in the visual cortex. For this reason, unilateral lesions in the visual cortex will usually spare central vision. Visual hallucinations are commonly reported by patients with visual cortex dysfunction.

Communicating axons from the calcarine cortex to the brain stem provide data for unconscious eye motions. Voluntary eye movements and fixation are directed by the eye centers of the frontal lobes of the cerebrum (area 8). Lesions in this area produce conjugate deviations.

Disorders of the Visual System

Impairment of the visual system may be the result of retinal disease or a lesion of the optic nerve, optic chiasm, optic tract, or occipital lobe. Loss of vision often accompanies a fracture through the sphenoid involving the orbital foramen.

Complete blindness of one eye invariably indicates a lesion of an optic nerve. Optic neuritis and tumors compressing an optic nerve are the most common lesions causing loss of the direct light reflex. Lesions of an optic nerve are especially noted with optic atrophy, optic neuritis, papilledema, and visual impairment. Thus, the optic nerves should be tested for visual acuity and fields of vision (refer to Fig. 4.5), and directly inspected by observing the condition of the fundi.

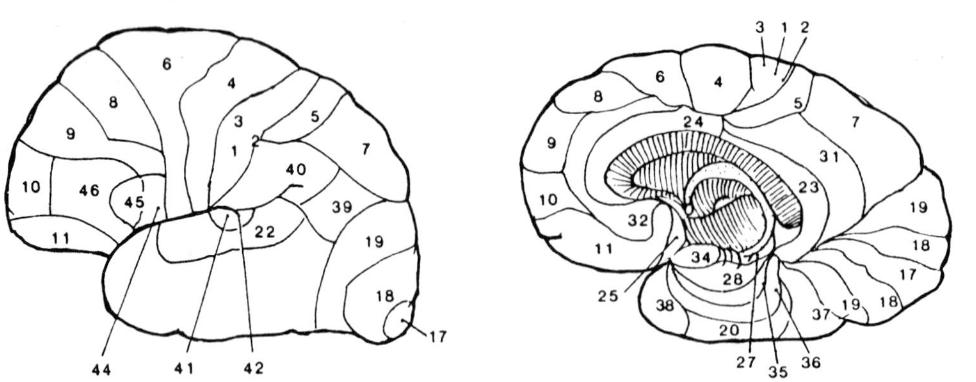

Figure 4.6. Brodmann's numbered areas of the cerebral cortex. *Left,* lateral view; *right,* medial view.

Homewood points out that, as the nasal mucosa, preganglionic fibers from T1—T4 which connect with postganglionic fibers of the superior cervical ganglion project to the dilator pupillae, part of the levator palpebrarum, the orbital Müller muscle, and the arteries of the eyeball and adnexia. Thus, upper cervical and upper thoracic subluxations may cause or encourage a wide number of motor and vasomotor syndromes of the eye. These same fibers, originating from T1—T4 and the superior cervical ganglion, supply many of the same tissues innervated by the oculomotor, trochlear, abducens, auditory, and spinal accessorycranial nerves. For this reason, visual, auditory, and equilibrium disturbances are frequency associated with whiplash injuries of the cervical and upper thoracic spine. Less frequently, but not rarely, vagal and phrenic syndromes may be related.

The Consciousness System

In 1909, Brodmann mapped the cerebral cortex on the basis of cortical cytoarchitectual patterns (Fig. 4.6). He numbered 47 distinctive areas of varying thicknesses. Since then, over 200 specific areas have been isolated, but Brodmann's original areas remain the basic reference (Table 4.2).

The major sensory pathways that provide the CNS with data from its external environment were described in Chapter 3. The highly complex *consciousness system* is another system. Its ascending portion runs parallel with other primary sensory tracts and provides stimuli for sensory discrimination and levels of wakefulness and attention.

Both systems, the primary sensory and the consciousness, terminate in the cerebral cortex, but they take different routes. The primary sensory system courses through specific thalamic nuclei and then extends to the sensory cortex. In contrast, impulses of the consciousness system travel over indirect, polysynaptic, multineuronal routes to nonspecific thalamic nuclei and then extend to all areas of the cerebral cortex.

It must be kept in mind when studying the sensory system that the only thing sensory nerves do is transmit impulse patterns. The consciousness system, however, does not interpret such signals as just impulse signals. The interpretation of receptor stimulation is experienced *subjectively* as feelings of

Table 4.2. Primary Brodmann's Areas

Area	Brodmann's Number
Auditory, association	20, 21, 22, 38
Auditory, primary	41, 42*
Cingulate gyrus	23, 24
Frontal association	9, 10, 11, 12, 46
Limbic	32
Motor, primary	4
Motor, supplementary	6 (premotor, extrapyramidal)
Orbitofrontal	11
Sensory, association	5, 7, 39, 40
Sensory, primary	1, 2, 3
Speech (Wernicke's area)	22
Speech, motor (Broca's area)	44, 45
Visual, association	18, 19
Visual, frontal eye field	8 (eye motion, pupil changes)
Visual, occipital primary	17 (striate cortex)

*Some authorities relate this area with auditory association.

touch, pain, temperature, or movement or as sensations of flavor, smell, sight, or sound. And beyond this, in consciousness, there is some mysterious "something" that witnesses all this and is apart from it. The processes of neural circuitry, convergence, summation, facilitation, inhibition, and divergence explain the "where" and "why" of some phenomena but fall far short of explaining the "what" and "how" of it all.

Anatomical Considerations

The major divisions of the consciousness system are the ascending reticular activating system (ARAS) and the final widespread terminations in the cerebral cortex. The ARAS is an aggragate of neurons that receives and integrates impulses from the sensory system, cerebral cortex, cerebellum, hypothalamus, and brain-stem nuclei and then projects them via modifying nonspecific nuclei of the thalamus to all areas of the cerebral cortex for connection with the sensory, motor, and autonomic systems.

The major structures of the ARAS are:

• *Portions of the brain-stem reticular formation.* The reticular formation (network) consists of complex clusters of diffuse and poorly organized large and small multipolar neurons and associated interneurons located in the central tegmental portion of the brain stem that extend from the decussation of the pyramids in the medulla to the thalamus. The *lateral receptive area* of the reticular formation receives afferent impulses from (1) collaterals from all ascending sensory pathways (eg, spinothalamic and lemniscal tracts); (2) the cerebral cortex (corticoreticular, corticospinal, corticobulbar fibers); (3) visceral afferents originating in the spinal cord and cranial nerves; and (4) the basal ganglia, hypothalamus, cranial nerve nuclei, and cerebellum. See Figure 4.7. The *medial projectional area* of the reticular formation gives rise to many efferent pathways (eg, thalamus, hypothalamus, cerebellum, and the visceral system). See Figure 4.8. With such diverse input and output, the reticular formation serves as a primary integrator, modifier, and regulator for various levels of the neuraxis.

• *The ascending projectional system.* Ascending fibers of the reticular formation are not located in specific tracts. They project diffusely from the brain stem (through the pons, midbrain, and diencephalon) to the hypothalamus and nonspecific nuclei of the thalamus.

• *Nonspecific nuclei of the thalamus.* The nonspecific nuclei of the thalamus are the (1) *reticular*, along the lateral margin of the thalamus; (2) *midline*, near the massa intermedia; and (3) *intralaminar*, along the internal medullary lamina.

• *Diffuse projections from thalamic nonspecific nuclei to the cerebrum.* The ascending thalamocortical reticular activating system offers diffuse projections from the nonspecific nuclei of the thalamus to all areas of the cerebral cortex. These pathways play an important role in modifying levels of

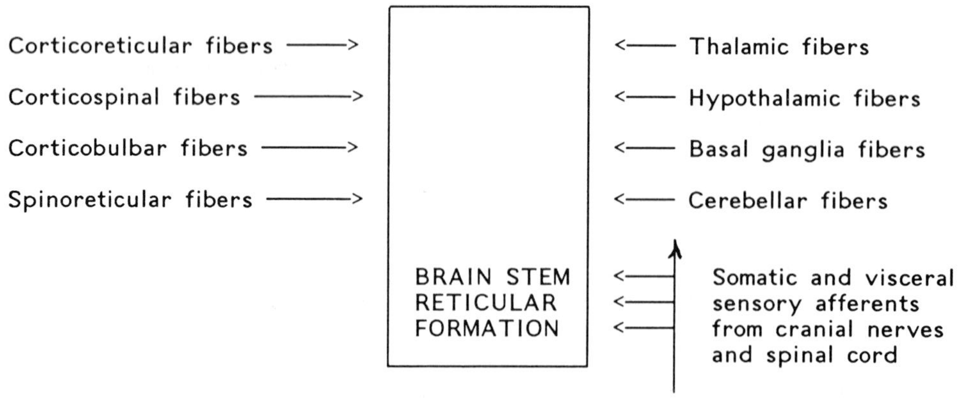

Figure 4.7. Diagramatic representation of input to the brain stem reticular formation.

consciousness and attentiveness by regulating the electrical activity of the cortex. An individual's degree of consciousness is not determined by a single area in the cortex such as seen in the primary sensory and motor systems; rather, consciousness is regulated by the quality and quantity of exciting, inhibiting, and synchronizing thalamocortical impulses to all areas of the cortex.

Physiologic Considerations

Because of their aggregate arrangement and multisynaptic connections, the neurons of the CNS do not function singularly. The electric activity of the cortical aggregates is the summed effect of the cortical action potentials occurring at the time. It is derived from (1) local activity, (2) input from specific thalamic nuclei, and (3) input from nonspecific thalamic nuclei. This summed effect produces an oscillating wave form of electric activity, rather than the simple spikes witnessed in the peripheral nervous system, that can be measured on an EEG.

EEG Tracings. The EEG tracing reflects the summed synaptic potentials of the dendrites lying near the periphery of the cerebral cortex, and the fluctuations represent the varied excitatory and inhibitory synaptic potentials impinging on the dendrites.

The activity of the cerebral cortex is modulated by two forces: (1) other cortical neurons, which play a minor role, and (2) neurons from the thalamus, which play a major role. Synchronizing "pacemaker" impulses from the thalamus determine the intrinsic resting frequencies of brain waves. Low-frequency thalamic impulses produce a synchronized rhythmic high-amplitude EEG wave pattern, while high-frequency impulses produce an opposite effect; ie, a desynchronized arrhythmic low-amplitude EEG wave pattern.

EEG patterns also vary according to which specific thalamic nuclei are stimulated. A rising and falling *recruiting response* is produced when nonspecific midline nuclei are stimulated. Their potentials are widely projected throughout the cerebral cortex. A diphasic *augmenting response* occurs when specific sensory nuclei are activated, and their potentials are projected to a specific sensory area of the cortex.

Consciousness. The faculties of consciousness such as alertness, perception, apperception, attention, memory recall, and the regulation of sleep are the primary responsibilities of the cerebral cortex and its input. These states can be viewed from two aspects: (1) The *degree of wakefulness*, which is the direct effect of emotions and ARAS input, and the indirect effect of corticoreticular, sensory, and motor stimulation. (2) *Content*, which is the product of cognitive mental activity occurring in the cerebral cortex.

Unconsciousness. There are two forms of unconsciousness: pathologic (eg, coma)

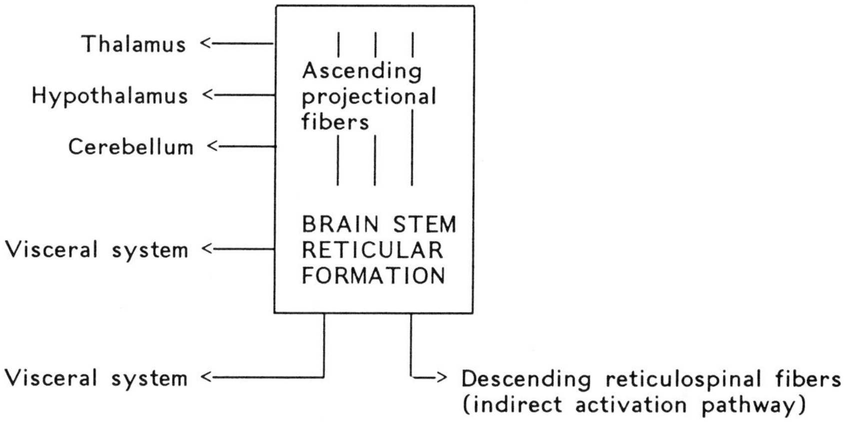

Figure 4.8. Diagramatic representation of output from the brain stem reticular formation.

and physiologic (sleep), and either may be transient or persistent. Transient states of pathologic unconsciousness are commonly associated with syncope, seizures, cranial concussions, and metabolic encephalopathy. The various pathologic states of unconsciousness were described in Chapter 3.

Mental Functions

The three primary attributes of the mind (a functional process) are *thinking* (intellectual thought development), *feeling* (the perception of sensation), and *choosing* (volition, the selection of voluntary action, will). Every mental action has one or more of these attributes as its foundation.

Presentative vs Representative Powers. While witnessing intellectual processes during daily activities, we can become aware that many relate to perceptions brought to conscious awareness by the specialized peripheral sensory receptors (eg, visible light waves striking the retinae, audible sound waves striking the ear drums, etc). It is in this manner that we become aware of objects within our external environment, here and now. When we come upon an animal, we see the animal, hear the animal, and possibly smell the animal. This ability to perceive sensations of objects present is called the *presentative power* of the mind and forms the basis of our conception of environmental reality.

The mind, however, not only receives impressions acting upon the peripheral sensors from external objects as here and now, it also can conceive of them during their absence and represent them to itself by mental images and thought forms. It also can relate one or more objects to other objects and to certain circumstantial actions and feelings. If we had at one time come upon a wild animal and the experience made a strong impression, we can remember how the animal looked, what the associated circumstances were, and how we felt at the time. This ability to perceive sensations of objects absent is called the *representative power* of the mind and forms the basis of simple recall, reflection, and situational memories.

Creativity Powers. Unlike either common presentation and representation of objects and situations experienced, the mind it also capable of imaging objects and situations completely different from any experienced (eg, a horseless carriage, a machine that can fly, a six-headed cow) to meet its fancy and ideals. This creative or inventive form of representative power, which is separate from that derived from sensory impressions, forms the basis of imagination as well as hallucination. With this ability, we can conceive of time, space, cause, effect, beauty, etc. Such conceptions may be suggested by sensed objects, but they are not conveyed to the mind through the senses. This ability is called the *originative (intuitive) power* of the mind.

Classification and Reasoning Powers. The mental functions described above encompass the abilities to present, represent, and create. Another important attribute is the ability to *generalize* and *classify* things, thoughts, and acts. That is, we may perceive certain common qualities, properties, and relations of objects rather that the objects themselves. Through such comparisons, we can group, stereotype, and catalog things such as by their visual impression (eg, color, size), audible impression (sounds), tactile impression (eg, texture, temperature), olfactory impression (smell), taste (eg, salty, bitter, sweet, spicy), proprioception (eg, weight), composition (eg, animal, vegetable, mineral components), function, etc. Such generalizations form the basis of our mental labels, codes, filing systems, and tabulations. They also form the basis of our likes, dislikes, and prejudices.

Rather than classifying certain objects by their like elements, we may reverse the process and analyze (inductively or deductively) the component properties and relations within specific things, thoughts, and acts. While such characteristics are the objects of thought and related primarily to sensible objects, the conceptions are not those presented by the senses. This involves the ability to perceive abstract properties and relationships, and the process is the basis of reasoning. *Reason* can be defined as the logical process of selecting associated ideas into an organized form. Thus, impressions of sense and discursive notions of understanding must be differentiated in order to maintain clear thinking.

Attention

In addition to its state of alertness, the consciousness system is also influenced by its attention toward or away from certain sensory input. That is, by enhancing or suppressing specific impulse transmission, the consciousness system can focus selective attention on the minute details of certain sources and patterns of input and ignore other stimuli. This is commonly seen when an individual is so absorbed in some type of work that various potentially distracting (but not harmful) environmental stimuli are completely blocked from consciousness. This is commonly witnessed when a person is concentrating on reading a book or watching a highly interesting event.

Attention span can be severely shortened by either physical or psychic mechanisms. It is commonly observed that concentrated effort is greatly limited in disorders associated with pain or fever. Likewise, emotional preoccupations can make it impossible to fix attention on a singular subject, regardless of its long-term importance to the individual. This should not be confused with simple habitual procrastination.

The attention span of a patient with an averge IQ or better can be simply tested clinically by the Serial Sevens Subtraction Test (Table 4.3). Patients with severe emotional distress (eg, acute anxiety) or paranoid tendencies frequently become highly threatened by such a test. Milstein and associates point out that patients with organic lesions make a large number of mathematical mistakes, but they rarely get overly disturbed with such errors. These errors are the result of impaired intellectual function and the inability to remember the last number vocalized. Patients with Korsakoff's syndrome, such as seen resulting from the organic brain lesions of chronic alcoholism, habitually give confabulatory responses.

Attention and the Alpha State

While it is generally held that the alpha-brainwave state cannot be obtained with the eyes open (because of the superimpingement of visual stimuli), distinct alpha states have been recorded while subjects are in a state of profound abstraction, meditation, imagery, or reverie (daydreaming) with the eyes open. Such a state may also occur when we become a witness to our own thoughts and actions. Thus, mental processes can be controlled to such an extent that attention can be focused in a one-directional manner to the point where impulses from the periphery will be ignored. This is not an unusual phenomenon. It occurs whenever we become completely engrossed in a book, a movie, or some other event to the degree that we become unconscious of potentially distracting environmental influences. During wartime, it is not unusual for soldiers to report that they were unaware of their wounds until the battle was over.

Such a mental focus or ability to think of one thing at a time is achieved from the faculty of *concentration* (intensified attention). It is the basis of all learning and achievement and is regulated by personal need, desire, sincerity, and motivation. We see this process manifesting constructively by watching a child learning to walk, by watching an adolescent learning to drive a car, or by watching someone master a complicated dance routine. We witness this steady focus by watching a child crippled with poliomyelitis perseveringly mold into an adult Olympic athlete or by watching an individual with meager educational, financial, or social advantages slowly attain to high status—not because of their advantages, but in spite of their handicaps. We also see this process manifesting destructively by watching the circumstantial fruits of the habitual pessimist. Thus, the faculty of *concentration* is a dual-edged sword.

Abstraction

A patient's ability to deal with abstract concepts is often impaired in mental illness of an organic nature. Psychotic patients and schizophrenics tend to become strikingly literal in their interpretation of speech and fail to understand the meaning of commonly used metaphors, proverbs, and other nonliteral expressions of speech. Thus, testing a patient's ability to understand abstractions is often helpful in differentiating the functional neurotic from the organic psychotic.

Thought Content and Association

Thought content may indicate such abnormalities as severe phobias, obsessions, morbid preoccupations, paranoia, or delusions. The patient with forebrain disease will be unemotional, mildly disoriented, and inattentive to personal details.

Thought association reflects the quality of interconnection between a sequence of ideas. When thought association is not orderly, such as speaking in disconnected sentenc-

Table 4.3. Cerebral Function Screening Tests

Function	Test
Attention	Attention span can be tested clinically simply by serial subtraction with a patient with an IQ over that of an average third-grade student. For example, the patient can be asked to begin with the number 100, subtract 7, then subtract 7 from the answer, and continue this process and give a verbal answer until zero nears. An occasional mistake can be attributed to carelessness.
Auditory-verbal comprehension	Watch if the patient carries out instructions or answers your questions correctly and adequately.
Automatic speech	Ask the patient to repeat a short poem or recite one or two familiar series such as the days of the week, months of the year, or counting.
Motor speech	Ask the patient to imitate several different familiar sounds and phrases of increasing difficulty. Note abnormal word usage in conversation.
Performance of skilled motor acts	Ask the patient to perform a complete simple motor act such as drinking from a glass, button a shirt or blouse, close a safety pin, or use common tools such as scissors, hammer.
Recognition of body parts and sideness	Ask the patient if he or she is aware of body parts; see if the patient knows right from left.
Sound recognition	Tell the patient to close the eyes, then recognize and identify similar sounds such as a bell, glassware ring, metallic sound, etc.
Visual object recognition	Ask the patient to identify familiar objects such as a pencil, a tie, a bracelet, or wristwatch.
Visual verbal comprehension	Ask the patient to read a short paragraph from a book and explain its meaning. If the person is mute, the practitioner should print instructions and determine whether the patient can carry them out.
Volitional speech	Does the patient answer questions relevantly?
Writing	Ask the patient to write name and address, a simple sentence, one word with the eyes closed, and then with the eyes open, and finally, the name of an object in the room.

es or offering an answer that is unparallel to a question asked, schizophrenia should be suspected. In schizophrenia and a few other mental syndromes, this inability to associate appears to be the result of impairment of various interrelated neuronal loops in the brain that serve to interconnect thought processes for an orderly sequence of thinking.

Body reactions indicate how completely the individual has entered a situation. Thus, an emotional response is a total measurement of mind, will, and body (including the endocrine system and all its ramifications). An individual's overenthusiastic emotions may alter one's psychic approach to life. Perception is changed, and values are amended. When under the influence of "hot" emotions, life appears different from that which is led by "cool" intelligence. The fading of an emotion is regretted if the associated feeling is pleasurable.

Gross impairment of judgment is characteristic of an organic lesion or severe psychosis. Minor impairments often signal the early stage of an organic lesion. This is often reflected in poor judgment of personal affairs (eg, personal relationships) rather than in nonpersonal affairs (eg, conceptual differentiation). A cursory estimation of a patient's quality of judgment can be obtained by discussing the patient's plans for the future and contingency plans if the ideal outcome is thwarted by some unanticipated obstacle.

Sleep States

When somatic or mental fatigue arises, the level of consciousness tends to decrease into a transient *sleep state.* This is not a passive phenomenon; ie, caused solely by decreased input to the cerebral cortex. Rather, it is a dynamic phenomenon and currently thought to be the result of activation of certain hypnogenic areas of the brain. These areas are believed to produce neurochemicals that actively promote inhibited cerebral activity and suppress the ARAS. Two hypnogenic areas have been isolated. One is located on the anterior aspect of the hypothalamus, and the other is in the upper medullary and lower pontine portion of the reticular formation. Lesions in these two areas will produce a constant state of wakefulness.

A more or less permanent deep sleep state (eg, coma) results if some of the consciousness system becomes impaired. The most frequent site for such a lesion occurs at the midbrain level of the ARAS, especially at the rostral portion of the brain stem and thalamus, above the trigeminal nerve entry zone. Bilateral lesions affecting the ARAS in the diencephalon produce a state of sustained somnolence with diffuse slow-wave EEG activity. A unilateral cortical lesion will not produce unconsciousness if the other hemisphere is functioning, but unconsciousness results if both hemispheres are impaired. A number of abnormal sleep states are defined in Table 4.4.

Sleep Patterns. Two distinct cyclic sleep states have been identified: those exhibiting rapid eye movement (REM) and those that do not (nonREM). Each of these states has distinct characteristics. About 50% of adult sleep and 80% of infant sleep is REM sleep. Upon falling to sleep, the first period is nonREM. It lasts about 60—90 minutes and is followed by a REM period, which lasts approximately 5—30 minutes. These cycles, thought to be the result of reciprocal release and inhibition of noradrenergic and serotonin mechanisms in the brain, continued to alternate 4—6 times during normal sleep.

REM Sleep. REM sleep, the sleep state in which dreams appear, features rapid conjugate motions of the eye, an increase in body movements and muscle twitches, fluctuations in respiratory and pulse rates, variations in blood pressure and body temperature, decreased muscle tone, and penile erection. EEG patterns reveal a fast wave similar to that of wakefulness with the eyes open but of much lower amplitude.

NonREM Sleep. NonREM sleep is characterized by a lack of rapid eye motion, fewer body movements and muscle twitches, more stable respiratory and pulse rates, and less variation in blood pressure or body temperature. NonRem sleep can be divided into three distinct EEG patterns:

• *Drowsiness*, exhibiting a low-amplitude pattern with slight fluctuations in rhythm.

• *Light—moderate sleep*, which features (a) frontal region EEG sleep spindles (ie, sinusoidal waves of 10—14 ips); (b) frontal and parietal region V waves (sharp high-amplitude waves); and (c) K complexes (combined spindles and V waves), common to partial arousal.

• *Deep sleep*, characterized by large groups of high- and low-amplitude slow waves.

Arousal from Normal Sleep. The normal physiologic loss of consciousness (sleep state) can easily be reversed by the activation of sensory or motor input to the cerebral cortex. When an individual is gently awakened from the sleep state, the EEG pattern changes from slow smoothly rhythmical waves to fast low-voltage waves.

Insomnia (Sleeplessness). The symptom of insomnia, the inability to sleep, should not be taken lightly. It may be the result of an organic lesion, and this commonly occurs at the midpontine pretrigeminal level, rostal to the trigeminal nerve entry zone and above the medullary and pontine sleep centers. If the lesion is severe, the state of wakefulness will be persistent. Milder forms of insomnia also may be due to other symptoms producing excessive sensory stimuli, a certain therapy, the patient's life-style, or various psychogenic factors. Cirrhosis of the liver, for example, often produces insomnia because of episodic nocturnal delirium. Overeating late at night may produce a reflux esophagitis, and overdrinking in the late evening may produce an alcoholic gastritis. The nocturia of renal or bladder disease, the palpitations and arrhythmias of heart disease, and the

Table 4.4. Abnormal Sleep-Related States

Cataplexy	A sudden loss of postural muscle tone, often precipitated by an emotional event, that may cause an individual to suddenly drop to the ground.
Hypnagogic hallucinations	False perceptions (visual or auditory) occurring just prior to falling asleep. They are often associated with sleep paralysis and narcolepsy.
Lethargy	A mild form of chronic drowsiness, torpor, or slugginess that resembles mild stupor.
Narcolepsy	A disorder (usually functional) of the sleep control mechanisms whose prominent feature are episodes of involuntary precipitation of sleep. Cataplexy, hypnagogic hallucinations, and sleep paralysis are often associated.
Sleep paralysis	Transient general paralysis that generally occurs during the transition between wakefulness and sleep.
Somnambulism	Sleepwalking, a subjective impulse that prompts a sleeping individual to unconsciously perform motor acts that naturally belong to the waking state. The term is also used to signify a form of hysteria in which behavior and purposeful actions are not subsequently remembered.
Somnolence	A slight disturbance of consciousness characterized by a marked tendency toward severe drowsiness or deep sleep from which the patient *can be* aroused by external stimuli. However, the patient drifts back to unconsciousness when external stimulation is removed. If the somnolence is an early stage of coma, its cause will be similar to that of coma. If it is not, it is probably the result of a disorder such as encephalitis lethargica, advanced atherosclerosis, or depressive narcolepsy.

dyspnea of pulmonary disease commonly cause insomnia. Coronary insufficiency frequently manifests only an early sign of nocturnal "heartburn." Any upper airway obstruction (eg, rhinitis, epiglottitis) will produce a fear of not being able to breathe during sleep that may maintain wakefulness. Hyperthyroidism, anemia of any type, heart disorders, and neurocirculatory asthenia are commonly associated with insomnia because of tachycardia. Brain tumors and inflammations frequently cause wakefulness and somnolence, and a large number of other neurologic disorders are associated with insomnia. The latter would include peripheral hypersensitiveness such as pressure on sensitive trigger points.

Sleep Theories. There have been several theories as to the causation of sleep that have now been discarded. They are briefly described below for historical interest only.

- *The Circulatory Theory.* Because vasculature changes were recorded during sleep, many believed that sleep was induced by a physiologic brain anemia. These changes were attributed to circulatory effects upon the cortex and vasoconstrictive centers of the brain stem.
- *The Histologic Theory.* This theory was based on animal studies that demonstrated CNS nerve cell changes after prolonged stimulation. It was thus hypothesized that sleep was the effect of such changes to allow for cellular revitalization.
- *The Hypoxic Theory.* This theory proposed that sleep was the result of accumulating hypoxia. The supposition was that brain cells during the waking state consumed a greater supply of oxygen than could be fully restored by the circulation. In time, this deficiency was thought to reach a point which induced sleep so that the CNS oxygen supply could be restored during the reduced metabolic state.
- *The Metabolic Theory.* At one time, some authorities held that sleep was induced by the progressive accumulation during wakeful activity of lactic acid, carbon dioxide, and associated metabolic debris.
- *The Psychobiologic Theory.* This theory held that sleep was an instinctive behavior that served to prevent the harmful effects of exhaustion.
- *The Psychoanalytical Theory.* Freud believed that sleep was an escape mechanism that involved a regression to an older, more primitive or infantile state.

The Hypnotic State. The word elements *hyp*, *hypno*, and *hypna* come from the Greek and mean sleep. Thus, the word *hypnosis* is a confusing misnomer as the state is much better described as a condition of profound highly alert concentration. The eyes need not be closed nor the sleep-resembling state acquired for "hypnotic" suggestibility to occur. This is demonstrated in the contagious atmosphere created by gifted orators and writers such as are utilized within the communications media, the mass hysteria of mob action, the tics and fads that spread throughout a school, subliminal messages, and the many psychosomatic disorders that are passed from one individual to another.

Dreams

Dreams are commonly defined as a more or less coherent train of partial conscious (preconscious) imagery occurring during sleep. They also may be induced in drugged or hypnotic states. It appears that during such sleep states thought residues from daily activities join with unconscious tendencies and memories that have been excluded from consciousness by the repression or suppression of painful ideas and form symbolic images of wishes, fears, or weaknesses. This allows some concept within the subconscious to express itself that would normally not be allowed to do so. These are the common wish-fulfilling dreams of some unsatisfied desire or dreams that reflect from a subconscious conflict.

There are also dreams that can be attributed to *physical* causes such as environmental noises, exposure to temperature extremes while sleeping, or indigestion. In addition, there are those extraordinary dreams that can be placed under the general category of *enlightenment* (eg, problem-solving, creative, spiritual).

The content of a dream (ideas expressed in a dream) is held to be of two fundamental types: (1) the *manifest content*, events occurring to the dreamer. The manifest content is usually a transformation, a disguise, and a distortion. It is usually the obvious incidents and circumstances of the dream. (2) The *latent content* (hidden residual thoughts), which must be revealed by the technique of psychoanalytic dream interpretation. This is usually achieved by having the patient free associate around the dream content and its symbols (repressed desires) until their wish-fulfillment nature and physical expression become apparent. Deeper than either the manifest or latent content there is a more impersonal symbolism that tends to relate the separateness and oneness of life.

Lucid Dreams. While all people dream during sleep, only some dreams can normally be recalled upon awakening. La Berge, who heads the Sleep Research Center at Stanford University has been directing investigations into the development of an inexpensive device that can be used by anyone who is interested in inducing lucid dreams (being aware of dreaming while dreaming). La Berge believes that the proper interpretation of lucid dreams can be used to facilitate creative problem solving, enhance self-image concepts, develop higher levels of consciousness, and improve mental, emotional, and perhaps physical health.

Supratentorial Disorders: Basic Considerations

The main objective of the neurologic evaluation is to determine (1) the presence or absence of nervous system function, (2) the location, type, and extent of lesions (if any), and (3) the degree to which the healthy portion of the patient's nervous system can be used for rehabilitation. Thus, the standard physical examination should be conducted prior to a more detailed neurologic assessment so that findings may be integrated to reach a conclusive diagnosis.

As many subjective tests are employed, the practitioner should make every effort to put the patient at ease and to explain unfamiliar procedures beforehand. In some instances, including the tests for general cerebral function, part of the examination can be conducted while taking the case history.

The effectiveness of therapeutic progress of a patient is often in direct proportion to the patient's psychologic acceptance of the doctor and the therapy. Kirby points out that it is therefore valuable in patient evaluation to judge the ability and willingness of the patient to follow the physician's orders and to create an atmosphere where the patient will have optimum confidence in the doctor's ability and offer optimal cooperation. Conversely, it is well to recognize certain types of patients who tend to be uncooperative and do not have the frame of mind necessary to achieve optimal results, even when the best diagnostic and therapeutic methods are applied.

When patients are obviously not responding adequately during the history interview in accordance with their background, occupation, and educational experience, a mental disorder should be suspected. During the early stages of mental illness, however, such faults may be extremely subtle.

A patient with a severe consciousness disturbance may require immediate surgical or psychiatric referral until the cause can be determined. Such situations are often urgent, and if the patient is conscious, uncooperativeness is the rule. Specialized experience, brain scans, EEGs, and CSF examinations are frequently required during the diagnostic process. For these reasons, the following descriptions for a conscious patient are brief.

Gross evaluation of the higher centers begins with a general mental and emotional evaluation during the case history process that extends throughout the examination—noting gait, carriage, handshake, gestures, facial expressions, grooming, cleanliness, and dress. Portrayed self-image, mood, judgment, response to simple requests, temporal and spatial orientation, memory, attention span, and language comprehension and articulation also can be generally appraised at this time. Language processing involves listening, comprehending, speaking, reading, and writing skills.

Once all examination data are collected, the practitioner should be able to determine whether the cerebral cortex is functioning adequately at its highest levels of integration. Typical syndromes likely to involve the cerebral cortex are listed in Table 4.5.

Agnosia

Agnosia is the inability to name, properly use, or comprehend the importance of sensory impressions although the sensory sphere and language capabilities are intact. There are seven types: (1) visual, (2) auditory (acoustic), (3) olfactory, (4) tactile, (5) gustatory, (6) digital (inability to count fingers), and (7) temporal (time duration). Four major types of agnosia are described by Tran/ Maori as follows:

- *Tactile agnosia* is a failure to identify objects by means of tactile and proprioceptive sensibilities when both are normal in that part of the body being tested. *Astereognosis* is the inability to recognize the form, size, texture, and identity of the object touched, due to sensory impairment at a cortical level. Tactile agnosia is related with lesions of the supramarginal gyrus (parietal lobe) of the left cerebrum.
- *Visual agnosia* is the inability to recognize objects not due to a defect of visual acuity or to intellectual impairment. Visual agnosia is associated with lesions of the lateral visual association areas of the occipital lobe in the dominant hemisphere.
- *Auditory agnosia* is the failure to distinguish different noises or sounds in a patient with normal hearing. It involves lesions in the superior temporal gyrus (area 22) in the dominant hemisphere. Refer to Figure 4.6.
- *Proprioceptive agnosia* is the inability to recognize body parts and relationships due to a lesion within the parietal lobe (posteroinferior regions).

Alexia and Agraphia

Alexia is the inability to read (word blindness) because of a central nervous system lesion. *Agraphia* is the inability to express thoughts in writing because of a lesion in the cerebral cortex. There are four main types of alexia: (1) *cortical alexia*, sensory aphasia due to a left gyrus angularis lesion; (2) *motor alexia*, inability to read a word aloud even though the patient understands the word when he sees it; (3) *musical alexia*, sensory or optic (never motor) inability to read music; and (4) *subcortical alexia*, alexia due to interruption of the connection between the gyrus angularis and optic center.

Alexia with agraphia is usually related to an infarction in the middle cerebral artery (parietal lesion). Alexia without agraphia is often the result of an infarction in the posterior cerebral artery or its distribution. Alexia with or without agraphia may be caused by the same disorder that causes aphasia. Stroke is the most common cause.

Aphasia

A normal educated person can understand and communicate in spoken and written language, as well as by gestures and other means. Any disorder that is characterized by receptive and expressive disturbances in the faculty of using symbols and signs to communicate is called *aphasia*. Aphasia can be caused by organic neural lesions that affect the cerebral memory mechanisms for lan-

Table 4.5. Common Syndromes Involving the Cerebral Cortex

Agnosia	Gerstmann's syndrome
Agraphia	Gliomas
Anxiety	Hysteria
Alexia	Intelligence impairments
Aphasia	Language defects
Apraxia	Mental retardation
Cerebral hemisphere disease	Metastatic neoplasms
Delusions and illusions	Nervous irritability
Dementia	Schizophrenia
Depression	Seizures
Dysarthria	Sensory and motor malintegration

guage without impairment of cortical or subcortical structures essential for the relay of impulses or the innervation of the speech organs. Although it is difficult to pinpoint the location(s) of such lesions, most researchers suggest that the dysfunction is associated with cerebral damages in the posterior temporoparietal region and Broca's area (pars opercularis and triangularis of the inferior frontal gyrus).

Aphasia is an impairment characterized by defective or loss of expression by speech, writing, or signs, or of comprehending spoken or written words because of a cerebral lesion or dysfunction (usually cortical, rarely subcortical), especially that of the left hemisphere. There are two main types:

1. *Expressive aphasia.* This is a motor aphasia caused by impairment or lack of ability to express thoughts in a meaningful way in speech or writing. It is the inability to utter words although the patient understands spoken and written words and knows what he wants to say. It is impossible for the patient to coordinate the muscles controlling speech because of a lesion or dysfunction of Broca's area. Frequently, both speech and writing (agraphia) are impaired. This aphasic condition is also called *aphemia, Broca's aphasia, motor aphasia,* or *ataxic aphasia.* The cause is a lesion of the inferior frontal gyrus, just anterior to Broca's area of the motor cortex.

2. *Receptive aphasia.* This is a sensory aphasia caused by impairment in the appreciation of the meanings of both spoken and written words; ie, the inability to comprehend written, spoken, or tactile communications. It is often called *sensory* or *Wernicke's aphasia.* The cause is a lesion that affects the postero-superior temporal gyrus and adjacent angular gyrus of the temporal lobe, disrupting the fibers which receive and integrate central impulses. The larger the area affected, the greater the degree of aphasia.

These two types of aphasia can be further divided into auditory receptive aphasia, visual receptive aphasia, expressive speaking aphasia and expressive writing aphasia. For example, other types of aphasia and related disorders include alalia, amnestic aphasia, auditory aphasia, conduction aphasia, fluent aphasia, gibberish aphasia, nonfluent aphasia, optic aphasia, paragrammatism, and paraphasia.

Isolated receptive or expressive aphasias are rare. Brain lesions that are large enough to cause speech impairment seldom produce pure effects.

The inability to articulate words properly (dysarthria) is a motor disorder and not an aphasia. Aphasic disorders are usually caused by the same diseases that cause hemiparesis; ie, infarct, stroke, trauma, tumor, aneurysm, infection, inflammatory disease, and degenerative disease. Alzheimer's disease and Pick's disease cause aphasia but not weakness.

Aphasia, agnosia, alexia, and apraxia are closely related. The etiologies of aphasia and agnosia, especially, are similar. The purpose of clinical and laboratory tests should be to confirm or exclude psychic, functional, and organic suspicions of causal relationships.

When aphasia is suspected, Heilman recommends five tests: (1) note spontaneity and fluency of patient's speech; (2) test comprehension of spoken and written words; (3) test ability to repeat sentences; (4) test ability to name familiar objects; and (5) test ability to write familiar words. The proper interpretation of these tests will help locate the site of the lesion.

Other common tests can be used in suspected agnosia, alexia, apraxia, and aphasia. Refer to Table 4.3.

Apraxia

Lesions in the cerebral cortex may involve the inability to perform certain learned complex movements in the absence of paralysis, sensatory loss, or disturbances of coordination. *Apraxia* is the inability to perform purposeful learned motor acts on command though physical ability and willingness are present; ie, motor and sensory impairments are not involved. The fault is within the neural pathways that retain memory of learned movement patterns so that willingness cannot be translated into physical action. Any structural or metabolic disease process that affects the brain diffusely and the frontal lobe in particular can produce apraxia. Selective apraxias exhibit loss of one or more specific movements. The disorder is classified into several types:

• *Kinetic apraxia* is characterized by an inability to perform precise acquired motor movements in the absence of paresis due to lesions involving the precentral cortex.

• *Ideomotor apraxia* is induced by an interruption of pathways between the center for formulation of a motor act and the motor areas necessary for its execution. The patient is unable to perform on command a voluntary movement he or she may know and want to fulfill. Ideomotor apraxia is commonly bilateral and is associated with lesions of the parietal lobe (supramarginal gyrus) of the dominant hemisphere.

• *Ideational apraxia* is characterized by the inability to formulate the conceptual plan for the execution of the components of complex movements. Simple isolated movements can be achieved by the patient with no difficulty. This has been implicated as the result of lesions of the dominant parietal lobe and/or corpus collosum.

• *Constructional apraxia* is a condition that features a loss of visual guidance, impairment of the visual image, and disturbance of revisualization. The patient is unable to reproduce simple geometric figures by drawing or by the arrangement of blocks. As a rule, the patient is unaware of the inability to perceive spacial relationships. The condition is associated with a lesion or interruption of pathways between the occipital and parietal cortex.

The Dominant Hemisphere

Often overlooked is whether the patient is right-handed, left-handed, or ambidextrous. This fact is important in analyzing the patient's complaints because (1) unilateral muscular development may be a factor in postural analysis, (2) the dominant hemisphere controls language functions, and (3) there are many functions that do not appear to be equally represented at a cortical level.

The left hemisphere is dominant in a right-handed person, and vice versa. According to Chusid, the dominant (major) hemisphere is mainly concerned with verbal, linguistic, arithmetic, calculating, and analytic functions. The nondominant (minor) hemisphere plays its major role in nonverbal, geometric, spatial, visual, pattern, and creative or other synthetic functions. Lesions of the corpus callosom will often reveal themselves in dysfunction of the nondominant hemisphere such as illegible writing, constructional apraxia, and the inability to match left-sided tasks easily conducted by the right side.

Heilman and associates list six conditions that can originate from a nondominant hemisphere deficit alone: (1) affective disorders, (2) inability to get dressed (dressing apraxia), (3) inability to perceive visual depth, (4) inability to produce musical sounds (amusia), (5) inability to recognize familiar faces (prosopagnosia), and (6) spatial disorientation when verbal clues are absent.

Cerebral dominance does not become established until about the 3rd or 4th year of life. Some physiologists have related dominance to cerebral asymmetries. Other psychologic studies have concluded that males tend to have a predominantly dominant hemisphere, while females tend to use both hemispheres more equally during conscious activities. Generalized differences in outlook between the sexes are sometimes attributed to this difference.

Gerstmann's Syndrome. This clinical picture strongly suggests parietal dysfunction of the patient's dominant hemisphere. Stroke is usually the cause. Gerstmann's syndrome is a symptom complex consisting of (1) acalculia, the inability to calculate; (2) agraphia, the inability to write; (3) finger agnosia, the inability to count fingers; and (4) right—left confusion, the inability to tell right side from left.

Cranial Entrapment Syndromes

Magoun, Upledger, DeJarnette, and others believe that slight cranial distortions and/or the loss of minute cranial bone mobility may readily lead to CNS dysfunction with expression at the terminals of involved pathways. They attribute many olfactory, optic, oculomotor, trochlear, and other cranial nerve disorders to tension or pressure on these nerves as the result of various direct or indirect effects from the bony components of the skull.

Some Current Subtle Energy Research

How subtle energies affect consciousness and the healing process has long been a mystery though many theories have been formulated. At one time, even speculations of the existence of such energies were placed in the realm of fantasy by most scientists; if they did exist, it was thought that they would be so minute in force that they would have no effect. During the last 2 decades, however, some important advances have been made by the scientific community in trying to determine how the mild stimuli of acupuncture can control pain via the release of endogenous opiate-like substances from CNS centers by directing or releasing such minute foci of energy. These studies also may bring forth new light on the role of subtle vertebral-related neurologic foci in disease processes.

From a viewpoint different from that of many of his medical colleagues, Pelletier, an associate clinical professor at the University of California School of Medicine, has focused attention on developing both a theoretical and a clinical model on how subtle energies (eg, those theorized to be used in acupuncture, homeopathy, and visualization) work in the healing process.

Studies focused on the effects of extremely diluted remedies have seen homeopathic concepts revisited in light of these new findings. Benson, director of the Division of Behavioral Medicine at Beth Israel Hospital at Harvard University is investigating the ancient Chinese practice of *chi-gong*, an ancient technique for eliciting the relaxation response associated with the alpha state. A joint United States—Chinese project is studying the usefulness of chi-gong and herbs in a number of neurologically related diseases.

Zimmerman has been conducting experiments at the University of Colorado on the interaction of living organisms in exterior and interior electromagnetic fields. A biomagnetic imaging system is being developed that will, hopefully, project the electromagnetic field of a living organism as a video image to allow investigation of the biomagnetic correlates of subtle energy healing intervention such as used in therapeutic touch and acupuncture.

At the School of Medicine of the University of North Carolina, Corless bases her project on the proposition that, if emotions are salient to disease onset and progression, they also may be significant to the resolution of disease. A prominent feature of her investigation is the inclusion of drawings, relaxation, mental imagery, and therapeutic touch.

THE POSTERIOR FOSSA LEVEL

This area contains all structures within the cranium that are situated above the foramen magnum and below the tentorium cerebelli. The major structures are the brain stem (medulla, pons, midbrain), proximal portions of cranial nerves III—XII, and cerebellum. The medulla is derived from the metencephalon; the pons, the metencephalon; and the midbrain, the mesencephalon. Those portions of the cranial nerves that are located outside the cranial vault are considered in this text to be part of the peripheral nervous system.

The posterior fossa is protected and supported by the temporal bones anteriorly and laterally and by the occipital bones at the base of the skull (Fig. 4.9). The structures within this area serve as the central cerebrospinal level for ascending and descending tracts traveling to and from the supratentorial structures, the brain stem cranial nerve nuclei, the cerebellum, and the spinal cord. As an overview, the major systems of concern are shown in Table 4.6. The posterior fossa area is also closely related to the aqueduct of Sylvius (midbrain), 4th ventricle (pons, medulla), and foramina of Megendie and Luschka of the CSF system.

It is unique to lesions at the posterior level that unilateral brain stem lesions produce disorders of the ipsilateral side of the face and the contralateral side of the body.

The Medulla Oblongata

The medulla (spinal bulb) serves as an organ of conduction for the passage of impulses between the spinal cord and the brain. It is continuous with the spinal cord, which, on passing into the cranial cavity through the foramen magnum, widens into a pyramidal shaped mass that extends to the lower aspect of the pons (Fig. 4.10). Externally, the medulla resembles the upper part of the spinal cord, but its internal structure differs considerably.

Basic Considerations

The nerve cells of the medulla are grouped into numerous nuclei, some of which are centers from which cranial nerves arise. The last four cranial nerves (IX—XII) originate from nuclei within the medulla. The motor fibers of the *glossopharyngeal* and *vagus* nerves and the cranial portion of the *accessory* nerve arise from the *nucleus ambiguus.* The *hypoglossal nerve* arises in the *hypoglossal nucleus.* From these and other fibers of the medulla, collaterals contribute to the reticular formation.

Some nuclei are relay stations of sensory tracts to the brain such as the *nucleus gracilis* and *nucleus cuneatus*, and some serve as centers for body function control such as the *cardiac, vasotonic* (vasopressor and vasodilator), *respiratory* (inhalation and exhalation), and *emetic* centers. There is also a *chemoreceptor trigger zone* at the

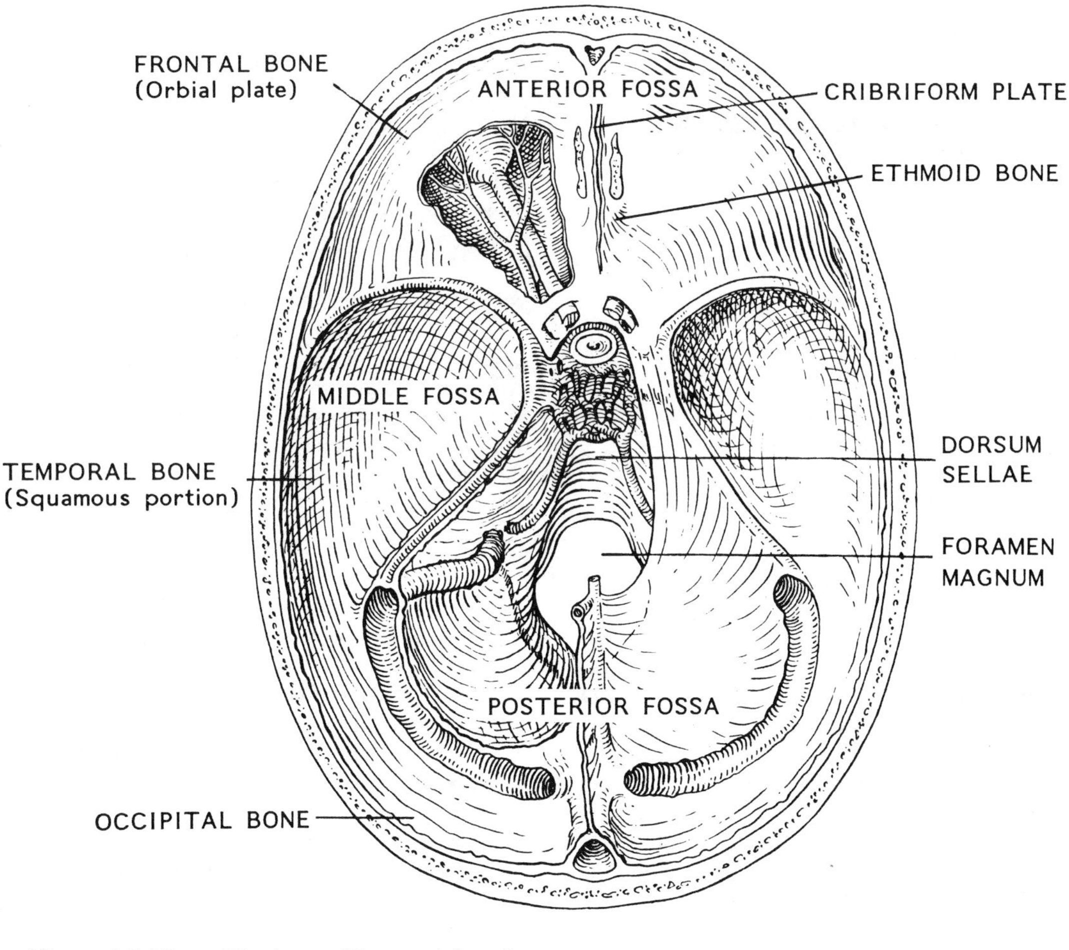

Figure 4.9. View of the base of the cranial cavity.

Table 4.6. Posterior Fossa System Components

Function	Structure
Consciousness System	
Mediation of consciousness, attention, wakefulness, sleeping states	Reticular formation
Motor System	
Many head, facial, and neck muscles; salivary and lacrimal glands; vasomotors	Final pathway of cranial nerves III—VII, IX—XII
Direct activation pathway	Corticospinal and corticobulbar tracts
Indirect activation pathway	Reticulospinal, rubrospinal, vestibulospinal tracts
Basal ganglia control circuit	Substantia nigra and red nucleus connections
Cerebellar efferents	Superior cerebellar peduncle connections
Sensory System	
Pain and temperature	Lateral spinothalamic tract
Touch	Anterior spinothalamic and medial lemniscal tracts
Conscious proprioception, discriminative sensations	Medial lemniscal tract
Unconscious proprioception	Anterior and posterior spinocerebellar, fastigiobulbar, and vestibulocerebellar tracts
Sensory receptors of head	Cranial nerves I, II, V, VII—X
Vascular System	Vertebrobasilar system
Visceral System	Cardiac, circulatory, respiratory, and vomiting regulatory centers
	Ascending and descending mediating tracts
	Cranial III, VII, IX, X preganglionic parasympathetic fibers
	Reticular formation

floor of the 4th ventricle that is highly sensitive to certain drugs and toxins. Besides these control centers, many other reflex activities are integrated in the medulla by the vagus and other cranial nerves. Such reflexes include several important acts such as swallowing, sneezing, coughing, vomiting, and the movements and secretions of the alimentary canal. The levels of integration of some major reflexes are shown in Table 4.7.

The Glossopharyngeal Nerve (Cranial IX). The glossopharyngeal is a mixed motor and sensory nerve that supplies the pharynx, posterior taste buds, parotid gland, and nociceptors of the middle ear. Its motor fibers arise from the nucleus ambiguus, project through the lateral medulla, and then pass with the sensory fibers. The sensory fibers arise in the superior and petrous ganglia, pass through the jugular foramen, and enter the medulla just behind the facial nerve.

The Vagus Nerve (Cranial X). The vagus is a mixed sensory and motor nerve that supplies the pharynx, larynx, esophagus, stomach, heart, lungs, and abdominal viscera, and serves as a pathway for multitudes of afferent and efferent reflex activities. Pharyngoesophageal swallowing, hunger, thirst, cardiac and respiratory rate, peristalsis, and the secretion of digestive juices are just a few examples. Vagal afferents arise from the jugular and nodose ganglia, located below the jugular foramen, pass through the jugular foramen, and enter the medulla just behind the glossopharyngeal nerve. Vagal efferents pass from the medulla and join the course of the sensory fibers.

The Spinal Accessory Nerve (Cranial XI). The multi-rooted accessory is a motor

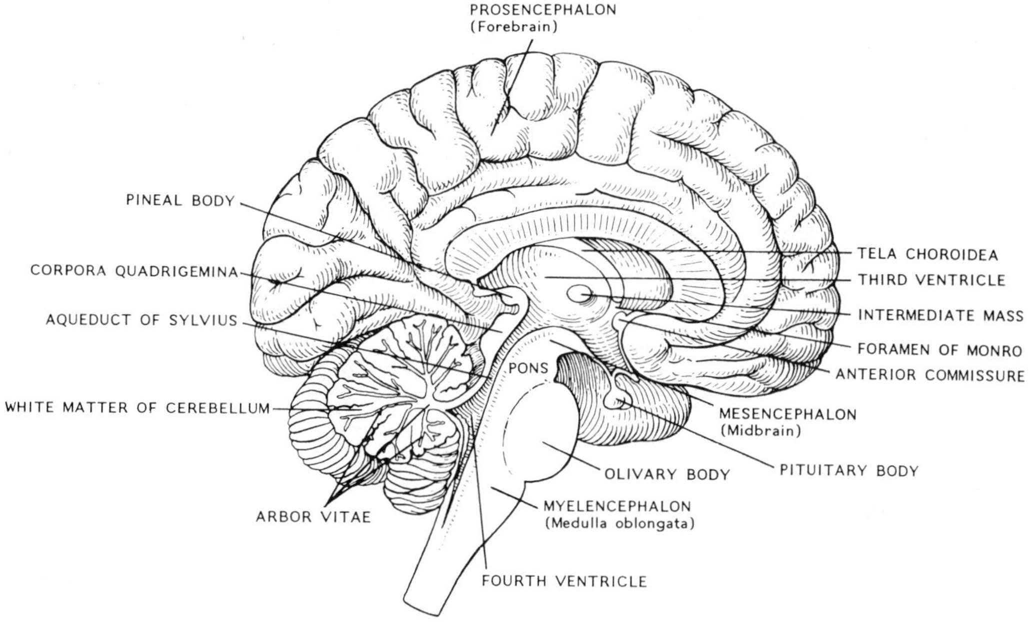

Figure 4.10. Sagittal section of the brain showing the brain stem, cerebellum, and cerebrum.

Table 4.7. Levels of Integration of Various Reflexes

Function	Level of Integration
Antigravity reflexes	Medulla
Blood pressure	Medulla
Body temperature	Hypothalamus
Conditioned reflexes	Cerebral cortex
Emotional responses	Hypothalamus, limbic system
Heart rate	Medulla
Initiative, memory, etc	Cerebral cortex
Locomotor reflexes	Midbrain, thalamus
Respiratory reflexes	Lower medulla
Righting reflexes	Midbrain
Spinal reflexes	Spinal cord
Vasculature tone	Medulla
Vomiting	Medulla
Wakefulness reflexes	Thalamus, limbic system

nerve to the sternocleidomastoideus and trapezius muscles. It differs only from a typical spinal motor nerve by its close connections with the vestibular system and other cranial nerves (eg, orientation of the eyes, nose, and ears toward environmental stimuli). The nerve's rootlets arise behind that of the vagus on the lateral surface of the medulla and upper cervical cord, and they exit the cranial vault via the jugular foramen.

The Hypoglossal Nerve (Cranial XII). The hypoglossal is a motor nerve to the intrinsic muscles of the tongue, thus involved in speaking, eating, and participating in the initial act of swallowing. Like the spinal accessory, the hypoglossal originates from several filaments. These filaments arise on the anterolateral sulcus of the medulla, quickly fuse into one nerve, and exit the posterior fossa of the cranium via the hypoglossal canal.

Basic Functions

Cardiac Center. This center consists of groups of bilateral cells in the medulla at the level of the nucleus of the *vagus* nerve. Fibers from this center accompany the vagi to the heart and unite with branches from the thoracic sympathetics to form the *cardiac plexus*, which envelops the ascending aorta and its arch. Vagal inhibitory and sympathetic accelerating fibers are true antagonists in terms of heart rate.

Respiratory Center. These bilateral groups of cells in the medulla have an inherent rhythmic activity similar to that of the cardiac center. These centers are especially sensitive to reflexes directed from the cranial and spinal nerves and all pathways between the cerebrum and medulla. Thus, almost any adequate sensory reflex impulses are likely to affect respiratory rate in an excitatory (pressor) or inhibitory (depressor) manner, depending upon the source and effect of the stimuli. Via collateral connections, neurons conveying these impulses affect vasculature tone, heart rate, and cardiac output.

Vasoconstrictor Center. From this bilateral group of cells in the medulla, fibers descend through the spinal cord, and at various levels they form synapses with spinal neurons in the anterior horns of the gray matter, which, in turn, project as preganglionic vasoconstrictor fibers that terminate in the sympathetic ganglia. Postganglionic fibers then extend to supply most of the peripheral vasculature. The vasoconstrictor center is normally in a state of continuous activity so that vasculature tone is constant, and different parts of the body are supplied by different paths (eg, skin, intestines). Its activity can be increased reflexly through many types of sensory stimulation to produce vasoconstriction and hypertension (pressor effects), or its activity can be decreased to produce vasodilation and lowered blood pressure (depressor effects).

Cranial Nerves IX—XII. See Table 4.8.

Medulla Dysfunction

All afferent and efferent tracts of the spinal cord are represented cephally in the medulla, and these tracts either end or decussate at this level. Thus, an isolated medulla lesion may exhibit motor or sensory dysfunction (somatic and/or autonomic) to a degree determined by the site and extent of the destructive process. Lesions of the upper central area of the medulala may involve vital nuclei in this area and produce a large variety of features. Lesions of the posterolateral area produce Wallenberg's syndrome; those of the anterior portion, hypoglossal hemiplegia alternans.

The glossopharyngeal, vagus, spinal accessory, or hypoglossal nerves may be damaged in the medulla or anywhere along their course to the periphery.

The Glossopharyngeal Nerve. Lesions of the glossopharyngeal nerve commonly arise as glossopharyngeal neuralgia, Bonnier's syndrome, Vernet's syndrome, or tympanic branch neuralgia of Jacobson's nerve. Symptoms of glossopharyngeal involvement include slight dysphagia and possible ear pain. General signs include an inhibited gag reflex, deviation of the uvula to the well side, loss of pharyngeal constriction during an "ah" test, diminished taste in the posterior third of the tongue, hypersalivation, tachycardia, and possibly associated nystagmus.

The Vagus Nerve. Partial destructive lesions of the cranial vagus exhibit as vagal,

Table 4.8. The Twelve Cranial Nerves

Number/Name		Type	Origin	Distribution	Basic Function
I.	*Olfactory*	Sensory	Nasal chamber	Nasal mucous membrane	Sense of smell and flavors except salty, sweet, bitter, and acid
II.	*Optic*	Sensory	Retina	Retina	Sense of sight
III.	*Oculomotor*	Motor	Midbrain	All ocular muscles except lateral rectus and superior oblique	Major down and out eye motion, pupil constriction
IV.	*Trochlear*	Motor	Midbrain	Superior oblique muscles of eye	Major down and in eye motion
V.	*Trigeminal*	Mixed	Pons and midbrain	Skin of upper face, ear, jaw, tongue, gums; teeth; muscles of mastication	Motor and chief sensory nerve of the face
VI.	*Abducens*	Motor	Pons	Lateral rectus muscle of the eye	Major abduction motion of eye
VII.	*Facial*	Mixed	Pons	Facial muscles, middle ear, anterior 2/3rds taste buds; lacrimal, nasal, sublingual, submaxillary glands	Muscles of expression, taste, salivation
VIII.	*Auditory*	Sensory	Pons	Middle and internal ear	Sense of hearing and balance
IX.	*Glossopharyngeal*	Mixed	Medulla	Posterior 3rd taste buds, pharynx, parotid gland, ear	Ear pain, swallowing, parotid parasympathetics, pharyngeal reflex
X.	*Vagus*	Mixed	Medulla	Pharynx, larynx, heart, lungs, esophagus, stomach, abdominal viscera	Swallowing, hunger, speech, epiglottal taste, breathing, heart rate, ear and throat pain, alimentary tract pain, peristalsis, digestive juices
XI.	*Spinal accessory*	Motor	Medulla and cord	Sternomastoid and trapezius muscles	Neck and shoulder girdle motion
XII.	*Hypoglossal*	Motor	Medulla	Intrinsic muscles of tongue	Speech, eating

recurrent laryngeal, or superior laryngeal paralysis; hysterical aphonia (laryngospasm); or superior laryngeal neuralgia. Caudally, irritative lesions manifest as visceral hyperparasympathicotonia and inhibited lesions as hypersympathicotonia. In lesions involving the distribution to the throat, symptoms include loss or weakness of voice, chronic cough, dysphonia, dysphagia, esophageal spasm, pharyngolaryngeal pain, salivation abnormalities, and possibly dyspnea and external ear pain. Overt signs include an inhibited gag reflex, an altered position of the vocal cords, bradycardia or tachycardia, and a dilated stomach.

The Spinal Accessory Nerve. Depending on the branch affected, irritative lesions manifest as trapezius and sternocleidomastoideus spasm; inhibiting lesions, as muscle weakness. These conditions can readily be appraised by noting the patient's ability to shrug the shoulders and rotate the head against resistance. In subtle cases, EMG studies may be necessary.

The Hypoglossal Nerve. Injury to the hypoglossal nerve frequently results in paralysis (flaccid or spastic), ataxic tongue, and dysarthria. The patient will complain of eating and speech difficulties. Examination will reveal weak tongue strength when the tongue is pushed to the side of the cheek against external resistance and possibly an atrophic tongue. In addition, lesions of the hypoglossal nerve are frequently combined with other cranial nerve involvement. See Table 4.9.

Table 4.9. Selected Syndromes Involving the Last Four Cranial Nerves

Disorder	Nerves	Features
Avells' syndrome	X, bulbar XI	Ipsilateral paralysis and anesthesia of soft palate, pharynx, larynx, contralateral dissociate hemianesthesia, dysphagia, dysarthria
Babinski-Nageotte bulbar syndrome	IX, X, bulbar XI, part of V	Ipsilateral paralysis of the tongue, pharynx, larynx; ipsilateral loss of taste (posterior third); ipsilateral Horner's syndrome; ipsilateral loss of pain and temperature on face; ipsilateral asynergia, ataxia, and tendency to fall toward side of lesion; contralateral hemiplegia of arm and leg; contralateral dissociate hemianesthesia
Bonnier's syndrome	VIII, IX, X	Paroxysmal vertigo, contralateral hemiplegia, transient somnolence, apprehension, tachycardia, weakness, and other variable manifestations of VIII, IX, and X involvement
Jackson's syndrome	X, XI, XII	Ipsilateral paralysis of the soft palate, pharynx, larynx, sternocleidomastoideus, trapezius, tongue, and atrophy of the tongue
Schmidt's syndrome	X, XI	Ipsilateral paralysis of the soft palate, pharynx, larynx, sternocleidomastoideus, trapezius (partially); palatal, pharyngeal, laryngeal anesthesia
Tapla's syndrome	X, XII	Ipsilateral paralysis of the pharynx, larynx, tongue, and tongue atrophy
Vernet's syndrome	IX, X, XI	Ipsilateral glossopharyngeal, vagal, and spinal accessory paralysis

The Pons

The pons (varoli) serves as a bridge between the two halves of the cerebellum and between the medulla and the cerebrum. It is in front of the cerebellum between the midbrain and the medulla oblongata and has interlaced transverse and longitudinal white nerve fibers intermixed with gray matter. The transverse fibers are those derived from the middle peduncles of the cerebellum and serve to join its two halves. The longitudinal fibers connect the medulla with the cerebrum. Within the pons are the nuclei of all or a part of the fibers of cranial nerves V—VIII. Their external origins are shown in Figure 4.11.

Basic Considerations

The Trigeminal Nerve (Cranial V). The three-branched trigeminal nerve contains a large sensory and a small motor root. It is the chief sensory nerve of the face and is distributed to the skin of the face, ear, jaw, tongue, gums, and teeth. Its motor fibers supply the muscles of mastication. The sensory root, which contains proprioception fibers from the TMJ and teeth sockets, arises from the gasserian ganglion in the lateral aspect of the cavernous sinus, passes posteriorly between the superior petrosal sinus and the tentorium, penetrates the middle cerebellar peduncle, and then enters the pons. Fibers of the *maxillary branch* exit via the foramen rotundum, and the *ophthalmic branch* leaves the cranial vault, via the superior orbital fissure, along with the oculomotor and trochlear nerves. Sensory fibers of the *mandibular branch* are joined by the motor fibers of the nerve, which leave the pons anteromedially to the sensory fibers and exit the skull via the foramen ovale.

The Abducens Nerve (Cranial VI). The abducens nerve supplies motor fibers to the lateral rectus muscle of the eye. When activated, the eyeball rolls laterally. It arises from the anterior surface of the brain stem at the groove that externally separates the pons

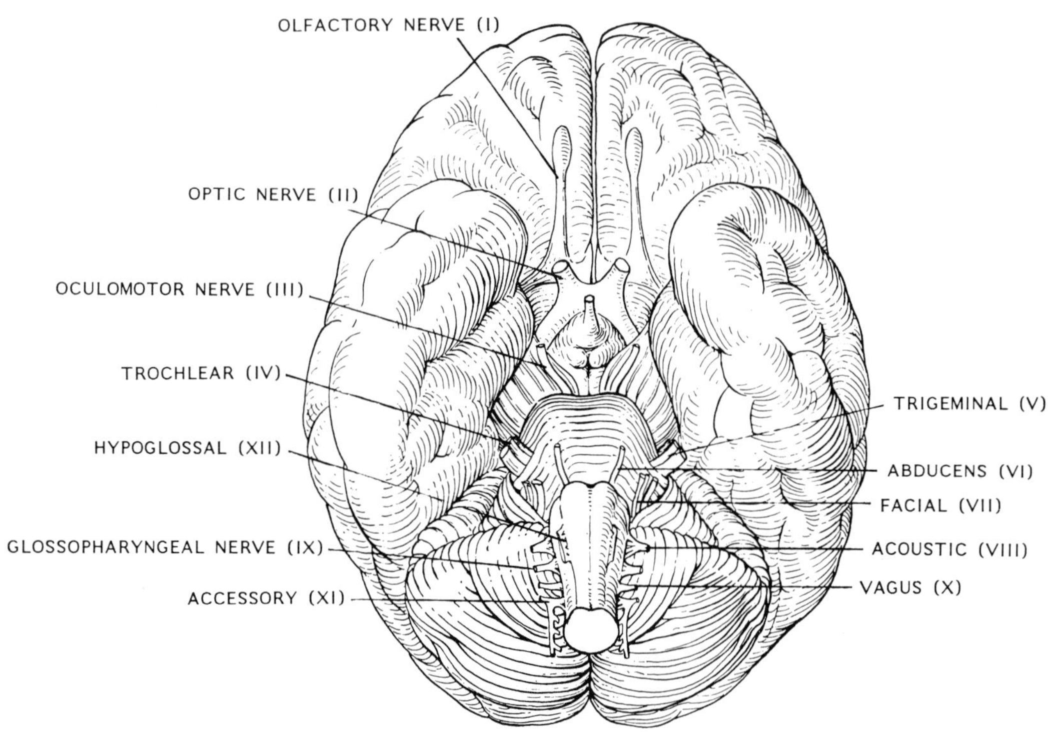

Figure 4.11. Basilar view of the origins of the cranial nerves.

and medulla. It then passes through the cavernous sinus and exits the skull via the superior orbital fissure, along with cranial III, IV, and V (ophthalmic branch) nerves.

The Facial Nerve (Cranial VII). The facial nerve is a mixed sensory and motor nerve that supplies the muscles of facial expression; the muscles necessary for hyoid elevation; the tongue's anterior taste buds; and the lacrimal, nasal, palatal, sublingual, and submaxillary glands. The sensory root originates from the cells of the geniculate ganglion, passes through the internal acoustic meatus and terminates in the medulla. The motor root projects from the posterior pons and exits the skull via the internal auditory meatus.

The Acoustic Nerve (Cranial VIII). The two-part acoustic nerve is the sensory nerve of hearing (middle ear) and balance (inner ear). The *cochlear branch* originates from the spiral ganglion, and the *vestibular division* arises from the vestibular ganglion (ganglion of Scarpa). The latter is in the posterior aspect of the internal auditory apparatus. The acoustic nerve enters the cranium via the internal acoustic meatus and enters the penetrates the brain stem just behind the posterior edge of the middle cerebellar peduncle.

Pontine Dysfunction

Lesions of the lateral pons (eg, pontocerebellar angle tumor) results in cranial nerve V—VII, IX—X, and XII dysfunction; alternating cranial V hemiplegia; ipsilateral ataxia,

Table 4.10. Lesions of the Pons

Syndrome/Lesion Site	Features
Foville's syndrome (crossed pontine hemiplegia)	Contralateral hemiplegia, ipsilateral cranial VII palsy, ipsilateral paralysis of lateral conjugate gaze
Millard-Gubler syndrome (facial hemiplegia alternans)	Contralateral hemiplegia, ipsilateral facial palsy
Pontine angle tumor syndrome	Ipsilateral facial anesthesia, loss of corneal and sneeze reflex, alternating trigeminal hemiplegia (V) Internal squint (VI) Ipsilateral facial muscle weakness (VII) Persistent tinnitus, progressive deafness, vertigo (VIII) Dysphagia (IX) Syncope (X) Ipsilateral tongue palsy, thick speech (XII) Papilledema (raised intracranial pressure) Ipsilateral ataxia, staggering, vertigo, arm/leg hypotonia (cerebellar peduncle) Contralateral hemiplegia and mild hemianesthesia (motor and sensory pathways)
Raymond's syndrome (alternating abducent hemiplegia)	Ipsilateral lateral rectus muscle paresis, contralateral hemiplegia
Raymond-Cestan syndrome	Anesthesia, nystagmus, quadriplegia

vertigo, hypotonia; contralateral hemiplegia, hemianesthesia; and general signs of increased intracranial pressure. Lesions of the anteroinferior pons frequently produce alternating abducent hemiplegia, Foville's syndrome, or Millard-Gubler's syndrome. The effects of common lesions in the pons are shown in Table 4.10.

The trigeminal, abducens, facial, and acoustic nerves may be damaged in the pons or anywhere along their course to the periphery.

The Trigeminal Nerve. Lesions of the trigeminal most frequently manifest as tic douloureux, paratrigeminal syndrome (Raeder's syndrome), or auriculotemporal nerve syndrome (Frey's syndrome). Symptoms of trigeminal involvement include anosmia (from nasal dryness), corneal anesthesia, hearing loss, numbness of upper face, pain, and possibly paresthesia. The signs of a trigeminal lesion include dental cavities, facial ulcerations, herpes simplex, jaw deviated laterally, inability to chew, masseter wasting, loss or inhibited reflexes (sneeze, lid, conjunctival, corneal, and jaw jerk), and neurokeratitis.

The Abducens Nerve. As the abducens is the motor nerve for ocular abduction, lesions produce paralysis of this function: medial in inhibiting lesions, lateral in irritating lesions. Both types will have associated diplopia.

The Facial Nerve. Lesions of the facial nerve most frequently exhibit as Bell's palsy, the nuclear or supranuclear types of facial palsy, geniculate neuralgia, facial spasm (paroxysmal facial hyperkinesia), bilateral facial palsy (facial diplegia), striatum lesions, Möbius' syndrome, and crocodile tears syndrome (paroxysmal lacrimation). Symptoms of facial nerve involvement include pain and facial motor abnormalities. The overt signs of a facial nerve lesion include the inability to smile or whistle, hyperlacrimation, facial twitching or paralysis (usually unilateral), facial asymmetry, and impaired taste on the anterior two-thirds of the tongue.

Cochlear Division of the Acoustic Nerve. The common symptoms of a lesion of the cochlear branch include deafness, tinnitus, hearing scotomas, and auditory hallucinations. The overt signs are diminished hearing acuity and sensory aphasia.

Vestibular Division of the Acoustic Nerve. Symptoms of a lesion of the vestibular branch include spatial disorientation, vertigo, and nausea. The major signs of vestibular nerve involvement are nystagmus, diaphoresis, hypotension, tachycardia, and vomiting.

The Midbrain

The midbrain (mesencephalon) is a short, constricted portion that connects the pons and cerebellum with the hemispheres of the cerebrum (refer to Fig. 4.10).

Basic Considerations

The midbrain is directed upward and forward, and its major structures are:

- A posterior portion (tectum), which contains four rounded eminences (corpora quadrigemina) arranged in pairs that hold important mediating centers and nuclei concerned with reflex coordination. The *superior colliculi* extend laterally to the *lateral geniculate body*, and the more prominent inferior colliculi project to the *medial geniculate body*. The former is associated with visual reflex activity; the latter, auditory reflex activity.
- An intervening passage or tunnel, the cerebral aqueduct (aqueduct of Sylvius) that joins the 3rd and 4th ventricles.
- An anterior portion, which contains a pair of cylindrical bodies (cerebral peduncles) that are made up largely of the descending and ascending fiber tracts from the cerebrum, cerebellum, medulla, and spinal cord.

The Oculomotor Nerve (Cranial III). The oculomotor nerve is a motor nerve to all ocular muscles except the lateral rectus and superior oblique. It contains fibers originating from the Edinger-Westphal nucleus. When activated, the pupil constricts and the eyeball rolls down and lateral. The nerve exits the brain on the medial side of the cerebral peduncle. It runs behind the posterior cerebral artery, anterior to the superior cerebellar artery, and lateral to the basilar artery. It then passes anteriorly in the cavernous sinus and exits the skull via the superior orbital fissure.

The Trochlear Nerve (Cranial IV). The trochlear nerve provides the major motor supply to the superior oblique muscle of the eye. When stimulated, the eyeball rolls down and medial. The nerve arises from the posterior surface of the brain stem, curves anteriorly between the posterior cerebral and superior cerebellar arteries, and continues forward (between the oculomotor and ophthalmic branch of the trigeminal) in the lateral wall of the cavernous sinus. It enters the orbit of the eye, along with the oculomotor nerve, via the superior orbital fissure.

Midbrain Dysfunction

The effects of common lesions in the midbrain are shown in Table 4.11.

The Oculomotor Nerve. Inhibiting lesions involving the oculomotor nerve affect the patient's ability to look nasally, up and nasally, up and temporally, and down and temporally. The pupil will be constricted in irritative lesions and dilated in nerve blocks.

The Trochlear Nerve. Inhibiting syndromes affecting the trochlear nerve prevent the patient from looking down and nasally.

The Cerebellum

The cerebellum develops embryologically as an outgrowth from the primary centers of the semicircular canals in the medulla. It is below the posterior portion of the cerebrum, from which it is separated by the tentorium cerebelli (a fold of dura mater), and behind the pons and upper aspect of the medulla (refer to Fig. 4.10). The oval cerebellum appears constricted in its center (vermis), flat-

Table 4.11. Lesions of the Midbrain

Area	Destructive Lesion Primary Effect
Cerebral peduncle (corticospinal tract)	Contralateral spastic paralysis
Corpora quadrigemina	Upward eye motion paralysis
Cranial III	Down and out eye motion paralysis, pupil dilation
Cranial IV	Down and in eye motion paralysis
Red nucleus, substantia nigra, reticular substance	Involuntary movements and rigidity
Syndrome/Lesion Site	**Features**
Benedikt's syndrome	
Cranial III nerve	Ipsilateral ophthalmoplegia
Red nucleus	Contralateral hyperkinesia (eg, tremor, chorea, athetosis)
Parinaud's syndrome	
Quadrigeminal plate	Conjugate vertical eye motion paralysis
Weber's syndrome	
Cranial III nerve, nucleus	Ipsilateral ophthalmoplegia
Cerebral peduncle and corticospinal tract	Contralateral hemiplegia

tened from above downward, and has lateral expanded portions (the hemispheres).

Structure

The cerebellum is divided into three lobes that have specific functions. The large *posterior lobe* is responsible for coordinated movements of the extremities, the *flocculonodular lobe* directs equilibrium and balance, and the *anterior lobe* is concerned with gait and posture.

The gray matter surface of the cerebellum is not convoluted; rather, it is transversed by numerous furrows (sulci). The gray matter contains cells from which fibers pass to form synapses in other areas of the brain and cells with which fibers entering the cerebellum from other parts of the brain form synaptic complexes. The internal structure of the cerebellum contains various important centers such as the dentate, emboliform, fastigial, globose, and interpositus nuclei.

The myelinated tracts of the cerebellum are connected with the cerebrum by the *superior peduncles*, with the pons by the *middle peduncles*, and with the medulla oblongata by the *inferior peduncles*. Afferent impulses from the motor centers of the cerebrum, the semicircular canals of the inner ear, the olivary body, and somatic muscles enter the cerebellum via the three peduncles (Table 4.12). Efferent impulses are transmitted to the motor centers in the cerebrum, to several cranial nerve nuclei, and down the brain stem and spinal cord to connect with somatic muscles. Synaptic connections occur at many levels.

Table 4.12 Major Cerebellar Tracts

	Sensory Pathways	Motor Pathways
Superior peduncle	General proprioceptors conveying muscle/joint proprioception via anterior spinocerebellar tract	From cerebellar cortex and deep nuclei (emboliformis, globosus, fastigii) to (1) contralateral red nucleus to influence rubrospinal tract and to (2) cranial nerve III, IV, VI, and XI nuclei
Middle peduncle	Frontal and temporal cerebral cortex conveying motion plans and data from eyes and ears	None known
Inferior peduncle	Fibers from olivary body	From cerebellar cortex and deep nuclei to vestibular nucleus to coordinate motion/position of head with postural tone
	Input from cutaneous receptors via nuclei cuntaneous and gracilis	
	Special proprioceptors conveying input from chochlear and vestibular tracts for head orientation	From cerebellar cortex and dentate nucleus to (1) premotor area of cerebral cortex via contralateral thalamus to influence voluntary motion and (2) contralateral red nucleus to influence rubrospinal tract
	General proprioceptors conveying muscle/joint proprioception via posterior spinocerebellar tract	

Function

Activities of the cerebellum do not enter normal consciousness. The cerebellum receives sensory impulses from the cerebral cortex, semicircular canals, body wall, and somatic muscles. It sends impulses into all somatic motor centers and helps to maintain equilibrium and the tone of voluntary muscles.

Dysfunction

Cerebellar lesions result in muscle weakness, loss of tone, and the inability to direct precise movements of skeletal muscle. There is usually difficulty in walking due to inability to control the muscles of the legs or difficulty in talking due to lack of coordination of the tongue and jaw muscles. The area of the body affected is determined by the location and extent of the damage. Only parts of the body on the ipsilateral side of the injury to the cerebellum are involved. If the damage is bilateral, then the lack of muscle tone and coordination may be so great that the patient is physically helpless.

Clinical Considerations

See Chapters 8 and 9.

THE SPINAL LEVELS

The spinal level is composed of spinal cord segments and those related neurologic tissues that extend outward from the spinal cord to slightly beyond the intervertebral foramina (IVFs). The neural structures of greatest concern are the spinal cord level, meninges, spinal nerves, and local vascular supply.

Functional Anatomy

The major structures within the vertebral canal are the spinal cord proper (central canal, gray matter, white matter, nerve root entries), blood vessels, CSF, nerve roots, and meninges.

The central gray matter of the spinal cord, which is composed of nerve cell bodies and supporting cells, is variably shaped as a crude H, and its design varies at different levels of the cord. When viewed unilaterally, the anterior portion (horn, column) contains cells of the origin of the anterior nerve roots. The lateral portion, which contains preganglionic cells of the autonomic nervous system, is most prominent in the upper cervical, thoracic, and midsacral levels of the spinal cord. The posterior portion, which extends to the posterolateral sulcus, provides an entrance for fibers within the posterior nerve roots (Fig. 4.12).

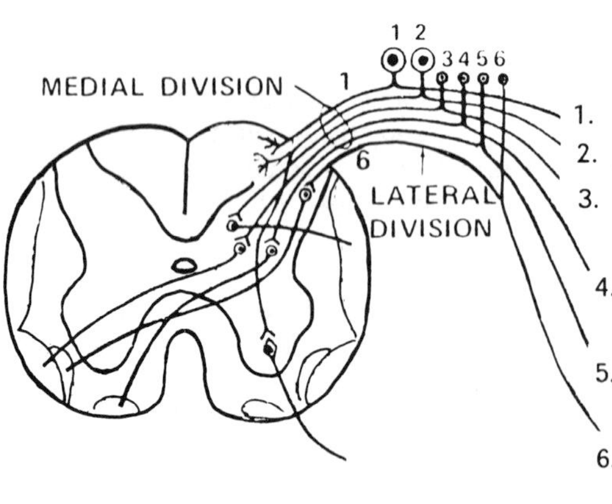

1. Pacinian corpuscles to posterior column.
2. Muscle spindles to posterior column.
3. Musculoskeletal impulses to the spinothalamic tract.
4. Musculoskeletal impulses to the spinocerebellar tract.
5. Musculoskeletal impulses to the ventral spinothalamic tract.
6. From nociceptors to the substantia gelatinosa of Rolando to connections with ipsilateral and contralateral tracts (especially spinothalamic).

Figure 4.12. Diagram of fibers entering a typical posterior root.

The white matter of the spinal cord consists of anterior, lateral, and posterior columns, which are composed of bare and myelinated nerve fibers within a network of neurolgia. Each of these columns contains ascending and descending tracts (Table 4.13).

Each segmental level (except the first and last) of the cord issues four nerve roots: an anterior and posterior root on each side. These roots are bathed in CSF. The posterior root at each side curves forward from the cord, enlarges (posterior root ganglion), then returns to its normal size, and finally becomes united with the ipsilateral anterior root by a sheath of dura mater as the ensheathed two roots exit the IVF as a spinal nerve (Fig. 4.13). Each spinal nerve then becomes part of the peripheral level and is distributed to a fairly well-defined area.

Within or just proximal to the IVF, the dura merges with the perineurium of the spinal nerve. It is primarily at this exit where the spinal nerve (and related veins and arteries) becomes most vulnerable to tension or compression from subluxations, posterolateral IVD protrusions, and apophyseal arthritic changes.

The posterior roots convey myelinated and unmyelinated sensory fibers originating in the periphery. Most of their cell bodies are in the posterior root ganglia. The anterior roots carry the (1) myelinated alpha, beta, and gamma neurons to somatic muscles and (2) myelinated preganglionic sympathetic neurons in the thoracic area and the preganglionic parasympathetic neurons in the sacral area.

Normal Reflex Activity

We frequently see the terms *sensory reflex* and *motor reflex*. These expressions of viewpoint can be misleading if the reader does not understand that all reflexes are cyclic processes (with numerous covert implications) that have an afferent (sensory) and an efferent (motor) component. For an action to manifest (whether it be a muscle contraction, a gland secretion, a thought perception, etc), the functional and structural integrity of both (afferent and efferent) components and their supportive elements must be operational. To study a reflex is to isolate a small aspect of one of many processes in a great chain of cause-and-effect processes.

General Considerations

Somatic and visceral body actions are modulated by several reflex activities, and these include all voluntary motor and involuntary autonomic actions and all sensory

Table 4.13. White Matter Tracts of the Spinal Cord

Column	Ascending Tracts	Descending Tracts
Posterior	Fasciculi gracilis and cuneatus (vibration, 2-point discrimination, passive joint motion)	Fasciculi interfasicularis and septomarginalis (association, integration)
Lateral	Anterior and posterior spinocerebellar (reflex proprioception) Lateral spinothalamic (pain, temperature) Spinotectal (reflex)	Lateral corticospinal (voluntary motion) Olivospinal (reflex) Rubrospinal (muscle tone, synergy)
Anterior	Anterior spinothalmic (light touch) Spino-olivary (reflex proprioception)	Anterior corticospinal (voluntary motion) Vestibulospinal (reflex balance) Tectospinal (audiovisual reflex) Reticulospinal (muscle tone)

perceptions, except the most simple local reflexes. Some reflexes are simple; many are complex. Some are conducted primarily at higher levels of the neuraxis, some involve multilevel integration, and some can be considered strictly horizontal (spinal and peripheral levels). It this latter type that will be described in this section.

Reflex activity is the basis of awareness, volitional activity, and homeostasis. To fail to understand the basics of reflex activity in the body is to fail to understand the science and clinical applications of chiropractic.

The efferent reflex response to a stimulus depends upon many factors such as the strength of the stimulus, the integrity of the afferent neuron, spatial and temporal summation at the spinal cord level, postsynaptic potentials at each synapse involved, longitudinal tract influences, the integrity of the final common pathway, the action at the nerve's termination, and the integrity of the straited or smooth muscles involved. Thus, a neuron does more than merely relay information; rather, it also processes (fractionalizes) that information according to these factors.

Basic Spinal Reflex Acts

The simplest form of motor control consists of a local reflex in which input from a specific sensory neuron induces output within a specific motor neuron. However, as Sherrington points out, the model of such a simple reflex is probably a purely abstract conception because all parts of the nervous

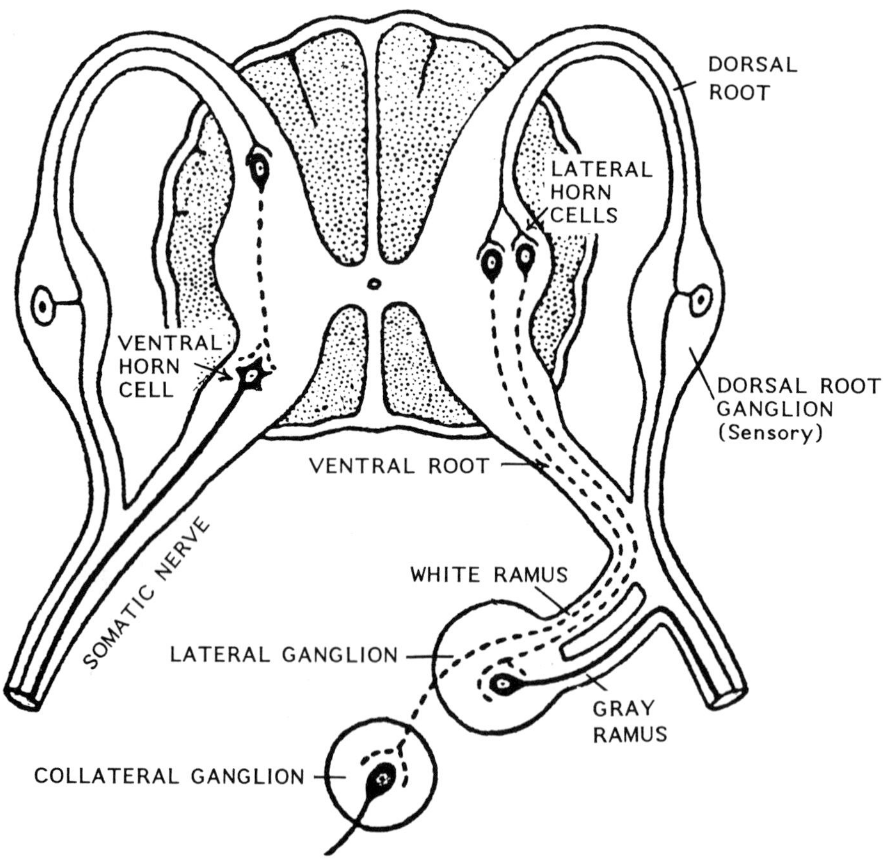

Figure 4.13. Diagram depicting the anterior and posterior roots. *Left,* somatic motor and sensory fibers; *right,* autonomic afferent and efferent pathways in and near the spinal cord.

system are connected. No part of it is probably ever capable of reaction without affecting and being affected by various other parts. It is a system never at rest.

Multithousands of such reflexes occur each minute whether the body is awake or asleep. There are three main categories of these local motor reflexes: (1) *stretch* reflexes, (2) *lengthening* reflexes, and (3) *nociceptive* reflexes. All use the final common pathway and alpha motor neurons. Refer to Table 3.4.

Reflex Modulation

Recent studies by Jankowska/Lundberg have shown that *interneurons* have a far more complex function than previously believed. Convergence of primary afferents and descending efferents appears to be the rule, with primary afferent control in multisensory and different higher centers contributing to the descending control of individual interneurons.

Flexor reflex habituation, acupuncture analgesia, and inhibitory build-up of spinal interneurons have several common characteristics in that they have a slow progressive onset and decay, are more readily induced by strong stimuli, are antagonized by strychnine, and depend upon descending influences from the brain. Pearson reports that, while the identity of the supraspinal structure which plays a part in the development of analgesia and spinal habituation has not been isolated, a likely candidate would appear to be the raphé nuclei of the brain stem. Stimulation of this area produces inhibition of the spinal interneurons and elevation of segmental pain threshold.

Stretch Reflexes

Any sudden pull on an unguarded muscle quickly stretches the involved muscle fibers. This stimulates the muscle spindle receptors (Fig. 4.14) so that action potentials are initiated in the afferent Ia fibers that are conveyed to the spinal cord and synapse with anterior horn motor cells. These activated efferent cells produce action potentials that are conveyed to the muscles of origin and the

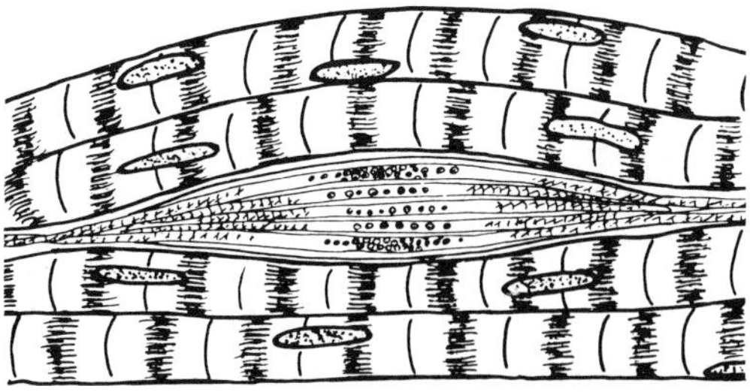

Figure 4.14. Longitudinal section representation of a neuromuscular spindle capsule lying in parallel with contractile muscle fibers.

muscles contract. It can therefore be stated that when a muscle is passively stretched by a load, the lengthening of its fibers compresses the spindles, the afferent annulospiral terminals become depolarized, and asynchronous impulses are relayed to the spinal cord via the sensory afferents. The heavier the load, the greater the stretching, and the more powerful the contraction to unload the spindles. This is one mechanism; another is that, concurrent with voluntary muscle contraction, the midfiber zone of the fiber can be stretched by contraction of the fiber's two polar segments.

There are two types of stretch reflexes: phasic (repositioning) and tonic (postural), both of which are monosynaptic and primarily involve axial and limb extensor muscles. *Phasic stretch reflexes* originate from receptors of primary endings in muscle spindles, are conducted by Group Ia (large, myelinated) afferent fibers, and usually induce a sharp transient muscle contraction and a relaxation of antagonists. *Tonic stretch reflexes* originate from receptors of secondary endings in muscle spindles, are conducted by Group II afferent fibers, and usually induce a slower and more sustained muscle contraction, a relaxation of antagonists, and activation of longitudinal motor neurons.

The large muscle afferents from muscle spindles synapse directly with motor neurons without assistance from cord interneurons. This always excitatory and always unilateral monosynaptic reflex arc serves as the basis of the stretch reflex that is restricted to the segments at the level of sensory input. This reflex becomes impaired whenever a lesion involves any part of the circuit (ie, the peripheral receptors, the distal portion of the sensory afferent neuron, the posterior root ganglion, the posterior nerve root, the ipsilateral gray matter of the spinal cord, the efferent limb of the circuit, the nerve-muscle junction, or the muscle itself. Hyperactive stretch reflexes (tendon jerks) unilaterally indicate upper motor neuron damage.

It should be noted that the myotatic stretch reflex uses a single sensory neuron and is initiated by elongation of the muscle spindle's annulospiral receptors. The effect is a protective contraction designed to protect against further stretch so that the muscle may maintain a constant length. This reflex action is many times more severe if initiated by a sudden stretch (eg, dynamic thrust) than by a slow stretch. In addition, inhibitory impulses are transmitted to the motor neurons of the antagonists (reciprocal inhibition) and facilitating impulses are transmitted to the synergists—both of which enhance the physical response. The stretch reflex is not normally initiated by voluntary contraction. If spasm occurs after trauma, the irritating focus can usually be attributed to irritating ischemia initially and blood debris later.

Stretch reflexes are often referred to clinically as *myotatic*, *tendon-jerk*, or *deep-tendon* reflexes. These latter two terms are misleading as they imply that the receptors are located within the tendon, which they are not. A tendon tap must stretch the muscle proper to activate a discharge of spindle afferents.

Role of the Neuromuscular Spindles in the Stretch Reflex. The complex muscle spindles, interspersed among skeletal muscle fibers, offer the most important sensory feedback from muscles. One large sensory annulospiral nerve fiber has branches that entwine around each muscle spindle, while other secondary flower-spray endings are sited near the extremities of the spindle (Fig. 4.15). Because they communicate messages of muscle fiber length (contraction magnitude), they are called *stretch receptors*. In addition, they also communicate information about the speed of fiber length changes (velocity). These afferent receptors have a low threshold to stretch, and their impulses excite a feedback stretch reflex that pro-

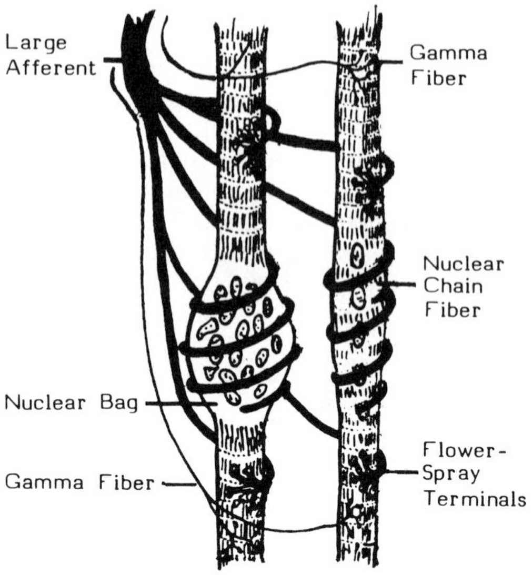

Figure 4.15. Diagram of a muscle spindle showing one nuclear bag *(left)* and one nuclear chain fiber *(right)*. The large afferent nerve fibers *(black)* end in annulospiral endings around the midzone of the muscle fibers. The smaller afferent fibers end in flower-spray terminals. Much smaller efferent gamma fibers supply both types of intrafusal fibers, as shown on the top and bottom of the diagram.

duces contraction of the same muscle.

Stretch Reflex Effects in Spasticity. Increased resistance to passive movement caused by increased tonic stretch reflexes is called *spasticity;* ie, a spastic resistance is a stretch reflex activity whose receptors are the muscle spindles that are scattered in parallel with the muscle fibers. In common spasticity disorders, the contracted muscles relax when the part is comfortably rested with support and become spastic with volitional movements, tendon tapping, and vibration, or sometimes even by startling noises.

If a constant stretch is applied to a spastic muscle and a tendon tap is applied, a sudden stretch is superimposed, and the result is a *series* of muscle contractions (clonus). It reflects a hypersensitive state of alpha motor neurons to synchronous afferent volleys.

Three hypotheses have been put forward by DeBacher to explain the hyperactive stretch reflexes that occur in spasticity:

1. Loss of corticospinal inhibition leaves the alpha motor neurons with a lower firing threshold so that they readily fire in response to any impinging sensory input, including that from stretch receptors.

2. A hyperactive gamma efferent system puts muscle spindles in a contracted state so that there is an abnormal response to stretch stimuli.

3. Spinal motor neurons normally exert a primarily inhibiting presynaptic modulating influence on afferent connections just proximal of the alpha motor neurons and damage to or dysfunction of the corticospinal pathways weaken this influence so that afferent impulses from stretch or other sensory receptors are more likely to increase the firing rate of alpha motor neurons even if the muscle spindles are not contracted.

Long-Loop Reflexes. According to Conrad/Meyer-Lohmann, long-loop reflexes may be thought of as analogous to segmental stretch reflexes. These reflexes are observed when externally perturbed volitional movements involve a transcortical route.

Lengthening Reflexes

Lengthening reflexes are sometimes called *Golgi tendon organs reflexes, inverse myotatic reflexes*, or *clasp-knife reflexes*. These reflexes are initiated at Golgi tendon organs, are conveyed by Group Ib (large, myelinated) afferents and interneurons, and produce a responsive relaxation of muscle, usually as a protective mechanism. The primary purpose of these reflexes, which effect a clasp-knife lengthening response, is thought to be to prevent overly intense contractions (that may produce muscle tears) induced by a stretch reflex.

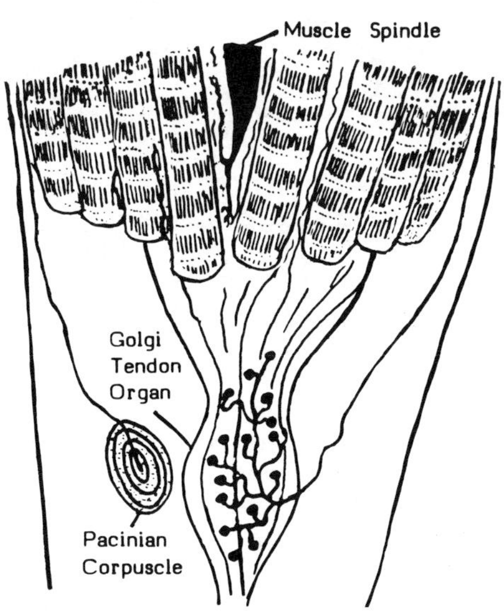

Figure 4.16. Site of a Golgi tendon organ at a musculotendinous junction.

Joint capsule and associated ligament and connective tissue afferent fibers originate from tiny areas of encapsulated collagen fasciculi. They are readily subject to movement, compression, depolarization, and firing when the tendon is stretched from muscle contraction. If the minute muscle fibers terminating in the collagen fasciculi at the musculotendinous junction are actively tensed, the Golgi organs increase their discharge of afferent impulses. Passive stretching, however, does not increase the discharge unless it is quite firm.

The more muscle fibers are passively stretched, the more powerful will be their contraction via the stretch reflex. However, this alert action by the low-threshold spindles is limited by the higher threshold Golgi tendon receptors that guard against an injurious reaction. These structures, unique to musculotendinous tissue, sense tension from either muscle contraction or extreme stretching. They have a much higher threshold to stretch than stretch receptors.

Golgi tendon organs are embedded in the musculotendinous area to protect against overstretch (Fig. 4.16). Each Golgi organ is penetrated by one or two terminal sensory fibers, and each communicates in series with several muscle fibers belonging to different motor units. Sensory input from Golgi tendon organs, pain receptors, and spindle flower-spray terminals to the spinal cord are transmitted to motor neurons via one or several interneurons and synapses that may have either an excitatory or inhibitory function. Through these multisynaptic routes, afferent impulses can be transmitted ipsilaterally, contralaterally, and inferiorly or superiorly to adjacent segments to excite accessory muscle groups or inhibit antagonists. Thus, each motor neuron is subject to numerous segmental influences as well as influences from higher centers transmitted via the descending pathways and long loops.

Reactions to Chiropractic Adjustments. A dynamic chiropractic adjustment, using a high velocity and low amplitude thrust, designed to increase the distance between muscle origin and insertion would quickly elongate the contracted muscle fibers and encourage relaxation via the *Golgi tendon organ reflex.* On the other hand, slow intermittent manipulation or traction would encourage resistance via the *stretch reflex.*

Nocifensive Reflexes

The primitive polysynaptic *nociceptive reflexes* are sometimes called withdrawal, cutaneous, or flexion reflexes (Fig. 4.17). The receptors of such reflexes originate from bare nerve endings within tissue (usually superficial) and are conveyed over small myelinated and unmyelinated (1) cutaneous A-delta and C afferents and (2) muscle Group III and C afferents to multisynaptic relays of the anterior motor neuronal pool, which has a residual after-discharge effect that outlasts the stimulus. The usual response is a quick ipsilateral flexion activation and extension inhibition (reciprocal innervation) withdrawal of the irritated limb, for example, and contralateral extension activation and flexor inhibition reaction (crossed extension) in the contralateral limb.

Abnormal nocifensive reflexes are diagnostic of CNS lesions. Babinski's plantar reflex in corticospinal tract disease is a classic example.

Sustaining Mechanisms

Reflexes such as stretch reflexes and inverse myotatic reflexes are self-limiting mechanisms whereby sensory impulses from muscle are transmitted to the same muscle via the afferent ——→ cord ——→ efferent reflex cycle. This type of activity, however, does not explain sustained activity such as seen in voluntary phasic movements. Voluntary activity is initiated and controlled by brain centers. It does not depend upon sensory stimulation, but it does include the segmental reflex centers, especially the stretch reflex circuits. Voluntary action involves loop coactivation of gamma and alpha efferents.

Gamma Neuron Reflexes

Movement can be initiated by activating either alpha or gamma motor fibers. When alpha motor neurons are stimulated, *extrafusal* muscle fibers contract and the length of the muscle spindles reduces. However, for a muscle spindle to respond appropriately to a change in tension, its length must be adjusted. This is accomplished by separate innervation (fusimotor system) via the plate and trail endings of gamma motor fibers. When the lower threshold gamma motor neurons are activated, the effect is on *intrafusal* muscle fibers of the muscle spindles. Gamma neurons receive their input segmen-

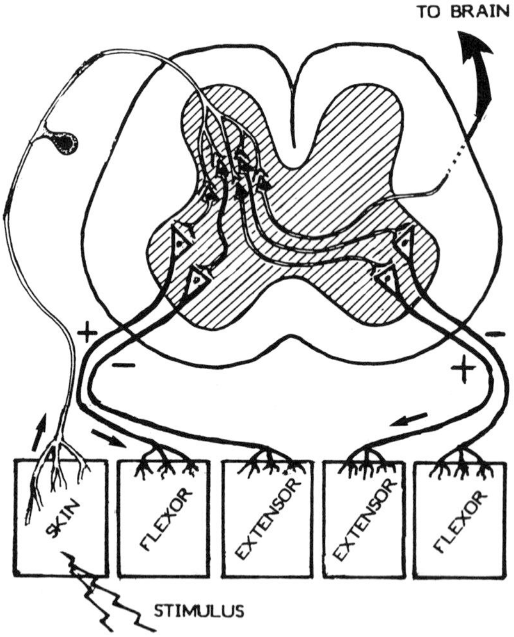

Figure 4.17. Reciprocal innervation mechanism, showing a single interneuron between the afferent and efferent fibers where there normally are many. In this example, a painful stimulus on the skin produces unilateral flexor excitation and extensor inhibition, and contralateral extensor excitation and flexor inhibition. This would be a typical nocifensive response.

tally and supraspinally from the corticospinal, reticulospinal, and propriospinal tracts.

Renshaw Inhibition

Renshaw cells are inhibiting interneuronal cells within Rexed's laminae VII and VIII of the anterior horn of the spinal cord. They project axons that interact with alpha motor neurons that innervate extrafusal muscles. When fast-twitch alpha motor fibers are activated, Renshaw cells become activated, which, in turn, temporarily inhibit the small alpha fibers of synergistic motor neurons (recurrent inhibition), thus acting as a stabilizer to subdue postural (tonic) stretch reflexes during phasic motor activity.

Righting and Placement Reflexes

Stretch reflexes, integrated in the spinal cord and medulla, are just one type of postural reflex; ie, an automatic response to keep the top side of the body or a body part properly positioned (eg, uppermost). *Optic righting reflexes* attempt to maintain the eyes on a horizontal level and depend on an intact occipital cortex. *Labyrinthine righting reflexes* attempt to maintain orientation of the head in space and require an intact midbrain. *Neck righting reflexes* arising *in* the neck attempt to maintain the body in proper relationship with the head and are integrated in the medulla. There are two types of *body righting reflexes:* (1) those acting upon the neck attempt to keep the

Table 4.14. Major Postural and Righting Reactions

	Stimulus	Receptor	Response
POSTURAL REFLEXES			
Stretch	Muscle stretch	Muscle spindles	Muscle contraction
Tonic labyrinthine	Gravity	Otoliths	Extensor rigidity
SUPPORT REFLEXES			
Hopping reaction	Lateral displacement while standing	Muscle spindles	Maintains legs in position to support body
Placement reaction	Visual, proprioceptive, and exteroceptive clues	Various	Foot or palm placed on surface to support body
Positive support	Sole or palm contact	Distal flexor proprioceptors	Foot extended to support body
Negative support	Muscle stretch	Extensor proprioceptors	Release of positive support reaction
RIGHTING REFLEXES			
Body-head righting	Lateral pressure on body	Exteroceptors	Head leveled
Body-body righting	Lateral pressure on body	Exteroceptors	Body righted even if eyes are not level
Labyrinthine righting	Gravity	Otoliths	Head leveled
Neck righting	Neck muscle stretch	Muscle spindles	Righting of trunk and pelvis
Optical righting	Visual data	Retina	Head leveled

head oriented in respect to the body and (2) body righting arising from surface receptors that act on the body in an attempt to maintain orientation in space. Both these types of body righting reflexes require an intact midbrain. These and other righting reflexes are described in Table 4.14.

Diagnostic Considerations

Part III of this book is directed almost exclusively to the study of clinical disorders originating at the spinal level. However, a few points are worthy of mention here.

At almost every level, the spinal level contains representatives of the CSF, motor, sensory, vascular, and visceral systems; thus, lesions will have widespread implications. Because the spinal level is the intermediary between the longitudinal and horizontal peripheral systems below the foramen magnum, a lesion at a spinal level may express longitudinal, peripheral, or combined manifestations.

Table 4.15. Major Signs of Spinal Level Lesions

Area Involved	Effect
Spinal Cord	
Anterior motor cell	Segmental atrophy, fasciculation, weakness, hypotonia.
Central processes of primary sensory neurons	Sensory loss.
Preganglionic fibers in the intermediolateral column	Sympathetic disturbances.
Spinal Nerve	
Autonomic fibers	Visceral and circulatory dysfunction.
Motor fibers	Flaccid weakness in a dermatomal pattern (later associated atrophy), possible fasciculation and fibrillation, with paraspinal changes related to posterior primary rami involvement.
Sensory fibers	Sensory loss (especially pain, temperature, touch) in a dermatomal pattern, with episodes of spontaneous pain (often referred), possible paresthesia or dysesthesia, and local tenderness.
Intersegmental Lesions	
Autonomic fibers	Signs of malfunction such as hypotension, perspiration disorders, or loss of bladder and rectal control.
Direct and indirect activation pathways	Inhibited abdominal, nociceptive, and crossed extension reflexes.
Long tract motor fibers	Spastic paralysis, exaggerated tendon reflexes, Babinski's plantar reflex.
Long tract sensory fibers	Signs of lateral spinothalamic and posterior column involvement.

Diseases at the spinal level can be classified into focal segmental (eg, IVF syndromes), focal intersegmental (eg, involving both segmental and longitudinal fibers), or diffuse (eg, meningitis, degenerative disorders). Typical signs are shown in Table 4.15.

Spinal Cord Injuries

Injuries to the lumbar cord or its tail occur from vertebral fractures, dislocations, or penetrating wounds in severe accidents. In rare instances, the cord may be damaged from violent falls with trunk flexion. The T12—L1 and L5—S1 areas are the common sites of injury, especially those of crushing fractures with cord compression. Neurologic symptoms develop rapidly, but the lower the injury, the fewer roots will be involved. More common than these rare occurrences are cord tractions, concussions, and contusions. Even a trace of sensory abnormality, objective or subjective, should immediately raise the suspicion of injury to the spinal cord or cauda equina.

Concussion of the Spinal Cord. Immediate signs of cord concussion are usually not manifested in mild or moderate injuries; but weeks later, lower extremity weakness and stiffness may be experienced. It takes time for nerve fibers to degenerate. Deep reflexes become exaggerated and originally mild sensory, bladder, and rectal disturbances progress. The picture is cloudy, often mimicking a number of cord diseases (eg, sclerosis, atrophy, syringomyelia). Life is rarely threatened, but a prognosis of full recovery should be well guarded.

Contusions of the Spinal Cord. Cord concussion usually complicates cord contusion. If laceration occurs, shock is rapid. Deep reflexes, sensation, and sphincter control are lost. The paralysis is flaccid. Obviously, a prognosis cannot be made until the shock is survived.

Pathologic Traction of the Spinal Cord. A scoliotic lumbar deviation is usually attended by a commensurate vertebral body rotation to the convex side. If this does not occur, it is atypical and most likely pain producing. If the vertebral bodies were not subject to the law of rotation during bending, the spine would have to lengthen during bending and its contents (ie, cord, cauda equina, and their coverings) would be subjected to considerable stretch. Thus, in a case of scoliotic deviation without body rotation toward the convex side, signs indicating undue tension within the vertebral canal should be sought. It also should be noted that atlanto-occipital, atlantoaxial, and coccygeal disrelation with partial fixation places a degree of traction upon the cord, dura, and dural sleeves in flexion-extension and lateral bending efforts.

Reflex Phenomena in Spinal Disorders

Sandoz believes that the main reflex phenomena associated with vertebral disarrangements and adjustments pertain to referred pain, the regulation of tonic and phasic activity of the innervated paraspinal musculature, the peripheral modulation of pain perception, and tonic neck reflexes.

THE PERIPHERAL LEVELS

The peripheral levels contain those neurologic structures exterior to the skull, vertebral column, and sacrum; and at each horizontal level, the sensory, motor, visceral, and vascular systems are represented.

Peripheral nerve histology and end-organs function have been described previously. Thus, mention of these subjects in this section will be brief. To review fiber class, diameter size, conduction velocity, and function, refer to Table 3.4.

The Peripheral Nerves

Each peripheral nerve has a well-defined course in textbooks. Such descriptions are averages, and it is not uncommon to see this course vary from 1 to 2 inches at various sites in individuals once they have extended well beyond their origins in the CNS. Things are not always as they should be, and to believe otherwise may lead to erroneous conclusions.

As each nerve progresses, it usually branches many times, and thick branches divide again and again, until a fine network of minute twigs is formed. This can be likened in many respects with the design of the tree, with the trunk of the tree representing the spinal column (Fig. 4.18). Within his 1925 text, Riley stated: "So completely are nerves distributed to parts of the body that were everything but the nerves removed, they alone would preserve the shape of the body in all its outlines."

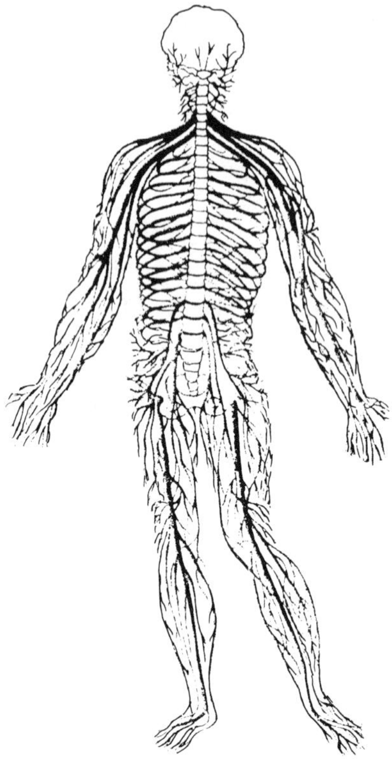

Figure 4.18. An artist's conception of the nervous system's extensive distribution.

The Peripheral Plexuses

A nerve *plexus* is a complex network of peripheral axons. There are three large somatic plexuses: the cervical, the brachial, and the sacral (lumbosacral). Refer to Table 3.12 for the neurologic signs exhibited in the cervical and lumbosacral radiculopathies. As weakness is a common sign in impairment of somatic effectors, testing distal muscle strength will often aid in localization (Table 4.16).

Table 4.16. Commonly Tested Muscles and Their Innervation

Muscle(s)	Spinal Nerves*	Muscle(s)	Spinal Nerves*
Neck flexors	C1—C6	Thigh adductor	L2—L4
Neck extensors	C1—C6	Quadriceps	L2—L4
Shoulder ext. rotators	C5—C6	Iliopsoas	L3—L4
Deltoid	C5—C6	Anterior tibial	L4—L5
Biceps brachii	C5—C6	Thigh abductor	L4—S1
Triceps	C6—C8	Hamstrings	L4—S1
Wrist extensors	C6—C8	Toe extensors	L4—S1
Wrist flexors	C6—T1	Peronei	L5—S1
Digit extensors	C7—C8	Posterior tibial	L5—S1
Digit flexors	C7—T1	Toe flexors	L5—S1
Thenar	C8—T1	Gastrocnemius	L5—S2
Hypothenar	C8—T1	Gluteus maximus	S1—S2
Interossei	C8—T1	Rectal sphincter	S3—S4
Abdomen	T8—T1		

*Spinal innervation varies somewhat in many people. The spinal nerves listed here are averages; eg, the abdominals may be innervated from T7-L1, T8-T12, or T8-L1 in a particular patient. Thus, an allowance of a segment above and below those listed should be considered.

The Posterior Rami

Shortly after the junction of the anterior and posterior roots, a typical spinal nerve divides into three divisions: (1) the rami commicantes, (2) a posterior primary division, and (3) an anterior primary division. See Figure 4.19. The fibers of the *anterior primary division* are most prominent in their formation of the cervical, brachial, and lumbosacral plexuses. The usually smaller *posterior primary division* consists of a medial branch and a lateral branch. The medial branch is sensory for the most part. The lateral branch is primarily a motor

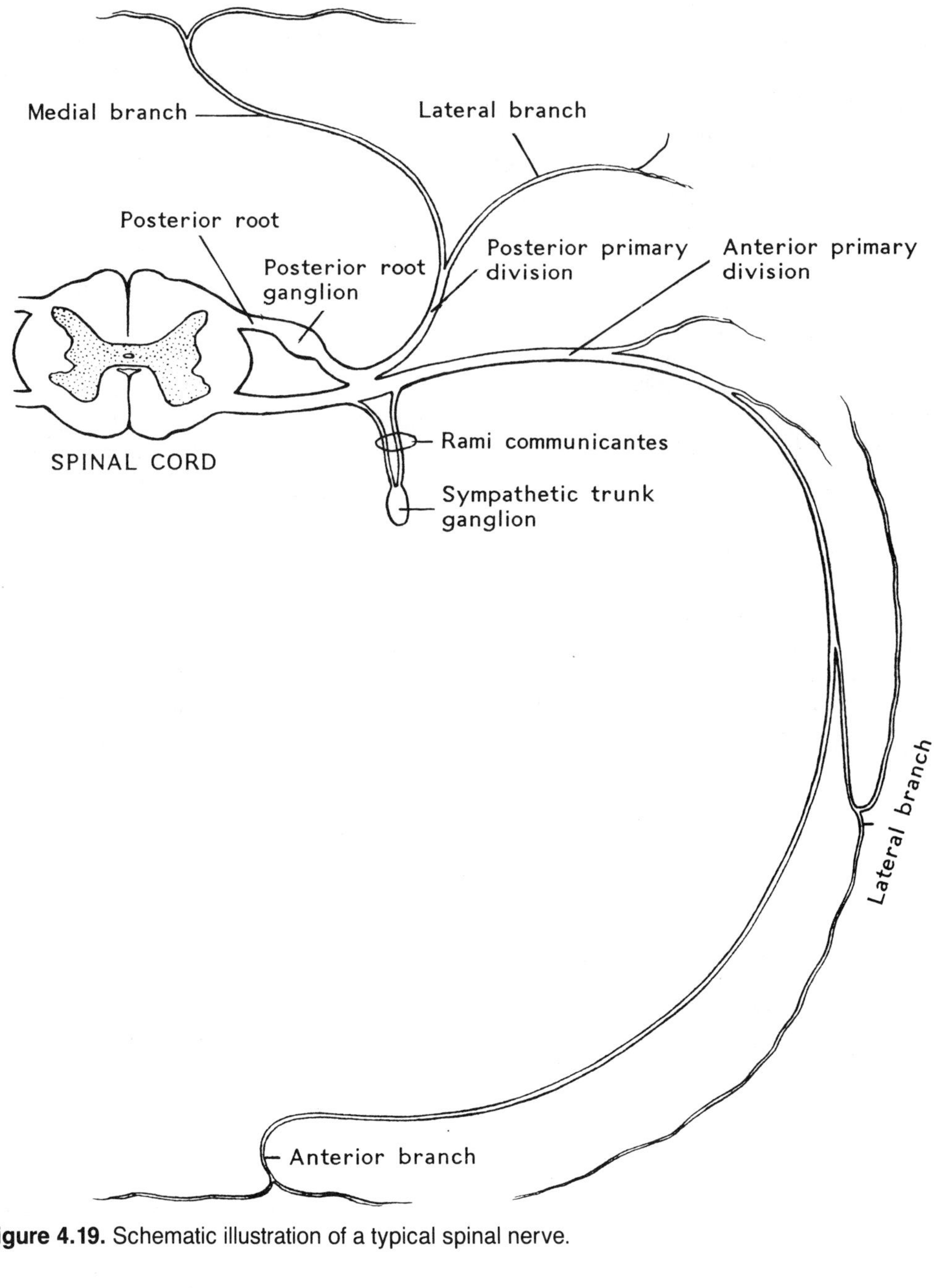

Figure 4.19. Schematic illustration of a typical spinal nerve.

nerve, but numerous sensory and autonomic fibers are present.

Significance of Tenderness. Tenderness over the rami of the posterior division has particular significance in the palpatory examination of the spine. The sensory distribution runs in a zone extending from the posterior scalp to the coccygeal area and then laterally to the greater trochanter.

Muscle Histology

Each cylindrical muscle fiber is covered with a specialized layer of *sarcolemma* that covers a peripheral longitudinal layer of nuclei and cylindrical myofibrils. Sacrolemma insulates each fiber from adjacent fibers so that excitation of one fiber does not affect its neighbors.

The basic functional unit of muscle is the *sarcomere*, many of which are connected end to end to form a single myofibril. About a thousand myofibrils, lying side by side, are contained within each muscle cell. Dispersed in a regular pattern among myofibrils is the sacroplasmic reticulum, which is an extensive membrane system of minute tubes; viz, the T-tubule system. This system is the major site of calcium sequestration within muscle tissue.

The tunnels of the T-tubule system, unique to muscle cells, extend completely through the cell and are continuous with the extracellular space at both ends. The fluid within them is primarily extracellular fluid that is thought to be altered by the interaction of its biochemical components with the extremely thin walls of the narrow tubules. Each tubule within a muscle cell is closely associated with several enlargements of the sacroplasmic reticulum (cisterns). Some unknown signal passes from the tubules to the cisterns during excitation during the contraction process.

Within each muscle fiber, there are a thousand or more longitudinal myofibrils arranged in bundles that constitute about 80% of fiber volume. Each myofibril contains many white *I bands* and many dark, short, thicker *A bands*, and each of these isotropic and anisotropic bands contains specialized zones. It is the stacking of myofibrils in register that gives voluntary muscle its microscopic transverse striations (Fig. 4.20).

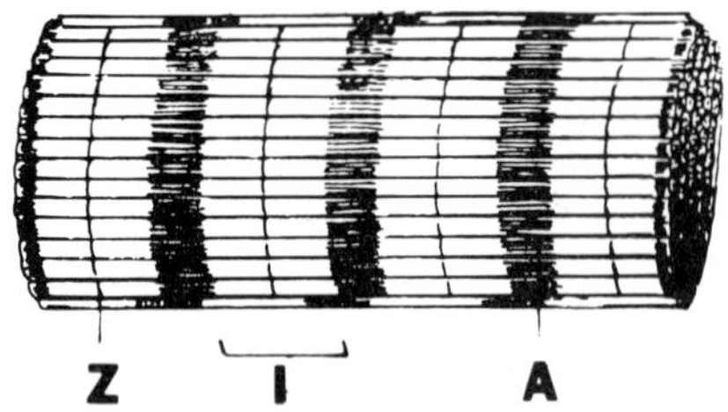

Figure 4.20. Muscle fiber schematic showing arrangement of dark A bands and light I bands.

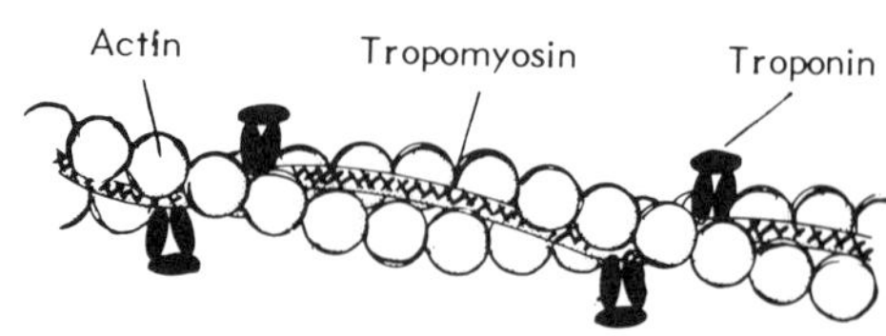

Figure 4.21. Diagram of the probable double helix arrangement of actin molecules along the minute strings of tropomysin (cross-hatched) and occasional troponin (black) within the thin I bands of a muscle fiber.

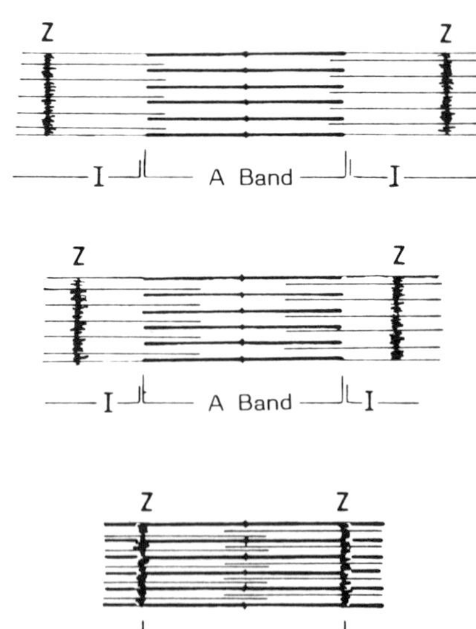

Figure 4.22. The probable arrangement of muscle filaments during stretch *(top)*, relaxation *(center)*, and strong contraction *(bottom)*.

The thin white bands of myofibrils contain smaller myofilaments composed of actin, tropomyosin, and troponin protein (Fig. 4.21); the thick dark bands consist primarily of myosin protein. An A band contains a central *H zone* composed solely of myosin filaments that interdigitate with the thin actin filaments on either side. The midpoints of the myosin filaments are secured to one another transversely by connections whose line of cross links is termed the M line at the middle of the H zone.

Gross muscle shortening should not be confused with filament shortening. During excitation, the contractile elements do shorten; however, whether the gross muscle shortens or not depends on the relation of the internal muscle force developed to the load. At the ultramicroscopic level, it is believed that the contractile elements (actin and myosin) also slide into an overlapping interdigitated arrangement upon excitation (Fig. 4.22).

The Neuromuscular Junction

The neuromuscular junction can be considered a specialized type of neuroeffector synapse. The myelin sheath of the terminal axon narrows and then ceases just prior to the motor end-plate. At the site of the end-plates, capillary anastomoses are especially well developed to maintain good nutrition.

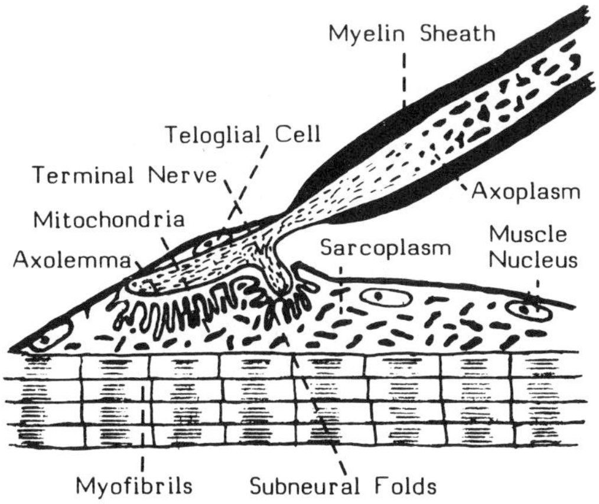

Figure 4.23. Diagram of a neuromuscular junction, its major components, and its relationship with myofibrils.

Nerve fibers enter the endomysium but do not penetrate the sarcolemma; their terminal branches appose the surface of the muscle fiber (Fig. 4.23). This site is a specialized area of axolemma and sarcolemma where the subneural apparatus is folded into clefts and the sarcolemma is abundant with mitochondria. It is a specialized area that serves as a minute structural barrier where the nerve impulse must be transmitted chemically.

Axon terminals contain mitochondria and numerous vesicles that store the chemical bridge acetylcholine which allows the nerve impulse to be transmitted across the synapse (Fig. 4.24). It is thought that the transmitter substance changes sarcolemma permeability to allow an influx of sodium ions which generates the electric potential to release the calcium necessary in turn for the acetylcholine release that allows the interaction of myosin and actin filaments to produce muscle contraction.

The enzyme cholinesterase has a dual function. It can activate nerve sheath acetylcholine into its active form or degrade it into acetic acid and choline. Thus, a lack of cholinesterase can either produce abnormal or

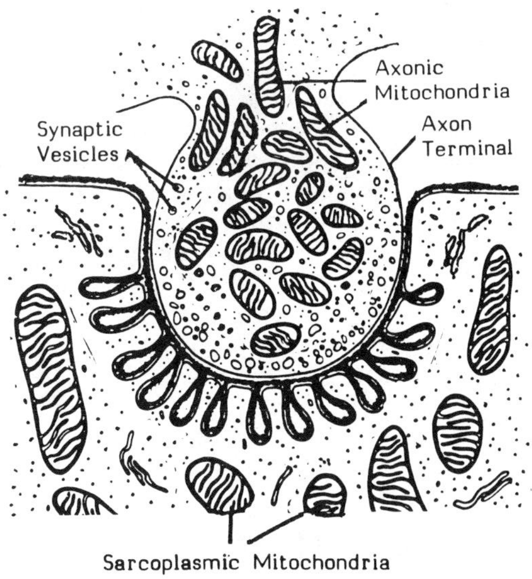

Figure 4.24. Illustration of the bulbous axon terminal, its vesicles and mitochondria, and its relationship to the subneural trough, clefts, and sarcoplasmic mitochondria.

subnormal function. This often manifests as jerking skeletal muscles just before or during sleep. This sign is thought to be due to a lack of cholinesterase that prevents residual acetylcholine from being properly inactivated. A complaint of frequently dropping objects involuntarily also may represent a shortage of cholinesterase failing to inactivate acetylcholine. Such signs may be a clue to otherwise subclinical riboflavin and/or niacin deficiency that may be expressed in neuromuscular biomechanical mechanisms.

Impulse Response

Nerves containing both motor and sensory fibers pierce muscle fascia at the site of the primary arterial branch (the neurovascular hila). These nerves then fan out to supply both motor and sensory nerve fibers to each muscle spindle.

With the arrival of nerve impulses, usually below 50/sec, all muscle fibers of a motor unit contract synchronously and contract to their maximum (all-or-none law). When several motor units are stimulated by asynchronous firings, the attached fibers contract, and voluntary body movement occurs. However, because motor units fatigue after several stimulations, other units must be called into play to allow for smooth movement. While it appears during normal muscle contraction that all muscle fibers are in a smooth continuous muscle contraction, they are not. This appearance results from the sum of a series of small groups of fibers contracting at the same moment.

All muscle fibers of a motor unit do not lie in an adjacent position. They are spread throughout the muscle belly so that excitation will produce a weak contraction in a broad area of the muscle, rather than a strong contraction at an isolated area. This allows delicate manipulations.

Muscle Spindles and Their Role in Motor Reflexes

It has been previously described that the alpha motor neuron must fire if a skeletal muscle is to contract; thus its designation as the "final common pathway" for motion. The major sources of input are the muscles spindles and the higher CNS centers related to voluntary movement. Muscle spindles also provide signals to the CNS about muscle stretch via Ia fibers and about steady muscle tension over group II fibers.

As described earlier, each muscle spindle contains a few muscle fibers whose purpose is *not* to help in contracting the whole muscle but to control the sensitivity of the muscle spindle to stretch. Spindle fibers are controlled by gamma motor neurons, while other muscle fibers are activated separately by alpha motor neurons. DeBacher has found that the more contracted muscle spindles become, the more sensitive they are to stretch stimuli.

If a tendon of an agonist muscle is tapped, the muscle and the spindle within it are lengthened and this excites the primary spindle receptors (the annulospiral endings) at the ends of the Ia fibers. This causes volleys of action potentials to course along many Ia fibers to the spinal cord wherein they excite many alpha motor neurons, whose action potentials, in turn, cause the muscle to contract. This concise explanation of these mechanisms by Prichard goes on to note that the synapse transmitter between the Ia terminals and the motor neuron pickup is unknown but thought to be of an electrical rather than chemical nature.

When the Ia volley stimulates motor neurons regulating its own muscle, it retards those regulating the antagonists through a disynaptic pathway. Again, the mode of impulse transfer to the inhibitory interneuron is unknown, but it is understood that the interneuron releases glycine which produces an inhibitory postsynaptic potential (IPSP) on the antagonist motor neuron.

The role of muscle spindles is to provide data to the CNS about muscle stretching *rates*. The spindles do this through the action potentials conveyed within the train of volleys conducted by the Ia fibers. Using this information plus signals concerned with limb position, the CNS computes the general position of the limb at some near future time. This calculated guess is necessary because without the element of anticipation, the time required for conduction from sensory receptors to cord, central processing, and conduction to muscle would be too long to regulate rapid motion.

The gamma (fusiform) motor neurons regulate the sensitivity of the spindle system by directing the shortening of the modified intrafusal muscle fibers. These fibers are in series with the central-receptor aspects of the spindles. As with alpha motor neurons, gamma fibers receive signals of many types and from various sources, including each other and the alpha motor neurons. It should be pointed out, however, that this complex segmental apparatus is only the lowest aspect of a highly integrated CNS system for central motor control.

The Contraction Process

When a decision is made at the supratentorial level to move a part (ie, contract the muscle fibers of specific motor units), a chain of command is invoked that has an action potential which is transmitted down the spinal cord and then peripherally to the appropriate neuromuscular junctions. From here, the action potential spreads from the end-plate area of the muscle cell along its plasma membrane, and acts upon the muscle cells to trigger the contraction process.

The action-potential process for muscle fibers is similar to that described for nerve fibers. The mechanism is initiated on the electrically excitable membrane surrounding the chemosensitive but electrically inexcitable end-plate by currents flowing through end-plate channels caused to conduct by acetylcholine.

When a nerve impulse reaches the neuromuscular junction, a transmitter is released that diffuses through the barrier to excite the muscle fiber. The energy potential enters the muscle fiber, via the minute T tubules, then travels to the A and I band junctions where it triggers the release of calcium, which initiates the process of fiber activity. Myofibril contractile elements tense as the action potential travels across the sarcolemma. The rate is 1—3 m/sec.

During rest, the thick myosin myofilaments only slightly overlap the thin actin myofilaments. During excitation, the A and I bands are thought to slide increasingly into an overlapping position to a degree proportional to the chemical interactions between filaments. The light bands appear to shorten and finally disappear as the thin filaments slide toward each other between the dark myofilaments. When the action potential ceases, calcium returns to storage, the elastic elements recoil, and the thin I bands draw back to their relaxed state (refer to Fig. 4.22).

Contraction Strength

Muscle power is equal to the load moved times the speed at which the load is moved. The amount of shortening (strength) of a muscle fiber following a stimulus depends on a combination of such complex variables as: (1) the number of nerve fibers employed in carrying stimuli to the muscle fibers, (2) the specific characteristics of the stimulus, (3) the speed at which the muscle is required to act, (4) the rate of flow of nerve impulses arriving from each active nerve fiber, (5) the degree of stretched fiber elongation at the beginning of contraction, (6) whether the muscle tissue is warm or cool, and (7) the state of local fatigue and nutrition. Although maximum effort may be applied to a task, biomechanical performance will be either enhanced or diminished by these conditions.

In addition to the above seven factors, the mechanism of the generation of motor nerve impulses in the brain is so susceptible to environmental and psychologic influences that the absolute strength of stimuli (number of nerve fibers and rate of nerve impulses) in two similar situations is unpredictable; eg, motivation affects work output. Different people respond differently to an identical stimulus.

Clinical Considerations

From a clinical standpoint, lesions of peripheral nerves are divided into disorders of nerve proper and disorders of their end organs. This is because impairments of nerves have different characteristics than do disorders of end-organs.

Focal and Diffuse Disorders

Diseases involving peripheral nerves may be either focal (involving one nerve) or diffuse (involving whole areas of peripheral nerves). See Figure 4.25.

Focal Disorders. Focal lesions are usually caused by trauma, entrapment, or an impinging mass. Nerves that pass through or near joints and dense soft tissues are particularly vulnerable to injury. Vertebral subluxation, carpal tunnel, tarsal tunnel, and other entrapment syndromes are common examples. Some nerves, are subject to trauma by being superficially exposed; eg, the peroneal nerve curves outwardly around the head of the fibula at the knee and thus is especially vulnerable to "clipping" injuries in football.

Diffuse Disorders. Diffuse lesions may be the result of poisoning, severe trauma, or a wide variety of degenerative, vascular, inflammatory, metabolic, endocrine, and neoplastic disorders. Either the myelin, the axons, or both may be involved, but in each instance, the clinical features are similar: (1) loss of most sensations distally; (2) paresthesia, dysesthesia, and hyperalgesia; (3) absent or diminished reflexes; and (4) distal muscle weakness leading to faccidness, atrophy, and deformity. Disorders involving primarily the axons feature early distal muscle fibrillation and severe atrophy. Disorders involving primarily the myelin are characterized by little or no early fibrillation and only minor atrophy.

Specific Peripheral Nerve Disease

Diseases involving peripheral nerves usually exhibit combined sensory, motor, and

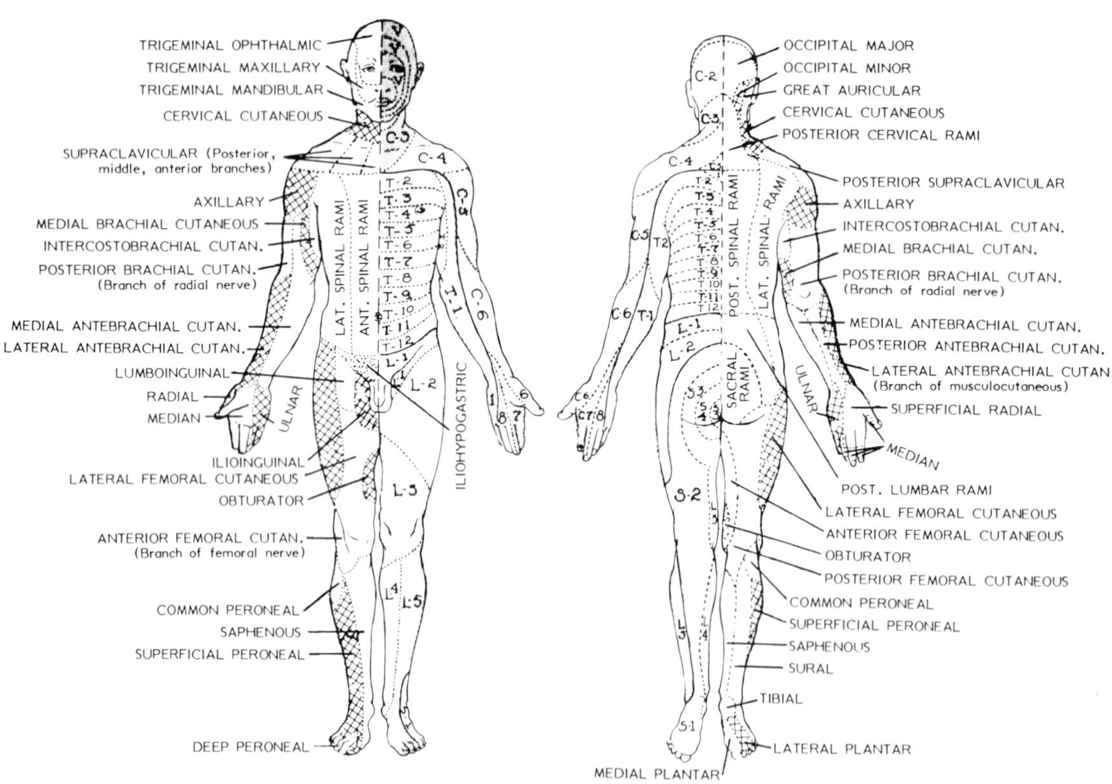

Figure 4.25. *Left,* anterior view of segmental and peripheral nerve distribution of the body. *Right,* posterior view. Peripheral distribution is shown on the right of each diagram; segmental (radicular), on the left.

autonomic signs and symptoms. Typical sensory/motor examples include segmental distal weakness and atrophy, absent or diminished sensations, and segmental loss or impairment of superficial and deep reflexes. If autonomic fibers are involved, temperature, perspiration, and trophic abnormalities will be exhibited. Causalgia also may be reported.

Neuronal Plasticity in the Healing Process: A Brief Review

When axons are injured by either trauma or a disease process, Bishop describes the process as an initial sealing of the cut ends. This is followed by orderly degenerative and phagocytic events in the segments lying distal and proximal to the lesion. Injured axons lose their dentrites and, thus, their synapses. Electrophysiologic and biochemistry properties are altered to prepare the injured neurons for synthesizing proteins needed for the formation of growth cones and regeneration of the fibers. During this period, the denervated muscle, if one is involved, undergoes dramatic atrophic changes that not only modify the electrical and chemical properties of its membrane but also reduce the diameter and weight of its fibers.

The response to injury of sensory axons depends on the site of the lesion. Cutting the fibers of a posterior root, for example, causes Wallerian degeneration of the primary afferents' central processes. Collateral sprouts from neighboring uncut root fibers are thought to take over the vacant synapses on the 2nd order neurons in the dorsal horn. Cutting a sensory axon peripherally eliminates the receptive field of the primary afferent initially, but in time, collaterals from neighboring cutaneous afferents provide the 2nd order neurons with a new receptive field. Synaptic reclamation and receptive field reorganization are but two dramatic examples of neuronal plasticity that lead to "rewired" neural circuitry.

Motor Axonal Impairments

A major sign of early motor impairment is *fasciculation*. Fasciculation (a small twitch under the skin) reflects a low-threshold firing somewhere in the motor unit (commonly in the efferent fiber), that is producing neuronal irritability and possible spontaneous firing. A similar hypersensitivity in a sensory fiber is perceived by the patient as pain if the small fibers are irritated or as a paresthesia (eg, tingling) if the large fibers are involved.

Axolemmal Blocks. Sole structural membrane blocks are rare. Physiologic blocks follow the effects of mechanical pressure, electrical shock, heat, ice, ethyl chloride, local anesthetics and certain other drugs. Transient, reversible paresthesia (numbness, pins-and-needles) is the major symptom.

Axoplasmic Disorders. A nerve's axoplasm and its flow is commonly disturbed by laceration, heavy pressure, or other types of severe injury. In some chronic slowly progressing disorders, the fibers tend to die distally (axonal atrophy) such as seen from local compression and in various deficiency, genetic, metabolic, and toxic states. Wallerian degeneration follows in both acute and chronic forms.

Note: In situations of local compression (eg, an entrapment syndrome), moderate narrowing of the axons involved results in a slowed conduction speed. Such axons will still transmit impulses but at subnormal rates. The higherfrequency impulses are affected most; thus, most noticeable will be impairments in (1) muscle spindle output, (2) rapid vibration perception, and (3) muscle contraction deficiency.

Myelin Disorders. A loss of myelin results in slowed conduction velocity as reflected in loss of reflexes and strong muscle contraction, and impaired vibration and proprioceptive sensations. As demyelinization progresses, action potentials will become completely blocked. Genetic, immunologic, and toxic disorders are the common causes.

Neuromuscular Trophic Impairments

Efferent nerves supplying muscles provide an important factor in muscle nutrition. Because of this, a denervated muscle will undergo membrane changes and atrophy. There are four common forms of this disorder:

1. In straited muscle trophic impairment, alpha efferents are involved and a spreading hypersensitivity of acetylcholine receptors results that starts adjacent to the end-plate. ***Fibrillation*** (rhythmic twitching of single muscle fibers) is an early finding.

2. In anterior horn cell involvement, one or more descending pathways are involved and hypersensitivity results from local sensory input. *Spasticity, hyperreflexia*, and *clonus* are early findings.

3. In destruction of postganglionic parasympathetic fibers of the oculomotor nerve, hypersensitivity to acetylcholine analogs results. ***Mydriasis*** (abnormal pupil dilation) is an early sign.

4. In destruction of postganglionic sympathetic fibers of the oculomotor nerve, hypersensitivity to epinephrine analogs results. ***Miosis*** (abnormal pupil constriction) is an early feature.

Neuromuscular Junction Disease

Neuromuscular junction disease (NMJD) mimics and differs from axonal disorders in several respects. There is no atrophy, reflexes and muscle tone are normal, sensory perception is intact, mental function is normal, and no signs are evident of longitudinal tract involvement. The major features of NMJD are fluctuating weakness upon exertion (usually in proximal or cranial muscles). See Table 4.17.

Peripheral Nerve Pinch, Stretch, and Compression Syndromes

Nerve "pinch" or "stretch" syndromes are especially common in sports. They are also seen after falls and industrial accidents, and the syndrome effects appear throughout the

Table 4.17. Differentiation of Multiple Sclerosis and Peripheral Nerve Disorders

	Major Signs and Symptoms	
Multiple sclerosis	Abdominal reflexes absent Deep reflexes increased Bilateral + plantar Babinski Nystagmus Intention tremor Slow staccato speech	Pain absent Optic temporal pallor Remittent episodic course Transient blindness or blurred vision
Radiculopathy	Boggy paravertebral tissues Dermatome, myotome, or sclerotome sensory changes Hyperesthesia Normal—subnormal deep reflexes Paresthesia, especially numbness	Paresis (late) Radiating pain, increased by certain motions and increased intrathecal pressure Segmental neuralgia Superficial tenderness Weakness (isolated)
Peripheral neuropathy	Atrophic flaccid paralysis Fasciculation (sometimes) Neuralgia Paresthesia Subnormal sensory changes	Subnormal stretch, superficial, and tendon reflexes Trophic lesions Weakness (distal)
Myasthenia gravis	Dysarthria Dysphagia Expressionless face Diplopia Ptosis Fasciculation absent	No sensory loss or wasting Hyperfatigue, rapidly recovering Normal tendon jerks, muscle tone, direct myotatic response, plantar reflex

cranium, spine, pelvis, and extremities. Hardly any peripheral nerve is exempt.

A *nerve pinch syndrome* may be due to direct trauma (contusion and swelling), subluxation, a protruded disc which results in nerve compression, sclerosis, or fracture (callus formation and associated posttraumatic adhesions). Any telescoping, hyperflexion, hyperextension, or hyperrotational force to the spine may result in a nerve pinch syndrome where pain may be local or extended distally. Peripheral nerve pinch syndromes are less common than nerve stretch syndromes but are usually more serious.

A *nerve stretch syndrome* is commonly associated with sprains, severe lateral cervical flexion with shoulder depression, or dislocations. Nerve fibers may be stretched, partially torn, or ruptured most anywhere in the nervous system from the cord to peripheral nerve terminals.

Table 4.18. Selected Nerve Entrapment Syndromes

UPPER-EXTREMITY SYNDROMES

Syndrome	Site	Nerve	Major Findings*
Anterior interosseous	Proximal forearm	Anterior interosseous	Abnormal pinch sign; normal sensations; flexor pollicis longus, pronator quadratus, and flexor digitorum profundus weakness; poorly defined ache in forearm.
Carpal tunnel	Wrist	Median	Pain, paresthesias, numbness, and poor two-point discrimination in thumb and radial 2-1/2 fingers; hypoesthesia especially on palmar aspect of second digit; thenar weakness and wasting; positive Tinel's and Phalen's signs.
Cubital tunnel	Elbow	Ulnar	Sensory loss in ulnar 1-1/2 fingers and ulnar aspect of the hand; weakness and wasting of ulnar intrinsic and flexor digitorum profundus; ache in medial elbow and forearm; little finger numbness; positive Tinel's sign.
Guyon's canal	Wrist	Ulnar	Sensory loss in ulnar 1-1/2 fingers; weakness and wasting of ulnar intrinsic muscles.
Postcondylar groove	Elbow	Ulnar	Sensory loss in ulnar 1-1/2 fingers and ulnar aspect of the hand; weakness and wasting of ulnar intrinsic and flexor carpi ulnaris muscles; elbow joint deformity.
Posterior interosseous	Proximal forearm	Posterior interosseous	Normal sensation; wrist drop; dull ache in dorsal forearm; difficult finger extension.
Pronator	Proximal forearm	Median	Proximal forearm pain and tenderness; flexor pollicis longus and abductor pollicis brevis weakness; paresthesias in thumb and radial 3-1/2 fingers; forearm and hand pain; positive Tinel's sign.

Table 4.18 continued

Syndrome	Site	Nerve	Major Findings*
Radial	Midarm, spiral groove	Radial	Sensory loss in radial side of dorsal hand; wrist drop; weak wrist and finger extensors; possible sensory impairment in web of thumb.
Crutch or sleep palsy	Axilla, humeral groove	Radial	Sensory loss of radial forearm; loss of elbow extension; wrist drop.

LOWER-EXTREMITY SYNDROMES

Syndrome	Site	Nerve	Major Findings*
Femoral	Inguinal area or pelvis	Femoral	Sensory loss of anteromedial thigh; weakness and wasting of quadriceps femoris; local tenderness in groin; impaired knee jerk.
Meralgia paresthetica	Inguinal area	Lateral cutaneous of thigh	Sensory loss, paresthesias, burning pain, and numbness in anterolateral thigh; no motor weakness.
Obturator	Pelvis	Obturator	Sensory loss of superomedial thigh; thigh adductor weakness.
Peroneal	Neck of fibula	Common peroneal	Sensory loss of dorsal foot and lateral leg; foot drop; steppage gait; local tenderness; anterior and lateral compartment atrophy.
Tarsal tunnel	Ankle	Posterior tibial	Burning pain and paresthesias of sole and toes; weakness of intrinsic foot muscles.

*Modified from Reddy

Peripheral Nerve Entrapment Syndromes

A peripheral entrapment syndrome represents a distinct type of neuropathy in which a single nerve is compressed at a specific site (eg, within fibrous tissue, a fibrous-osseous tunnel, or a muscle), either by external forces or by normally surrounding tissues. Local impairment of blood supply may further damage the entrapped nerve if associated vessels become stretched, kinked, or compressed. Thus, two factors must be considered: (1) the effects of pressure upon nerve fibers and (2) the effects of ischemia upon nerve fibers. These factors may exist separately or in combination.

So that a patient may avoid unnecessary pain and disability, it is important to identify a peripheral entrapment syndrome rapidly through careful examination and appropriate diagnostic studies such as EMGs, nerve conduction evaluations, and diagnostic imaging. Severe impairment of nerve function is usually only reversible in its early stages.

The major features of upper- and lower-extremity nerve entrapment syndromes are shown in Table 4.18. Spinal entrapment syndromes are described throughout Part III.

Bibliography

Abdel-Maguid TE, Bowsher D: Interneurons and proprioneurons in the adult human spinal gray matter and in the general somatic and visceral afferent cranial nerve nuclei. *Journal of Anatomy*, 139(1): 9-19, 1984.

Arbuckle BE: Reflexes. *Journal of the American Osteopathic Association*, 46(7), July 12, 1946.

Bartocci PA: The psychological self, the ego, and personality. *American Psychologist*, 10:191-198, 1955.

Benson H: Chinese project. Department of Medicine, Division of Behavioral Medicine, Beth Israel Hospital, 330 Brookline Avenue, Boston, MA 02215.

Berger PA: Medical treatment of mental illness. *Science*, 200:974-981, 1978.

Bishop B: Neural plasticity. *Physical Therapy*, part 1, 62(8):132-134; part 2, 62(9):1275-1282, 1982.

Bizzi E: The coordination of eye-head movement. *Scientific American*, 231(4):100, 1974.

Blacker HM: Evaluating sensory and motor systems. *Patient Care*, 17(16):121-136, 1983.

Bleuler E. *Textbook of Psychiatry;* translated by Bull AA. New York, Macmillan, 1924, pp 1-48.

Bradley KC: The posterior rami of segmental nerves. In Glasgow EF, Twomey LT, Scull ER, Kleynhans AM, Idczak RM: *Aspects of Manipulative Therapy*, ed 2. New York, Churchill Livingstone, 1985, pp 59-63.

Brzozowske WT: Mental health. *The Texas Chiropractor*, March 1974.

Buhler C: Maturation and motivation. *Personality*, 1:185, 1951.

Calbe DB, Eisler T: The pathogenesis and medical treatment of extrapyramidal disease. *Medical Clinics of North America*, 63:715-727, 1979.

Carmichael L (ed): *Psychology*. Boston, Houghton Mifflin, 1946, pp 243-262.

Chusid JG: *Correlative Neuroanatomy & Functional Neurology*, ed 19. Los Altos, CA, Lange Medical, 1985, pp 19-36, 37-63, 87-107, 134-161, 180-187, 239-243.

Conrad B, Meyer-Lohmann J: The long-loop transcortical load compensating reflex. *TINS*, 3(11):269-272, 1980.

Corless IB: Mind/body interventions in healing. School of Medicine, University of North Carolina, Carrington Hall, 214 H, Chapel Hill, NC 27514.

Daube JR, Sandok BA: *Medical Neurosciences*. Boston, Little, Brown, 1978, pp 127-128, 138-154, 160-169, 221-222, 262-287, 296-320, 324-371, 376-417.

DeBacher G: Biofeedback in spasticity. In Basmajian JV (ed): *Biofeedback: Principles and Practice for Clinicians*. Baltimore, Williams & Wilkins, 1979, p 61.

DuBois JM: Cranial nerve testing. *The Chirogram*, May 1975.

Eisen A, Hoirch M: The electrodiagnosis evaluation of spinal root lesions. *Spine*, 8(1):98-106, 1983.

Fitz-Ritson D: The anatomy and physiology of the muscle spindle, and its role in posture and movement. *Journal of the Canadian Chiropractic Association*, 26(4):144-150, 1982.

Friedman HH: *Problem-Oriented Medical Diagnosis*, ed 2. Boston, Little, Brown, 1979, pp 15-17.

Green EE, et al: Voluntary control of internal states: Psychological and physiological. *Journal of Transpersonal Psychology*, II, 1970.

Guyton AC: *Textbook of Medical Physiology*, ed 6. Philadelphia, W.B. Saunders, 1981, pp 577-587, 684-709, 724-762.

Haldeman S: Interactions between the somatic and visceral nervous systems. *ACA Journal of Chiropractic*, V:57-64, August 1971.

Haldeman S: Neurophysiological concept of importance to chiropractors. *Journal of the Canadian Chiropractic Association*, 18(3):6, 1974.

Hanning JM: The role of the emotions in clinical practice. *The Chirogram*, February 1974.

Heilman KM, Watson RT, Greer M: *Handbook for Differential Diagnosis of Neurologic Signs and Symptoms*. New York, Appleton-Century-Crofts, 1977, pp 114-122.

Hodge JR: *Practical Psychiatry for the Primary Physician*. Chicago, Nelson-Hall, 1975, pp 15-22, 51-96.

Holmes TH, Masuda M: Psychosomatic syndrome. *Psychology Today*, April 1972.

Homewood AE: *The Neurodynamics of the Vertebral Subluxation*, ed 3. Place of publication not shown, published by author, 1981, pp 112-117, 122-125, 132-146, 250-260, 278-281.

Hooper EW: The usefulness of screening for mental illness. *Lancet*, 1:33, 1984.

House EL, Pansky B, Siegel A: *A Systematic Approach to Neuroscience*, ed 3. New York, McGraw-Hill, 1979, pp 215-216.

Houston JC, Joiner CL, Trounce JR: *A Short Textbook of Medicine*, ed 6. Philadelphia, J.B. Lippincott, 1979, pp 10-55.

Janda V: Muscle and joint correlations. In Lewis K, Gutmann G (ed): *Rehabilitácia, Proceedings of the IVth Congress Prague International Federation of Manual Medicine*, Supplement 10-11:154-157, 1975.

Janse J: A concept: The neurological element as it relates to clinical chiropractic. *The Chirogram*, December 1975.

Jankowska E, Lundberg A: Interneurons in the spinal cord. *TINS*, 4(9):230-233, 1981.

Jewett DL, Rayner MD: *Basic Concepts of Neuronal Function*. Boston, Little, Brown, 1983.

Kimber DC, Gray CE, Stackpole CE: *Textbook of Anatomy and Physiology*, ed 11. New York, Macmillan, pp 199-207, 218-250.

Kirby JD: Evaluating the problem patient. *The Chirogram*, March 1976.

Krupp MA, Chatton MJ, Werdegar D: *Current Medical Diagnosis & Treatment—1985*. Los Altos, CA, Lange Medical, 1985, pp 19-20, 521-527, 610, 631-685.

Kuntz A: Anatomic and physiologic properties of cutaneo-visceral vasomotor reflex arcs. *Journal of Neurophysiology*, 8:421-429, 1943.

Kuntz A: *The Autonomic Nervous System*. Philadelphia, Lea & Febiger, 1949, pp 22, 486.

La Berge S: Lucid dream project. P.O. Box 2364, Stanford, CA 94305.

Lewis MMcD: Muscle spindles and their function: A review. In Glasgow EF, Twomey LT, Scull ER, Kleynhans AM, Idczak RM: *Aspects of Manipula-*

tive Therapy, ed 2. New York, Churchill Livingstone, 1985.

Lico MC, Hoffman A, Covian MR: Influence of some limbic structures upon somatic and autonomic manifestations of pain. *Physiology and Behavior*, 12(5): 805-811, 1974.

Luria AR: *Higher Cortical Functions in Man*. New York, Basic Books, 1966, pp 432-439.

MacDonald ML, Stanish WD: Neuromuscular system. In Scott WN, Nisonson B, Nicholas JA: *Principles of Sports Medicine*. Baltimore, Williams & Wilkins, 1984, pp 15-24.

McNaught AB, Callander R: *Illustrated Physiology*, ed 4. New York, Churchill Livingstone, 1983, pp 214-218, 224-240, 242-243, 257-259.

Milstein V, Small JG, Small F: The subtraction of serial sevens test in psychiatric patients. *Archives of General Psychiatry*, 26:439-441, 1972.

Magoun HI: Entrapment neuropathy in the cranium. *Journal of the American Osteopathic Association;* part I, 67(6): 643-652; part II, 67(7):779-787, 1968.

Morgan WP: Selected psychological considerations. *Research Quarterly*, 45:374, 1974.

Nideffer RM: *Test of Attentional and Interpersonal Style*. Rochester, NY, Behavioral Research Applications Group, 1977.

Olson WH, Brumback RA, Gascon G, Christoferson LA: *Practical Neurology for the Primary Care Physician*. Springfield, IL, Charles C Thomas, 1981, pp 1-32.

Otto HA: *Explorations in Human Potentialities*. Springfield, IL, Charles C. Thomas, 1966, pp 53-62.

Palmer DD: *Textbook of the Science, Art and Philosophy of Chiropractic*. Portland, OR, Portland Printing House, 1910, pp i, 7.

Patterson MM: The reflex connection: History of a middleman. *Osteopathic Annals*, 4(9):357-367, 1976.

Pearson JA: The modulation of reflex activity in the spinal cord. *Journal of the Canadian Chiropractic Association*, 20(3):12-13, 1976.

Pearson KG: Interneurons and locomotion. *TINS*, 4(6):128-131, 1981.

Pelletier KR: Experimental data regarding subtle energy—homeopathy project. School of Medicine, A-405, Parnasus Avenue, San Francisco, CA 94143.

Penfield W, Rasmussen T: The Cerebral Cortex of Man: *A Clinical Study of Localisation of Function*. New York, MacMillan, 1950.

Pottenger FM: *Symptoms of Visceral Disease*, ed 6. St. Louis, C.V. Mosby, 1949, pp 31-32, 76-78, 134-135, 225.

Prichard JW: Nerve. In Albright JA, Brand RA (eds): *The Scientific Basis of Orthopaedics*. New York, Appleton-Century-Crofts, 1979, pp 399-400, 403-404.

Quigley WH: Self-concept, mental health, and chiropractic. *ACA Journal of Chiropractic*, March 1971.

Reddy MP: Peripheral nerve entrapment syndromes. *American Family Physician*, 28:5, November 1983, pp 133-143.

Redman S, Walmsley B: The synaptic basis of the myosynaptic stretch reflex. *TINS*, 4(10):248-251, 1981.

Riley JS: *Science and Practice of Chiropractic with Allied Science*. Washington, DC, published by author, 1925.

Rosse C: Muscle action and its control. In Rosse C, Clawson DK (eds): *The Musculoskeletal System in Health & Disease*. Hagerstown, PA, Harper & Row, 1980, pp 64-65, 70-75.

Sandow RW: Some reflex phenomena associated with spinal derangements and adjustments. *Annals of the Swiss Chiropractors' Association*, 7:45-65, 1981.

Schafer RC: *Clinical Biomechanics: Musculoskeletal Actions and Reactions*. Baltimore, Williams & Wilkins, 1983, pp 131-137.

Schafer RC: *Physical Diagnosis: Procedures and Methodology in Chiropractic Practice*. Prepublication manuscript, chapters 4 (Clinical interpretation of pain), 7 (Basic neurologic considerations), and 10 (Basic evaluation of mental and emotional status). Arlington, VA, American Chiropractic Association, 1989.

Schafer RC: *Symptomatology and Differential Diagnosis*. Arlington, VA, American Chiropractic Association, 1986, pp 23-44.

Seltzer B, Sherwin I: Organic brain syndromes: An empirical study and clinical review. *American Journal of Psychiatry*, 135:13-21, 1978.

Sherrington C: *The Integrative Action of the Nervous System*. Cambridge, England, Cambridge University Press, 1947, pp 7, 148.

Skully RL: The nervous system and its disorders. *ACA Journal of Chiropractic*, January and February 1972.

Smart A: Conscious control of physical and mental states. *Menninger Foundation Perspective*, April-May, 1970.

Tran TA, Maori TT: Essentials of the neurological examination: Tests for cerebral function. *The Chirogram*, July 1975.

Tran TA: The motor system: A general look at its components and their clinical correlations. *The Chirogram*, October 1976.

Upledger JE, Vredevoogd JD: *Craniosacral Therapy*, Seattle, Eastland Press, 1983.

Walker HK, Hall WD, Hurst JW (eds): *Clinical Methods*. Woburn, MA, Butterworth Publishers, 1976, 686-717.

Witkovsky P: Peripheral mechanisms of vision. *Annual Review of Physiology*, 33:257, 1971.

Zimmerman J: Bio-electro-magnetics project. University of Colorado, Health Services Center, 4200 East Ninth Avenue, Box C268, Denver, CO 80262.

Part III: Clinical Neurology

Chapter 5

Neuroconceptual Models of Chiropractic

Gary C. Johnson, DC

This chapter offers a summary review of the highlights of preceding chapters that concern subluxation syndromes and forms a foundation of thought for following chapters.

INTRODUCTION: EXPLANATION OF CONCEPTUAL MODELS

Conceptual models are collections of ideas, principles, facts, philosophy, and experiences setting our attitudes and directing our behavior. *Ideas* and *principles* include hypotheses and theories (whether right or wrong) that generate new attitudes and behavior, the spirit of invention, and the accessibility to important facts.

Scientific facts and our philosophical hierarchy of importance (priority) provide selective (choice) groupings of knowledge and thoughts, comfortably placed in support of our experiences. How we perceive what we do, why we do it, why the results, and how the results occur set attitudes and practice activities and change our minds and activities as new concepts are developed and tested.

CLASSIC CONCEPTS OF THE CHIROPRACTIC SUBLUXATION

The structural spinal fault, the associated nerve involvement, and the ensuing functional alterations comprise *classic chiropractic subluxation concepts*. In contrast, limited concepts of spinal biomechanical faults, modes of possible nerve involvement, and etiologic rationales of functional changes promote narrow viewpoints, disciplines, and therapeutic approaches, as well as foster empiricism and dogma. Awareness of the varied concepts of structural lesions, neuroinsults, and the causes of abnormal functional changes promote wider perspective for intuitive practices, multifaceted observations, and fewer practices with reliance on empiricism that is dictated by dogmatic frameworks.

To illustrate the variations of concepts on structual spinal faults, the term *subluxation* can be defined in the areas of static juxtapositions of vertebrae (eg, lateral flexion subluxation, rotation subluxation, anterolithesis subluxation, etc). Another category is spinal "dyskinesia" with all its potential faults (eg, fixation, altered range of motion, hypermobility, etc). The focal points of structural stress in different postural attitudes can be considered as subluxations or they may produce structural compensations that manifest as subluxations.

The multiple concepts of possible nerve involvement include the subluxation as an intrinsic source of irritation (excitation), a source of impulse generation, a source of interference in impulse conduction, a source of segmental neuronal pool facilitation, and a source of impedance of axoplasmic flow. In the following sections of this chapter, facts and ideas will be presented to support the development of the many conceptual models possible for the "chiropractic subluxation."

The Stimulus—Response Phenomenon

Life has classically been described as a stimulus—response phenomenon. External and internal changes of the environment act as stimulants that evoke reactions in response to the change. The reactions of the response are meant to keep the organism in harmony with itself and its dynamic external and internal environmental elements. Within certain parameters of the rate and magnitude of responses afforded by the organism, the harmony and equilibrium are usually expected and insured. However, a major class of variables in higher forms of life is also present and can play a major role in the stimulus—response phenomenon and the quality of life.

The changes occurring with the stimulus *should* excite some tissues that, in turn, *should* excite some afferent neuronal elements. The afferent neurons *should* transport this information to the CNS for awareness, recognition, and the selection of priority of importance. The CNS *should* process the stimulus-generated information and initiate and direct a selected afferent patterned response. The afferent neurons, in turn, *should* transport the demand information to proper reactive target tissues. To complete the process, the reactive tissue *should* be acceptable and responsive to the demand and be capable of performance as directed. This response should be timely, accurate, and be of exact duration in harmony to the stimulus.

The "shoulds" in the above scenario suggest the many variables and possible alterations of the elements and mechanisms involved to produce such a stimulus—response phenomenon and to the extent that, if the response is appropriate and accurate, it is an astonishing phenomenon in itself!

A given stimulus (ie, an environmental energy change within the parameters of enough magnitude to excite and not too great as to injure the organism) should excite (stimulate) receptor cells of lower threshold to the specific type of energy change. After the stimulus depolarizes the receptor membrane, the generated action potential (impulse) should initiate conduction of the impulse via afferent fibers to the CNS. On arrival, the afferent firings should produce patterns of impulses through multiple synapses and resulting pathways at different rates within the spinal cord and brain. The final destination of these sensory patterns of impulses in the brain greatly determines the conscious or unconscious perception of the stimulus. This perception of the stimulus should be accurate concerning the stimulus (ie, touch should be perceived as such and not as pressure or pain). The message received at the cortex is a pattern of impulses dispersed in time and space and not just that of a single fiber of a special sensory modality.

Classically, this phenomenon of stimulus—sensory perception was simplified by the *doctrine of specific nerve energies* by M. Muller (1801—1858). This explanation theorized that there were specific receptors of lowered threshold to one particular modality of sensation. In turn, the special receptor activates a neuron having a "private line" to a specific point in the sensory cortex. Excitation of this specific point by a specific fiber in the spatial organization of the cortex identified the type of stimulus perceived more than the character of the actual stimulus.

We are now confronted by more difficult concepts of neurophysiology, moving from the simplistic to the more involved variables present in the stimulus perception phenomenon.

Variables Between Stimulus and Perception

The most obvious variables between peripheral activation and central perception deal with the state of the receptors, the state of the peripheral afferent nerves and their fibers, the state of the cord level sensory neuronal pools, the state of the cord sensory tracts, and the state of the cerebral sensory cortex.

The response of the receptor and the following perception, within limits, depend upon the strength of the stimulus, the rate of stimulus application, and the duration of stimulation. Multiple factors of adaptation, phasic receptors, tonic receptors, recruitment, habituation, sensitization, ionic concentrations, inflammation, degeneration, undifferentiation, and fatigue can alter receptor function and the physiologic role between stimulus and perception.

The role of peripheral afferent nerves and fibers in transmission of messages to the CNS is variable in performing responsibility by biochemical changes, direct stimuli, mechanical deformation, degeneration, regeneration, inflammation, ischemia, and ionic concentrations. Interference with patterned afferent impulse conduction can obviously alter the perception of the stimulus, even to the degree that with no stimulus present at receptor site, midfiber stimulation produces perception of the receptor site plus antidromic depolarization inhibition of the involved receptors to true stimulation.

Perception is affected by attention with over 90% of stimuli suggested to be ignored as unimportant. The selection of priority perception through a learned process depends on the perception of past experiences. Some experiences develop greater attention to certain stimuli; others may block attention. The state of sensory perception also can be altered by fatigue, chemical imbalances, disease processes or their remnants, drugs, and advanced aging processes.

Variables Between Perception and Response

The transfer of information from afferent sensory input through the sensory cortex or lower centers and levels of perception of the stimuli affect the motor cortex or lower centers as patterns of impulses that excite efferent elements of response. Again, memory patterns of learned responses selectively direct the nature of the reaction. Accuracy, precision, and appropriateness of the response depend on the level(s) of perception, the selection of perception, and continued attention as priority awareness of higher brain levels, as well as the state of the descending tracts, motor neuron pools, anterior spinal nerve roots, peripheral efferent nerves, and the target (reactive tissues).

Altered states of the neuromotor system result in inaccurate, inappropriate, crude, diminished, or exaggerated responses. Timeliness, synchronization, duration, magnitude, and coordination of responses are also variables.

The responses in the simple, primitive concept are reflexes. Many of these simple responses are cord-level controlled. Sensory stimuli enter the cord, diverge, ascend to the brain, or initiate cord-level motor response as reflexes. The descending motor impulses have the major responsibility to either facilitate or inhibit cord-level reflexes. By facilitation and inhibition reactions, reflexes of multiple-unit reactions become body system activities. This is illustrated by pyramidal tract lesions producing hypotonicity by loss of facilitation and by extrapyramidal tract lesions followed by hypertonicities with loss of inhibition, and spontaneous, aimless, unintentional movements.

Patterns of responses are classically identified as innate reflexes, habitual responses (preferred group of reflexes), special learned responses (practiced reflexes with special directions of responses), and pathologic responses (loss or altered physiologic reflexes and actions).

The variables involved in reflexes and responses are characterized by the state of facilitation or inhibition of the higher centers of the CNS such as motor loss after stroke and the altered state of cord-level neuronal pools with internuncial facilitation and inhibition. The state of the peripheral efferent motor neurons is altered by stages of degeneration or regeneration, mechanical deformation, inflammation, ischemia, and changing ionic concentration. The state of the neuromuscular junctions are dependent upon the production and release of neurotransmitter substances, ionic ratios, frequencies of repetitive nerve stimulation and stages of fatigue. Finally, the state of the reactive gland or muscle target tissue can be changed as witnessed in ischemic conditions, myositis, and degenerative states.

DISEASE AND THE STIMULUS—RESPONSE PHENOMENON

Neuroinsult and the Origin of Disease

Life can be explained as a stimulus-response phenomena when in a homeostatic range of interactions. However, from the preceding explanation of the variables between stimulus and response, it can be concluded that homeostasis is not automatic or guaranteed, or the result of simple phenomena.

"Disease in its beginning is abnormal function. Abnormal function is function out of time and phase with environmental need. Disease, whether of the heart, kidney or brain, is disturbed function, not merely disordered structure," stated William Boyd, the father of modern pathology. The functions related to in this quotation are groups of responses related to the descriptions previously made. Some diseases can be explained by abnormal responses (functions) to stimuli; others can be attributed to normal responses to abnormal stimuli or sensory perceptions (processing).

Stimuli may be too great for an appropriate response (shock), for adequate psychologic adaptation (sudden loss of a loved one with neurotic anxiety and depression), for physiologic response (frost bite), or they may become irritants above the resistance at a given time (resistance fluctuates with many variables).

As it mediates between stimulus and response, the nervous system, with all the variables identified, may not perceive and process sensory signals adequately or correctly. The responses may be directed inaccurately and/or be malcoordinated. The control of various functions in response to changes may not be appropriate. "Many pathological processes, the cause of which had been regarded as absolutely foreign to nervous influences, have been found to be in reality entirely dependent on the latter for their origin," wrote Speransky.

Because a given stimulus can be altered by the sensory system (eg, amplified, diminished, diverged, inhibited, facilitated, perceived, or ignored), and a designated response can be altered by the motor system (eg, exaggerated, weakened, synchronized, unsynchronized, prolonged, or shortened) the nervous influences on life processes, functions, structural integrity, biophysics, and energy utilization of the body may seriously compromise the health and welfare of the individual.

Any situation, phenomenon, or condition that interferes with the mediating functions and responsibilities of the nervous system could be initiating or sustaining causes of disease and the associated clinical signs and symptoms of altered functions.

Stimuli and Pseudostimuli

A *true stimulus* initiates sensory signals at a receptor that produces impulse generation and subsequent afferent conduction. A *false stimulus*, on the other hand, does not affect a receptor but initiates impulses somewhere proximal to the receptor, along the course of the afferent fiber. This is allowed by an action potential being reached anywhere on the surface of a neuron that results in impulses being generated and transmitted. Impulses thus generated are transmitted in dual directions: (1) toward the CNS (orthodromic) and (2) back (distally) toward the receptor (antidromic).

The antidromic impulses, in the sense of going against "normal traffic," interfere with conduction of true sensory information that is being generated at the receptor. In such a situation, the depolarization of antidromic impulse meets the depolarization of the true impulse and cancels both transmissions (Fig. 5.1). Unimpeded antidromic impulses reaching the receptor terminals do not produce resultant changes or effects, simply because they are receptor organs and not effector organs.

The false orthodromic impulse is transmitted in the normal direction (centrally) to the CNS. On reaching its destination in the sensory cortex or other interpretive centers, false signals are perceived as any other information and recognized as true or real data. The CNS cannot differentiate between actual stimulus-receptor impulses and pseudostimulus (nonreceptor) impulses. Therefore, the false information is processed as true information and passed on to the motor centers to evoke responses to possible nonexisting stimuli of any modality, both somatic or autonomic.

Even if the false sensory information is too weak to produce a response, the impulses thus generated may produce a state of facilitation in the pattern of sensory neuron pathways at the spinal cord and/or higher levels. This inevitably produces lowered thresholds to other subsequent real or false sensory impulses, which results in exaggerated or prolonged responses.

Functional Alterations

In the same manner that false sensory information can be generated midneuronally, so also can response-directed motor efferent impulses be generated and transmitted. Again, these false demand impulses are conducted in opposite directions, orthodromic and antidromic. However, in the case of efferent neurons, the antidromic direction is toward the CNS and the orthodromic is the normal course (directed peripherally) toward reactive target tissue for muscle or glandular action.

The antidromic false impulses (moving

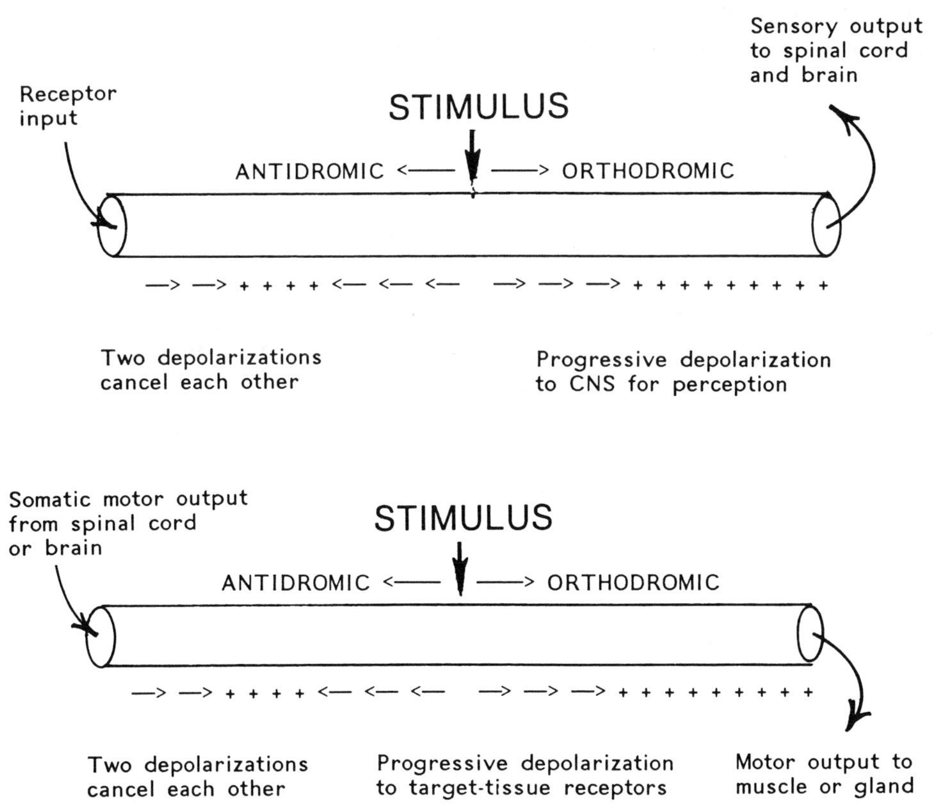

Figure 5.1. Midneuron stimulation.

against traffic) can either interfere with normal efferent impulses by predepolarization or terminate at the next synapse with no effect. It is presently thought that antidromic impulses cannot jump synaptic clefts or continue to the next higher motor neuron.

False orthodromic efferent impulses travel the same course and produce the same responses as would true motor impulses. The potential tragedy is the exaggeration of responses to no true stimuli and the misdirected responses from the CNS. The normal neurologic influences of inhibition, facilitation, coordination, and timeliness on function may be absent. The resultant unchecked reactions may produce the syndromes of signs and symptoms of many disease stages. This state could represent the abnormal function referenced by Boyd as the beginning of disease. Abnormally low function could be false inhibitory reactions. Conversely, excessive activity could be the result of false excitatory reactions going unchecked.

Causes of Disease: Traditional and Current Concepts

The chiropractic pioneers of D.D. Palmer's time considered the causes of disease to be essentially trauma, poison, and autosuggestion. In more modern times, the terms physical trauma, chemical irritation, and psychologic stress might be used.

Current pathology broadly classifies the causes of disease as either environmental or constitutional. Environmental factors of external origin include physical injury (frank trauma or progressive microtrauma), infectious agents (parasites, bacteria, fungi, viruses, etc), harmful inanimate objects (eg, inert foreign bodies or chemical toxins), diet abnormalities (deficiencies or excesses in various ingested substances), psychologic irritants (emotional trauma, stresses, and behavioral restraints).

The constitutional factors of internal origin include inherited genetic abnormalities (eg, inborn errors of metabolism), remnants of developmental anomalies (eg, osteogenesis imperfecta), changes from previous disease states (eg, postmeasles problems), physical conditioning (eg, muscle strength and mass), sex (eg, menopausal changes), and age (eg, senile osteoporosis).

In the concept of environmental and constitution factors of disease, the ideal approach to prevention and treatment would be to remove or control the sources of irritation in the patient's environment while at the same time building resistance through an improved constitutional health status.

The Irritation—Resistance Concept

An individual's health status can be viewed as the overall state of function in respect to the presence of irritation and the level of resistance. Stimuli become irritants with increased magnitude, duration, quantity, and concurrent combinations. *Irritants* are stimuli endangering or detrimental to the individual. *Resistance* is the recruitment of functions (responses) designed to lessen the irritant to a stimulus or to remove the threatening source completely or develop functions of adaptation that reduce the impact of the irritant on body parts, functions, and systems.

Stimuli also become irritants at different degrees in different individuals and in the same individual at different times. Levels of resistance also vary between individuals and within the same individual at different times. Systemic equilibrium is the key, and the nervous system is its major mediator. Within limitations, irritations can be recognized and proper responses can be used to resist the insult and normalize functions.

In recognition of the responsibilities of the nervous system to play the role of mediator, the ideal approach to prevention and treatment of disease now goes beyond environmental controls and constitutional status to the necessity of maintaining sustained neurologic integrity.

Habitual Responses

In review of the stimulus-response phenomenon and all the variables previously listed between sensory recognition and motor reactions, the mediating activities of the nervous system are not as simple as they may have initially appeared. The processes of recognition and reaction are complicated by the nervous system, which, in reacting to irritations, may establish certain neurologic patterns of response. These patterns may become habitual or self-perpetuating to the extent of producing physiologic and/or structural alterations.

The alterations thus produced, in tandem with the initial neurologic patterns of response, become intrinsic sources of neurologic irritation, generating additional patterns of response with more functional and/or structural alterations. This condition may persist or progress long after the original stimulation (irritation) has ceased. Via positive feedback reflexes and recruitment, the condition may even worsen after removal of the causative factors.

First-stage resultant functional and/or structural alterations can become constitutional stimuli (irritants) demanding awareness and reaction by way of sensory and motor activities. This internal (intrinsic) source of sensory stimulation (irritation), in turn directing motor responses, may be the etiologic factor in the production of signs, symptoms, functional changes, and morphologic alterations associated with various disease entities. See Figure 5.2. As disease processes progress, the positive feedback circuit continues with the development of more intrinsic sources of sensory stimulation. Thus, more motor responses with chronic syndromes result.

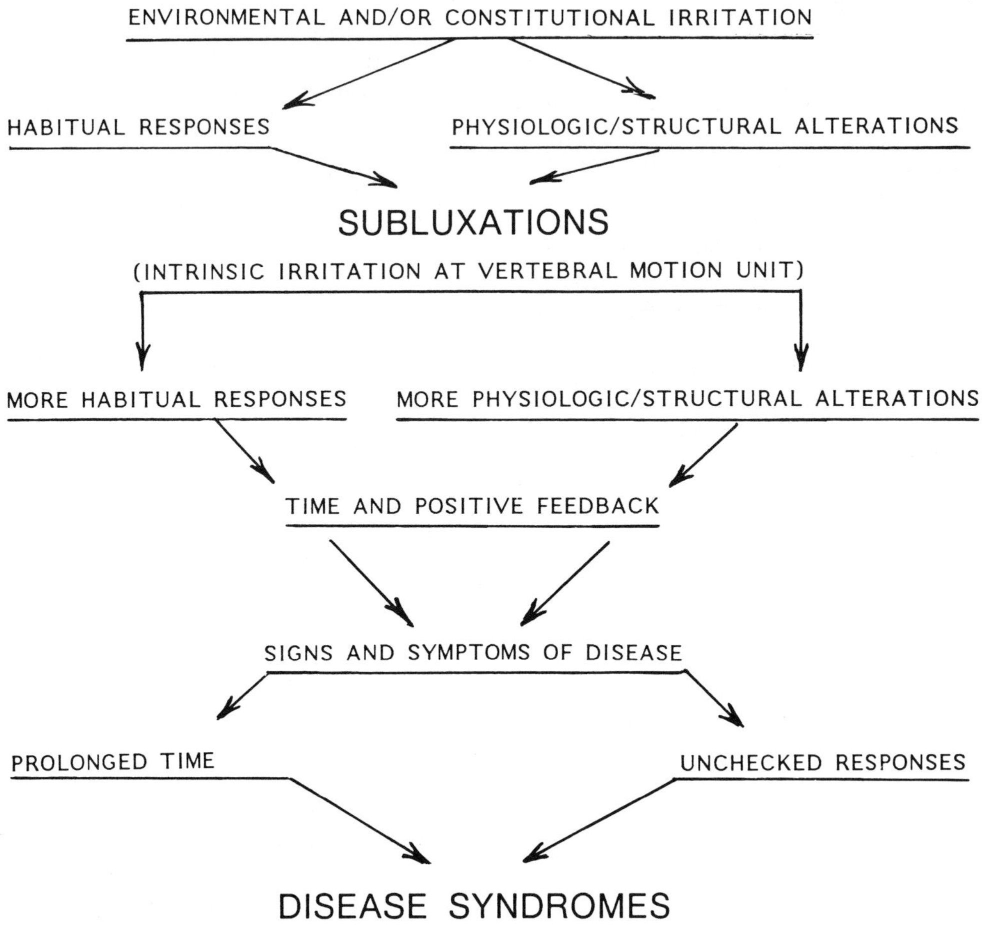

Figure 5.2. Model of the role of subluxations in disease processes.

Reactions at the Vertebral Motion Unit. A major site of a secondary internal source of sensory stimulation due to and producing physical and functional changes is the *vertebral motion unit* and its closely associated neurologic components. The motion unit can show evidence of physical changes subsequent to the original stimulus-response reactions and become a mechanical source of neuropathologic reflexes and referrals. The primary source may diminish or vanish, leaving the secondary vertebral source actively propagating functions out of time and phase with environmental need. The motion unit also can show evidence of physical changes in normal ranges of daily activity and become a primary internal source of reflexes and referrals with similar adverse effects.

THE INTRINSIC FACTOR (SUBLUXATION)

The vertebral motion unit, with physical changes produced as explained, is the *intrinsic factor* recognized in chiropractic as a *spinal subluxation.* A subluxation, more specifically, is an intrinsic factor of abnormal biomechanical relationships between adjacent anatomical structures that is eliciting and/or contributing to neurologic responses which may clinically manifest as signs, symptoms, functional changes and morphologic alterations of a disease state.

The abnormal biomechanical relationships of the motion unit in subluxation may anatomically exist as a static malposition of related structures (counter rotation, etc) or as an alteration of the biokinetic range of motion of the motor unit (hypomobility, etc).

The *intrinsic factor* may be neurogenic in origin, participating as a habitual response to a distant source of irritation. The subluxation also may originate as a simple biomechanical fault, self-irritating and self-perpetuating. In either case, the effects are similar in potential harm and in need of corrective attention.

Definitions of Subluxation

Following are some selected references that define the term *subluxation.*

• Palmer DD: *Textbook of the Science, Art and Philosophy of Chiropractic.* Portland, OR, Portland Printing House, 1910.

"A vertebra is said to be displaced or luxated when the joint surfaces are entirely separated. Sub-luxation is a partial or incomplete separation; one in which the articulating surfaces remain in partial contact. This latter condition is the one so often referred to and known by Chiropractors as sub-luxations.

"A vertebra racked from its normal position ever so little, is rotated around its axis, thereby displacing all its parts proportionately. The relationship existing between bones and nerves are so nicely adjusted that any one of the 200 bones, more especially those of the vertebral column, cannot be displaced ever so little without impinging upon adjacent nerves.

"A sub-luxation does not restrain or liberate vital energy. Vital energy is expressed in functional activity. A subluxation may impinge against nerves, the transmitting channel may increase or decrease the momentum of impulses, not energy.

"A subluxation consists of two or more bones, whose articular surfaces have *lost in part* their natural connection—or in which the articulating surfaces *remain in partial contact*—those which partly preserve their connection."

• Stephenson RW: *Chiropractic Textbook.* Davenport, IA, published by author, 1927.

"A subluxation is the condition of a vertebra that has lost its proper juxtaposition with the one above or the one below, or both; to an extent less than a luxation; which impinges nerves and interferes with the transmission of mental impulses."

• Homewood AE: *The Neurodynamics of the Vertebral Subluxation,* ed 3. Place of publication not shown, published by author, 1981.

"The disrelation of a vertebral segment in association with the contiguous vertebra, or vertebrae, is not visualized as a partial dislocation, as the term implies, but, rather, as a disturbance of normal function of a vertebral segment, which would be better expressed by the term 'Fixation'. Thus, the vertebra in question is within its normal range of motion with its facets continuing to articulate with those of the vertebrae above and below. Such a fixation does not alter the size of the associated intervertebral foramina materially, yet the disrelation, or disturbed function, does have profound significance for the neuromere and nerve trunk."

• Janse J: History of the development of chiropractic concepts: Chiropractic terminology. In Goldstein M (ed): *The Research Status of Spinal Manipulative Therapy.* Bethesda, MD, NINCDS Monograph No. 15, US Dept of HEW, 1975.

"Subluxation: D.D. Palmer insisted that the word subluxation be applied to the intervertebral disrelationships amounting to less than a locked dislocation. He maintained at the same time that there is a functional response within the nervous system resulting from this structural disrelationship."

• Schafer RC (ed): *Basic Chiropractic Procedural Manual*, ed 4. Arlington, VA, American Chiropractic Association, 1984.

"Subluxation: A subluxation is the alteration of the normal dynamics, anatomical or physiologic relationships of contiguous articular structures."

• Suh CH: Biomechanical aspects of subluxation. In Goldstein M (ed): *The Research*

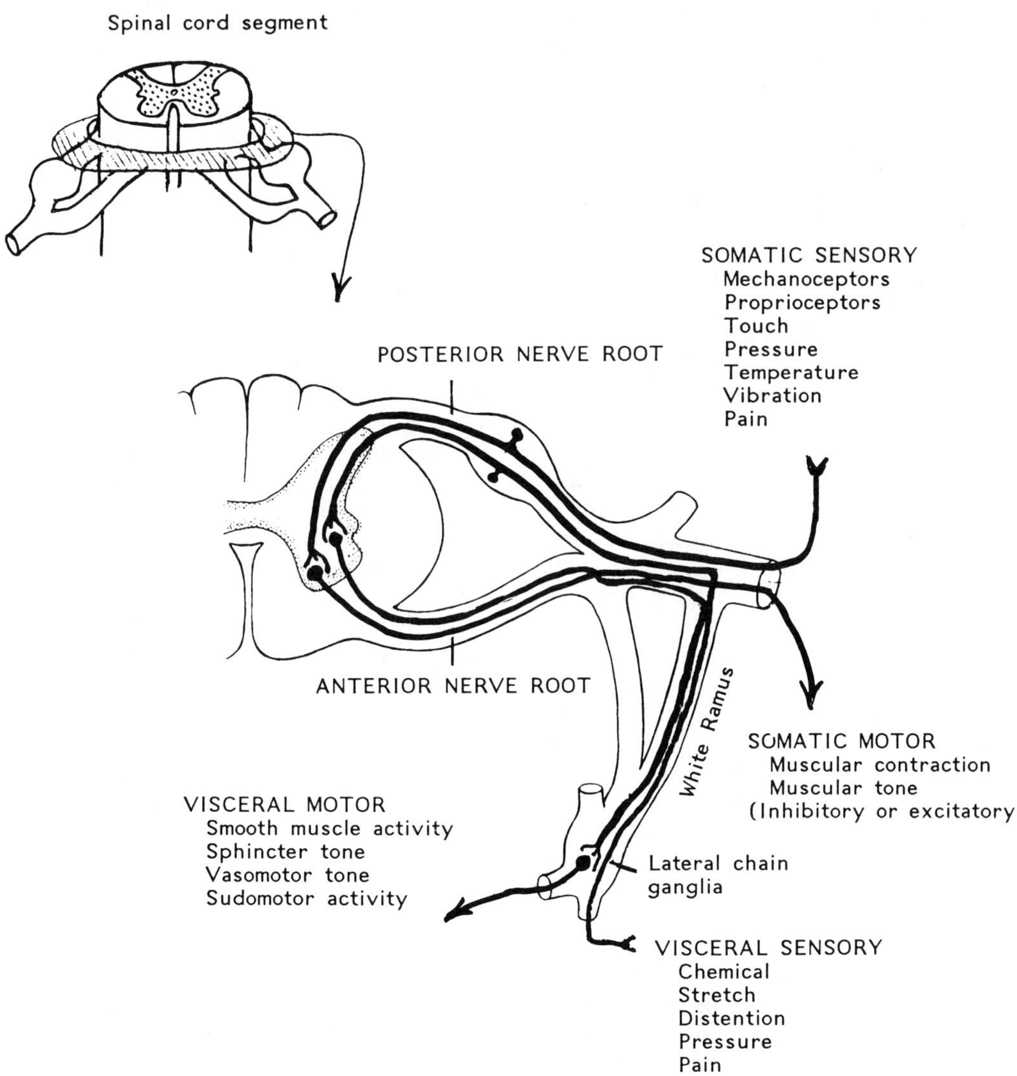

Figure 5.3. Patterns of sensation and selection.

Status of Spinal Manipulative Therapy. Bethesda, MD, NINCDS Monograph No. 15, US Dept of HEW, 1975.

"Next to the word 'chiropractic,' the term 'subluxation' or 'spinal subluxation' is perhaps the most important and most frequently used word employed by chiropractors. The definition of 'subluxation' varies, depending on whether it is viewed from a chiropractic or medical point of view.

"The major difference between the medical and chiropractic viewpoint is that chiropractic includes 'neurophysiological disturbances' in the definition of 'subluxation'. This implies that 'subluxation' has a living character which includes both biomechanical and neurophysiological abnormalities. Therefore, any conclusion regarding subluxation that is based solely on the study of cadavers is not acceptable."

Irritation—Subluxation—Disease

As a simplistic overview of this section, the following tour of events is offered.

Environmental or constitutional irritation received, transmitted, and mediated by the nervous system produces patterns of habitual responses. This patterned activity can alter function and structure. A primary site of alteration is the vertebral motion unit, demonstrating abnormal position, faulty kinetics and segmental neurologic changes. The altered motion unit is a spinal subluxation and an *intrinsic factor* of irritation and reaction, producing a second generation of habitual responses.

The subluxation complex is a site of both stimulation and response. Later responses may continue from the intrinsic factor after the original environmental or constitutional irritations cease. In addition to persisting, these secondary patterns of responses may produce an additional set of functional and structural alterations. With prolonged time and continued cyclic positive-feedback-dominating activity, signs, symptoms, malfunction, and morphologic changes of disease states may become apparent. When left unattended for a long duration, these adverse processes may recruit more abnormal responses and become packaged into the manifested syndromes of chronic disease states.

Patterns of Sensation and Selection

Because the triad of the nervous system (sensory, motor, and autonomic) is segmentally organized, the subluxated segment will exhibit clinical evidence of the signs and symptoms of subluxation; eg, segmental tenderness; spontaneous pain; altered activity of segmentally innervated muscles; and vasomotor, sudomotor, and visceral changes of segmental sympathetic innervation (Fig. 5.3).

CAUSES OF SUBLUXATION

The Intrinsic Factor Has Physical Properties: Two Major Categories

In view of the variables of phenomena from stimulus to response as mediated by the nervous system, the initial causes of subluxation are often difficult to identify. However, subsequent to all the possible initiating factors producing the *intrinsic factor* (the structural/functional deviation of the vertebral motion unit), there are two major classifications of causes.

The first category is an active one of muscular effort. Abnormal muscular responses, usually directed by the nervous system, produce and sustain abnormal positions and motions of the vertebral motion unit. The presence of these abnormal responses generate sensory irritation and motor deviations of the nervous system. Referral, reflexes, and unequal, asymmetrical, excessive, deficient, untimely, aphasic muscular efforts thus can produce all three criteria of subluxation: malposition, dyskinesia, and neuroinsult.

An appreciation of subluxations caused from abnormal muscular efforts is more readily developed in view of spinal muscle responsibilities in support of spinal functions. Spinal functions are commonly identified to include motion, support, and protection. Allowing and generating motion, within certain parameters, of gross movement, sectional movement and segmental activity are obvious spinal functions of design.

Spinal motion is directed by muscular efforts, ligamentous restrictions, osseous architectural forms, and intervertebral disc plasticity. Structural support of form (postural attitude) is a spinal function afforded by muscular efforts, ligamentous restrictions, osseous density, and the intervertebral disc. The protection of the delicate elements of the nervous system is provided as a spinal function of muscular guarding, ligamentous absorption of forces, osseous armature, confinement by the associated IVD, and cushioning by the meninges and CSF.

Muscular Responsibilities

Muscular efforts in support of spinal column function include the following:

1. Muscle activity provides, along with ligamentous elasticity, postural tone. The ligamentous spine is unstable and unable to maintain erect postural attitudes. Changes in postural attitude (eg, a shift in center of gravity) must be counterbalanced by active muscular efforts perceived and directed by the nervous system. This ongoing muscular activity may result in observable motion or a state of hypertonicity (viz, a muscular resistance to effects of other forces). These muscular efforts to maintain posture also provide spinal preload forces to segments of much larger magnitude than the physiologic loads of motion that occur during normal activity. Preload forces provide support through stiffness and motion through flexibility. Postural tone and preload, as products of muscular activity, provide for a degree of inactive symmetry. This symmetry of posture provides for added spinal structural support and, in tandem, more protection of the neurologic elements. Postural tone is also important in providing preparedness of the muscular state for active movement. The strength of contraction is affected by previous activity. Muscular efforts provide direct sensory information generated by contraction and indirectly provide sensory information from resulting changes in muscle fiber tone and length. Combined, this information provides a status report on spinal functions and a data supply for further reactions.

2. Muscle activity generates and directs spinal actions of movement. Muscular efforts perform the work that produces movement. Under the direction of the nervous system, the work done provides accurate, adequate, and prompt activities of spinal movement. Muscular efforts also provide for asymmetrical static or motion positions during or following an activity. Within a normal range of motion, a state of active equilibrium is provided by excitation and inhibition of muscular efforts within myotatic units of function. Muscular efforts are also required in maintaining asymmetrical postural positions for as long as is necessary.

3. Muscle activity returns parts to symmetrical perfection when desired or after activity is performed. Muscular efforts provide precise and prompt return of symmetry to re-establish spinal stability, regain maximum spinal support, protect the nervous system, and prepare for the next activity. In this context, Steindler reports: "In the ability of the spine to revert to symmetry at will from all asymmetrical positions with promptness and precision lies the characteristic earmark of the normal spine. The inability to do so makes the spine abnormal. The normal spine can, at any point within its range of motion, establish an active equilibrium, can maintain this position at will as long as necessary, and can return to the position of perfect symmetry again, whenever it is desired."

Muscular efforts in support of the spinal functions just outlined may be altered by the following:

1. *Acute frank trauma.* Trauma may result in damaged muscle tissues releasing excitatory substances to pain receptors and initiate an inflammatory reaction. Muscle inflammatory changes in myositis, myofibrositis, and fibromyositis, along with pain, exhibit muscular guarding, edema, circulatory changes, metabolic changes, toxic metabolic end-products, fatigue, scar-tissue formation, and calcium infiltration. During the early stage, there is nociceptive domination of sen-

sory and motor impulse direction over proprioceptive signals and reactions.

All the above changes occur at various degrees posttrauma and alter the ability to perform normal contraction functions. Proprioceptive block and dominant-pain-directed guarding results in the inability to maintain static equilibrium of the postural tone (segmentally, sectionally, or totally) of the spinal system. Muscular reactions also result in the inability of segments and spinal sections to perform in normal ranges of motion (axial rotation, lateral bending, flexion, extension). The inability of the spine and its parts to return to perfect symmetry also is presented with altered muscular efforts and activities. The malpositions of spinal elements, the altered spinal kinetics of segments and sections, and the neuroinsult to sensory awareness and motor attempts at correction of the muscular reactions to trauma combine to produce such intrinsic factors as "segmental subluxations," "sectional towers," and "spinal distortions."

2. *Microtrauma.* Trauma of less magnitude and longer duration may produce the same alterations of spinal muscular efforts as does acute trauma. The process is slower with aches instead of pain and tonicity changes in muscles instead of active guarding, and the overt manifestations may remain subclinical over a long period.

Prolonged stresses of faulty postural attitudes, habitual activities, and altered spinal biomechanics can manifest as inflammation, edema, circulatory changes, metabolic activity, fatigue, scar formation, and calcium infiltration of muscular tissue. As with acute trauma, altered spinal muscle efforts produced by prolonged microtrauma can produce such intrinsic spinal factors as malposition, dyskinesia, and neuroinsult—collectively identified as the "segmental subluxations," "sectional towers," and "spinal distortions," described above.

3. *Postural compensations.* Postural adaptations to minor mechanical faults of support, minor dyskinesia in the ranges of motions, and minor instability of asymmetry of position may produce spinal muscular efforts of self-correction. Proprioceptive sensory awareness to minor structural faults of sectional or segmental deviation prompts spinal muscle activity in an attempt to remove the fault. If successful, the spinal muscle efforts cease with no more proprioceptive irritation. If the effort is unsuccessful, the proprioceptive demands continue and adaptive (compensatory) changes in the spine follow with continued muscular efforts. These on-going muscular efforts along with efforts to perform normal daily activities fragment the spinal system, reducing the activity of some levels or segments while recruiting more activity in other levels or segments. The minor mechanical faults, dyskinesias, and instabilities initiating unequal muscular efforts may progress through these continued efforts to become intrinsic factors of malposition, altered kinetics, and neurologic irritants of segmental spinal subluxations.

Segmental dyskinesia may be amplified by the starting position of the vertebral motion unit. When at rest, the motion unit exhibits a minor fault in resting position, rotation, flexion, extension, and lateral bending, and it is then called on to perform a motion. The predisposed attitude may limit final performance or shift the responsibility to perform to another level. For example, the L5 vertebrae may be rotated 5° to the left at rest. Axial rotation of the lumbar spine is necessary in a movement and L5 may not be able to contribute without damage to restricting elements or without placing the responsibility at higher levels of the lumbar spine. The abnormal muscular efforts involved in diverting the responsibilities of motion to higher levels may cause the altered position, deranged kinetics, and neuroinsults commonly associated with spinal subluxations.

Segmental biokinetics may be altered by spinal preload. The presence of forces of weight-bearing and the tonic muscular action associated with normal resting and active posture is *spinal preload.* The weight-bearing forces on a spinal segment are more than the weight of the body above that segment because of spinal ligament and muscular activity or tone. Preload is responsible along with other elements (eg, strapping ligaments) for segmental stiffness. The spinal stability provided by preload may alter the kinetic range of motion of the vertebral motion unit by an excessive or a diminished amount of preload. The following altered range of motion may result in unequal muscular efforts to induce motion in a stiff segment, or it may add stability to an overly relaxed segment. These muscular efforts may cause spinal subluxations that exhibit segmental juxtaposition, neuroinsults, and the obvious kinetic faults.

Segmental ranges of motion may be altered by osseous architectural asymmetries of facet tropism or wedged-shaped vertebral bodies, for example. Attempts to perform spinal motions with such structural deviations present may lead to unequal spinal muscular efforts to produce and maintain vertebral subluxation at the level of the abnormal bone position or remote from it.

Habitual motion patterns of the spine or sections of the spine may alter segmental ranges of motion in several ways. Motion patterns may lead to changes in ligamentous resistance sectionally and segmentally, allowing for altered muscular efforts and the various ranges of motions. Unilateral motion patterns may produce muscular hypertrophy of required muscles and atrophy of unused muscles. Unequal use and subsequent unequal strength of spinal muscles may reduce the responsibilities of those muscles in maintaining position and performing other activities of a segment and thus lead to subluxation.

The transfer of normal spinal forces and added loads to other areas of the spine may result in abnormal ranges of motions as suggested in the case of spinal preload. Segmental forces of shear, compression, tension, and torsion change in different postural attitudes at all levels of the spine. Different combinations of these loads at various levels produce proprioceptive sensory information, which elicit spinal muscular activity in an attempt to reduce focal points of stress, disperse the forces over larger areas, and redirect the potentially more harmful forces to vectors that produce loads to which the spinal elements are more resistant.

The ensuing muscular efforts to normalize segmental loads may produce the triad of a subluxation in the process. Segmental position, kinetics, and neural neutrality could therefore be easily compromised.

Muscular efforts are also influenced by mechanoreceptor signals from all segments of the spine. Motion and the resultant changes in segmental positioning are constantly producing sensory data. This information is used to analyze angle, velocity, direction, and amplitude of joint displacement by awareness to the amount of or changes in tension. Dyskinesia of a spinal section or segment produces patterns of mechanoreceptive information and subsequent patterns of spinal muscle reactions. Assuming these patterns of muscular responses are present in a given area and additional activity is required that involves that area, the potential of unequal, asymmetrical, and inappropriate muscular efforts could produce vertebral position changes, kinetic changes, and unnecessary neurologic reflexes or referrals common to the subluxation syndrome. Sensitization, accommodation, denervation, degeneration, or a degree of regeneration of mechanoreceptors also may alter sensory information, motor responses, segmental motion, and produce subluxations.

Spinal motions accompanied by pain perception may lose mechanoreceptive input centrally because of the dominance of pain signals. Muscular efforts, in turn, are primarily concerned with guarding of painful motion. Thus, segmental subluxations may follow the loss of appropriate muscular activity.

Postural compensations to minor spinal instabilities caused by fatigue, incomplete responses to changes in forces and loads, proprioceptive lesions, prolonged static stress, habitual stress patterns of motion, and altered ligamentous tension may incorporate profound muscular efforts of adaptation. The minor instabilities, with time and active muscular responses, may produce major spinal instabilities of subluxation.

In summary, spinal muscle efforts involved in postural compensations to minor biomechanical faults may result in the inability to maintain static equilibrium of postural tone, inability to perform in the normal ranges of motions, and the inability to return to resting symmetry. These deficiencies of function may allow for segmental malposition, aberrant motion, and neuropathologic reflexes and referrals. Segmental deviations become the intrinsic factors of subluxations. Spinal subluxations become intrinsic sources of irritation with special patterns of responses. The presence of subluxation may precipitate major postural compensations, distortions, and health liabilities.

4. *Biochemical changes.* Biochemical alterations can alter muscular efforts of the spine that are required for normal spinal functions. Ischemia of spinal musculature due to functional constriction or actual obstruction of vessels results in varying degrees of circulatory deficiencies in delivery and removal. Heat, oxygen, carbon dioxide, glucose, lipids, buffers, phagocytes, calcium, potassium, and sodium concentrations and their availability to muscle tissue can have profound effects on contractability and relaxation. Abnormal concentrations may change peak tension, periods of contraction and relaxation, the rate of tension change in contraction and relaxation, and the period of latency.

The most obvious changes in spinal muscle activity would be expected in myotatic units where muscle members are interdependent mechanically. Changes in length or tension of a particular muscle should have a direct effect on its synergists and antagonists. Biochemical changes in a particular muscle could alter its functional relationship within the myotatic unit and thus alter spinal efforts enough to produce segmental subluxations. On a larger scale, myotatic units of spinal sections could be altered as well as gross spinal distortions from myotatic units of the trunk muscles.

5. *Psychologic Stressors.* Vertebral efforts can be altered by states of psychologic and emotional stress. This is illustrated in the classical posture of profound anxiety. The "worry muscle," the trapezius, is innervated by the spinal accessory nerve (cranial XI). The hypersympathetic activity aroused by stress or fear produces generally increased spinal muscular tone and stiffness and especially targets the trapezius muscle. Prolonged anxiety coupled by hypersympathicotonia (sympathetic dominance) and excessive motor activity could well be an initiating factor altering spinal muscular efforts and the etiology of subluxations.

6. *Primary neuromuscular disease.* Primary diseases of the neuromuscular system, either active or inactive with remnants of altered function and structure, can affect spinal muscle efforts. Muscular imbalances at the vertebral motion units, deviations in tone or strength, and proprioceptive embarrassments following disease processes may ultimately alter vertebral position and the quality of motion, and initiate the pathologic reflexes and referrals common to spinal subluxation.

7. *Secondary motor reactions.* Secondary motor reactions of the vertebral motion unit musculature to sensory stimulation or irritation of either somatic or visceral origin arising anywhere and having afferent neurons enter the CNS at or near the corresponding cord level may alter spinal muscle efforts. Stimulation of somatic or visceral sensory neurons that enter a given neurologic segment and elicit somatomotor or visceromotor responses may cause responses throughout the various ramifications of that segment as defined in dermatomes, myotomes, sclerotomes, and rudimentary visceral innervations. These visceral or somatic motor responses may affect motion unit musculature via somatic reflexes and referrals, resulting in altered muscular tone or activity. The motion unit also may be affected by visceral reflexes and referrals, producing vasomotor responses that can alter muscular activity by ischemia or hyperemia. Vertebral position, motion, and neurointegrity could be consequently reduced to the state commonly associated with a subluxation syndrome.

Supporting-Tissue Responsibilities

The second major category of causes of segmental subluxations is inequality of supporting tissue of the vertebral motion unit. In recognition of the significance of this cause of subluxation, the following review of supportive tissue responsibilities in assisting normal spinal functions of motion, stability, and protection of the neurologic elements is provided.

The four most important supporting tissues of the spinal motion units are the paraspinal ligaments, the intervertebral discs, the posterior facets, and the vertebral bodies.

1. *The spinal ligaments.* Spinal ligament

responsibilities are recognized to include allowance for adequate motion, support for static postural attitudes, protection of the spinal cord by restricting motions within well-defined limits, and protection of the spinal cord from trauma of high loads applied at fast speeds. The elastic nature of ligaments provides spinal support and stability with a minimum expenditure of muscle energy. The ligaments readily resist tensile forces and absorb large amounts of energy that are suddenly applied to the spine. Assisted by muscular efforts, they provide a degree of tone and contribute to spinal preload forces. However, when taken beyond normal elastic limits, tone may be lost with resulting lengthening and laxity; and if damaged, scaring and shortening results.

2. *The intervertebral discs.* The IVDs have responsibilities of absorbing shock, dispersing forces, providing a fulcrum of balance, bearing weight, adhering vertebral bodies together functionally, limiting ranges of motions, separating vertebral bodies, maintaining height of the IVFs, and contributing to the normal A-P spinal curves. Degenerative changes and aging reduce the passive role of the IVDs in many of these responsibilities.

3. *The apophyseal joints.* Restricting the ranges of motions within normal limits, sharing compressive loads of weight bearing, and adding to torsional stiffness are the responsibilities of the posterior facets. By their shape, size, plane of articulation, density, and other joint properties, the facets play important roles in spinal function. Trauma, degenerative joint disease, tropism, and edema adversely affect normal support properties.

4. *The vertebral bodies.* The vertebrae centra, along with the IVDs, give structural height, help form the A-P spinal curves, and share the compressive loads of weight bearing. Malformations, compression fractures, and degenerative changes with aging may compromise the responsibilities of the vertebral bodies in spinal functions.

Subluxations following structural alterations of these supporting tissues may be augmented by musculature efforts the vertebral column or be clinically reduced by successful accommodations of response. As the supporting tissues allow subluxations to occur, evidence of segmental malposition, altered kinetics, and neuroinsult may become apparent.

The "chicken or egg" argument can lead to academic debate on the sequence of events that lead to the presence of the *intrinsic factor* (subluxation). It is a clinical exercise because indifference to the initiating role of muscular efforts, supporting tissues, or neuropathologic reflexes and referrals promotes multiple recognition of simultaneous factors in the genesis of subluxation and multiple approaches to eradication or reduction of these somatic faults through manipulation and adjunctive therapy.

An interesting concept that is parallel to the supporting functions of vertebrae described in this chapter is suggested in the following report by Drum in *An Introduction to the Study of Postural and Spinal Mechanics:*

"Mechanical stress is converted to an electrical stimulus by piezo-electric elements within the bone; this stimulus affects pH and ion population, the alignment and probably the aggregation pattern of extracellular macromolecules and also cell behavior; through these cellular and extracellular influences the electrical stimulus produces change in the osseous architecture appropriate to resist the deforming force and shut off the initiating signal. Astronauts, subjected to the weightlessness of space, rapidly become osteoporotic because they loose a major portion of three of the four mechanical stimuli to bone. This should make it clear that stress is essential for the maintenance of a strong skeletal architecture; that the ideal approach to combat disease is not the search for a stress-free environment, but rather a strengthening of the body's inherent defense mechanisms so they can adequately cope with a level of stress commensurate with an exciting productive life."

The various processes, outlined above, are not limited to the vertebral column or its paravertebral tissues. Similar conditions may exist in other musculoskeletal tissues producing similar intrinsic factors (subluxations) and self-perpetuate neuropathic responses. However, in respect to the vertebral column, the effects may be more evident and crucial because of the close anatomical relationships and the functional importance of normal mechanical integrity to the closely associated delicate elements of the nervous system.

Stoddard states that the effects of mechanical irritation to especially vulnerable neurologic areas are:

• The anterior and posterior nerve roots are affected by abnormal tensions in the ligamentum denticulatum.

• The posterior nerve root ganglia in the cervical IVFs and the combined nerve roots in the IVFs can be irritated by pressure from osteophytes, disc protrusion, arthritis, apophyseal synovitis, fibrosis, and edema.

• More distally, the nerves can be affected by abnormal tensions in muscles; eg, the scalene and piriformis muscles.

• The first rib may be elevated by anomaly or lesions of the first costovertebral joint, causing traction on the lower portion of the brachial plexus.

• Mechanical irritation of the ulnar nerve at the medial epicondyle.

• Mechanical irritation of the median nerve in the carpal tunnel.

• Mechanical irritation of the radial nerve in the spiral canal posterior to the humerus.

• Mechanical irritation of the lumbar nerves as they traverse the psoas muscles.

• Mechanical irritation of the lateral cutaneous nerve of the thigh as it passes under the inguinal ligament.

• Mechanical irritation of the peroneal nerve coursing around the head of the fibula.

• Mechanical irritation of the plantar nerve medial to the os calcis.

• Mechanical irritation of the digital nerves between the metatarsal heads.

BASIC EFFECTS OF SPINAL SUBLUXATION

The effects of subluxation may be divided into three major categories: immediate local effects, mechanical effects, and neurologic effects.

Immediate Local Effects of Subluxation

Immediate local responses of any tissue to irritation, degeneration, or changes resulting from disease processes may occur within and around the vertebral motion unit tissues. Inflammatory reactions of redness, swelling, heat, and pain may follow precipitating injury, degeneration, or proliferative reactions and processes of repair, healing, and regeneration. Local effects also may include edema, circulatory and pH changes that adversely affect joints, muscles, and nerve roots.

Mechanical Effects of Subluxation

Mechanical effects are alterations in biokinetic ranges of motions, balance, or position of local segments, or include the effects upon the musculoskeletal system elsewhere, due to compensatory distortions and alterations as the proprioceptive-directed mechanisms attempt to correct their mechanics to the segmental presence of structural imbalance.

Neurologic Effects of Subluxation

Neurologic effects of subluxation are manifested in alterations of the neurologic triad: sensory, motor, and autonomic. Some neurologic effects are a result of direct physical pressure (compression) and stretching (tension) of the nerve. Other effects may follow circulatory changes supplying the cord and nerve roots, meningeal irritations, impedance of CSF flow, direct proprioceptive insult, and propagation of facilitated segments.

THE EFFECTS OF BIPEDISM

An individual's postural attitude is continually unstable; ie, constantly changing; going through adaptations, compensations, alterations, and long-range and short-term reactions.

Postural deviation demands and elicits complex responses of interrelated parts (postural components) organized by the CNS. The stimulus-response of proprioceptive mechanisms is mediated from mechanoreceptors to spinal muscles. These complex responses are initiated by insult or excessive demand placed on any tissue or organ. Through spinal reflexes and/or referrals, the initial stimulus alters input and reaction of the proprioceptive mechanisms.

The responses are essentially the same for all tissues, depending on which part of the nervous system is involved. Each level will show responses in proprioception, sensory, motor and autonomic changes directed by the level of the insult. The more levels involved, the more complex the syndrome of alterations.

Involvement of somatic musculoskeletal components, especially of the axial structure, has a high incidence in man. They manifest as disturbances intensified by gravitational stresses and as initiating factors in the syndromes of complex responses. Vertebral subluxations are the musculoskeletal components of the spine initiating sensory, motor, and autonomic alterations. Their presence and significance are magnified and prolonged by focused gravitational stresses.

Once the responses are organized and initiated by the CNS, the total postural response to gravitational factors is altered, producing new compensations, new stresses, and new more-complex responses. The presence of a vertebral subluxation, with its sustained responses, alters its ability to participate in normal postural responses, shifting responsibility to other components that react with new compensations, stresses, and responses.

The recruitment of overtaxed musculoskeletal components that are reflexly organized and sustained by stress, foci irritations, and excessive demands become sustaining or exacerbating factors in the complex responses of postural accommodation (even if secondarily induced). Such inability for vertebral subluxation self-correction results in sustained responses, exaggerated responses, and the recruitment of other responses that perpetuate patterns of postural reaction (distortions of structure).

Pain, tenderness, muscular rigidity, and motor, sensory, and autonomic disturbances are interrelated components of this syndrome of response. The gross evidence of spinal structure distortion leads to obvious evidence of vertebral subluxations with identifiable characteristics of sensitivity changes, reaction alterations, and autonomic visceral changes segmentally patterned. It is not coincidence to find a somatic component and to find visceral components as they are interrelated by design, development, and function. They individually represent the two different sides of the same coin.

Musculoskeletal stress is an extremely frequent initiating factor to complex responses of the nervous system associated with and contributory to many different chronic and acute functional disorders to which humanity is peculiarly susceptible. Erect posture is an active defiance toward gravitational forces. Compliance to gravitational forces becomes a matter of choice. The correct choice is often not made because of lack of sensory information, priority options, socioeconomic demands, or unawareness of consequences.

The concept of cause (an initiating etiologic idea) finds soundness as it directly guides successful diagnostic implications and therapeutic applications. The inability to identify the responses and the lack of suggested therapeutic direction strongly suggest that the etiologic concept is deficient or incorrect in rationale.

Implied Etiology

1. The local, discrete somatic component of the *vertebral subluxation* is a reflexly organized and sustained biomechanical response to stress, irritation, and excessive demands placed upon the axial structure by the environment and by the total activities, responses, and adaptations of the individual. The differences in our environments, our elected and demanded activities, our patterns of responses, and our special adaptive mechanisms result in individual evidences of stress.

2. The musculoskeletal component of the *vertebral subluxation* elicits a complex response organized by the CNS that is basically the same for all and extends, to some degree, to all tissues (somatic and visceral) directly related to the corresponding part of the nervous system. The singular stimulus of the somatic component's presence excites sensory elements of proprioception, muscular activ-

ity, ligamentous tension, tissue damage, and excessive forces. Culmination of this sensory information is received via the CNS with a complex group of responses organized and directed (requested) through the CNS.

3. The organization of the responses to *vertebral subluxation* by the CNS involves sensory, motor, and autonomic responses that interfere with the organization of normal responses to the impact of life situations and environmental factors. The result is that ordinary life situations become stressful and taxing, demand costly reserved bioresources, and reduce protective responses. The triad of nervous system responses is designed to redirect sensory attention, specifically designate motor responses, and focus functional changes. Because the vertebral subluxation receives this attention from the CNS, other situations and environmental changes encountered during daily activities are either given less attention than would normally be required or they are given excessive attention of alarm by an overly alert CNS. Either way, additional stimuli, may evoke (elicit) abnormal responses (excessive or inadequate), both of which adversely affect the body's bioresources and protective responses.

4. Initiating factors arise most frequently in the musculoskeletal system because of man's incomplete adaptation to the vertical stance and as part of each individual's postural adaptation to gravitational factors. The segmented vertebral column provides many vulnerable sites for focused stress as it provides the means for postural adaptations. Ideal dispersion of gravitational stresses would occur with total spinal adaptations. However, segmental adaptations are the rule rather than the exception. Segmental adaptations focus stress over the level of tolerance and resistance.

5. Whatever the mode of initiation of subluxation, its presence sensitizes every disease process to the influence of *gravity*. The primary subluxation and the secondary subluxation both, by their presence and affect on the nervous system triad, are focal points of stress. Continual or additional gravitational demands magnify the complex responses associated with each subluxation, accelerating the abnormal processes involved.

6. Local or segmental neurologic and neurovascular disturbances contributing to chronic and acute diseases appear to be a significant part of this general process. The subluxation syndrome includes less stimulus of deep pressure to elicit discomfort, less stimulus required to produce muscular responses, and the recognition of vasoconstriction in tissues innervated by the affected segment.

7. The rate and degree to which disease develops through the subluxation complex will be determined by the total demands upon the individual and the other determining factors of physical configuration (eg, age, attitude, nutrition, exercise, habits, etc) that influence the total "adequacy to cope." The subluxation inevitably impairs human (resistance) adequacy to some extent, while the importance of the subluxation to the individual is determined by the *total* adequacy to the *total* environment and to the life situations encountered and created. The subluxation increases the importance of *every* stress and *every* defect; ie, *every* stress and *every* defect renders the subluxation more critical.

The presence of the subluxation may vary in the degree of the associated complex responses. Subclinical responses may stay within physiologic limits and not be of assistance in locating the subluxation. The degree of subluxation malposition, altered kinetics, and neurologic insult are also factors in directing the magnitude of responses and clinical significance.

The subclinical "dormant" subluxation may be elevated in clinical importance by additional stresses produced by new or continued demands upon the individual. Along with the degree of subluxation and its responses is the variable factor of the number of subluxations in the system as well as the levels or groupings of subluxation patterns.

Environmental stress may increase and lower resistance through the subluxation or resistance may be lowered through subluxation so that environmental stresses that would not ordinarily be taxing become overwhelming, producing pathologic responses and syndromes. The duration of the subluxation complex also may be a determining factor as to its clinical significance relative to the amount and degree of degenerative changes, the amount and degree of accommodations and compensations, and the amount of tissue changes that have occurred progressively over time.

8. Since the neurologically directed response to local stress, irritation, or excessive demand is basically the same for all subluxations, the potential clinical manifestations will be determined by the segment level (and its associated tissues) involved rather than by the nature of how the subluxation was produced. However, the nature of how the subluxation was produced will help to determine the procedures necessary for its reduction, removal, and prevention of its return. The same process, acting through different levels of subluxation, produces a variety of syndromes. The location and nature of the subluxation determine the target organs and therefore the potential pathology effected.

The location of the subluxation, arising in adaptation to the erect posture, is significantly influenced by habitual postural attitude along with the additional factors of age, physical configuration, etc, with suggested relationships between grouped factors and the incidence of various disease processes. Knowledge of the patterns of postural distortions and subluxations associated with increased incidence of various diseases allows for prediction of possible liabilities. Conversely, various diseases that become clinically evident may strongly suggest levels and patterns of distortion and subluxations.

Implied Diagnosis

1. On the basis of the etiologic significance of the subluxation complex just outlined, the finding of a subluxation marks a segment in which or through which the probability of disease is relatively high. The potential probability of adverse effects varies with the subclinical changes, its chronicity, the effects of remissions and exacerbations, and the obvious manifestations (which may be only the effects of exacerbation).

2. At best, the subluxation is only a vulnerable segment, demanding compensations from the entire organism. Where resources and reserves are adequate for directed accommodations and compensations of response, the subluxation remains only vulnerable.

3. At worst, the presence of subluxation indicates compensation has already been overtaxed and spent resources and reserves are not available for additional responses of accommodation and compensation or resources and reserves are no longer available to support or maintain the responses of long-standing accommodation and compensation.

4. Recognition of a vertebral subluxation can reveal early invasion of physiologic reserves and predisposition to disease. With potential probability and subclinical presence of disease, preventive measures can be identified and therapy (subluxation reduction, postural correction) can be initiated in advance of the clinically proven presence of disease.

5. Spinal subluxations appear to be the silent insidious problems, which leading medical thinkers have concluded need to be sought in apparently healthy people and which are some of the earliest clues to chronic disease. Postural distortions of compensation may be the more silent insidious problem that produce, allow the presence of, or perpetuate the presence of spinal subluxations. Postural distortions then become an even earlier clue to chronic disease, preceding spinal subluxations. The earliest clue may exist before postural distortions are evident in patterns of excessive, prolonged gravitational stresses even before these stresses produce postural compensations with subsequent spinal subluxation.

The Diagnostic Recognition Hierarchy

Five points should be noted:

1. Recognition of habitual, excessive gravitational stress in an individual's daily activities.

2. Recognition of postural compensations in response to gravitational stresses.

3. Recognition of the presence of spinal subluxations in postural compensations.

4. Recognition of the depletion of physiologic reserves by subluxations.

5. Recognition of disease processes as a result of loss of or misdirection of reserves and resources.

Implied Therapeutics

1. Along with the relief of pain and discomfort, therapeutic attention must obviously be given to all the controllable factors in and around each patient that influence total fitness and resources. This therapeutic approach directs itself to all diagnostic implications (hierarchy of recognition), whereas subsequent implications are directed to the *spinal subluxation.*

2. Because of the neuropathology associated with the subluxation increases the vulnerability of the individual to all factors, decisive, critical importance should be directed to the reduction of vertebral subluxations (no matter what level of recognition or stage of involvement).

3. Since existing subluxations impair the resources of the ill patient for further resistance and recovery, regardless of their apparent etiologic relation to the illness, no therapy can be complete without the maximum liberation of those resources (plus the provision for additional resources).

4. Treatment of the vertebral subluxation offers a specific approach to the local neurologic disturbance that is associated with many chronic diseases. Diagnostic implications of subluxation and diseases lead automatically to therapeutic implications in the reduction of subluxation and disease.

5. The direct participation of the subluxation in basic responses to disturbing influences, its accessibility, and its responsiveness to appropriate chiropractic adjustments render it a direct and strategic factor through which to modify the response (the disease process) and to augment the patient's capacity for response, resistance, recovery, and adaptation.

6. Since the spinal subluxation both reflects and influences the adequacy of the individual's resources and reserves, responses to the demands of life, vulnerability, and predisposition, early detection and treatment to reduce subluxation offer a direct and systematic approach to the prevention of chronic disease.

The origins of subluxation, the processes with which they are associated, and their implications to health have yet to be fully explored or understood. This is the major challenge before us now.

SPINAL SUBLUXATION'S CLINICAL SIGNIFICANCE

1. Subluxated segments of the spinal column occur in all individuals, including apparently healthy persons, and the presence of spinal subluxations is universally apparent in all individuals. The variability among individuals is in the number, degree, duration, level, grouping, and peculiarity of the subluxations as well as the individual's ability to accommodate and compensate in respect to their resources and reserves.

2. Subluxated segments are abnormal in their activity and in their response to various stimuli. Biomechanically, the vertebral subluxation is an alteration in the normal kinetics of the vertebral motion unit as well as a level of focused stresses of abnormal tension, torque, shearing, compression, and other forces affecting the unit's ability to provide required support as a segment in the column.

The presence of the subluxation also alters the segments' role of responsibility in providing protection for the neurologic elements of that level. Decreased protection allows for neural insult from external stimuli and also from internal stimuli (of which the subluxation is an intrinsic source because of aberrant position and motion).

Because they are abnormal in their activity, subluxated segments can no longer play normal roles in desired or demanded activities; ie, otherwise normal responses become exaggerated or diminished. Because of the persistent neuroinsult involved, the segment is also unable to receive stimuli adequately, because a normal excitation is unable to generate or direct a normal corresponding response.

3. Subluxated segments affect some neurons mediating sensory, motor, and autonomic function by altering their state of excitability. This results in abnormal re-

sponses to impulses reaching them from many sources. A vertebral subluxation decreases the function of spinal column to provide protection of the neurologic elements, allowing neural insult at the level of the subluxation. The nature of the resulting neurologic insult can categorically be identified by the effects on various activities under the control of the specialized elements affected.

The subluxation may allow insult to the sensory elements (neurons) in many variable patterns depending on the nature of the insult, the spatial location of the insult, the area or numbers of sensory neurons involved, and the modalities of sensation transmitted by the involved neurons. The classic patterns of effects of sensory insult are hyperesthesia, paresthesia, hypesthesia, anesthesia, discomfort, and pain (especially pain with *no* evidence of tissue damage).

The subluxation also may allow insult to the motor elements (efferent neurons) in the same variable patterns as above. The classic involvement of motor neurons is hypertonicity, hypotonicity, atony, and spastic or flaccid paralysis.

In addition, the subluxation may allow insult to the autonomic afferent and/or efferent neurons in variable patterns depending on the same variables as above in relation to either sympathetic or parasympathetic motor and sensory activities. The classic patterns of effects of autonomic insult are increased or decreased glandular secretion, motility, and sensitivity, constriction or dilation of innervated organs, and vasotonic disorders.

Further complexities of neural insult are possible with the involvement of a nearly infinite combination of elements involved. Clinical manifestations become most evident when a predominant involvement is present.

4. Subluxated segments are susceptible to sustained and exaggerated activity under conditions of daily life. In the state of maximum rest of the body, with no activities occurring and a minimum of sensory stimuli present in the environment, the vertebral subluxation continues to be a source of intrinsic stimuli and generated responding efforts (including efforts to self-correct). The complex responses even in this state are spending resources and taxing reserves of the individual when normal energy consumption should be minimal and body parts should be recuperating and repairing.

The obvious continual stress and demand associated with subluxation in this state are greatly amplified by restlessness and by added irritating stimuli from the environment. Added to this state of restlessness are the activities of daily life at home, work, play, and even during leisure periods. The stresses at rest are magnified many times with sustained and exaggerated activity. Activities for which one is unaccustomed are even greater sources of stress and usually demand new accommodations and compensations. Habitual activities become more stressful with extended duration, increased loads or demands, coupled activities, and unpleasant environmental changes.

5. Subluxated segments alter the normal influence of the neurons on the tissues they innervate and, in turn, the activity of those tissues is altered. The stimulus-response phenomenon mediated by the nervous system depends on the integrity of that system and all its parts. The normal mediating influence can not occur with any degree of diminished integrity of the system or any of its parts.

6. Subluxated segments are evidence of postural weight-bearing adaptations and compensations. The resulting muscular efforts due to adaptation and compensation are above and beyond the efforts required for normal activities and responses of motion units. Supportive tissues of the motion unit change in response to postural adaptations and compensations. The resulting unequal muscular efforts and changes in the supportive tissue allow or actively produce vertebral subluxation.

7. Subluxated segments result in the inability to provide adequate support and normal motion in the axial skeleton and inadequately protect the delicate elements of the nervous system from insult. The recruitment of muscular efforts for compensations alters the availability of muscular efforts required for normal motion patterns. Changes in supportive tissues in compensatory responses alter the reliability of support for stability, and the normally allowed ranges of the various motions and the unit's stability are shift-

ed one way or the other. With either excessive motion or stability, the potential of function necessary for protection of the mediating nervous system is compromised.

8. Subluxated segments displace weight-bearing forces, producing points of focused stress. The requirements for weight-bearing transfer forces from one segmental level to the next and direct the roles of muscular efforts and supportive tissues.

9. Subluxated segments have altered kinetic patterns that affect the normal range of motion in spinal activity. The normal vertebral segment is allowed activity patterns with normal ranges of axial rotation, lateral bending, flexion, and extension to participate in gross spinal column mobility. When the segment is already in a state of axial rotation, lateral bending, flexion, or extension prior to activation of the spine, the additional demands may be out of normal ranges resulting in excessive stress damage and/or referral of participation to other elements or segments.

A given vertebra, for example, in the preactive state of the spine is in axial rotation to the limits of its normal range of that level. A subsequent active state of the spine for a given movement normally requires axial rotation of the involved segment. During the effort to participate in the spinal activity, the segments that produce excessive stress in abnormal range of axial rotation may damage elements of restraint designed to maintain the range of motion or may transfer its response to another level—with that level now responsible for its own normal participation as well at that of one of its fellows. The final product will be faulty spinal motion because of faulted biomechanical function.

10. Subluxated segments induce spinal accommodations and compensation responses, eventually producing subluxated segments at other levels. In the preactive state of the spine, the vertebrae in a state of rotation, bending, flexion, or extension (subluxated) alter their support base to the vertebrae above and alter their transfer of forces to the vertebrae below. In response, the vertebrae above accommodate or compensate to or for the altered support base. Also in response, the vertebrae below accommodate or compensate to or for the altered transfer of forces from above. Continued or progressive responses above and below produce muscular reactions and changes in supporting tissues of other segments of the spinal column, resulting in subluxation of those segments with all the clinical significant potentials as the originally involved vertebra.

In the active state of the spine performing a daily activity, the subluxation producing excessive stress, damaging restraining elements, and/or transferring activity to other elements. The result is altered muscular activity and changes in supporting tissues of other segments of the spine, which then become subluxated. These subsequently subluxated vertebrae possess all the potential of the initial subluxation. The vicious cycle involved in subluxations is, in itself, of extreme clinical significance that is often overlooked in studies of axial skeleton disorders.

11. Subluxated segments misdirect and tax the individual's bioresources, resulting in diminished reserves. *Neurologically, the subluxation can adversely misdirect the effects of the utilization of bioresources for abnormal muscular activity of self correction or accommodation. Statically,* the subluxation requires use of reserves to supply additional responses for altered base support and to transfer forces to other supportive tissues. *Stressfully,* the subluxation places more demand intrinsically for compensation by the system. *Pathologically,* the subluxation results in damage to overstressed tissues that require repair resources. *Physically,* the subluxation transfers responsibility of responses to other tissues, increasing their consumption of bioresources. *Collectively,* the subluxation is a potential ecological disaster!

Facilitation and the Subluxation: Segmental Rheostats of Lowered Thresholds

The various definitions of facilitation all support the effect produced in nerve tissue by the passage of an impulse. The resistance of the nerve is diminished so that a second application of the stimulus evokes the reaction more easily. The *law of facilitation* specifically addressed, according to *Dorland's Medical Dictionary,* is "when an impulse has passed once through a certain set of neurons to the exclusion of others, it will tend to take the same course on a future occasion, and each time it transverses this path, the resistance in this path will be smaller."

Sensory impulses traveling via afferent neurons to a spinal cord segmental sensory neuronal pool causes facilitation of that pool, and sensory stimulation terminating in a segmental motor neuronal pool of the spinal cord causes facilitation of that pool. Descending motor impulses over efferents from higher motor centers of the brain to a segmental motor neuronal pool cause facilitation of that pool.

Sensory origins include both somatic afferents and visceral autonomic afferents, and descending efferents may originate in somatic brain centers or autonomic visceral centers. Motor neuronal pools facilitated by sensory afferents or descending efferents are both somatomotor and visceromotor pools.

When a segmental neuronal pool is in a state of facilitation, afferent impulses have a greater than normal effect on the neuronal pool; thus, they produce increased sensitivity. Efferent impulses are more easily generated; thus, they produce increased motor activity. This increased sensitivity and motor activity includes the autonomic pools and functions. Musculoskeletal stresses of subluxation initiate or are associated with an unbalanced stream of impulses entering the CNS. This, in effect, upsets the delicate balance of that part of the nervous system with which it is most intimately connected.

The debate rages on (chicken or egg). The theoretical possibility of segmental facilitation producing spinal subluxation is just as popular as that of spinal subluxation producing segmental facilitation. Even without settlement, the presence of subluxation as an intrinsic source of sensory irritation and the state of facilitation altering muscular activity of a vertebral motion unit warrants further thought.

Segmental Facilitation and Subluxation

Subluxated segments meeting the criteria of malposition and altered biokinetics have lowered motor reflex thresholds. The more clinically evident the subluxation, the lower the threshold.

Research has demonstrated that lesioned segments, as determined by clinical criteria, were distinguishable by physiologic criteria of motor activity. Segmental motor reflex thresholds were determined by measuring the amount of pressure applied to the spinous process of each segment that just evoked contraction of the paravertebral muscles at that segmental level. Muscle contractions were detected and evaluated by EMG recordings. Denslow found that lesioned segments invariably required weaker stimuli to produce reactions than did normal segments.

A later study demonstrated that diffuse and remote stimuli, including those from higher centers, and stimuli that occur in normal daily life, preferentially excited the pathways of paravertebral muscles of the facilitated segments. Other segments remained quiescent. Under conditions in which there was generalized muscular contraction, the activity in the facilitated segments was relatively exaggerated. The easier opening of the motor pathways, the motor facilitation, had its origin in a sustained afferent bombardment by impulses from some segmentally located source, according to Denslow, Korr, and Krems. It is suggested, therefore, that lowered segmental motor reflex thresholds, in a state of segmental facilitation, would result in exaggerated activity of those innervated postural muscles when only postural tone is required. The resultant activity, out of phase with need, could perpetuate existing subluxations or generate new subluxations.

Since postural spinal muscles function in myotatic units (together or in opposition) and are mechanically interdependent, any change in the activity of one muscle has direct effects on its synergists and antagonists. When facilitated, excitatory motor efferents elicit exaggerated muscle contractions of that muscle directly innervated as well as its synergists, and the facilitation will increase inhibition of the antagonists. This exaggerated reaction and increased antagonistic inhibition further alters the ability to stabilize posture by imbalanced postural tone and postural activity. This also may suggest that kinesiologic testing of a myotatic unit innervated by a subluxated segment would establish a weak (inhibited) muscle component and a strong (exaggerated) muscle component. Which muscle is inhibited and which is exaggerated may be dependent on the source originating the facilitory state. From a clinical viewpoint, the weak component has the same significance as the strong component.

Subluxated segments also exhibit a state of hyperirritability to sensory stimuli. Sensory components were measured and evaluated through cutaneous pain thresholds in various dermatomes and through mapping areas of cutaneous and deep hyperesthesia. Evidence gathered by Korr for hyperirritability of sensory pathways found the presence of persistent areas of lowered pain thresholds and of tenderness.

When using pressure on the spinous processes to elicit paravertebral contractions, it also was suggested that the involved segment with a demonstrated lowered segmental motor reflex threshold would also be hyperirritable to a pressure stimulus applied to the spinous process. Denslow found that the product of a lowered motor threshold plus a lowered threshold to sensory stimuli further exaggerates the motor activity associated with the abnormal segment.

Also suggested through hyperirritability and hypersensitivity in subluxated segments is the facilitated reception of all modalities of sensation with innervation through the sensory components of a given segment. In addition to cutaneous pain, lowered thresholds to sensations of somatic temperature, vibration, touch, proprioception, pressure, muscle stretch, and visceral pressure, distention, and pain also may be altered in the facilitated segment.

Skin Resistance Findings

Studies, limited to the sympathetic division because of segmental distribution, were evaluated through measurement of the activities of the sweat glands and blood vessels of the skin. These cutaneous visceral structures served as physiologic indicators of activity of sympathetic outflow to the corresponding areas or segments. Sweat gland activity was measured by electrical resistance of the skin (ERS). Skin resistance is lowered by increased sweat secretion and elevated in its absence. Also used were thermal readings of the skin. Cool skin with higher vascular tone suggests increased sympathetic motor innervation, as does increased sweat. Segments of sympathetic hyperirritability showed low ERS recordings and comparatively cool skin. There was also segmental lowering of the red (hyperemic) response to mechanical stroking of the skin.

Findings of a low ERS, low skin temperature, and feeble red response suggest increased irritability of both sensory and motor sympathetic pathways in affected spinal segments. Other studies have suggested relationships among a diagnosed pathologic organ or structure and areas of low ERS, especially where there was also a pain component present. After exploring large numbers of apparently healthy persons, it was found that in a growing number of such individuals the signs and symptoms of visceral disease appeared months and years after the demonstration of prominent areas of low electrical resistance in dermatomes related to the involved viscera. Some of these symptom-free subjects who later developed visceral disease had pre-existing ERS patterns resembling those found on patients with similar diseases. In other subjects, it was shown that new and prominent areas of low ERS could be induced experimentally by acute stresses and myofascial irritations, and accidentally as a result of trauma.

Conceptual Models

Some interesting conceptual models of subluxated segments and the facilitated state are offered below:

1. Facilitated segments of the spinal cord occur in most individuals, including apparently healthy persons.

2. These segments are abnormal in motor activity and in response to various stimuli.

3. In these segments, at least some neurons mediating sensory, motor, and autonomic functions are in a state of hyperexcitability with easier, exaggerated, and pro-

longed responses to impulses reaching them from many sources.

4. These segments are susceptible to sustained and exaggerated activity occurring in normal daily life.

5. The influence normally exerted by these neurons on the tissues that they innervate may thereby be exaggerated.

6. The antagonists of those muscular components that are in a state of facilitation are correspondingly inhibited, and the synergists are excited.

7. The state of facilitation effected by a subluxated segment refers to the tissues innervated by that segment; thus, the individual as a whole, through imbalance of homeostatic controls, is sensitized to all the influences operating within and without.

8. Facilitation of the sensory pathways in a subluxated segment means there is easier access to the nervous system through which environmental changes (especially stressful, noxious, or painful stimuli) have exaggerated impact on the individual.

9. Facilitation of motor pathways leads to sustained muscular tensions, exaggerated responses, postural asymmetries, and limited and painful motion. Positive feedback occurs because the muscles have rich sensory innervation, and under these conditions, the related muscles, tendons, ligaments, joint capsules, and articular surfaces become sources of intense and unbalanced afferent streams of impulses that perpetuate the state of facilitation.

10. Local sympathetic hyperactivity secondary to segmental facilitation subluxation that is reflected in the skin may be associated with sympathetic hyperactivity in the viscera. The cutaneous manifestations are associated with disturbances elsewhere in the segment, and this local sympathetic activity is an important factor in the production of disease processes. Hyperhidrosis and lowered ERS in dermatomes related to pathologic viscera have been demonstrated.

Autonomic Imbalance

Many serious clinical entities may be associated with local autonomic imbalance in the direction of *sympathicotonia*. Symptomatic relief, lasting improvement, and even "cures" have been achieved through surgical, pharmacologic, and other blocks of the sympathetic pathways to the involved organs.

A number of visceral and other chronic diseases appear to begin as ischemic states of the involved tissues due to local neurogenic vasospasm. This vasospasm seems to be of sympathetic origin and is also associated with vasospasm, pallor, and hypothermia in related segments of the skin. Vasomotor responses in the skin and viscera are quite parallel; ie, stimuli that elicit vasoconstriction in one, commonly do so in the other. This is exemplified in diffuse sympathetic activation under intense environmental or emotional stress, with blood being shunted from the viscera and skin to skeletal muscles. The ensuing visceral ischemia of the gut produces abdominal "butterflies," and the patient's ischemic skin gives an "as white as a ghost" appearance.

Normal sympathetic activity is intermittent and comparatively brief in response to emergency situations. When sympathicotonia is sustained, reduction in visceral blood flow, inhibition of secretion and smooth muscles activity, and spasm of sphincters will eventually result in some damage and dysfunction of the affected organs and thus the entire body's economy.

Summary. Under conditions of normal daily life, there may be steady streams of impulses flowing out of facilitated subluxated segments through sympathetic pathways to structures that they innervate. These impulses and the reactions to them may be beyond or conflict with the demands of homeostatic mechanisms. Under circumstances in which sympathetic activity normally occurs, the "drive" through facilitated segments is initiated earlier, reaches higher intensities sooner, and is sustained longer than in unfacilitated segments. With conditions of chronic environmental and emotional stress, the potentially dangerous influences will be preferentially focused upon and channeled through the facilitated segments. Whether overt disease processes develop depends on the total resources and resistance of the individual and demands of daily life. The greater the demands made by the total environment or the individual in relation to available resources, the more likely the following may be realized.

1. The greater the invasion of physiologic reserves, the higher the probability that the subluxation will become the decisive factor that limits the adequacy of or misdirecting the use of available resources.

2. With altered bioresources, the certainty that associated tissues will be impaired and damaged by exaggerated demands is greater.

3. The greater the sum of altered resources and tissues, the greater probability that disease will start in or through the facilitated segment and/or in the mechanisms that carry the burden of compensation for the altered functions and structures.

It is important to recognize that the early and progressive manifestations of subluxation may change with time. Prolonged activity may *fatigue*, resulting in changes from hyperhidrosis to hypohidrosis and vasospasm to vasomotor atonia.

It appears that segmental sympathetic hyperactivity originates as a part of a highly organized reflex response that is organized at the spinal cord level. It is initiated by certain forms of sustained irritation arising in one or more tissues innervated from or by the corresponding segment; manifesting sustained and exaggerated impulse traffic in the sensory, motor, and autonomic pathways that originate in this segment. This state of facilitation may be maintained by impulses reaching this segment from any source. The factors that evoke these segmental responses arise with high frequency in the weight-bearing or axial portion of the musculoskeletal system. One culprit may be the sustained impulses from proprioceptive insult caused by minor biomechanical faults.

Most visceral structures and functions are under both sympathetic and parasympathetic influence at least by a tonic level of activity. By either increasing or decreasing the influence of one system, the result will be an alteration of the influence of the other through antagonistic actions. Hypersympathicotonia thus could result, in effect, from either increased sympathetic activity or inhibited parasympathetic activity. Hyperparasympathicotonia, conversely, could result, in effect, from constant parasympathetic activity or inhibited sympathetic activity.

The centers controlling the sympathetic system can determine to a great degree whether they discharge selectively or totally. Under basal conditions, selective tonic and reflex activities occur; but under stress or in anger, the system can and does discharge as a whole.

Autonomic fibers are not essential to the functioning of all visceral tissues. However, overaction of this innervation has major physiologic consequences and underaction also impairs normal function, at least until the tissues recover from their dependency on this innervation.

Low vasomotor tone produces orthostatic hypotension. Overactivity of vasomotor nerves can result in hypertension. In Raynaud's disease, there is a spasmodic contraction chiefly of the blood vessels supplying the digits.

A general conceptual model is that the parasympathetic system has a conserving, protective function and tends to promote emptying of the hollow organs. The sympathoadrenal system functions in emergency situations, during stress, fear, anger, and rage, or when suffering with pain. Both systems tend to preserve an essential homeostatic balance of body functions, correct imbalances, and support behavioral activities.

Hypersympathicotonia may be involved in the following changes: pupillary dilation and protrusion of the eyeball in exophthalmos, constriction of gland cells with immediate increased secretion, vasoconstriction of glands with later decreased production and secretion, cardiac acceleration of pacemakers and increased strength of contraction with dilation of coronary arteries, dilated bronchi with decreased secretion and mild constriction of blood vessels of the lungs, decreased peristalsis and tone of lumen in the GI system with increased tone of sphincters plus inhibited secretion and vasoconstriction, vasoconstriction of renal vessels with decreased output, increased output of both epinephrine and norepinephrine from the adrenal medulla, increased adrenal cortical secretion, vasoconstriction of cutaneous vessels and vasodilation of blood vessels of skeletal muscles, piloerection and increased secretion of eccrine sweat glands, (but not the approcrine glands, which are humorally influenced), inhibited gallbladder contraction, increased glycogenolysis and increased liberation of glucose by the liver, reduction in blood clotting time, and contraction of the spleen to discharge red blood cells.

Reflex and Referral Models

In the following conceptual models, reflexes are defined as sensory activity producing motor responses. Referrals are defined as sensory activity referred by divergence of synapses to excite other sensory activities. In other words, reflexes are sensory to motor patterns and referrals are sensory to sensory patterns. Both should originate at sensory receptors, but they may originate anywhere along the course of an afferent fiber.

The various reflexes and referrals of initial stimuli that exist within and between individual components of the sensory, motor, and autonomic systems may exhibit the neurologic effects of subluxation. The ramifications and complexities of various reflexes and referrals and the countless number of signs, symptoms, and pathologic changes arising from these neurologic activities are even more challenging when considering not one but the interactions of many of these mechanisms that occur simultaneously in various degrees, overlappings, and combinations.

For ease in presentation of "the big eight" reflexes and referrals, each will be identified singularly:

1. *Somatosensory⟶somatomotor reflexes.* The simple reflex arc shows a somatosensory stimulation synapsing in the cord to a somatic motor neuron, with consequent somatic muscle reflex actions. This is illustrated by the simple stretch reflex (Fig. 5.4).

2. *Somatosensory⟶somatosensory referrals.* Somatosensory neurons may diverge to other somatic afferent fibers on route, causing their facilitation or stimulation and a resultant interpretation of sensory awareness in a somesthetic area some distance from the original stimuli; therefore, a somatosensory to somatosensory referral of sensation (Fig. 5.5).

Somatosensory neurons are those afferent fibers that carry sensory information to the cord from all somatic structures innervated by that cord segment; particularly, dermal sensations, muscle stimuli, and musculoskeletal-related proprioceptive sensations of motor activity, vibration, and position. *Somatomotor neurons* are those efferent fibers that innervate skeletal muscles at

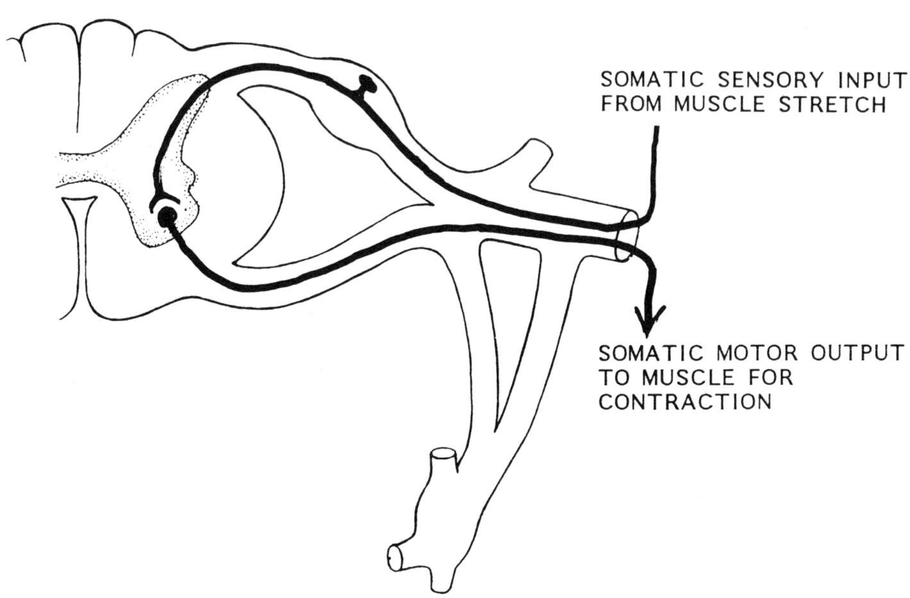

Figure 5.4. A somatosensory to somatomotor reflex (simple stretch reflex).

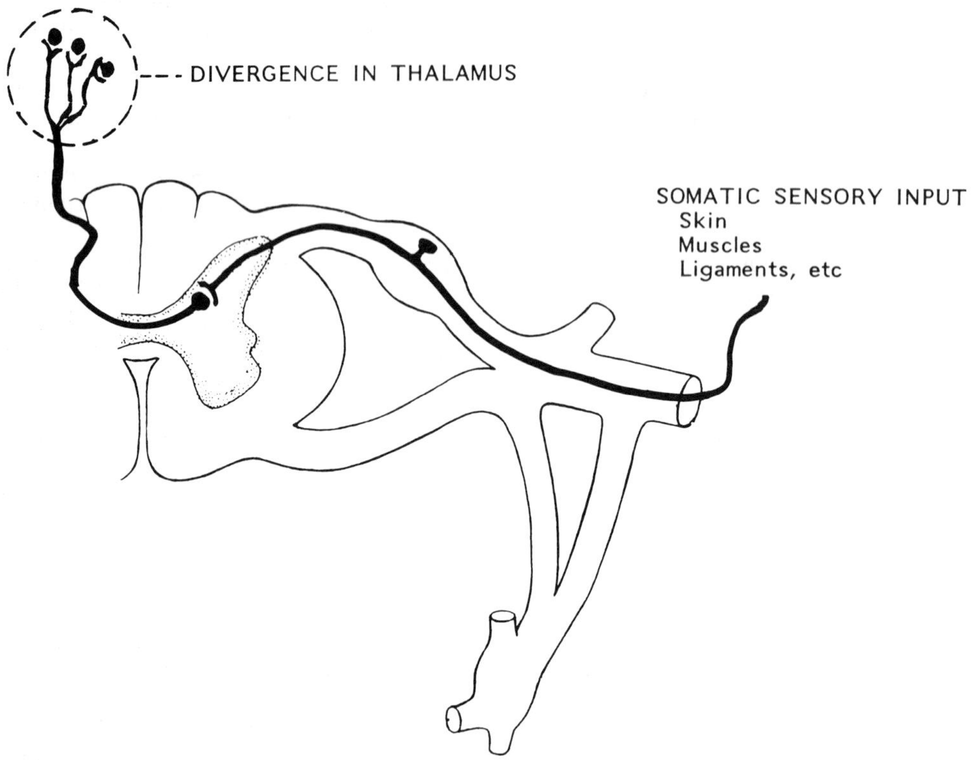

Figure 5.5. A somatosensory to somatosensory referral.

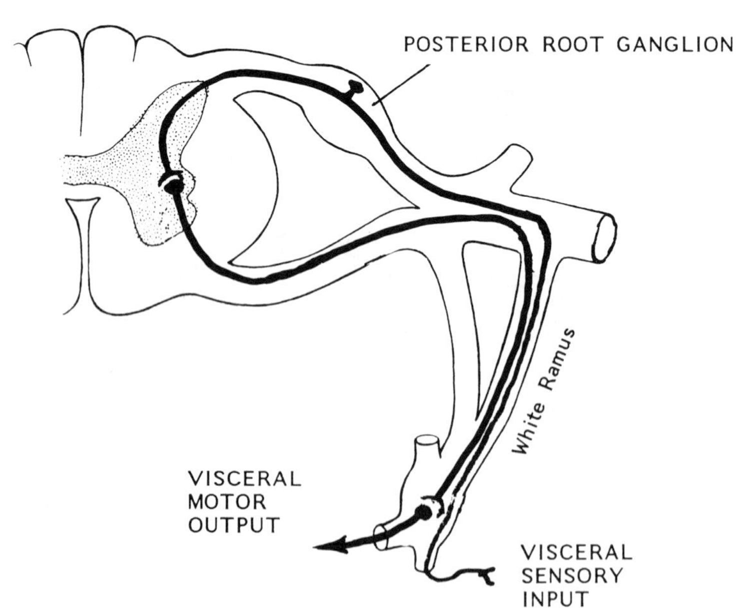

Figure 5.6. A viscerosensory to visceromotor reflex.

a given cord level and control tonus or contraction of the related somatic elements.

3. *Viscerosensory ⟶ visceromotor reflexes.* Afferent visceral sensory neurons arise from internal organs and tissues or from the visceral components of skin, muscles, tendons, ligaments, or other somatic structures that contain viscerosensory receptors (Fig. 5.6). The visceromotor activity that occurs reflexly is dependent upon the nature of viscerosensory stimulation. One simple example might be the presence of a bolus of food in the esophagus exciting stretch receptors of viscerosensory neurons producing visceromotor reflexes of peristalsis, secretion and sphincter contractions.

The sympathetic visceromotor response may occur throughout a specific neuromere. Therefore, a viscerosensory stimulus may elicit a vasomotor response of constriction or a smooth-muscle contraction in a specific organ. It also may cause a vasoconstriction of blood vessels of the somatic structures, musculature, skin, ligaments, etc, depending on the divergence of collaterals of the visceromotor neurons affected.

4. *Viscerosensory ⟶ viscerosensory referral.* There may occur within the cord a referral of viscerosensory stimuli to afferent fibers from other visceral sources that, in turn, elicit visceromotor responses other than those produced reflexly. This is similar to somatosensory to somatosensory referral See Figure 5.7.

5. *Viscerosensory ⟶ somatosensory referral.* This is commonly accepted as the mechanism of referred pain, with the afferent viscerosensory fibers diverging to internuncial or first-order neurons of a somatosensory nature, causing their stimulation and the perception of pain in a somatic area or structure (Fig. 5.8). Once initiated, this referral may cause additional areas to become involved through somatosensory to somatosensory referrals so that referral of conscious pain may occur in other areas than that of the segment involved (cord, medulla, or thalamus level). A classic ex-

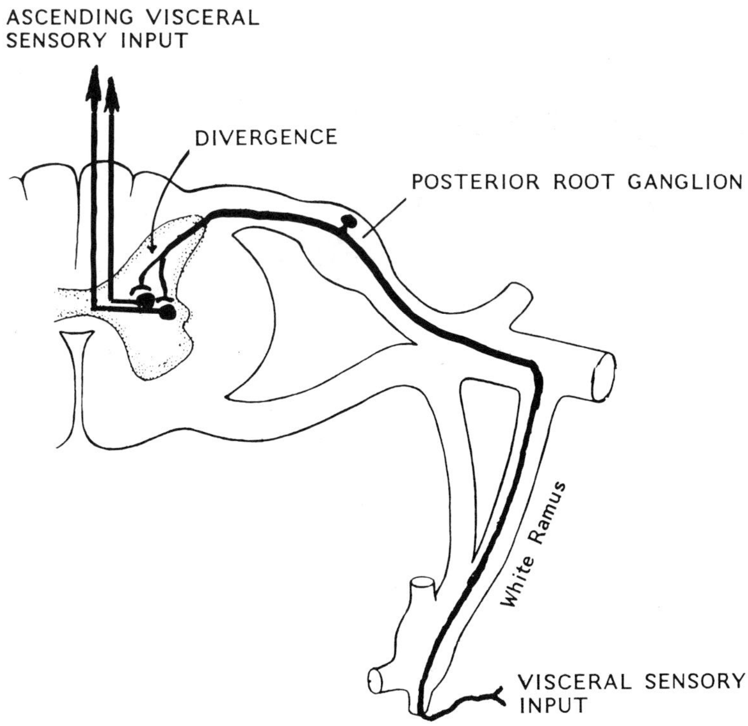

Figure 5.7. A viscerosensory to viscerosensory referral.

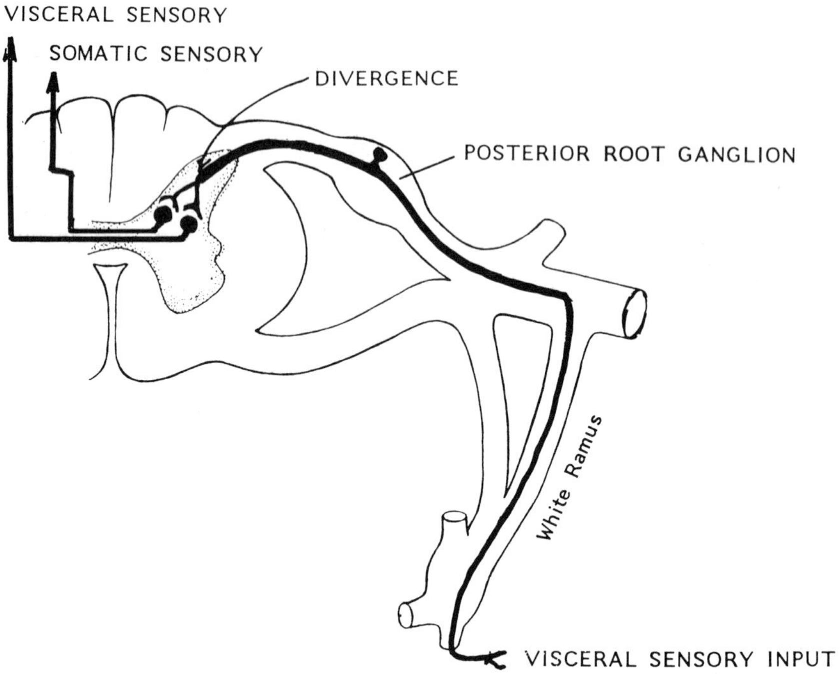

Figure 5.8. A viscerosensory to somatosensory referral (referred pain).

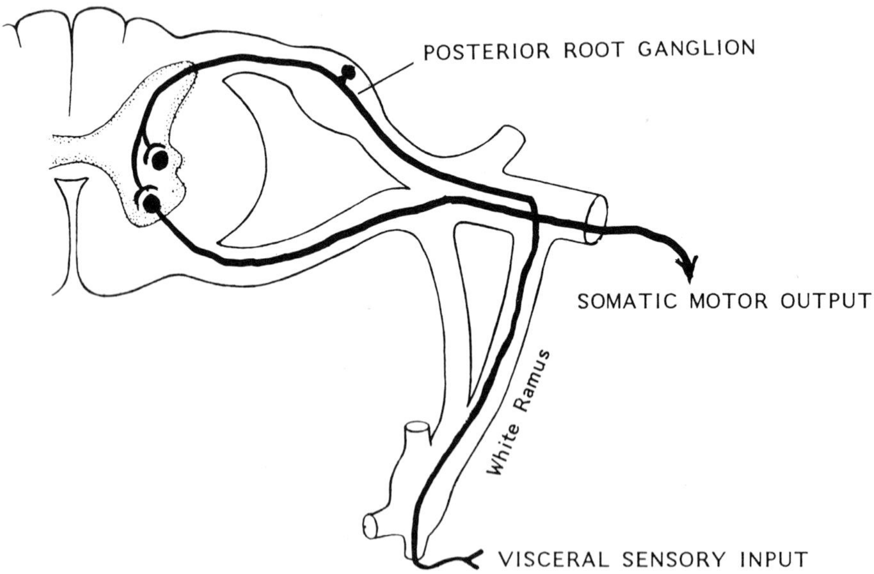

Figure 5.9. A viscerosensory to somatomotor reflex.

ample is the angina of ischemic heart muscle with viscerosensory impulses of the heart being perceived as somatic sensitivity of the left shoulder and arm.

6. *Viscerosensory ⟶ somatomotor reflexes.* Somatic muscular spasm is in response to viscerosensory afferents in appendicitis with abdominal cramps (Fig. 5.9). This may involve viscerosensory to somatosensory referral that, in turn, sets up the somatosensory to somatomotor reflex.

7. *Somatosensory ⟶ visceromotor reflexes* (Fig. 5.10). Ussher states: "In general, afferent impulses from the skin, the dorsal musculature, or the articulations of the vertebral column are relayed through the cord and emerge as impulses to the viscera." An example might be subluxation of the T6 vertebra that produces somatosensory irritation, resulting in spastic closure of the cardiac sphincter by visceromotor reflexes producing achalasia. This reflex also explains the red response of stroking the skin and various systems of reflexology. Somatic stimulation of a vertebra (manipulation, percussion, etc) also may alter visceral motor responses. Subluxation is a somatic lesion and through somatosensory irritation of its presence may reflexly alter segmental visceral functions.

Another example needs mention because somatic-tissue irritations may directly induce the inflammatory reflexes of vasculature.

8. *Somatosensory ⟶ viscerosensory referrals.* The distribution of, as well as the character of, referred visceral pain may not only have its origin in an internal viscus, it also may arise from the stimulation of somatosensory, proprioceptive, and pain-conducting fibers in ligaments, musculature, fascia, or other somatic sources (Fig. 5.11).

Korr states that injection of the C7—T1 interspinous ligament with hypertonic saline solution produced a perfect facsimile of an angina attack, not only pain distributed substernally, pain and radiation to the ulnar surface of the arm, but also hyperalgesia areas, muscular rigidity, and a sense of compression of the chest. Injection of the first lumbar

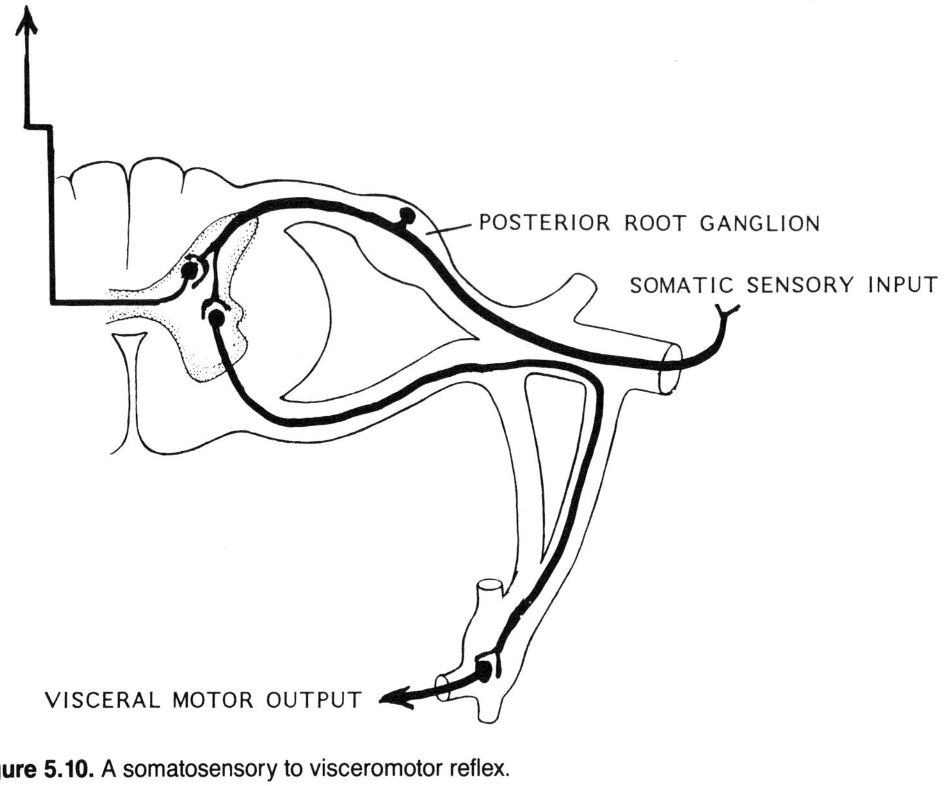

Figure 5.10. A somatosensory to visceromotor reflex.

interspinous ligament produced pain of renal colic.

Somatomotor or visceromotor effects through reflexes and somatosensory or viscerosensory referrals may be initiated by either a visceral or somatic stimulus. But the synaptic area (neuronal pools) subserving these processes, both in the spinal cord and/or brain centers, may, because of repetitious activity or previous stimulation (activation), have lowered thresholds (eg, be in a facilitated state). Even if the initiating cause of this process is removed, the minimal thresholds for eliciting a neurologic response is reduced so that what was previously subthreshold stimuli may now elicit or maintain the signs, symptoms, and pathophysiologic processes involved. In such a situation, previously irrelevant stimuli evoked by daily environmental or constitutional stress may now maintain (sustain) or exacerbate (amplify) these processes through facilitated reflexes and referrals.

Korr states: "Because of the sustained facilitation of sensory, motor, and autonomic pathways, the lesioned segment acts as a neurological lens, focusing and exaggerating the effects of impulses from many sources upon the tissues innervated from that segment; through the segment the individual is subject to the exaggerated impact of life situations and environmental factors."

In view of the basic tenets of D.D. Palmer's chiropractic philosophy and the concepts presented thus far, it is strongly suggested that a system of healing based on that philosophy, incorporating these concepts, must be as liberal as its therapeutic applications. Further suggested are methods and procedures necessary for the removal and/or correction of mechanical, chemical, and psychic irritations (environmental and constitutional factors of disease) as related to the nervous system as well as removal of the subluxations, which maintain or amplify the neurologic aberrations thus initiated.

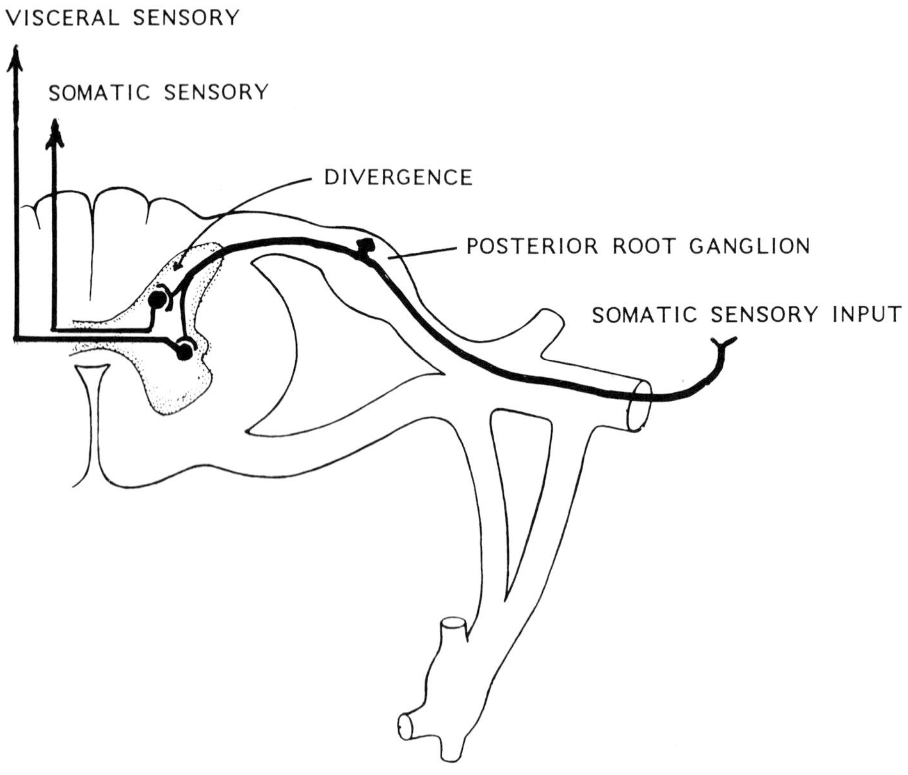

Figure 5.11. A somatosensory to viscerosensory referral.

The "Garden Hose" Theory

Historically, this concept suggests that pressure on a nerve, produced by subluxation, decreases its ability to transmit impulses. This author has not found scientific evidence to support such a phenomenon in all neurologic tissue. The research findings of Suh indicate that spinal nerve roots are far more susceptible to compression block than peripheral nerves. Large rapidly conducting fibers are more susceptible to compression block than small slowly conducting fibers. Inhibition of trophic nerve flow is also suggested by the "garden hose" theory.

In peripheral nerves, some fibers are blocked by pressure as low as 30 mm Hg. Reduction of compound action potential to at least half required at least 100 mm Hg. A pressure of 150 mm Hg was required to produce a complete block of the sciatic nerve within 3 minutes. In contrast, with pressure applied to spinal nerve roots, slight impairment could be observed with 10 mm Hg and was reduced to half size by only 20 mm Hg.

Denny-Brown and Brenner report that "Sensory fibers are more resistant to pressure than motor fibers." Suh states that "Fibrotic and thickened ligaments may, in the extremes of motion, press on spinal nerves where they exit from the IVFs. Protruding discs may encroach on spinal nerves. Thinning discs and other disorders may result in narrowing of the foramina and pressure on spinal nerves. The compression of spinal nerves presumably results in aberrant neuronal activity which alters the operating characteristics of reflex mechanisms within the cord."

Most biologists would agree with Crelin that the vertebral column of man is marvelously engineered to protect the delicate spinal nerves. Through a wide dynamic range and while supporting large loads, the spinal column normally performs well, IVFs normally remain spacious, and nerves normally need not endure sustained compression effects. Nevertheless, the literature provides ample evidence that the spinal nerves can be compressed during certain pathologic conditions, including disc protrusion or thinning, fibrosis or thickening of spinal ligaments, osteoarthritis, neoplasms, hemorrhage or swelling, etc. Between the extremes of normal functioning and those of gross pathology such as are associated with medically diagnosed nerve compression syndromes, there must exist various degrees of abnormality in which forces transmitted to spinal nerves can exceed the normal level. Under such conditions, subtle impairment of nerve function may occur that are not easily diagnosed as a nerve compression syndrome. Such impairments might, however, respond to manipulation provided by chiropractic treatments and be recognized as significant phenomena of the subluxation syndrome.

With *compression block*, two factors have been implicated: (1) anoxia, with resulting effects on the microvasculature of the nerve, and (2) mechanical deformation or rupture of nerve fibers. Both could be involved, especially in chronic nerve compression. Recent studies of nerves subjected to chronic constriction indicate that the most peripheral fibers undergo the earliest degeneration.

Causey/Schoepfle state: "The maintenance of the normal structure and function of peripheral nerve fibers depends on an adequate blood supply to nerve trunks. The importance of the blood supply is illustrated by the observations that for the first 6—8 hours after section of a nerve, the metabolic activities associated with the recovery from fatigue induced by stimulation are more dependent on the blood supply to the fiber than on its connection with the cell body."

According to Moldaver: "It can be accepted as a generalization that, during the development of a compression block, the different modalities are lost in the following order: proprioception, touch, temperature, and pain sensibility."

The Melzak/Wall Gate-Control Theory

In view of the *law of specific nerve energies*, impulses conveyed to the CNS by nociceptive afferent fibers would be interpreted as painful, and those conveyed by contact-sensitive fibers would be interpreted as non-injurious mechanical stimulation. But Melzak/Wall point out that the signals often seem confused or inhibited. Neuralgia and causalgia are examples of excruciating pain being produced by gentle touch or vibration. Pain generated by tissue damage may diminish or disappear in emotional excitement or in the presence of "counterirritants."

Theory. Impulses in large mechanoreceptive fibers and those in small nociceptive fibers converge on specialized nerve cells (T-cells) in the posterior horn of the spinal gray matter. Somatosensory information is processed here and relayed to the brain through ascending tracts.

When the activity in T-cells reaches a high level, it is interpreted as a sign of potential tissue damage and reacted to as if it were painful or threatening (a demand for awareness and action). If this were all, any intense somatosensory stimulation would be painful, but this theory assumes the existence of a "sensory gate."

Both large and small fiber input (both nociceptive and nonnociceptive input) can be blocked by the activity of inhibitory interneurons in the substantia gelatinosa area of the dorsal gray matter. These inhibitory neurons act directly on the sensory endings of the afferent neurons to reduce their effectiveness and inhibit transmission to the T-cells. These inhibitory neurons, partly because of descending influences from the brain, are always active, tending to hold the sensory gate partly closed (centrifugal influences).

The large, mechanoreceptive fibers activate the inhibitory cells, tending to close the gate. The small, nociceptive fibers, on the other hand, retard the substantia gelatinosa inhibitory cells, and by this "inhibition of inhibition" open the sensory gate (Fig. 5.12).

In the subluxation-free segment, large mechanoreceptive fibers carry continual impulses to the cord and maintain the gate in the closed position. With the addition of a subluxation that has a compression factor on the spinal nerve root and that compression selectively blocking large mechanoreceptive fibers, the symptoms of pain may appear as a result of an opening effect of the sensory gate. Conversely, removal of compression-causing subluxation may allow return of the large mechanoreceptive fiber impulses, closing the gate and relieving the symptoms of pain.

Trophic Influences of Nerves

The trophic influence of nerves on the organs and tissues they innervate has long been recognized as a mysterious innate phenomenon in chiropractic philosophy and practice.

We are now approaching an understanding of how nerves exert long-term influences that cannot be ascribed to impulse conduction. Research suggests that there are certain proteins (not yet identified), and possibly other highly specific substances of large complex molecular structure, that are synthesized in peripheral nerve cells (so-

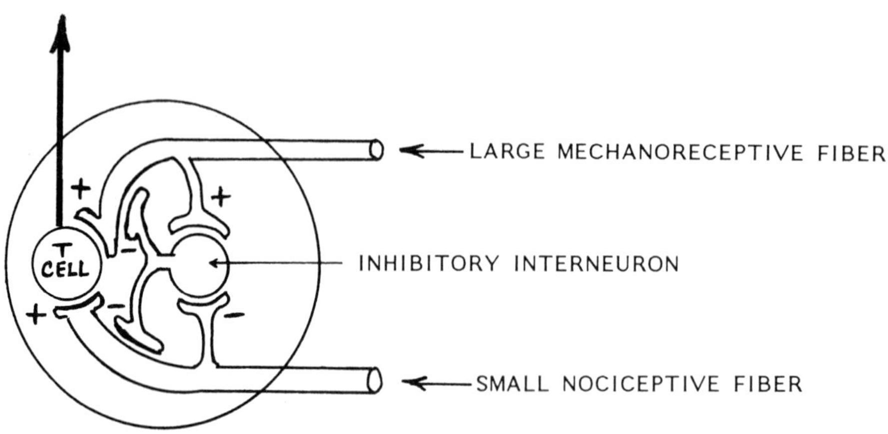

Figure 5.12. Schematic of the theoretical pain gate.

mas) and that these neuronal components (trophic substances) are transported through the length of the fiber (neuronal peristalsis) and cross the junctional barriers into tissue cells.

Interruption of the Neurotrophic Flow

Korr reports that "The atrophy of denervation (interrupted neurotrophic flow) and the atrophy of disuse (interruption of motor nerve impulses) in the structural, functional, and biochemcial aspects of muscle are quite different in nature and in course, though the former does naturally include aspects and components of the latter. What seems involved is not so much interruption of impulses (and therefore contractile activity), but disconnection between nerve cells and muscle cells."

Confirmation of this concept can be approached several ways:

1. Atrophy of denervation is due to disconnection between neuron and organ rather than the arrest of impulse traffic as seen in cutting the glossopharyngeal nerve on one side. The taste buds (sensory organs and receptors) on the same side of the tongue soon began to dedifferentiate back into nonspecific epithelium, eventually disappearing completely. On reinnervation, redifferentiation was triggered, and complete normal gustatory apparatus was restored. The fact that sensory receptors do not rely on impulse arrival (antidromic impulses) suggests that the degeneration and dedifferentiation were secondary to interruption of neurotrophic flow and that the subsequent regeneration and differentiation was also under the influence of neurotrophic substances.
2. Atrophy of disuse (diminished impulse traffic) in a muscle can be avoided or corrected by synthetic electrical stimulation of that muscle. However, the atrophy of denervation is not reversed or avoided by synthetic electrical stimulation and continues its course of degeneration and dedifferentiation.
3. A hair-size string tied around a fiber may act as a node of Ranvier, not interfering with impulse conduction (may even facilitate impulse conduction) but, rather, interrupting neurotrophic flow. Impulses (orthodromic) continue to arrive at the end organ. Dedifferentiation and degenerative changes occur in the end organ with interrupted neurotrophic flow. The atrophy of disuse, a result of interruption of impulses, has been found much less severe, much more readily reversed, and different in many ways than the atrophy occurring following axonal interruption.

Conditioning Influences of Nerves

Nerves exert a conditioning effect on the functional properties of some tissues and on responses to other influences; ie, denervation of skin augments its susceptibility to the action of carcinogenic agents. Denervation also affects responses of various organs to certain hormones.

Morphogenetic Influences

If the nerve supply to one kidney is interrupted in a puppy before the 10th or 11th day of life, the development of the kidney is also interrupted at that point. This is also suggested in muscle differentiation and growth.

Role of Nerve in Regeneration

Nerves are capable of regenerating entire limbs after amputation. If the nerve is removed from the amputated stump, regeneration does not take place. Resection of the sensory fibers in the stump allowed for regeneration. Healing and regeneration are influenced by nerve supply in wounds and repair of defects in skin, bone, and other tissues, in all mammalian species, including man.

Regulation of Gene Expression

Skeletal muscle is commonly classified into two categories: red and white. *Red fiber* is slowly contracting and relaxing with twitches of long duration, and sent into sustained tetanic contraction with low-frequency stimulation; ie, tonic, postural muscle. *White fiber* is phasic, rapidly contracting muscle, with brief twitches, and requires high-frequency stimulation to produce tetanus. Red muscle is largely aerobic (oxidation metabolism), while white muscle is capable of a high degree of anaerobic glycolytic metabolism.

When the nerves to red and white muscle cells are switched (by cross-reinnervation) and time is allowed for neural regeneration, an important generalization emerges: A remarkable degree of cross-transformation takes place, which includes structure, chemical composition, metabolic pathways, and enzyme activity. The nerve, in effect, instructs the muscle (muscle is pluripotential) by determining which genes of the muscle cells will be repressed and which will be expressed.

Over time, any factor altering the metabolism and protein synthesis of a neuron or impedes axonal transport could interfere with the neurotrophic influences on the innervated structures or cause an adverse or detrimental effect, thereby contributing to disease processes. The most likely factor is the vertebral subluxation, with compressive forces and mechanical stresses occurring where the nerves pass, the accompanying chemical changes in these tissues, and the associated aberrant sensory input and motor activity.

Bibliography

Boyd WA: *A Textbook of Pathology*. Philadelphia, Lea & Febiger, 1961.

Denslow JS: Evidence of the osteopathic lesion: Data on what is known, what is not known, and what is controversial. In Goldstein M (ed): *The Research Status of Spinal Manipulative Therapy*. Bethesda, MD, NINCDS Monograph No. 15, US Dept of HEW, 1975.

Homewood AE: *The Neurodynamics of the Vertebral Subluxation*, ed 3. Place of publication not shown, published by author, 1981.

Janse J: History of the development of chiropractic concepts: Chiropractic terminology. In Goldstein M (ed): *The Research Status of Spinal Manipulative Therapy*. Bethesda, MD, NINCDS Monograph No. 15, US Dept of HEW, 1975.

Janse J: A concept: the neurological element as it relates to clinical chiropractic. *The Chirogram*, December 1975.

Janse J: The integrative purpose and function of the nervous system: a review of classical literature. *Journal of Manipulative and Physiological Therapeutics*, 1(3), September 1978.

Korr IM: Discussion: papers of Sidney Ochs and David E. Pleasure. In Goldstein M (ed): *The Research Status of Spinal Manipulative Therapy*. Bethesda, MD, NINCDS Monograph No. 15, US Dept of HEW, 1975.

Korr IM (ed): *The Neurobiologic Mechanisms in Manipulative Therapy*. New York, Plenum Press, 1978.

Korr IM: The spinal cord as organizer of disease processes: Some preliminary perspectives. *Journal of the American Osteopathic Association*, September 1976.

Melzack R, et al: Neurophysiological foundations of pain. In Sternbach RA (ed): *The Psychology of Pain*. New York, Raven Press, 1978, pp 1-26.

Melzack R, Wall PD: On the nature of cutaneous sensory mechanisms. *Brain*, 85:331-356, 1962.

Palmer DD: *Textbook of the Science, Art and Philosophy of Chiropractic*. Portland, OR, Portland Printing House, 1910.

Schafer RC (ed): *Basic Chiropractic Procedural Manual*, ed 4. Arlington, VA, American Chiropractic Association, 1984.

Speransky AD: *A Basis for the Theory of Medicine;* translated by C.P. Dutt. New York, International Publishers, 1943.

Steindler A: *Kinesiology of the Human Body Under Normal and Pathological Conditions*. Springfield, IL, Charles C. Thomas, 1955.

Stephenson RW: *Chiropractic Textbook*. Davenport, IA, published by author, 1927.

Suh CH: Biomechanical aspects of subluxation. In Goldstein M (ed): *The Research Status of Spinal Manipulative Therapy*. Bethesda, MD, NINCDS Monograph No. 15, US Dept of HEW, 1975.

Suh CH: Computer-aided spinal biomechanics. In Haldeman S (ed): *Modern Developments in the Principles and Practice of Chiropractic*. New York, Appleton-Century-Crofts, 1980.

Wall PD: Gate control theory of pain mechanisms: a reexamination and re-statement. *Brain*, 101:1-18, 1978.

Chapter 6

General Causes and Potential Effects of the Subluxation Complex

This chapter reviews the concepts underlying chiropractic articular therapy, with emphasis placed on neurologic implications. General etiology, manifestations, terminology, pertinent anatomical features, and applications are described.

SPINAL SUBLUXATION: CAUSES AND EFFECTS

Until the last 2 decades, most evidence about the success of chiropractic adjustments on the correction of vertebral subluxations and their related functional disturbances was empiric. The gap between controlled research documentation and frequent clinical observation still exists, but it has greatly narrowed in recent years. The greatest concern today is not *is it effective* but *why is it effective* and *why is it effective in some cases but not in others that appear almost identical?* Added to these can be the questions: *what causes the positive effects in a specific body area that result from spinal adjustments that cannot be explained on an anatomical basis* and *what causes the indirect, far-reaching, diverse improvement in function so often witnessed?*

It is widely recognized that the predisposition to dysfunction is created by definite combinations of internal nervous relations and not merely by an undermining of the general state of health. Present clinical state-of-the-art holds that any nerve point, including the peripheral nerve structures, may become the initiator of neurodystrophic processes and serve as a temporary or permanent originator of such processes. Speransky stated: "...neurodystrophic processes are not confined to a limited sphere, they enter into the composition of all pathologic processes without exception, are not separable from them, and consequently, do not constitute and cannot constitute a separate chapter in pathology." There is hardly a known function that can be realized without a change in the state of some organ, except possibly memory. Thus, the external manifestations of complex human nervous processes are extremely diverse.

General Causes of Spinal Subluxations

Several authorities describe the general causes of vertebral subluxations as including mechanical irritation, overt trauma (eg, blows, whiplash, lifting, falls, birth injuries), chronic spinal strain or sprain, somatosomatic and viscerosomatic reflexes, IVD protrusions and distortions, postural tension due to balance faults (eg, scoliosis, pregnancy, visceroptosis) and the stress of bipedism, chemical and toxic irritation, and psychologic or environmental stress—all which may result in asymmetric muscle spasticity leading to articular malalignment and/or fixation. Susceptibility is thought to increase in states of chronic fatigue, anemia, erosive arthritides, systemic toxemia, and hereditary predisposition because of anomalous development.

Many spinal subluxations have more than one immediate cause and effect. For example, a developmental abnormality may be complicated by degenerative joint disease, retrograde changes, inflammation, or muscle splinting. The effects may be direct upon blood vessels and nerves, reflex in nature, etc. Therefore, a complicated and far-reaching series of interacting and interdependent changes occur that may be designated as a subluxation syndrome.

The extent of dysfunction of a bony segment within its articular bed may vary in effect from a microtrauma to one that is macroscopic and quite readily discernible. It is always attended to some degree by articular dysfunction, neurologic insult, and stressed muscles, tendons, and ligaments. Once produced, the lesion usually becomes a focus of sustained irritation from which a bombardment of impulses stream into the spinal cord where internuncial neurons receive and relay them to motor and/or sensory pathways. The muscular contraction that provoked the subluxation originally is thereby reinforced, thus perpetuating both the structural subluxation and the pathophysiologic processes involved.

Priority subluxations are often specific positional errors originating from alterations in the integrity of the paraspinal supporting tissues of the involved joint itself. As such, they are beyond the capacities of the muscular system to correct by its own functional adaptations.

Precipitating Factors of Spinal Subluxations

Vertebral subluxations may be either causes or effects, and the immediate causes may be divided into two major categories: the unequal or asymmetrical muscular efforts upon the joint structures and the inequality in the supporting tissues of a particular joint such as the cartilage, IVD, ligaments, etc. Some form of internal or external stress is usually necessary to produce a fixation to a degree sufficient to cause a state of dysfunction.

An inequality in muscular balance (ipsilateral weakness and compensatory contralateral contraction) may be initiated by (1) trauma, (2) postural distortion phenomena, (3) psychomotor responses, (4) somatic and visceral responses, and (5) paralytic effects. Two other causes not previously described in previous chapters are (6) biochemical reactions and (7) stress factors, both of which may overtly manifest biomechanically. Typical examples would include those shown in Table 6.1.

Biochemical Reactions

A state of acute or chronic hypo- or hypertonicity of musculature may be due to various biochemical changes within related tissues. This may be brought about by either local or general disorders that may cause anoxia, ischemia, toxicity, etc, by foreign bodies, systemic fatigue-producing activities, nutritional deficiencies or excesses, caustic chemical exposure, ingestion of harmful chemicals, inhalation of noxious gases, microorganism toxins, abnormal glandular activity, excessive heat or cold, or electric shock affecting the chemical environment of cells.

Stress Factors Producing Subluxation

Any internal or external stress factor can involve the nervous system directly or indirectly, depending on the degree of stress produced. This may result in decreased mobility of the vertebra of the involved neuromere, and the decreased mobility may be the result of (1) muscle splinting, especially on the side of greatest stimulation according to Pfluger's law or (2) from abnormal weight distribution to the facets and other weight-bearing structures of the vertebrae involved.

Pfluger's law states that if a stimulus received by a sensory nerve extends to a motor nerve of the opposite side, contraction occurs only from corresponding muscles; and, if contraction is unequal bilaterally, the stronger contraction always takes place on the side that is stimulated. When affecting one or more vertebrae, this state of decreased mobility of the motion unit encourages nerve dysfunction, leading to pathologic processes in the areas supplied by the affected nerve root or neuromere depending upon the degree and chronicity of involvement.

Physical Diagnosis Criteria

The most commonly used criteria in physical diagnosis of determining the existence of vertebral subluxation-fixation are (1) asymmetry such as paraspinal soft-tissue changes (spasticity, contractures, or flaccidness) and palpable osseous malposition (often misleading); (2) restricted segmental mobility in one or more planes; (3) dermatomal skin abnormalities such as altered texture or color, bogginess, and vasomotor disorders with resultant temperature, thermographic, and electrical resistance changes; and (4) possibly altered reflexes. Differential diagnosis by exclusion is frequently applied. See Appendix, Figures A.1—A.3.

General Effects of Spinal Subluxations

As a primary concept of chiropractic science, spinal subluxations may result in the development of disease states locally within the vertebral motion unit itself or throughout specific areas of the body. These primary and secondary effects of subluxations may be classified into three major categories:

1. The mechanical effect, motion, and balance of the local segment, or the effect upon the skeleton elsewhere, due to compensatory distortions and alterations as proprioceptive mechanisms attempt to correct the mechanics in the presence of structural imbalance.
2. The effect of any localized condition occurring within the articulations due to interarticular stress and trauma (often microtrauma) such as irritation, inflammation, swelling, necrosis, and other degenerative changes.
3. The neurologic scope of subluxation effects may be grossly differentiated as nerve pressure, nerve stretch, nerve torsion, circulatory changes, meningeal irritations, cerebrospinal fluid flow alterations, alterations of proprioceptive responses and reflexes, traumatic insult to the rami communicantes or sympathetic ganglia, among many others.

Table 6.1. Precipitating Factors of Spinal Subluxations

Muscular overload or weakness		
Abnormal glandular activity	Exposure to drafts	Somatospinal reflexes
Biochemical imbalance	Nutritional deficiencies	Toxic states (endogenous or exogenous)
Caustic chemical exposure	Paralytic effects	Trauma, frank/acute
Electric shock	Postural distortion phenomena	Viscerospinal reflexes
Excessive heat or cold	Psychomotor responses	
Structural imbalance		
Connective-tissue diseases	Osseous pathology	Strain
IVD pathology	Postural fatigue	Structural anomalies
Kyphosis	Scoliosis	Trauma, cummulative/repetitive microtrauma/overuse syndrome
Lordosis	Short-leg etiologies	
	Sprain	

The neurologic effects are undoubtedly the more important of the three from a clinical aspect.

Spinal subluxation syndromes may have more than one immediate cause and effect. Abnormality of development may be complicated by degenerative joint disease, retrograde changes, inflammation, and muscle splinting, for example. The effects may be direct upon nerve roots and their blood vessels, reflex in nature, etc. Therefore, a complicated and far-reaching series of interacting and interdependent changes occur that may be designated as a subluxation syndrome.

Potential Scope of Reactions

When dysfunction manifests clinically, it can be assured that some degree of pathology is present. It also can be appreciated that any point in the complex nervous system can produce changes in the body when stimulated. These changes may manifest not only in adjacent parts but also in areas far remote from the site of irritation. If an irreversible change occurs at any point as a result of local irritation, the effect is some loss of a particular function and the establishment of new pathologic excitations that draw other parts into the process. Pathologist Boyd boldly states, "Disease is function gone wrong."

The neurons are the anatomical and functional units of the nervous system; and *localization of effect* does not exist in the nervous system. This is not to say that every active means of producing a transformation of the normal nervous state will be reflected in the same manner in the various pathologic progressions because the neurologic element is highly complex in its overt and covert functions. The nerve impulse creates a multitude of cellular reactions and responses besides those of the most intricate, subtle, and variable sensations and motor activities. Once this is recognized, the diagnostician must add the complexities of:

Abnormal cerebrovisceral interreactions
Abnormal viscerocerebral interreactions
Biochemical affinities
Disintegration of synaptic thresholds
Facilitation patterns
Genetic neurologic diatheses
Input of the ascending and descending reticular activating mechanisms
Neuroendocrine interrelations
Neurologic spread and buildup
Predisposition to sensorial aberration
Proprioceptive buildup
Psychosomatic overtones
Reflex instability
Summation increments
Synaptic overlaps
Trophic effects

To these can be added those many phenomena that science is only beginning to appreciate or are beyond our present understanding. This underscores the fact that the quality of nerve function relates directly or indirectly to practically every bodily function and contributes significantly to the beginning of physiologic malfunction and the development of pathologic processes.

Functional Alterations

It is a basic premise of chiropractic that a relationship exists between dysfunction of the nervous system and many diseases. It is also fundamental that some aberration within the spinal column produces the nerve dysfunction, or more specifically, that a malpositioned vertebra is at fault. Bergmann reminds us that, besides this malposition, it must be clearly understood that the nerve dysfunction results from more than the structural misalignment. There are neuropathophysiologic, kinesiopathologic, myopathologic, histopathologic, biochemical, and possibly somatopsychic effects involved. Correction of the articular fixation tends to restore normal physiologic processes, and the pathologic processes involved subside to the degree that they are reversible.

It is likely that several overlapping processes are involved in the typical subluxation complex and its reduction by adjustive and manipulative therapy. Individually, the three most popular hypotheses currently being investigated to determine the effects of chiropractic primary therapy are:

1. *The impulse-related theory:* eg, improving the transmission or expression of neurologic impulses.

2. *The nonimpulse-related theory:* eg,

improving the transmission of axonal transport mechanisms.

3. *The biochemical theory:* eg, decreasing the local sensitivity of joint afferents and discouraging the production of metabolic debris, including bradykinin, and/or stimulating the production of CNS endorphins.

Local Pathophysiologic Effects of Subluxation

A working hypothesis regarding spinal subluxations states that the vertebral displacement fixation will cause adjacent articulations of the spine to become hypermobile, resulting in stress of these motor units. Frogley believes that neurologic feedback causes the elicitation of ACTH and a resulting increase in the production of corticosteroids as an adaptive mechanism, according to the Hans Selye stress syndrome, and this also may be reflected by possible blood sugar changes.

Irritation at the site of misalignment and hypomobility will cause an inflammatory reaction with edema leading to a disturbance in the normal exchange of nutrients and waste products between capillary and extracellular fluid. Added to this stasis is the probable factor of lactic acid buildup in the area as a result of the release of the acid from the surrounding hypertonic musculature.

While toxic metabolic end-products (eg, urea, uric acid, creatinine, lactic acid) accumulate in stagnant tissue and congested capillary beds, there is also a corresponding decrease in nutrient and oxygen concentration in these fluids. Thus, the nerves emitting from the involved area will be deficient in necessary nutrients and quite possibly hypoxic as well. This situation along with the toxicity effects upon the nerve may well result in a disorder in membrane permeability leading to dysfunction and disease. When toxicity occurs in the central and peripheral nervous systems, the formation of acetylcholine at the level of involvement will be interfered with and result in further neural disturbances due to an increased impairment of conduction.

Spondylosis and Related Disorders

The Phases of Vertebral Unit Degeneration

The degenerative process has been divided by Kirkaldy-Willis into three phases (dysfunction, instability, and stabilization) into which a patient may pass into, out of, and return, depending on various circumstances such as degeneration progression and recurrent trauma (intrinsic or extrinsic). The *phase of dysfunction* following trauma exhibits somewhat minor pathologic changes in the involved vertebra's disc and posterior facets, and there are few, if any, residual symptoms following recovery. The *phase of instability* features segmental hypermobility as the result of lax facet capsules and weakened anular structure. The *phase of stabilization* is characterized by a return of segmental stability as the result of area fibrosis, apophyseal osteophytes, and centrum osteophytes within the disc and at the disc's periphery. Table 6.2 outlines a summary of findings, with some modification, described by Kirkaldy-Willis.

Disc Degeneration

Disc degeneration can be either a cause or an effect in a subluxation syndrome. Nuclear shifting or asymmetric thinning of physiologic, traumatic, or pathologic origin may readily lead to vertebral malposition. Likewise, subluxation (which inevitably results in some degree of asymmetrical weight imbalance, muscle tension, or muscle weakness) will have a deforming effect upon disc symmetry.

Spinal Trauma

Sunderland points out that nerve trunks are usually protected from physical deformation (short of luxation) by the anterior course of the nerve trunks, the slackness of the nerve trunks, the elasticity of the neurons, the cushioning effect of the epineurium, the specialized arrangement of the dura in the IVF, the mobility of the nerve complex in the IVF, and the attachment of certain nerves to the transverse processes. However, the nerve trunks are vulnerable to deformation as they have poor tensile strength because of the absence of perineurial tissue, they are highly susceptible to compression because of the lack of epineurial packing, the nerves within the IVF are highly subject to adhesion formation, and the fact that injured nerves are more susceptible to physical deformation and ischemia.

Prevalent Theories of Spinal Pain

Although there are many good theories, the actual cause of common spinal pain remains unknown unless gross pathology can

Table 6.2 Phases of Vertebral Unit Degeneration

Features	Dysfunction ⟶	Instability ⟶	Stabilization
History	Strain/sprain	Strain/sprain with likely history of previous injury	Chronic episodes of pain
Signs and symptoms	Perivertebral muscle splinting, pain (usually local, unilateral) that is aggravated by certain movements (eg, "catches"), tenderness of hypertonic erectors, lateral flexion unilaterally restricted, painful extension from flexion, antalgic scoliosis with muscle contraction on concave side of lateral bending	Similar to those of dysfunction, except feelings of weakness and periodic tendency toward collapse are usually reported; a segmental shift may be seen during extension from flexion	Radicular pain, area stiffness, incapacitating attacks after minor trauma, muscle weakness
Biomechanics	Rotation or compressive overstress leading to subluxation	Hypermobile joint motion with frequent subluxation, facets likely open and malpositioned	Hypomobile joint motion
Pathology	Small anular disc tears, possible disc bulging or herniation, possible nuclear displacement, synovitis leading to facet fixation due to intra-articular adhesion and/or articular cartilage degeneration, probable facet displacement (subluxation)	Lax anulus and posterior joint capsules, coalesced disc tears, degenerated nucleus with probable displacement, circumference bulging of disc at periphery, probable abrupt change in pedicle height, possible A-P shift of unit during flexion and extension, possible tilt of unit on rotation, possible nipping of a synovial fold	Fibrosis, loss of nuclear substance severe disc-space thinning, apophyseal osteophytes, centrum osteophytes, possible ankylosis, probable root entrapment

be demonstrated. There is no one type of subluxation picture or abnormality that is associated with all forms of spinal pain, nor does the presence of a subluxation or abnormality mean that the patient will have pain. Diagnosis must be approached with caution because of the many structural, functional, and psychologic mechanisms that may be involved. Common factors influencing spinal pain are shown in Figure 6.1.

It is known that mechanical forces (traction or compression) on axons or nerve trunks *inhibit* rather than excite. This blocking effect would appear to contraindicate spinal manipulation whose aim is to relieve *pain* caused by stretched or compressed IVF contents. However, rapid transient mechanical distortions, such as would be aggravated during normal motion, depolarize nerve trunks and mechanoreceptors and produce impulse bursts of short duration. Other explanations include (1) soft-tissue receptors as the source of pain impulses, (2) vascular pulsations offering repeated transient mechanical stimuli to tensed or compressed roots, or (3) inflammatory foci responsible for a sustained neural discharge rather than that of mechanical forces.

Pain perceived in the spine may be the result of either intrinsic or referred causes. Common disorders associated with spinal pain are shown in Table 6.3. Some selected

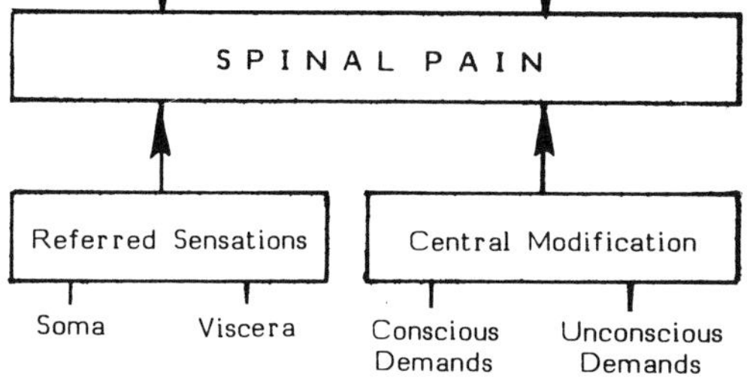

Figure 6.1. Common factors that influence spinal pain.

diseases referring pain to the spine are shown in Table 6.4. The anticipated pain pathways of subluxations are shown in the Appendix, Figure A.4.

SUBLUXATION TERMINOLOGY

Abnormal spinal biomechanics clinically relate to subluxations and other spinal malfunctions that result in structural and physiologic inadequacies of the spinal column. This state is the condition of a vertebral motion unit that has lost its normal structural and/or functional integrity and is, therefore, unable to move from its normal resting position, to move properly through its normal range of motion, or to return to its normal resting position after movement.

There are numerous methods of classifying vertebral subluxations. Each has its own rationale and each has certain validity that has been a contribution to our understanding of this complex phenomenon. In chiropractic, the general term *vertebral subluxation* refers to any alteration of the normal dynamic, anatomical, or physiologic relationships of contiguous articular structures. There are 115 diarthroses within the spine and pelvis vulnerable to the abnormal movement related to subluxation. Each of these articulations is a site of proprioceptive sensitivity that, when under articular strain, is provoked to express pathophysiologic sensory and motor impulses.

Fundamental Considerations

During the course of the clinical picture of a related pathophysiologic process, an altered vertebral motion unit may be a predisposing factor, a primary factor, a concomitant factor, an attenuating factor, a complicating factor, or a consequential factor. Thus, a complete description of vertebral subluxation syndromes would be voluminous and far beyond the capacities allotted here. Thus, the following should be considered only basic information.

A fixated subluxated vertebral motion unit (Fig. 6.2) has lost its normal structural and/or functional integrity and is, therefore,

Table 6.3. Typical Disorders Possibly Related to Spinal Pain (Acute/Chronic)

Type	Examples	
Degenerative process	Apophyseal osteoarthritis Cauda equina disorders Disc degeneration Hyperostosis Joint instability	Nerve root compression Spinal cord disease Spinal stenosis Spondylolisthesis Spondylosis
Developmental deficit	Bastrup's disease Hypermobility Kyphosis Lordosis Scoliosis	Short-leg syndrome Spondylolisthesis Various anomalies (eg, hemivertebrae)
Iatrogenic origin	Ill-advised manipulation Misplaced spinal tap Myelography	Poorly fitted support Postsurgical adhesions Prolonged use of support
Infective arthropathy or neuropathy	Actinomycosis Brucellosis Icterohemorrhagica Influenza Leptospirosis Meningitis Osteomyelitis Paratyphoid fever Poliomyelitis	Smallpox Staphylococcal infection Subarachnoid hemorrhage Syphilis Syringomyelia Tetanus Tuberculosis Typhoid fever
Inflammatory arthropathy	Ankylosing spondylitis Fibrositis Focal sepsis Muscular rheumatism Osteochondritis Panniculitis Polarteritis nodosa Polymyalgia arteritica	Psoriasis Regional ileitis Rheumatoid arthritis Reiter's disease Secondary spondylitis Systemic lupus erythematosus Ulcerative colitis
Metabolic deficit	Gouty rheumatism Hyperparathyroidism Osteomalacia	Osteoporosis Paget's disease of the spine
Spinal tumors	Aneurysmal bone cysts Hodgkin's sarcoma Myelomatosis	Neurofibroma Secondary carcinoma
Trauma	Disc protrusion Dislocation Facet syndrome Fracture Obesity Postural fault Short-leg syndrome	Spondylolisthesis Sprain/strain Subluxation Trauma, cummulative/ repetitive microtrauma/ overuse syndrome

unable to move from its normal resting position, to move properly through its normal range of motion, or to return to its normal resting position after movement. Thus, consideration must be given to a vertebral subluxation's static and dynamic structural position and related functional abnormalities.

The biomechanical element of the vertebral motion unit subluxation is classified by Hildebrandt/Howe according to its static or kinetic aspects and with the number of vertebral motion units involved.

Static Vertebral Motion-Unit Subluxations. Examples are:

Anterolisthetic subluxations
Costotransverse subluxations
Costovertebral subluxations
Decreased interosseous space subluxations
Extension subluxations
Flexion subluxations
Foraminal encroachment subluxations
Increased interosseous space subluxations
Lateral flexion subluxations
Laterolisthetic subluxations
Retrolisthetic subluxations
Rotational subluxations
Sacroiliac subluxations

The titles listed in the above list refer to the primary position involved. As a vertebral motion unit has five planes of motion, all movements are *biomechanically coupled* to some extent.

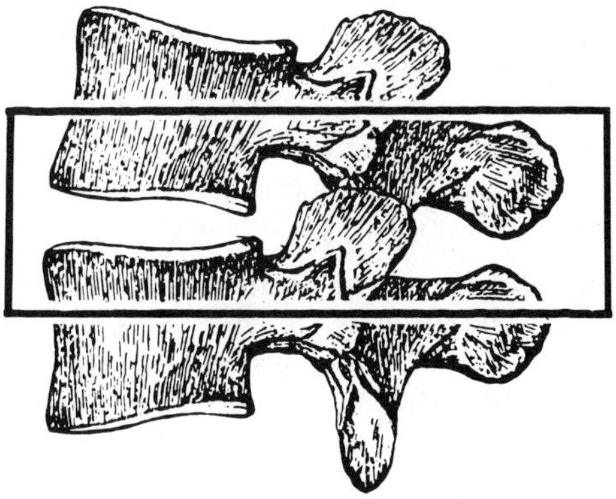

Figure 6.2. The functional area of an intervertebral motion unit.

Table 6.4. Selected Pathologies Simulating Spinal Pain

Type	Examples	
Cervical pain	Malignant lymphadenopathy Pancoast tumor	Subarachnoid hemorrhage Vertebral artery syndrome
Thoracic pain	Aortic aneurysm Bronchial carcinoma Cardiac enlargement Coronary artery disease	Gallbladder disease Herpes zoster Hiatus hernia Pulmonary disease
Lumbar pain	Aortic obstruction Colon carcinoma Disseminated sclerosis Endometriosis Hip disease Miscellaneous pelvic carcinoma Obstruction of iliac arteries	Pancreatic carcinoma Peptic ulcer Prostatic disease Rectal carcinoma Renal disease Short-leg syndrome Spinal cord tumor
Miscellaneous	Central nervous system diseases such as meningitis, poliomyelitis, syringomyelia, tetanus, spinal subarachnoid hemorrhage Iatrogenic manifestations Psychogenic causes Visceral diseases causing referred pain to the spine or pressure erosion	

The common clinical picture is one of segmental fixation during motion relative to the vertebral segments above and below. The commonly associated "off centering" is usually far less in extent than the incomplete dislocation referred to by allopathic orthopedists. In chiropractic semantics, this "off centering" may not even exist in the static spine as seen in the "subluxation" of fixation that produces an abnormal pivot within the normal physiologic range of motion or in the hypermobile segment that returns to a centered position in the neutral position. In addition, an "off centered" vertebra that is not interfering with function is rarely considered a "subluxation" in clinical chiropractic.

Kinetic Vertebral Motion-Unit Subluxations. The three major types are: (1) aberrant movement subluxations, (2) hypermobility subluxations, and (3) hypomobility subluxations.

Clinical Classes of Subluxation

The seven commonly recognized clinical types of subluxation are: (1) *functional subluxation*, a functional and slight "off centering" with partial fixation in an otherwise normal articular bed; (2) *pathologic subluxation*, an "off centering" derangement in an articular bed that has become deformed as the result of degenerative changes; (3) *traumatic subluxation*, in consequence to an extraneous or intrinsic force and the associated muscle spasm; (4) *reflex subluxation*, "off centering" induced by asymmetrical muscle contraction from aberrant visceral or somatic reflexes; (5) *defect subluxation*, subluxation of an anomalous or developmentally defective spinal or pelvic segment; (6) *fixation subluxation*, hypomobile fixation in which a spinal or pelvic segment that is in a neutral position of mobility

Table 6.5. Cervical Motion-Unit Dysfunction

Criteria	Nature of Acute/Chronic Cervical Subluxation-Fixation Complex: Common Examples	
Etiologic agent	Abnormal structural support Contractures Unequal muscle balance Paralysis	Poor sleeping postures Somatic or visceral response Sprain Strain
Symptoms	Articular grating Headaches Neuralgia Numbness Pain (especially on motion) Possible remote somatic effects	Possible remote visceral effects Stiffness Tenderness Tension Upper extremity pain Weakness
Signs	Altered normal reflexes Boggy tissues (focal) Electromyographic signs Fibrosis Hyperemia Hypertonic/flaccid muscles Segmental atrophy	Skin electro-resistance alterations Skin temperature alterations Skin texture alterations Thermographic signs Trigger point development Visual postural imbalance
Anatomical alteration	Palpable malalignment Roentgenographic signs	Segmental motion alterations

fails to participate fully in movement; (7) *hypermobile subluxation*, pathologic segmental increase in movement consequent to the loss of integrity of the retaining mechanism caused by trauma or degenerative pathology.

The Subluxation Complex as a Disease Entity

In Greenman's opinion, which is shared by many, "Manipulative therapy is not utilized just to treat a specific disease, but rather to maximize the structural-functional integrity of the total human organism to cope with its internal and external environmental stresses which have resulted in the patient's disease." This statement is generally true from a broad viewpoint.

From a more restricted viewpoint, an osseous disrelationship or an abnormal degree of physiologic segmental motion is generally considered a finding and associated soft-tissue aberrations are considered part of the syndrome. It may be either a contributing cause or an effect. Thus, in this context, describing a subluxation would not be a diagnosis. However, some may consider the spine as an organ; ie, a part of the body exercising a specific function, and the spine readily meets this definition. In this context, it would be difficult *not* to consider a specifically defined primary subluxation complex as a diagnosis in that it arrives at the determination of the nature of a disease (ie, a disorder of body function).

A disease entity is characterized usually by at least two of the following criteria: (1) a recognized etiologic agent (or agents), (2) an identifiable group of signs and symptoms, or (3) consistent anatomical alterations (*Illustrated Stedman's Medical Dictionary*, ed 24, 1982). Rarely does a subluxationfixation entity have difficulty in meeting these criteria. Examples for cervical motion-unit dysfunction are shown in Table 6.5.

It should be noted that the American Chiropractic Association has adopted the policy that the chiropractic use of the term *subluxation* in reporting is usually valid as an objective descriptor, but it is not acceptable as a diagnostic term unless demonstrable as a scientifically acceptable and classified entity. Refer to "Subluxation," *Indexed Synopsis of ACA Policies on Public Health and Related Matters*, 1987, p 18.

THE APOPHYSEAL JOINTS

The articulating processes of the spine have weak synovial joint capsules that are strengthened by two strong anterior and posterior ligaments, with fibers running perpendicular to the facet plane. They attach just beyond the margin of the facets. They are quite loose and elastic in the cervical region to allow greater mobility without capsule stretch. They are tighter and stronger in the thoracic and lumbar regions.

The surfaces of the articular facets are covered by tough hyaline cartilage and separated by meniscus-like tabs of synovium that originate from the synovial lining. These tabs glide in and out of the joint during motion but are rarely nipped during joint jamming. The tabs appear to allow a degree of extra shock-absorbing and pressure-absorbing protection for the articular cartilage.

The vertebral tilting that is seen in subluxations with disc wedging exhibits an alteration of the relationship of apposing articular surfaces. This produces a change in the direction of compressive forces on these joints. In contrast, severe rotation produces a jamming compression on ipsilateral facets and contralateral facet opening. When continuous compression is applied to any active and mobile joint, cartilaginous erosion followed by arthritis can be expected. Possible pain-provoking mechanisms at the facet joints include capsular ligament sprain, facet jamming or fixation by subluxation, pinching of a synovial fringe, entrapment of a loose cartilaginous body in the joint, and cervical or lumbar meniscoid entrapment.

The posterior articular facets of the spine possess the histologic capability to account for many of the various phenomena found in the subluxation syndrome. Their proximity to the IVF is of special interest because both structural and functional changes in these facets have been shown to affect the nerve-root sheath and contents.

Structural Changes in the Subluxation Complex

Following experimental research on the apophyseal joints, especially that of normal joint structures and their reaction to injury, Reiter reports an anatomical study of 75 postmortem spines that revealed significant changes, many of which would not be visible on x-ray. Capsular changes included edema, granular ossification, calcification, and adhesion between the capsule and the meningeal covering of the nerve root adjacent to it. Intra-articular changes included hypertrophy of the menisci up to four times their normal size, occasional chondrification and ossification of the menisci, detached bodies, ulcerated areas of denuded hyaline cartilage, cartilage thinning, fibrillation, and osteophytic marginal proliferation.

Spinal Joint Locking

Good defines spinal joint blocking within a subluxation syndrome as an actively maintained, reversible, biomechanical phenomenon in which paravertebral spasm (especially unilateral multifidus and rotatore contraction) physiologically locks one or more motion segments, causing a shift of the axes of motion toward an apophyseal joint to the degree that the unsynchronized segment is unable to articulate about the new axis. Thus, any method that assists relocation (normalization) of the axes of movement that releases the nociceptor feedback or relaxes the segmental spasm will be effective in reducing acute joint hypomobility whose initial origin was that of strain.

ARTICULAR NEUROLOGY

Wyke points out that, with few exceptions, any type of adjustive or manipulative technique imposes static and dynamic forces across the joint or joints being treated. This is as true for soft-tissue massage as it is for dynamic thrusts. Thus, the general principles of receptor neurology must be recognized if diagnosis and therapy are to be directed in a scientific manner.

Receptor Types

The synovial joints of the body, including the apophyseal joints of the spinal column, are provided with four types of receptor terminals that have variable characteristics. The major features of articular receptor sensory systems are shown in Table 6.6. Types I—III are corpuscular proprioceptive mechanoreceptors that serve as organic transducers. They are stimulated by increased tissue tension such as that induced by any type of active or passive mobilization.

Type I receptors are dynamic articular mechanoreceptors that have an extremely low threshold and are slowly adapting. They are found in the superficial fibrous layers of capsules and respond whenever the joint capsule is stretched; thus, they are active almost continuously. These superficial receptors signal the direction, amplitude, and velocity of joint movement. The frequency of discharge is proportional to the forces applied to the capsule.

Type II receptors are also dynamic articular mechanoreceptors that have a low threshold, but they adapt faster than Type I receptors. They are found in the deep subsynovia of joint capsules. They are normally inactive in resting joints but respond whenever capsule tension is increased. The primary purpose of these deep receptors is merely to signal (by a brief burst of impulses) that joint movement has been initiated.

Type III receptors are commonly found in peripheral joint ligaments, but they are absent in paraspinal ligaments. They have a high threshold and adapt slowly, responding only when capsule tension is extremely increased.

Type IV receptors are widely dispersed pain-conducting nonproprioceptive bare nerve endings within many joint tissues that are normally inactive but become excited when exposed to a high degree of mechanical stress or chemical irritants. They are located in the superficial layers of joint capsules as fine plexuses, in the collateral and intrinsic ligaments of a joint as a fine meshwork, and distributed within articular fat pads and vascular sheaths. Type IV receptors are *not* found within synovial lining, menisci, or articular cartilage.

Table 6.6. Characteristics of Joint Receptor Systems

Type	I	II	III	IV
Resembles	Ruffini corpuscles	Pacinian corpuscles	Golgi end-organs	
Location	Outer layers of joint capsule, grape-like clusters (3—8)	Sparsely found in deep layers of joint capsule and in fat pads, grape-like clusters (2—4)	Joint ligaments, grape-like clusters (2—3) or found individually	Joint capsule (except synovia), joint ligaments, fat pads, periosteum; absent in articular fibrocartilage
Endings	Encapsulated	Thickly encapsulated	Thinly encapsulated	Bare nerve-ending plexus
Fiber type and size	Myelinated, small (6ɥ—9ɥ)	Myelinated, medium (9ɥ—12ɥ)	Myelinated, large (13ɥ—17ɥ)	Myelinated and unmyelinated, variable size (92ɥ—2ɥ)
Threshold	Very low	Low	High	High
Conduction	Slow	Medium	Rapid	Slow
Adaptation	Slow	Rapid	Very slow	Nonadapting
Action	Mechanoreceptor	Dynamic mechanoreceptor	Dynamic mechanoreceptor	Nociceptor
Function	Signals static position of joint, speed and direction of joint movement; constantly firing; aids in regulating postural tone and muscle tone during joint motion.	Signals only rapid changes in movement: acceleration, deceleration; helps to initiate momentum; does not signal joint velocity, amplitude or direction.	Signals direction of movement; guards against excessive joint movement by regulating muscle tone (braking mechanism).	Signal noxious changes: mechanical or chemical.

*Adapted from data of Kessler/Hertling and Wyke.

Clinical Considerations

Knowledge of the function of the various types of joint receptors is important to any physician directing physical therapy because of the threefold effect produced when these mechanoreceptor impulses enter the spinal cord as the result of active motion, therapeutic mobilization, traction, or vibration.

Reflex Effects

Like the sensory fibers projecting from mechanoreceptors of the skin, the afferent impulses emanating from joint mechanoreceptors take a polysynaptic course. The primary fibers terminate with the *fusimotor neurons* (but not alpha neurons) in the motoneuron pool within the gray matter of the spinal cord. Thus, they contribute to monitoring muscle spindle activity such as *muscle tone* and *stretch reflex excitability.*

In addition, to this primary course, mechanoreceptor afferents also send collaterals that are distributed intersegmentally throughout the neuraxis. Because of this extensive intersegmental system of communication, any motion produced in one joint will tend to inhibit the motor-unit activity and facilitate the tone of the muscles near the joint and often some quite remote (even contralaterally) from the joint stimulated.

Pain Suppression

Unlike the sensory fibers from joint mechanoreceptors, impulses of the primary nociceptor afferents from Type IV receptors course to the *alpha neurons* in the motoneuron pool within the gray matter of the spinal cord. The effect is abnormal reflex activity in the muscles supplied segmentally.

Like the sensory fibers from joint mechanoreceptors, collaterals are given off in the spinal cord that synapse in the "gateway" of the basal nucleus of the gray matter, ascend via the anterolateral spinal tracts, and ultimately end in the limbic region of the cerebral cortex. However, this flow of pain-provoking impulses can be inhibited presynaptically in the substantia gelatinosa by superimposed impulses from the mechanoreceptors whether they originate from joint mechanoreceptors *or* cutaneous mechanoreceptors. It is in this manner that Wyke and others believe joint-pain suppression is achieved by massage, vibration, stretching, traction, TENS, compression, mobilization, rocking, or mild exercise. This theory suggests that the degeneration of peripheral mechanoreceptor pathways commonly associated with the aging process might explain why physical therapy is less effective in relieving pain in the elderly than in the young.

If central input from all joint receptors is blocked, the effect would mimic joint-infiltration anesthesia and feature a diminished joint-pain threshold, absent kinesthetic sensations, postural abnormalities, movement impairments, and gait disturbances.

Conscious Perception

Mechanoreceptor afferents course polysynaptically in their upward ascent, via the posterior and posterolateral columns, to terminate in the paracentral and parietal cerebral cortex. Types I and III (but not Types II or IV) afferents are primarily responsible for initiating kinesthetic perceptions. For this reason, the decrease or loss of kinesthesia is one of the first symptoms to appear when joint disease blocks or destroys Types I and III mechanoreceptor afferents. Pain may stubbornly persist, however, as long as Type IV impulses can reach the brain stem and cerebral cortex. Degenerative, inflammatory, and traumatic disorders of joints commonly result in a loss of Types I—III mechanoreceptor input but not of Type IV nociceptor input.

THE INTERVERTEBRAL FORAMEN

An intervertebral foramen (IVF) is generally bounded above by the inferior pedicle notch of the superior vertebra, below by the superior pedicle notch of the inferior vertebra, anteriorly by the intervertebral disc (IVD) and parts of the two vertebral bodies, and posteriorly by the superior and inferior articular processes (refer to Fig. 6.2).

Vertebral segments normally move in the planes of their articulations (unless the motion is blocked), and it is at the level of the apophyseal facets that most subluxations occur and influence the IVFs far more than any other articulations of the spinal column. Changes in the diameter of normal IVFs result in an abnormal channel between spinal and peripheral levels of the nervous system, which predisposes to malfunction as well as being a direct factor in altering the curves of the spine in which this structural defect is found.

The nerve roots of the *cervical spine* are located anteriorly and inferiorly to their facets. In the *thoracic spine*, they lie directly anterior to the facets. In the *lumbar spine*, the nerve roots are located anteriorly and superiorly to the facets, beneath the pedicles.

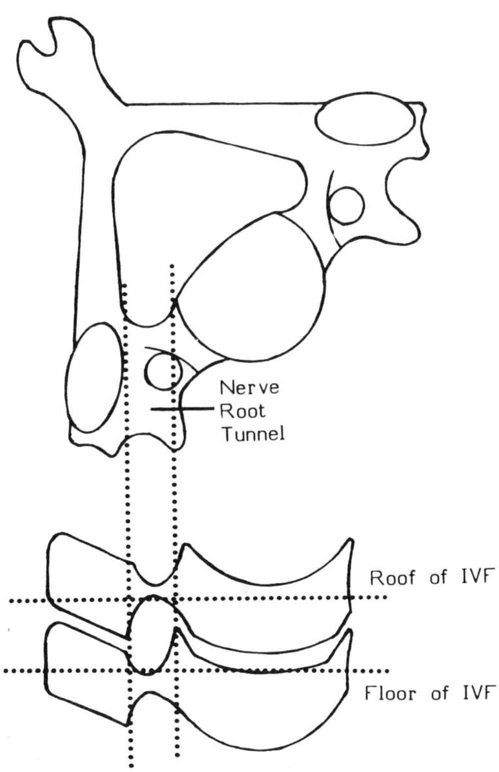

Figure 6.3. Schematic of the structural relationships of the intervertebral tunnel. *Top*, from above; *bottom*, sagittal section.

Size and Shape Considerations

When viewed laterally, an IVF is generally elliptical in shape, with the diameter of its vertical axis about double its A-P dimension. See Figure 6.3. Because of this, there is usually adequate space for changes in vertical dimension (eg, dynamic axial traction or compression, moderate disc flattening) without injury to the IVF contents as long as there is adequate fat and fluid present. However, reduction of an already short transverse diameter can produce many noxious effects. For this reason, complete disc collapse vertically is often asymptomatic, while a slight posterolateral herniation may protrude upon the IVF and produce severe symptoms.

The Cervical Area

The cervical foramina are designed more in the shape of rounded gutters than orifices, averaging 1 cm in length. There is no IVF between the atlas and the occiput or between the atlas and the axis. The C1 nerve exits over the superior aspect of the posterior arch of the atlas in the vertebral artery sulcus. The C2 nerve exits between the inferior aspect of the posterior arch of the atlas and the superior aspect of pedicle of the axis. It then dangerously transverses the lateral atlantoaxial joint, anterior to the ligamentum flava. The C3—C8 nerves exit through short oval canals, which increase in size as they progress caudally. Cervical nerves, especially, fill the transverse diameter of their IVFs. Thus, any disorder that reduces this dimension (eg, subluxation, osteophytes, disc herniation, edema) will undoubtedly compromise the integrity of the IVF contents. See Figure 6.4.

The Thoracic Area

The pedicle notch of the vertebra above is quite deep in the thoracic region, while that of the vertebra below is relatively shallow. The result is a pear-shaped canal with sharp bony edges that predispose to fibrotic changes from chronic irritation. The vertebral body and the disc of the superior vertebra form most of the IVFs anterior boundary.

The Lumbar Area

A lumbar IVF is shaped like a kidney bean. It takes considerable posterolateral disc protrusion to encroach the nerve exiting at the same level because the lumbar IVFs are comparatively large. When herniation does cause trouble, it is usually due to pressure on the laterally placed nerve root on the vertebra above. Sunderland stresses the fact that the passage of the medial branch of the lumbar dorsal ramus and its accompanying vessels through the osseofibrous tunnel and the intimate relationship of the neurovascular bundle to the capsule of the apophyseal joint represents a potential site of fixation and entrapment following pathologic changes involving the joint. The general anatomy of this area, as view from the posterior, is depicted in Figure 6.5.

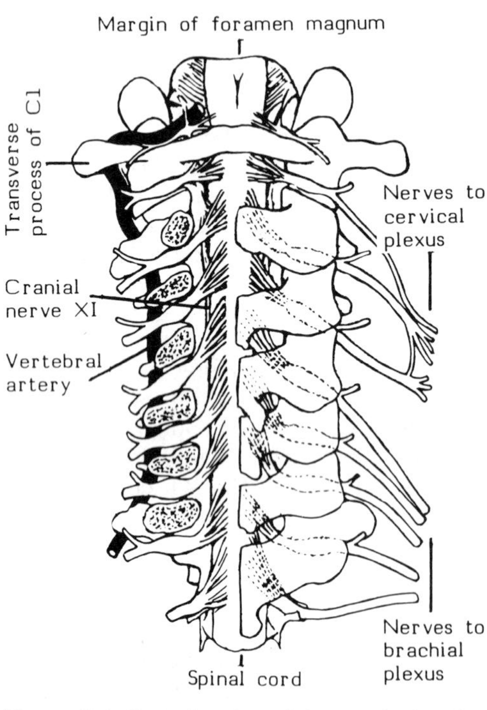

Figure 6.4. Posterior view of the cervical region. *Left,* the laminae have been removed to expose the precarious position of the intervertebral contents.

Contents and Size Alterations

Each IVF of the spine is dynamic; widening and expanding with each spinal motion, serving as a channel for nerve and vascular egress and ingress, and allowing compression and stretching of the lipoareolar bed. From one-third to one-half of the foraminal opening is occupied by the spinal nerve root and its sheath, with the remaining portion filled primarily by fat, connective tissue, and the various vessels.

The following structures are found in the IVF:

- The anterior nerve root
- The posterior nerve root
- A portion of the dorsal nerve root ganglion
- A bilaminar sleeve of dura and arachnoid membrane, extending to the ganglion

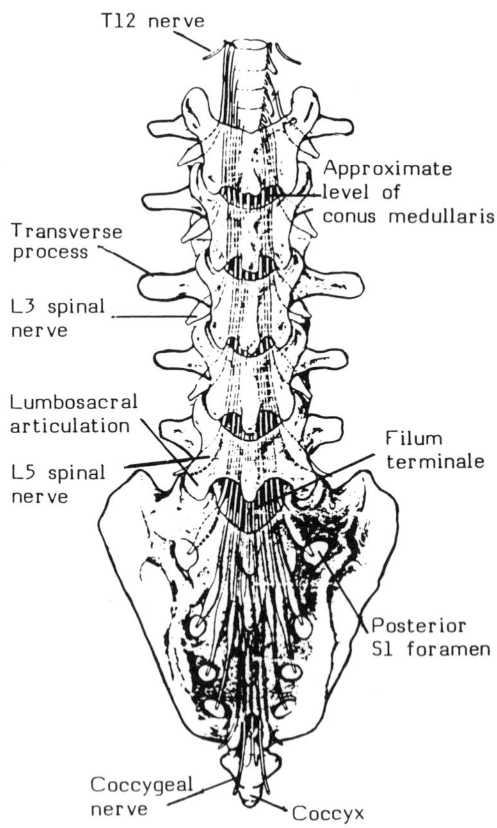

Figure 6.5. Major architecture of the lumbar area as view from the back.

• A short continuation of CSF-containing subarachnoid space, which ends just after the ganglion

• The recurrent meningeal nerve
• The spinal ramus artery
• The intervertebral vein
• Lymphatic vessels.

Factors That Change IVF Diameter

The typical factors modifying the diameters of the IVFs are (1) the disrelation of facet subluxation, (2) changes in the normal static curves of the spine, (3) the presence of induced abnormal curves of the spine, (4) degenerative thinning, bulging, or extrusion of the related IVD, (5) swelling and sclerosing of the capsular ligaments and the interbody articulation, and (6) marginal proliferations of the vertebral bodies and apophyseal articulations.

Consequences of IVF Diameter Alteration

The above factors can insult the viable contents of the IVF and subject its contents to physiologic compromise that results in nerve root pressure, traction, or torque; constriction of the spinal blood vessels; intraforaminal and paraforaminal edema; induration and sclerosing of the periarticular ligaments with incarcerating insult upon the contained receptors; forcing of the foraminal contents into protracted constriction and altered position; and other consequences. Nerve tissue tolerates slow compression without offering obvious symptoms. Acute phenomena are usually the result of friction, severe or repeated trauma, and encroachment from degenerative thickening or exostosis.

Subluxation Effects At the Intervertebral Foramina

Normally, the cross-sectional area of an IVF leaves ample room for its neural contents during the dynamics of daily life. The IVF narrowing that occurs during spinal extension movements has little if any adverse effects in the normal spine. The channel contents are normally free to adjust to movements throughout the normal range of regional motion. Pathologic changes in and near the foramen may reduce its dimensions and lead to compression, but, as Sunderland points out, friction over osseofibrous irregularities or traction on a nerve or nerve roots fixed in the foramen by an adhesion is much more likely.

When under constant stress, a vertebral motion unit normally adapts so that changes occur in adjacent IVDs, ligaments, membranes, muscles, and other associated tissues that produce some degree of fixation. Because of this segmental fixation, adjacent IVFs are altered in size. As a rule, two of them become smaller than normal, and the other two become larger than normal. Nerve roots and other contents of the affected IVFs become subjected to insult at the smaller foramina and stretching at the larger foramina.

Possible intervertebral events as a result of a subluxation complex are shown in Table 6.7.

Effects of Microtrauma

The zygapophyseal articular complex of a subluxated vertebral motor bed is initially subjected to the stress of "off centering" and is attended by the following aspects of microtrauma: (1) minute hemorrhage, transudation, and arteriovenous stagnation from the sluggish circulatory flow resulting from the motion unit's decreased mobility and arterial backup, (2) para-articular and paraforaminal traumatic edema, (3) eccentric compression stress upon the IVD and the apophyseal cartilages, (4) possible separation of minute fasciculi of the retaining fibers of the anulus, joint capsule, dural root sleeve, and nerve root sheath, (5) stress insult of the proprioceptive bed, (6) minute crushing of the periosteal margins with resultant proliferative irritation, and (7) minute tearing of the attachments of the dural root sleeves if they attach to the lining of the IVF.

The following pathologic changes typically occur:

1. Extravasation and edema, along with the precipitation of fibrinogen into fibrin, result in interfascicular, foraminal, articular, and capsular thickening and adhesions that restrict fascicular glide, ingress and egress of the foraminal contents, and the competent movement of the vertebral segment within its articular bed. Whenever there is extravasation, mineral salts are precipitated and infiltration and sclerosing commonly result.

2. Binding adhesions may develop between the dural root sleeves and the nerve roots within the interradicular foramen and between the spinal nerve root sheath and the inner margins of the IVF. When subjected to microtrauma, mesenchymal connective tissue undergoes a relative rapid and extensive degenerative change that is character-

Table 6.7. Possible Intravertebral Events as a Result of Subluxation

Articular and Para-Articular Changes
- Bony foraminal encroachment
- Changes resulting from mechanical deformation
- Eccentric zygapophyseal cartilage compression
- Joint capsule overstress, resulting in capsule thickening, reduced mobility
- Trauma to periosteal margins producing proliferative changes
- Traumatic edema

Circulatory Changes
- Arteriovenous stagnation
- Cerebrospinal fluid flow alterations
- Changes resulting from ischemia
- Interference with IVF interstitial fluids
- Interference with nerve root intracellular fluid
- Sluggish lymphatic flow

IVD Changes
- Anular fiber overstress
- Eccentric compression
- Nuclear displacement
- Protrusion or herniation

Paraforaminal Soft-Tissue Changes
- Adhesions
- Altered nerve root level
    - Encroachment symptoms
    - Traction symptoms
    - Pedicle kinking
- Atrophy
- Contractures
- Ganglionic compression or irritation
- Hyper- or hypo-tonicity
- Meningeal traction
- Minute hemorrhages
- Minute tearing of dural root sleeve attachments in or near IVF
- Paravertebral pain and tenderness
- Pedicle kinking
- Sclerosis
- Transudation
- Traumatic edema

Proprioception and Autonomic Changes
- Reflexes to motor components
    - Abnormal or subnormal somatomotor reflexes
    - Abnormal or subnormal visceromotor reflexes
- Stimuli interpreted as peripheral sensory stimulation
    - Misinterpreted somatosensory reflexes
    - Misinterpreted viscerosensory reflexes
- Visceromotor reflexes
    - Circulatory dysfunction
    - Smooth muscle dysfunction
    - Secretory dysfunction
    - Trophic dysfunction
        - Musculoskeletal
        - Visceral

Toxic Metabolic Products and Effects of Venous Stagnation from Arterial Backup
- Acetylcholine inhibition
- Cellular malnutrition
- Creatinine
- Hypoxia
- Inflammatory residues
- Ionic imbalance
- Lactic acid buildup
- pH changes
- Urea
- Uric acid

ized by a loss of functional integrity and substance.

Proprioceptive Responses and Reflexes

The most significant effect is likely that of proprioceptive irritation. The musculoskeletal tissues and particularly the ligaments and paravertebral or intervertebral musculature of the spine are richly endowed with proprioceptive receptors. First, when overly stimulated by stretching, these neurons interpret the stimuli as somatic sensory stimulation that may be perceived as pain. Second, they also may send reflexes to their motor components to produce changes within the paravertebral muscles or elsewhere in the soma supplied by the segment. Third, they may be interpreted as viscerosensory stimuli, whose visceromotor response alters circulatory changes, smooth muscle activity, glandular secretions, or trophic activity in the musculoskeletal tissues or viscera supplied. It is this vast ability of the proprioceptive sensory beds to influence motor changes, both of a somatomotor or visceromotor nature, that is perhaps the most universal effect of vertebral subluxation.

Direct Nerve Pressure

Nerve roots are normally well protected from trauma by the bony border of the IVF and the tough fibrous dura. However, Schaumburg shows that when distorted by degenerative bone and joint disease or a variety of space-occupying lesions, these same protective layers may damage the delicate neural structures. Direct nerve pressure may come from the misaligned osseous segment itself or from various soft-tissue pathologies causing or affected by the mechanical fault such as contractures, adhesions, inflammatory residues, atrophies, cysts and tumors of related tissues. Direct physical nerve pressure may be responsible for motor alterations and sensory disturbances within this particular nerve and its innervated structures or cause other ramifying reflexes.

Research findings described by Sharpless indicate that the posterior nerve roots are about five times more susceptible to compression block than a peripheral nerve. As little as 10 mm Hg pressure held for 15—30 minutes reduces the compound action potentials of posterior roots to about half their initial value. This effect is thought to be due to mechanical deformation rather than ischemia since the larger fibers are blocked first. It is believed that anoxia affects the small fibers first.

Ganglion Irritation/Compression

Because of its juxtaposition to the IVF, another important factor to be considered is that of irritation/compression of a posterior root ganglion. The ganglion of each spinal nerve generally lies within the upper medial aspect of the IVF, a precarious position. Whenever the transverse diameter of the IVF is modified, the ganglion may be subject to compression and irritation. This is especially true at the cervical level where it tends to occupy the medial limits of the IVF and is thus vulnerable to and most likely to become involved in any changes in IVF diameter on any event of trauma or the manifold processes of spondylosis. For example, an acute whiplash-like mishap to the cervical spine, especially of the hyperextension type, may force the vagus and the superior cervical sympathetic ganglion against the transverse processes of the atlas and axis, often provoking bizarre autonomic reactions.

Intraneural Effects

It is probable that any interference with or abnormality of the interstitial fluids in which the nerves lie and/or the intracellular fluid of the nerve body itself or the nerve axoplasm will cause a breakdown of the sodium pump mechanism that will prevent the normal flow of impulses along the nerve fibers concerned. These abnormal impulses refer to an overaction or underaction in the rate of impulse frequency along the nerve. Once a threshold stimulus has been reached, a nerve will fire according to the all-or-none law.

Meningeal Irritations

Biomechanical errors in motion and position may place compressive or tractional forces upon the meningeal coverings of the cord or dural root sleeves that may produce mechanical pressure upon the neurons and CFS flow emanating from the cord itself. These may, therefore, cause the elicitation of abnormal neurologic motor effects or sensory interpretations.

Altered Nerve Root Level

Any induced disrelationship between position level and course direction of nerve root origin (spinal cord) and nerve root exit (IVF) is an important factor to consider. Whenever there is subluxation, changes in normal curves, or the presence of abnormal curves, the relative levels of points of nerve root origin and exit are altered and the nerve root becomes vulnerable to encroachment compression or irritation. This results whenever the normal curves of the spine are grossly modified (eg, kyphotic deviation of the cervical spine, lordotic exaggeration of the lumbar spine, scoliotic deformity especially at the cervicobrachial area and lumbosacral junction), the nerve root is forced to assume an unusual approximation to one or the other walls of the IVF. Thereafter, the least additional deviation may precipitate a nerve root irritation syndrome. In addition, a vertebral column affected with partial fixation of several segments when subjected to flexion, extension, and circumduction efforts will suffer marked tension upon the dural root sleeves and the related spinal nerve radicles, especially the cauda equina.

If one or more vertebral segments are functionally embarrassed for any reason by abnormal motor action, added articular and proprioceptive responsibility is imposed upon the segments above and below the involved area. Thus there is an extension of harmful effects that may have noticeable complications. In addition, the phenomenon of bipedism neurologically necessitated the development of an ascending and descending reticular activating mechanism. It can be assumed that spinal and pelvic interosseous disrelation may overstimulate the ascending portion of the reticular activating mechanism. On the other hand, excessive psychic stress may, by means of the descending portion, provoke overstimulation of the cellular elements in the anterior and lateral horns and provoke abnormal somatic and autonomic reactions.

Paraforaminal Adhesions

Paraforaminal adhesions as the result of stress and traumatic edema often result in a painful restriction of the normal back-and-forth glide (¼—⅓ inch) of the nerve root within the IVF. Symptoms simulate a low-grade radiculitis: increased pain on movement, straining, and stretching; pain on changing positions and when placing the involved part in extension.

Circulatory Changes

Restricted mobility (eg, vertebral fixation) of a motion unit within its normal physiologic range of movement may cause sluggish lymphatic or vascular circulation that is further influenced by mechanical pressure. This can cause chemical or physical changes within tissues such as anoxia, toxicity, swelling, edema, etc, and the consequent derangement of normal function brought about by these disorders. Local irritation at the site of misalignment and a decreased ability to move produce an inflammatory reaction with edema leading to a disturbance in the normal exchange of nutrients and waste products between capillary and extracellular fluid. Added to this stasis is the probable factor of lactic acid buildup in the area as a result of leakage from the surrounding hypertonic muscles.

Local Toxicity Effects

Venous stagnation from arterial backup can produce local toxicity at the spinal level. While toxic metabolic end products (eg, urea, uric acid, creatinine, lactic acid) accumulate in the stagnant tissue and congested capillary beds, there is also a corresponding decrease in nutrient and oxygen concentration in these fluids. Thus, the nerves emanating from the involved area will be deficient in necessary nutrients and quite possibly hypoxic as well. The buildup of metabolic waste products in the area of the IVF, also may alter the normal pH of local fluids causing a breakdown of the Krebs cycle, due to decreased oxygen and toxicity, which causes a partial breakdown of the sodium pump mechanism, resulting in an ionic imbalance. As the sodium pump can no longer maintain a normal ionic balance, the imbalance can result in a degree of erratic nerve conduction and edema in the tissues of the immediate area. This erratic nerve conduction may be exhibited in all fibers passing through the involved IVF and immediate area. When toxicity occurs in either the central or peripheral nervous systems, the formation of acetylcholine at the level of involvement will be interfered with and result in further disturbances due to increased nerve conduction impairment. This situation along with the toxicity effects upon the nerve may well result in abnormal membrane permeability leading to dysfunction.

Cerebrospinal Fluid Flow Alterations

This category of disturbances relates to the mechanical effect upon the flow of CSF within the CNS and perhaps within the nerve roots. CSF stagnation possibly occurs in association because of the intimate relationship between spinal fluid and venous

Table 6.8. Possible Distal Manifestations of Vertebral Subluxations

- Acroparesthesia
- Angioneurotic edema
- Cutaneous discolorations
- Cutaneous flushing or pallor
- Decreased electrical resistance of skin
- Dermatographia
- Fasciculation
- Formication
- Gastrointestinal sphincter spasm or inefficiency
- Hyper- or hypo-esthetic areas
- Hyper- or hypo-hidrotic areas
- Hyper- or hypo-peristalsis
- Hyper- or hypo-reflexia
- Hyper- or hypo-thermic areas
- Hyper- or hypo-tonicity
- Hypertrophy or atrophy
- Increased flare to scratching
- Increased or decreased gastrointestinal secretions
- Increased or decreased glandular secretions
- Increased or decreased strength
- Local swelling
- Malcoordination
- Mucous membrane congestion or blanching
- Myocardial spasm or inefficiency
- Neuralgia and neurodynia
- Pain and tenderness
  - Cutaneous and subcutaneous
  - Deep muscular
    - Somatic
    - Visceral
  - Periosteal
- Postural fatigue
  - Abnormal somatospinal reflexes
  - Abnormal viscerospinal reflexes
  - Diaphragmatic dysfunction
  - Gait disturbances
  - Lymphatic traction or compression
  - Mediastinal displacement
  - Nerve traction or compression
  - Organic displacement
  - Respiratory inhibition
  - Sustained postural stress
  - Vasculature traction or compression
  - Visceral support stretching or shortening
  - Visceral traction or compression
  - Visceroptosis
- Proliferation or degeneration
- Sluggish movements
- Tics
- Tingling
- Tremor

blood, contributing to toxicity in the nerve root area. According to some researchers, minute pressure on meninges alters the flow of CSF and interferes with its ability to remove wastes and provide nutritional substances to the cord and nerve roots. This may be either the effect of direct mechanical pressure or impairment of motion necessary for proper intake and outflow of this nutrient material.

Distal Neurologic Manifestations of Subluxations

Because of the effects of the subluxation's microtrauma and the consequent pathologic changes involved, the neurologic insult may result in (1) modification of the basic chronaxie; (2) alteration of normal impulse amplitude, wave length, and force intensity; and/or (3) extension of the refractory period.

The neurologic manifestations of a subluxation are not always indicated by the response the nervous system makes to irritation not external to it (ie, discernible in its immediate area), but rather from within the body. Thus, it can be an intrinsic source of neurologic irritation. This altered state of nerve-fiber threshold and the impulse proper leads to dysfunction of the sensory, motor, vasomotor, and spinovisceral responses.

Possible distal manifestations of vertebral subluxations are shown in Table 6.8.

Somatosensory Responses

Dysfunctions in the somatosensory system include varying degrees of discomfort and pain, tension, superficial and deep tenderness, periosteal tenderness, hyperesthesia or hypesthesia, haptic sensations, acroparesthesia, formication, flushing, numbness, coldness, and postural fatigue. Dysfunctions in the somatomotor system include painful muscle spasms (especially proximal); abnormal muscle tone (from hypotonicity to spasm), weakness, atrophy, or degeneration in long-standing cases; sluggish and uncoordinated movements; paralyses; and fasciculations, tics, and tremors.

Visceromotor Responses

Visceromotor responses of the nervous system may be exhibited in several ways. For example:

1. Dysfunctions in the vasomotor field include angioneurotic edema, flushing, mucous membrane congestion, urticaria and dermatographia, vasospasm, and blanching. Minor changes in the circulation of the skin can be crudely measured indirectly by various heat sensitive devices, thermography, or infrared photography. Such changes often parallel circulatory changes in the deeper tissues as they too are affected by similar vasomotor responses.
2. Changes in the ability of the skin to secrete oils or perspiration can be measured by various electrical resistance instruments. These secretory errors also may be indicative of similar changes in deeper visceral tissues. Hyperhidrosis or dryness, as well as hyperesthesia or hypesthesia, in a local area near the spine implies altered vasomotor activity in the subsequent spinal segment. Hyperesthesia and hyperhidrosis are usually associated with an increased flare (red response) from scratching and a decrease in electrical skin resistance.
3. Dysfunction in the spinovisceral field may include visceral smooth-muscle abnormalities, glandular and mucous membrane secretory malfunctions, and sphincter spasms of the detrusor muscles and myocardium.
4. Alterations in the quality of tissue may result from trophic disturbances such as atrophies, degenerations, thinning or discoloration of the skin, or other changes that reflect viscerotrophic abnormalities.

THE SPINAL NERVES

A sole spinal nerve trunk is a mixture of several posterior sensory (afferent) and anterior motor (efferent) rootlets. The anterior fibers arise from cell bodies in the spinal cord's ventral gray horn, while the posterior fibers are from cell bodies in the spinal dorsal root ganglia that lie outside the cord and partially within the IVF. The ganglion usually

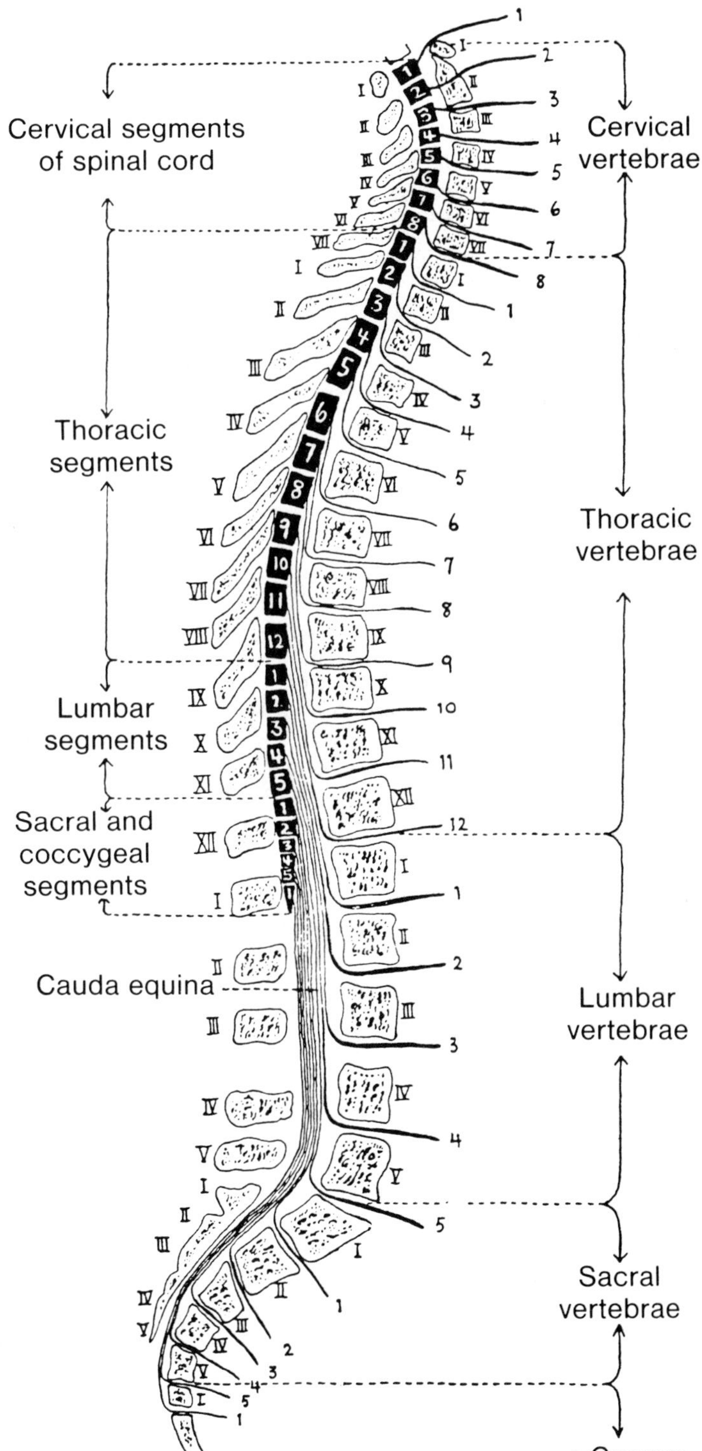

Figure 6.6. Illustration of spinal segments depicting the bodies and spinous processes of the vertebrae, the place of origin of the nerve roots from the spinal cord, and the root exits from the corresponding IVFs.

rests against the pedicle. Except for C1 and C2, which do not have IVFs, the common trunk forms just outside the IVF, where it quickly divides into anterior and posterior rami. See Figure 6.6.

Nerve roots are not normally firmly attached to the margins of their respective IVFs and thus can move about quite freely during spinal motions. However, fibrotic changes following the granulation tissue of irritation frequently fix the sleeve(s) at one or more points, which contributes to traction on the sheath and its contents during movement. These attachments increase in strength with aging and other degenerative changes.

Sensory Manifestations

Segmental Sensory Supply

Figure 6.7 depicts most pain-sensitive tissues of the vertebral motion unit. Each vertebral motion unit derives high-threshold sensory fibers from:

1. The usually two fine branches of the recurrent (sinuvertebral) meningeal nerve, running anterior to the spinal nerve in the IVF. An autonomic branch from the paravertebral plexus accompanies the recurrent spinal nerve, usually within the same sheath. These supply the anterior dura, blood vessels of the spinal canal, posterior longitudinal ligament, cortex of the vertebral bodies, and the surface of the posterior anulus. Fibers rarely enter the central IVD. Communicating and linking branches extend across, up, and down at least one segment, and frequently produce radiating or referred symptoms.

2. The medial branch of the posterior primary ramus. These fibers supply the ligaments and muscles of the posterior aspect of the vertebral unit. As in all synovial joints, the capsules of the articular processes, their fat pads, and their intrinsic and extrinsic ligaments are richly endowed with pain and proprioception receptors. This nerve also sends communicating and linking branches across, up, and down a few segments.

The vertebral joint proper receives innervation from rostral and caudal segments besides those from the local segment. This means that a segmentally arranged nerve supply (with its specific dermatomes, muscles, and reflexes) is not available to evaluate a particular specific vertebral motion unit with certainty.

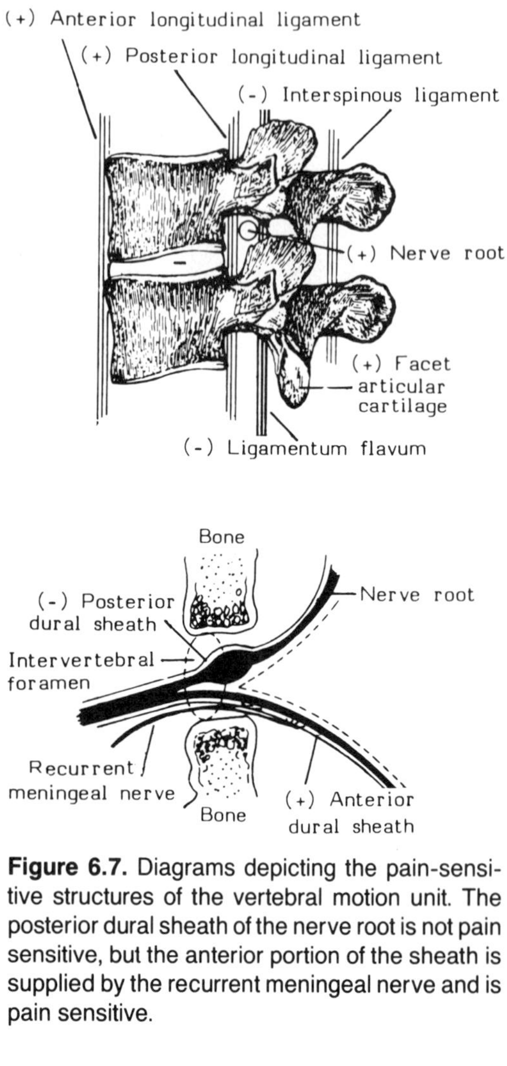

Figure 6.7. Diagrams depicting the pain-sensitive structures of the vertebral motion unit. The posterior dural sheath of the nerve root is not pain sensitive, but the anterior portion of the sheath is supplied by the recurrent meningeal nerve and is pain sensitive.

Nerve Fiber Proportions

There are about three times more sensory fibers than motor fibers in the cervical area, one and a half more in the thoracic region, and twice as many in the lumbar area. This thought should be kept in mind during palpation.

Pain Distribution

When the *anterior root* is irritated, pain is felt in the muscles supplied (ie, with *myotomal* distribution) and often becomes self-perpetuating from the focal spasm produced (eg, a trigger-point syndrome). When the *posterior root* is irritated, the pain is usually perceived in a *dermatomal* distribution.

The Autonomics

As the autonomic nerve pathways innervating musculoskeletal tissues are intimately connected with the spinal nerves, it can be recognized that these systems do not operate in isolation. Structural disorders in the spine frequently cause, contribute to, or mimic such "functional" disorders as Meniere's disease, causalgia, shoulder-hand syndrome, asthma, sphincter spasms, cluster headaches, angina, and a large variety of referred pains.

Nerve Root Insults

As described previously, disturbances of nerve function associated with subluxation syndromes can manifest as abnormalities in sensory interpretations and/or motor activities. These disturbances may be through one of two primary mechanisms: (1) direct nerve or nerve root disorders, or (2) of a reflex nature.

If direct involvement occurs on the posterior root of a specific neuromere, it manifests as an increase or decrease in awareness over the dermatome; ie, the superficial skin area supplied by this segment. Such manifestation is usually tested with a cotton wisp and pinwheel. Typical examples might include foraminal occlusion or irritating factors exhibited clinically as hyperesthesia. For example, abnormal sensitivity often occurs on the posterior and lateral aspects of the thumb and radial side of the hand, when involvement occurs between C5—C6. At other times, this root involvement may cause hypertonicity and the sensation of deep pain in the musculature supplied by this neuromere; eg, C7 involvement, with deep pain in the triceps and supinators of the forearm. In addition, direct pressure over the nerve root or its distribution may be particularly painful.

Cyriax gives the cardinal signs of nerve pressure as (1) pain on stretching the nerve, (2) the provocation of paresthesia (eg, pins and needles) on motion, (3) swelling and tenderness over the nerve sheath, (4) postural deformity, and (5) evidence of secondary parenchymatous changes in the nerve (eg, impaired conduction during electrodiagnosis).

Prolonged and/or severe nerve root irritation may also produce evidence of trophic changes in the tissues supplied. This may be characterized by apparent atrophy, but such a sign is particularly objective when the circumference of an involved limb is measured at the greatest girth in the initial stage and this value is compared to measurements taken in a few weeks later. It is for this reason that the circumference of the thigh, leg, forearm, and upper arm are measured and recorded during many standard examinations.

Motor Manifestations

Nerve root insults from subluxations also may be evident as disturbances in motor reflexes and/or muscular strength. Examples of these reflexes include the tendon reflexes such as seen in the reduced biceps reflex when involvement occurs between C5 and C6, the reduced triceps reflex when involvement occurs between C6 and C7, or the reduced patella and Achilles tendon reflexes when involvement occurs between L4 and L5. These reflexes must also be compared bilaterally to judge whether hyporeflexia is unilateral; unilateral hyperreflexia is pathognomonic of an upper motor neuron lesion.

Muscle strength may be tested in various manners, depending upon which muscles are involved; the primary purpose being to compare the isometric strength of resistance against counterpressure. For example, the strength of the biceps (C6—C7), triceps (C6—C7), anterior tibialis (L4—L5), and gastrocnemius (L5—S1) muscles are commonly tested.

The Posterior Rami

The posterior rami turn sharply backward to supply the spinal muscles and skin of the back. Sunderland emphasizes that the passage of cutaneous branches through the muscles and fascia of the back should not be overlooked as potential sites of entrapment. Such entrapment is most frequent of the greater occipital nerve and the cutaneous branches of the posterior rami of L1—L3 nerves.

A few posterior rami intermix branches, but most remain segmental. The anterior rami run ventrally and laterally, and most enter plexuses or connect with sympathetic fibers via the rami communicantes, whereafter their specific identity is difficult to determine. In the fused sacral region, the anterior and posterior rami, respectively, exit the bony canal through the anterior and posterior foramina.

Tenderness of the rami of the posterior division has particular significance in the palpatory examination of the spine. The sensory distribution runs in a zone extending from the posterior scalp to the coccygeal area and then laterally to the greater trochanter. See Tables 6.9 and 6.10.

THE VERTEBRAL CANAL AND RELATED TISSUES

The spinal cord, continuous with the medulla oblongata at the foramen magnum, is protected within the spine anteriorly by the posterior aspect of the vertebral body and IVD, posteriorly by the bony laminae, and laterally by the pedicles. Further protection and stability are provided by the cord's three membranes, the two fluid-filled spaces, the ligamentum flava and dentate ligaments, and the nerve root sheaths. To accommodate necessary innervation for the limbs, the spinal cord is enlarged at (1) the cervical segments (C4—T1) to supply the brachial plexus, and (2) the lumbosacral segments (L2—S3) to supply the lumbar and sacral plexuses. The average sagittal diameter of the adult cervical vertebral canal is 18 mm.

Cord-Canal Relationships

Relative to the origin of the 31 pairs of spinal nerves, a spinal cord "segment" does not necessarily correspond in height or location to its corresponding numbered vertebra and disc, spinal nerve, or the level of the spinous process. The cervical spine contains eight cord segments; the thoracic spine, about 20 segments; and the lumbar spine, probably only a few sacral and coccygeal segments. The adult spinal cord can generally be considered to occupy only the upper two-thirds of the vertebral canal. Exact depth is quite variable.

In the embryo, the spinal cord and vertebral canal are about equal in length until about the 10th week. Because the vertebral column grows faster than the spinal cord, this relationship does not persist. The cord ends near the level of the L3 disc at birth; the L2 disc at age 5; and higher in the adult. This is usually near the level of the L1 disc. Occasionally, it is seen at surgery to terminate in the adult as high as T12 or as low as L3. As the lower third of the vertebral column is approached, the length and obliquity of the nerve roots must progressively increase to reach their respective IVFs (refer to Fig. 6.6).

The vertebral canal increases in length during spinal flexion and lateral bending, and decreases in length during extension. Illi has shown that the amount of linear change is considerably reduced because of the flex-

Table 6.9. Comparatives Sizes of Typical Adult Posterior Rami Nerves

Nerve	Average Diameter
C1	1 mm
C2	2½ mm
C3—C8	1¼ mm
T1—	
T12	1½ mm
L1—L4	2 mm
L5	⅓ mm
S1	1 mm
S2	½ mm
S3—S4	¼ mm

Table 6.10. Distribution of Spinal Nerve Somatic Rami

Rami	Distribution
C1	Adjacent muscles, filaments to capsule of atlanto-occipital joint and connections with the anterior branch of C2.
C2	The posterior branch supplies and overlying skin, adjacent muscles, and adjacent facet joints. The anterior branch (greater occipital nerve) passes horizontally across the inferior oblique muscle beneath the semispinalis capitis as it transverses vertically and then proceeds within the fascia of the trapezius to the scalp where it divides into numerous twigs that extend as far anterior as the coronal suture. Filaments supply the occipital and superficial temporal arteries. Impulses initiated at the C2 level of the cord in the greater occipital nerve merge with those of the C2 level spinal nucleus of the trigeminal. Thus, this nerve is often involved in suboccipital pain and occipitofrontal headache.
C3	The posterior branch supplies overlying skin and superficial musculature. The anterior branch divides with one branch winding around the facets of C3 and another communicating with the greater occipital nerve.
Posterior cervical plexus	This plexus is formed by the posterior rami of C1—C3 and sensed as a mass of neurovascular tissue lying beneath the semispinalis capitis muscle and as such is quite vulnerable to cervical strains, whiplash-type trauma, and subluxation syndromes.
C4—T1	Medial branches essentially supply overlying skin and superficial muscles, and the lateral branches essentially supply the deep muscles of the cervical region. As the nerves cross around the faces of the articular masses between the superior and inferior articular facets, these nerves are quite vulnerable to entrapment. The posterior rami of C8 follows a groove in the superior aspect of the 1st rib and is often involved in a cervical rib or scalenus anticus syndrome.
T2—T6	The posterior branches of the upper thoracic nerves are accompanied by the posterior arterial branch of the thoracic aorta as they pass posteriorly via an osseofibrous canal located about 2 cm from the midline. A shorter segment lies transversely between the costotransverse ligaments prior to dividing about 2.5 cm from the midline into terminal branches. The medial branches pass medioinferiorly, send twigs to nerves above and below, and supply adjacent muscles, ligaments, and joint capsules. Cutaneous branches must pierce the trapezius (3—4 cm from the midline) and pass laterally to supply the overlying skin. Thus, numerous areas of possible entrapment occur in the course of these nerves.
T7—T12	The posterior divisions of the lower thoracic nerves differ somewhat from those of the upper thoracic nerves. The medial branches are essentially muscular and supply the supraspinous and interspinous ligaments, but they have no cutaneous twigs. The larger lateral branches take an oblique course, emerge from the sacrospinalis, and follow the thoracolumbar fascia.

Table 6.10, continued

Rami	Distribution
T7—T12, continued	Small, short trunk *sinuvertebral* nerves enter the canals and are distributed to the vertebral arches and posterior facets, veins, sheath surrounding the dura matter, and communicate with the sympathetic chain. Thus, these nerves have two components: one from the spinal nerve and the other from the sympathetic chain. The spinal nerve portion arises just lateral to the posterior root ganglion and is often double. The fine sympathetic twigs arise from the rami communicantes.
L1—L5	The relatively small posterior division of lumbar nerves splits from the anterior division at almost a right angle as it projects backward and enters the posterior compartment via an osseofibrous tunnel as it forms partnership with other members of the neurovascular bundle. Some branches quickly course medially (about 5 mm from their origin) and divide into a medial branches and lateral branches: 1. Medial twigs to supply structures around the apophyseal joints such as the multifidus, interspinales, and erector spinae muscles; articular capsules; and the ligamentum flava, interspinous, and supraspinous ligaments. This supply covers an area that extends about 3 cm from the midline. Collaterals extend to communicate with two or more segments above and below. During their course, the medial fibers become flattened against the osseofibrous tunnel. This tunnel is about 6 mm long and is located at the inferior border of the transverse process at the root of the articular process. Thus, this is a common site of irritation and entrapment in which pain is referred to the tissues supplied. 2. Lateral limbs course obliquely inferolaterally over the back of the blunt transverse processes and project to supply the muscles lateral to the apophyseal joints and the intertransverse, iliolumbar, lumbosacral, and posterior sacroiliac ligaments. The lateral branch of the posterior ramus of L5 nerve descends vertically in a groove on the sacral ala just lateral to the S1 articular process to join the lateral branch of S1. The medial branch of L5 curves medially under the lumbosacral apophysis and sends branches medioinferiorly and posterior into the local multifidus muscles and lumbosacral ligaments.
S1—S4	These nerves form a plexiform arrangement on the back of the sacrum. The lateral branch of S1 joins with that of L5. The lateral branch of S2 projects downward over the sacrum just lateral to the 3rd and 4th foramina and joins the lateral divisions of S3 and S4. All these nerves lie between the interosseous and overlying sacroiliac ligaments, which are supplied by the lateral branches of the L5—S3 posterior rami. The fine medial branches of S1—S4 supply the multifidus muscle.

Note: Above data adapted from Bradley with modifications.

ion-rotation coupling that occurs. Because of its substantial degree of flexibility, the cord readily adapts to normal lengthening and shortening of the canal during motions.

The Meninges

The spinal cord is sheathed by three cylindrical membranes that extend from the foramen magnum to the midsacral region: the internal pia mater, the middle arachnoid, and the exterior dura mater (Fig. 6.8). These membranes tightly invest the spinal roots and cord, and their extensions surround the cauda equina and fuse at the external terminal filum.

The Dentate Ligaments

The 20 or 21 dentate (sawtoothed) ligaments derive from thickened pia mater. They are inferiorly inclined and extend bilaterally between the anterior and posterior nerve roots from the foramen magnum to the T12—L1 area, penetrate the arachnoid and its fluid-filled spaces, and fix to the inner surface of the dural membrane (Fig. 6.9). They provide a unique pretensed suspension system against sudden jars. It is because of the dentate ligaments that the spinal cord and its roots, but not the rootlets, are put under tension during spinal movements.

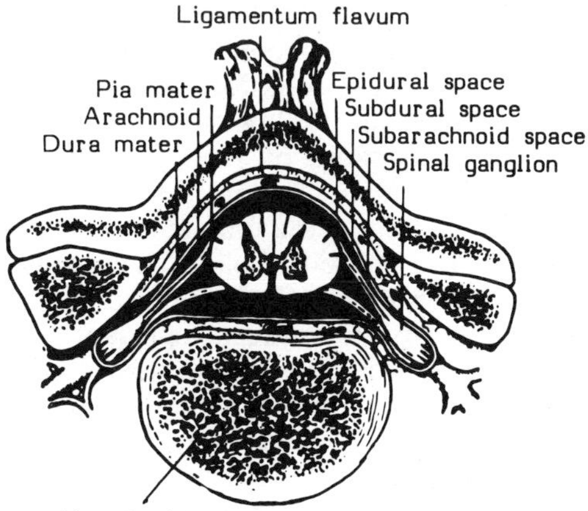

Figure 6.8. Schematics of the spinal cord membranes and their related spaces.

The Spinal Cord Proper

Cord Flexibility

Although dentate ligaments help to stabilize the spinal cord in a central position in the canal and help to protect against undue stretch, the cord is still flexible enough (10% of length) under small loads to move as much as ⅜ inch. The cord is quite elastic when deformed axially, but prone to severe damage if a vertebra is displaced horizontally. A space-occupying sclerotic or fibrotic lesion will restrict the cord's mobility and extensibility and thus increase tensile, torsion, and compression stresses. The symptoms thus produced can be alleviated if the cord can be relaxed.

Grieve proposes that if a biomechanical evaluation could be conducted at the microscopic level routinely in clinical practice, many neurologic disorders in which no mechanical component is suspected would be shown to have their origin in tension of nervous and vascular microtissues that produce a reduction of conduit diameter that interferes with function. We should be reminded here that the founder of chiropractic stated before the turn of the century that "chiropractic as a science is founded on tone."

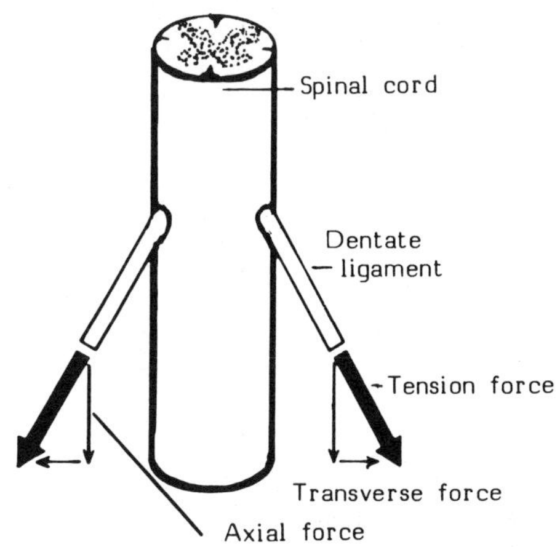

Figure 6.9. A unilateral diagonal dentate ligament would provide the spinal cord with axial and transverse pretension, but the bilateral pair offers the added benefit of resistance against axial tension.

Cord Folds

In its neutral state, the cord possesses accordion-like folds that flatten on stretch (flexion) and increase on relaxation (extension). This folding and unfolding mechanism is responsible for about three-fourths of the cord's change in length from full flexion to full extension. Once these folds have flattened during flexion, the cord is subjected to direct tensile forces. As a rubber band, the diameter of the cord then reduces on stretch and increases on relaxation.

The Cervical Cord

As maximum cervical movement is at the C5—C6 level and the spinal cord snugly fills the cervical canal, arthritic changes and disc herniations in this area may encroach upon the canal contents. As the cervical cord is at its maximum width at this level, injury may readily lead to neurologic damage.

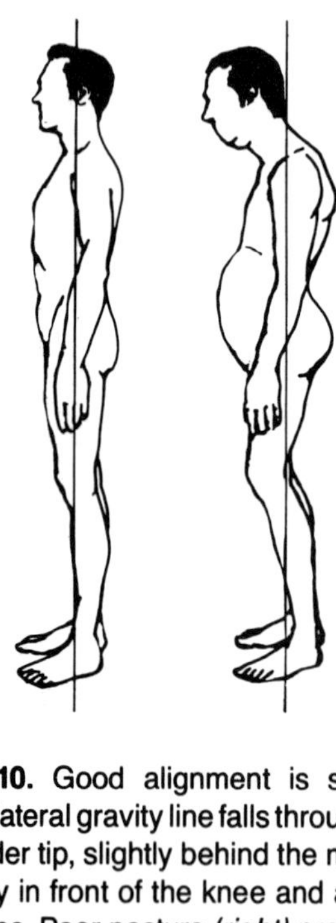

Figure 6.10. Good alignment is shown *(left)* where the lateral gravity line falls through the dens and shoulder tip, slightly behind the mid hip joint, and slightly in front of the knee and ankle joints' vertical axes. Poor posture *(right)* predisposes to spinal subluxations due to the abnormal load carriage.

The Lumbar Cord

The spinal cord ends near the L1 disc. Below this, the elements of the cauda equina are within the vertebral canal of the lumbar spine (refer to Fig. 6.6). The mobility of the cauda equina roots in the relatively large canal provides a safety factor not found in the cervical or thoracic regions. This safety factor, however, is minimized in spinal stenosis.

POSTURAL AND STRUCTURAL EFFECTS

An individual's posture can be defined as the relationship of each body structure to the entire structure (Fig. 6.10). Normal posture is that posture which best suits individuals according to their internal and external environmental conditions.

The Effects of Bipedism

An adult discless spine would resemble that of the newborn. Since animals that walk on four legs and infants prior to assuming the erect position do not have the physiologic curves of the erect adult, it is assumed that these curves are the result of bipedism. In the erect position, the lower lumbar area is especially subjected to considerable shearing stress.

The biped stance requires recognition of certain anatomical considerations to recognize that the spine and pelvis are of clinical importance because of their intimate involvement with the nervous system. In the human biped, there is a unique relationship between the musculoskeletal mechanism and the neurologic bed. The neurologic factors that relate to bipedism represent a rationale of clinical chiropractic that is often readily portrayed during dynamic postures.

Human architecture is much like a triad of three superimposed inverted triangles in which strain and stress are greater at certain points than at others (Fig. 6.11). Within the zone of these points of primary function and stress, there is a relatively heavy deposition of sensory nerve endings and motor end plates. When these areas, heavily populated with neuronal and vascular ramifications, are subject to trauma, occupational stress, the strains of postural fatigue, and abnormal viscerospinal reflexes, the process of transudation, fibrin precipitation, and adhesion formation ensues to establish an intramuscular and myofascial trigger point. To this must be added the principle of neurologic fascilitation and spread. Not uncommonly, there is a musculoskeletal syndrome complex that challenges the reserves of the most healthy.

Bipedism underlies the clinical concern of gravity and weight bearing, postural faults, strains and stresses of occupation, play, and trauma. Because of such stress, the articular, syndesmotic, and myologic proprioceptive complex is often disturbed. This results in the development of many common spinosomatic and spinovisceral syndromes. A deranged spinal or pelvic segment within its motor bed will invariably result in disturbance of the proprioceptive bed with facilitation of the discomfort/pain phenomenon.

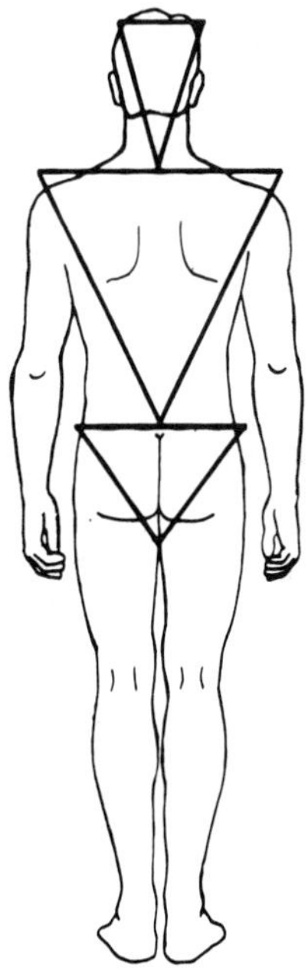

Figure 6.11. The inverted pyramid design of the body predisposes its potential instability and chronic stress to maintain balance.

Pelvic Posture Considerations

When erect, body weight and any extrinsic loading of the upper body are transmitted from L5 to the sacral base, the sacroiliac joints, ilia, and ischia. Impact forces from below arise from the foot through the tibia and femur. These axial forces meet at the acetabulum and are primarily dissipated transversely, to be absorbed by the cartilages and ligaments of the hip joints, sacroiliac joints, symphysis pubis, and the spongiosa of pelvic bone. The gross effect is locking of the involved joints by opposing forces traveling around each side of the pelvis anteriorly and posteriorly from the acetabulum. If these counterdirected axial forces are not equalized, the pelvis would not be in a state of equilibrium according to Newtonian principles. When the force from below is greater, the head of the femur tends to jam within the acetabulum. If the force from above is

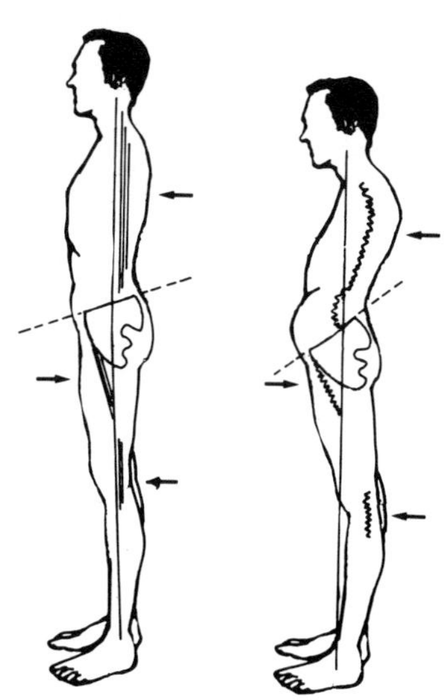

Figure 6.12. *Left,* the major ligaments involved in maintaining static balance are the anterior longitudinal ligament of the spine, the anterior iliofemoral ligaments of the pelvis, and the posterior ligaments of the knees. *Right,* typical posture of severe ligament laxity. Note loss of height, flattened chest and thoracic kyphosis, pot belly and lumbar hyperlordosis, anterior rotation of pelvis, and genu recurvatum. This posture exhibits biomechanical failure (sinking) from the pull of gravity.

greater, the L5 and S1 end plates or sacroiliac joints tend to displace.

Structural-Functional Relationships

Research data strongly suggests that sensory afferent impulses may play an important role relative to the maintenance of dynamic equilibrium of the human body to its environment. Overstress of muscles, tendons, and ligaments brings about a change in patterns of afferent nerve impulses that are fired from their nociceptors and mechanoceptors and transmitted to the CNS. It can be hypothesized that, because of these changes, stress develops that affects not only the body's dynamic equilibrium with the forces of gravity but also possible visceral dysfunction, and, in turn, visceral disorders influence the body's dynamic equilibrium (Fig. 6.12).

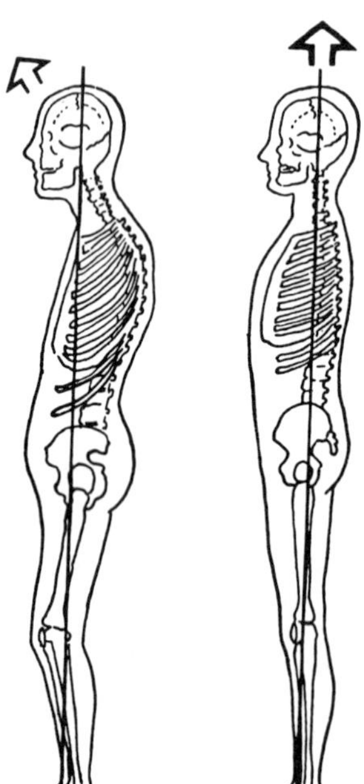

Figure 6.13. *Left,* poor posture from excessive sagging, producing joint centers out of alignment and resulting in increased muscle activity. *Right,* good postural alignment of body centers (with permission of Behavioral Research Foundation).

Balance Considerations

No two individuals react in an identical manner to actual or potential loss of body balance. All vary somewhat in the accommodation process, depending upon one's gross structure and functional capabilities, the momentary potential for redistributing body mass, and the visual efficiency necessary to guide correct accommodations (Fig. 6.13). Irregularities of postural control can be expected to result in deviations from normal standing values.

The symptomatic picture of balance defects is often unclear because individuals vary so much in response to mechanical insult. Some people present with immediate symptoms upon slight deviation, while others offer no symptoms until pathologic changes are in progress. Much of this is determined by how the body is used; eg, occupational and athletic considerations.

Within normal parameters, according to Fernie/Holliday, healthy people have a slightly variable mean speed of postural sway and range of movement in the sagittal and coronal planes. Vision also affects these values significantly, as shown in differences between eyes-open and eyes-closed tests. Studies of normal subjects and amputees show that postural sway increases with age, but the visual dependence for the control of sway is unaffected by age.

Spinal subluxations are often the forerunners of balance defects brought through the effort of the spinal column to compensate for the stress and thus to reduce the more serious effects. Balance defects also may originate from habitual faulty postures in standing, sitting, and lying, as well as from activities that constantly employ the forces of the large muscles in asymmetrical action (Fig. 6.14). When created, such defects serve to lessen the power of the body to withstand shock and are, in turn, the precursors to subluxations.

Additional causes of defects in balance are found in the frequent occurrence of unequal lower extremities, in faulty development of vertebrae and the sacrum, and from the effects of abnormal reflexes. The least common causes of balance defects can be attributed to inheritance and disease. Constitutional stress, visceral malfunction, nutritional status, fatigue and debility, neuromuscular tension, a large variety of psychologic factors, height, weight, and body type all combine to express themselves in one's posture, body balance, and motor ability.

Most balance faults witnessed in practice will be within "physiologic" limits without obvious structural deformity, yet it should be appreciated that abnormal function leads to reduced performance capabilities early and to pathology later if left uncorrected. Isolated muscle weakness should be suspected especially in situations of head or pelvic tilt, trunk imbalance, scoliosis, and uneven gait or limp.

The major adverse influences on posture are shown in Table 6.11. Some recognized clinical disorders having an adverse effect on posture are shown in Table 6.12.

Functional Stress and Fatigue

The physiologic stress and fatigue of chronic balance defects cannot be discussed in unrelated terms. Tension arises when the body is forced to be used in a position that is not favorable to muscle balance or when the joints are at their physiologic limit of articulation. Thus, pull comes from ligaments rather than muscles. The result is tissue insult leading to edema, pain, and physical deformity that is referred to (1) the structures upon which the strain is imposed, or (2) the cutaneous branches of the spinal

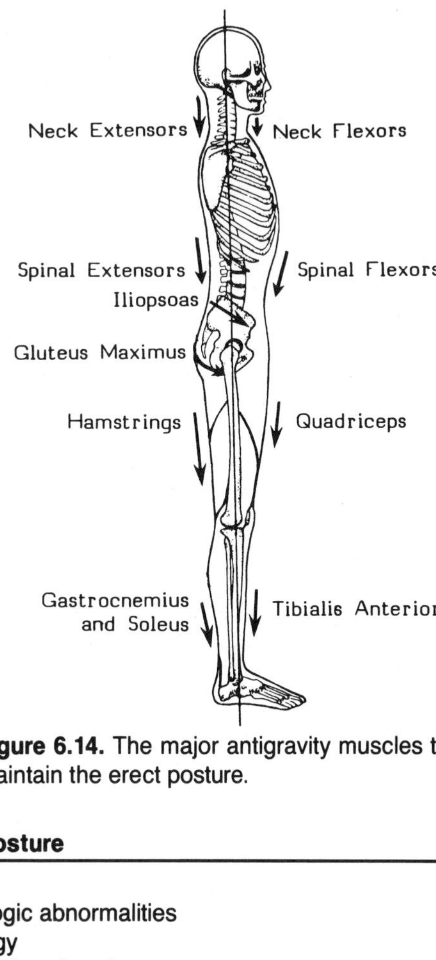

Figure 6.14. The major antigravity muscles that maintain the erect posture.

Table 6.11. Major Adverse Influences on Human Posture

Conditioned reflexes	Physiologic abnormalities
Gravity	Pathology
Emotional states	Endocrine disorders
Anxiety	Joint disorders
Depression	Myopathy
Joy	Neuropathy
Environment	Structural anomalies
Clothing	Lower extremities
Occupation	Organs and tissues that attach to or are suspended from the spinal column
Social customs	Pelvis
Weather	Upper extremities
Ground angle	Vertebral column
Ground surface	Structural malpositions
Heat and cold	Dislocations
Wind	Fractures
Fatigue	Subluxations
Pain	

nerve root supplying the strained tissues. Long-term muscle strain results in adaptive changes in the joints and ligaments to meet the needs of the malaligment. Thus, low-key chronic sprain is a part of the picture. Abnormal fatigue is the result of wasted energy.

The more pronounced an abnormal spinal curvature, the greater becomes the mechanical disadvantage to which the supporting structures are subjected. Thus, the process is a vicious cycle. Along with chronic stress and fatigue, constant pull causes small tears in ligamentous attachments. This results in a series of subperiosteal hemorrhages that may later calcify into exostoses, becoming extremely painful upon further stress. Such a situation may occur in any joint that is subjected to prolonged strain, but it is especially common in the spine and other weight-bearing joints.

Raphael points out that, besides postural stress, the effects of cummulative or repetitive trauma should not be neglected in any discussion of functional stress and fatigue. "Not only is poor posture a predisposing factor to subluxations but also overuse of muscles which lead to myofascial pain syndromes and subluxations."

Neurologic Considerations

There usually is some degree of IVF insult present in spinal malalignment effected by improper balance. Exaggerated cervical or lumbar lordosis, for example, decreases the size of the IVFs and frequently leads to chronic radiculitis. Neuralgic pains in the thorax and legs are common. Less common is intercostal neuralgia. If originating in the cervical region and associated with hypertrophic changes, pain is often referred about the shoulders and down the arms, frequently being mistaken for angina pectoris. Similar neuralgic pains in the chest wall can be mistaken for pleurisy, pleural adhesions, or pulmonary lesions. Auscultation will serve in differentiation. Narrowing of the IVF also may cause severe pain that has a segmental distribution perceived in the skin, muscle, or parietal peritoneum. This condition can be misleading as to origin as it mimics the presence of some intra-abdominal disorder.

Trigger Points

Concurrently with postural stress-related neuralgia, myositis, and the development of intrafascicular adhesions, similar events occur in the myofascial planes at points of major tensile stress, leading to the development of "trigger points" and the resulting delta or spread effect. All muscles have their fascial encasements (epimysium, perimysium, endomysium); and, as muscles lie and move one upon the other, the myofacial planes are described. The amount of fasciculi involved in the all-or-none contraction effort determines the tone or strength of muscle contraction. Furthermore, a muscle usually does more work at one point of its composite than at another.

Circulatory Implications

Disturbances of vascular flow are rarely absent when postural distortions are gross.

Table 6.12. Common Clinical States That Affect Normal Posture

Aerophagia	Fatigue	Myalgia
Albuminuria	Gait disturbances	Neuralgia
Anorexia	Increased energy requirements	Pseudoemphysema
Arthralgia	Intolerance to stress	Reduced endurance
Circulatory impairments	Intrafascicular adhesions	Respiratory inefficiency
Constipation	Irritability	Trigger points
Digestive disturbances	Lowered immunity	Visceral dysfunctions
Drainage impairments		Visceroptosis
Dysmenorrhea		

The low diaphragm results in venous congestion in its failure to assist blood returning to the heart. Sagging viscera stretch mesenteric vessels and narrow their lumina. Duodenal stasis may be attributed to increased tension on the superior mesenteric vessels. Thus, circulatory symptoms may manifest throughout the body. Researchers have recorded the relief of eye strain and mild myopia in children by postural correction alone. They explain this as a relief of venous congestion in the head.

Such impaired circulatory inefficiency in extreme cases may be sufficient to produce a marked fall in blood pressure and loss of consciousness. This is said to be the result of general muscle relaxation with pooling of blood in the venous reservoirs, especially in the abdomen, thus reducing the practical blood volume. More often, it causes only dyspnea and weakness, sometimes accompanied by palpitation. Precordial pain resembling angina pectoris is not uncommon. Even when heart disease exists, part of the symptomatic picture may be the result of a postural defect that tends to aggravate the pathologic defect. The marked kyphotic "stoop" of the chronic cardiac case is frequently seen.

Drainage Impairments

Faulty posture mechanics may cause the liver to rotate anteriorly and to the right. Traction is thereby exerted on the common bile duct and in some cases seriously interferes with biliary drainage. Ptosis of the kidneys, especially the left kidney, results in traction on the renal veins that may obstruct venous outflow to cause passive congestion and albuminuria.

Respiratory Considerations

Respiratory balance and the maintenance of proper intra-abdominal pressure depend on good body mechanics. In the ideal attitude, the position of the well-poised head with the chest held high is important because the anterior mediastinal ligaments attached to the diaphragm originate in the deep cervical fascia and are attached to the lower cervical vertebrae. See Figure 6.15. When postural mechanics are poor, a lowered diaphragm is the rule and proper coordination of the muscles of respiration is lost. This abnormal position may decrease vital capacity by more than half. This is commonly recognized. What is not commonly recognized is the importance of the diaphragm in venous and lymphatic circulation.

Venous and lymphatic return is greatly assisted by the rhythmic contractions of the diaphragm. When the diaphragm has been lowered, it has a much shorter range of excursion and is thus much less effective as a circulatory aid. In poor body mechanics, there is always some degree of circulation retardation and improper oxygenation that results in a diminished supply of impoverished blood.

It has been shown that the respiratory difficulty of emphysema is largely due to the low position of the diaphragm (associated with the higher intrathoracic pressure), which limits diaphragmatic excursions. Thus, dyspnea is greatly relieved by a supportive device that increases the extent of diaphragmatic movements. Because of the

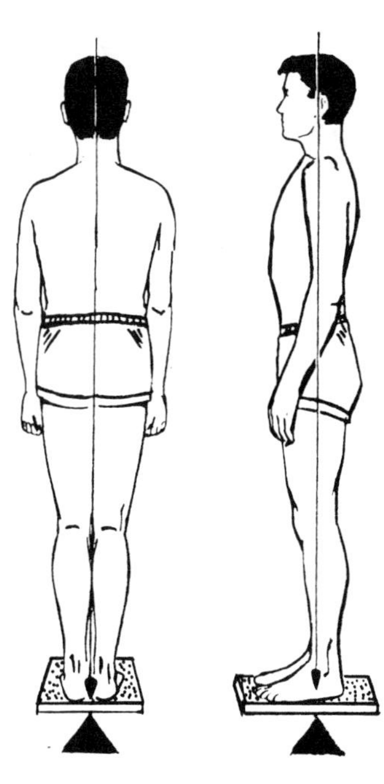

Figure 6.15. *Left,* lateral gravity line. *Right,* anterior-posterior gravity line.

depressed rib angles, decreased chest diameters, and low diaphragm associated with poor posture, respiration may be deep and slow. However, it may be shallow and fast in a sitting slumped posture that causes the diaphragm to be raised by viscera pushing upward.

Digestive Disturbances

Mild digestive symptoms may exist in the apparently healthy person. This is sometimes traced to a degree of visceroptosis, which results in dysfunction of the displaced organs. Abdominal dilatation and motility disturbances are not infrequent occurrences. This is most likely the outcome of stretching of the sympathetic nerves. Pottenger points out that stretched nerves within involuntary or voluntary muscles usually produce a temporary paralysis. In addition, when the abdominal cavity becomes shortened longitudinally, the viscera become crowded as do the glands of internal secretion and the nerve ganglia as well. Thus, orthostatic albuminuria, dysmenorrhea, and constipation may be associated.

Gynecologic Considerations

Slouching while sitting plays a dual role in its effect upon the female pelvic organs. The flattening of the chest walls and the restricted chest motion decrease the thoracic capacity to the extent that active inspiration is only permissible by forcing down the diaphragm. The result is an increase in intra-abdominal pressure that forces the intestines into the pelvis and upon the uterus, tubes, and ovaries. This is partly compensated for by abdominal protrusion; but in time, the supporting ligaments of the uterus lose their elasticity, become elongated, and displacements follow. Pioneer chiropractors were often quite skillful in correcting such prolapses.

Janse describes an article by F.N. Miller that appeared several years ago in the *Journal of the American Medical Association.* Miller, while professor of gynecology at the School of Medicine of the University of Iowa, showed a correlation between poor posture and such gynecologic disorders as dysmenorrhea, leukorrhea, chronic backache, constipation, amenorrhea, and complaints of pain in the sides. According to Miller, "The fact that exercise, manipulative therapy, and body development have reduced the frequency of many of the more common female disorders (where traditional methods have failed) would indicate that the cause for these conditions may be found in faulty spinal balance rather than essentially in local lesions."

Goldthwait and other investigators have shown that spinal imbalance definitely distorts the innervation to the reproductive organs and blood vessels within the female pelvis, leaving them prone to congestion, lack of tone, and irregularity of function. In addition, poor posture permits a sagging of the abdominal viscera and their encroachment upon the pelvic contents, which in turn results in a tensile stress upon the nerves and plexuses as well as the blood vessels and organs proper, leading to a large number of functional ailments that are especially common in the female.

Postural Analysis

Gravitational forces create subluxations and spinal distortions by the constant pull of body structures toward the center of the earth. Such distortions are exaggerated by increasing the distance of the vertebrae from the center line of gravity and are decreased by decreasing the distance of the vertebrae from the center line of gravity. Thus, during spinal and pelvic analysis, it is imperative that spinal mechanics and structural deviation are interpreted from the gravitational center line, along with their neuromuscular implications, if the body is to be returned to its normally balanced position.

McDowall offers the hypothesis that primary muscle imbalance leads to vertebral instability and thus subluxation. His findings indicate that studies authorized by B.J. Palmer considered this phenomena prior to 1934. Okubo reports that posturography was initiated in 1908 to analyze body motion in cases of cerebellar disease, cerebral disease, and hysteria. Allopathic research during the 1940s was primarily concerned with orthopedics, while the examination of posture through photographic and goniometric means was the trend during the 1950s.

Anatomists and neurologists no longer question the significance of the entire proprioceptive bed disposition in the ligamentous and myologic elements of the spine and pelvis. As a diagnostic aid during the evaluation of postural faults, pioneer chiropractors used a simple plumbline (refer to Fig. 6.15). In more recent years, a number of more sophisticated devices have been invented to measure postural distortions and therapeutic effects. Several types are briefly described below.

The Posturometer. While posture is an ever-changing phenomenon, some reliable baseline of measurement must be devised if postural assessment is to be considered as an integral component of chiropractic spinal analysis. In a study conducted by Vernon, 80 male subjects were assessed with a *posturometer*. The level of intra- and inter-observer correspondence was calculated to be in the 75% range, indicating that, with minor exceptions, a significant level of reliability was reached to provide a standard of reference for postural assessments.

An earlier posturometer survey of two beginner judo classes was conducted by Homewood. It produced data indicating typical posture. Almost all subjects demonstrated a posterior gravity line. A right-tilted and rotated pelvis and a right low shoulder corroborated earlier studies that showed excessive weight on the right side in most subjects. A recheck after judo instruction and practice showed an improved gravity line but little change in other indicators. It was concluded that judo exercise was inferior to chiropractic in terms of correcting structural distortions.

The Gravity Stress Analyzer. This instrument (GSA) is designed to measure degrees of rotation and lateral flexion of the head, shoulders, and pelvis as they deviate from perfect alignment in the sagittal plane. In addition, deviations of C7 and L5 vertebrae in both the coronal and sagittal planes are recorded. Anderson/Winkler's evaluation of the GSA showed that it was a lightweight, quick to use (5 min or less) instrument. These investigators state that it is essential that studies be carried out to determine: (1) the accuracy of measures recorded and (2) the ranges of measurement that characterize normal nonpatient populations.

Photographic Imaging. The development of a static posture analysis instrument with direct application as an objective screening procedure was investigated by Hadden. It allows photographic recording of a patient's static posture and center of gravity vector. The overall accuracy was found to be N4.2 mm on a 360° protractor for the center of gravity vector and an overall error of N5.3 mm for measuring spinal distortion as compared to roentgenographic analysis. Hadden suggests that the device can be used as a pre-x-ray screening instrument to (1) determine static biomechanics, (2) reduce the clinical need for roentgen examination, or (3) suggest the specific type of films required. It also can be used to evaluate immediately the effect of orthopedic appliances on static posture.

The Four-Quadrant Weight Scale. A unit to analyze posture was developed to evaluate weight-bearing in the sagittal and coronal planes. A report by Vernon/Grice found that the 4QWS instrument may assume a useful role in the chiropractic analysis of the locomotor system.

Integrated Systems. A video-integrated measurement (VIM) system was investigated by Spector and associates that incorporated the use of various noninvasive diagnostic procedures (moiré contourography, electromyography, posturometry, infrared thermography, etc) used individually or in combination for the evaluation of musculoskeletal and other disorders and their management with biofeedback and other therapeutic procedures. The system provides for measuring individual diagnostic and therapeutic modes on a video monitor, or multiple modes by split-screen superimposition, of real time (actual) images of the patient and idealized (ideal normal) models, along with analog and digital data graphics in color, and other transduced symbolic information. It was concluded that the system (1) provided an innovative method by which the therapist and patient could interact within biofeedback training-learning processes and (2) holds promise for more effective measurement and treatment of a wide variety of physical and behavioral disorders.

The reader should be alerted that specific procedures, techniques, or devices described by the author within this publication do not necessarily imply the approval or the endorsement of the American Chiropractic Association. It is recommended that doctors of chiropractic consult with their respective State Board of Chiropractic Examiners concerning the use of any specific procedure, technique, or device.

Visceroptosis

Nature provides good support for the abdominal organs when the body is normally erect. In the ideal attitude, tissue ledges and shelves exist that partially support the abdominal organs. However, if the lumbar and dorsal curves increase and the abdominal wall relaxes, these vital supports are lost (Fig. 6.16).

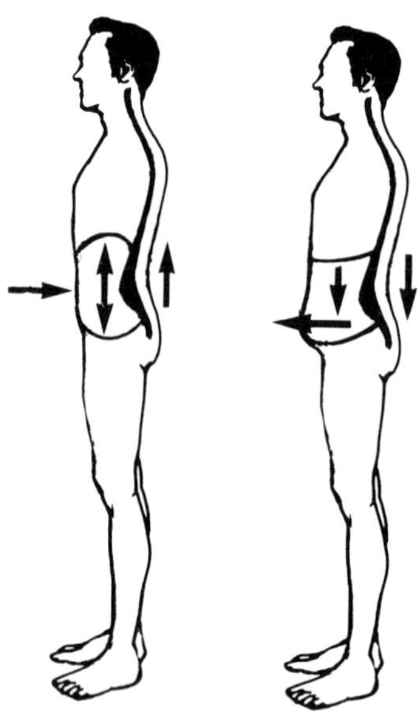

Figure 6.16. *Left,* the abdominal cavity serves as a hydraulic sac. Firm abdominal muscles tend to keep the diaphragm up, the pelvic floor down, and to elongate the lumbar spine. This tends to reduce added stress to the weight-bearing lumbar vertebral segments by seating the weight of the viscera within the pelvic basin. *Right,* conversely, weakened abdominal muscles allow the diaphragm to descend, the viscera to protrude anteriorly, and the lumbar curve to increase anteriorly. This adds to lumbar stress and hypertonicity of the posterior musculature. Most back pain is exacerbated not a weak back, but by a weak abdomen.

Basic Considerations

Abnormal body mechanics affecting the thoracic and abdominal cavities can interfere with normal function by (1) abnormal efferent visceral stimuli reaching organs from the facilitated segment, (2) abnormal tensions and stretching of visceral supports, nerves, blood and lymph vessels, (3) venous pooling as the result of inactivity, diaphragm dysfunction, organ displacement, and sustained postural stress, or (4) abnormal vasomotor impulses to blood vessels. Blocking stress or irritation of blood vessels leads to ischemia or congestion.

There are many general effects to the body as a whole besides these local effects because each abnormal stress results in abnormal discharges of afferent impulses to the CNS, with consequent hormonal reactions that are systemic in character. Also to be considered should be the associated psychic stress that contributes to the clinical picture.

Extreme curvature and malalignment produce physiologic changes and are considered pathologic, but how much deviation is possible without causing severe impairment of health? The effect on function varies in research literature. Most all agree, however, that poor body mechanics predispose to certain visceral disorders; ie, the viscera are held in their optimum position for function in good body mechanics.

Implications

If body mechanics are good, the abdominal cavity is shaped like an inverted pear with adequate space above L4 for the abdominal viscera of an intermediate body type. Anatomical ledges and shelves exist that partially support the abdominal organs. However, if the lumbar and dorsal curves increase and the abdominal wall relaxes, these vital supports are lost (Fig. 6.17).

With the *stomach* lying mainly to the left of the spine and supported by a diaphragmatic attachment behind the transverse sagittal plane, there is little tendency for downward displacement of the stomach if there is no rib-cage deformity or abdominal muscle weakness. The *liver* is generally posterior to the transverse sagittal plane. It is partly supported by the surrounding organs and its attachments to the diaphragm, but most of its weight is borne by the concave space at the side of the spine and by the curves of the lower ribs. The *spleen* is well back and held in place by peritoneal folds, and the *pancreas* depends chiefly on the surrounding organs for support. The *kidneys* normally rest in definite depressions that begin around the level of L4 and are supported by the psoas muscle, quadratus lumborum, and retroperitoneal fat. The attachments of the hepatic and splenic flexures of the *colon* are external to the kidney and attached to the posterior surface of the abdominal cavity. About seven-eights of the weight of the abdominal organs is borne by the psoas shelf and the muscles of the abdominal wall.

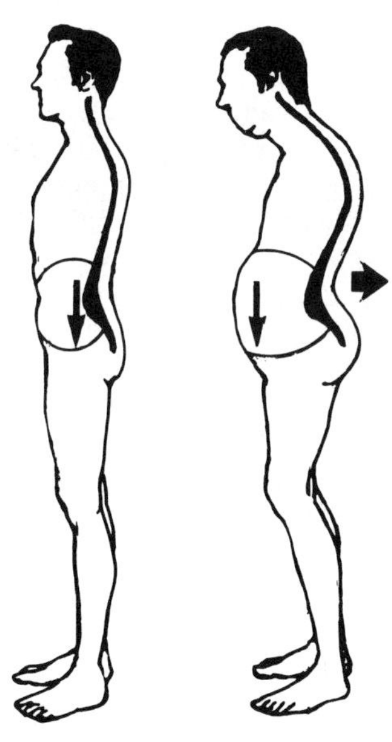

Figure 6.17. *Left,* in good posture and weight balance, gravitational forces fall slightly anterior to the sacrum. *Right,* in obesity with weak abdominal muscles, the center of mass is shifted anteriorly, causing an increase in the sacral angle and hyperextension of the lumbodorsal area.

Postural visceroptosis results in dysfunction of the displaced organs. Goldthwait observed that a faulty posture causes the liver to rotate anteriorly and to the right. Traction is thereby exerted on the common bile duct and sometimes seriously interferes with its drainage. Abdominal dilatation and motility disturbances are also frequent occurrences. This is most likely the outcome of stretching of the sympathetic nerves. Stretched nerves within voluntary muscles usually produce a temporary paralysis. In addition, when the abdominal cavity becomes shortened longitudinally, the viscera become crowded but so do the glands of internal secretion and the nerve ganglia as well. Thus, orthostatic albuminuria, dysmenorrhea, and constipation may be seen. Visceroptosis also causes an abnormally low pressure in the upper abdomen. If this pressure is sufficiently below atmospheric pressure, air is drawn into the stomach during respiration (aerophagia).

Because of visceroptosis, a compensating lumbar lordosis, and the insult at the IVFs, symptoms can be diffuse and subtle. It has been previously described that duodenal stasis may be attributed to increased tension on the superior mesenteric vessels. One study showed that postural correction relieved 65% of cases exhibiting a picture of duodenal obstruction and 75% of cases presenting with gastric distress, nausea, and abdominal pain associated with visceroptosis.

Postural Effects of Pregnancy

Several years ago, studies by Goldthwait demonstrated the ill effects on spinal posture during pregnancy and visceroptosis. These effects were attributed to the increased tension on nerves and vessels. Browde showed that prolonged experimental increase of intra-abdominal pressure results in neurodegeneration of the end plates and terminal nerve fibers. A similar picture is seen during pregnancy wherein it has been shown histologically that degeneration of nerve fibers precedes changes in the musculature of the diaphragm and abdominal wall. These degenerative changes in the fibers appeared to be the result of increased intra-abdominal pressure, yet they differed from that of typical wallerian degeneration.

SEGMENTAL HYPERMOBILITY

The phrase *spinal instability* refers to that state of a vertebral segment in which it cannot maintain its normal relationships with its contiguous structures under normal loading conditions for the individual. The results are likely chronic irritation of the nerve, root, or cord; intolerable pain; and degenerative structural alterations.

Basic Considerations

Segmental hypermobility is allowed by ligamentous laxity, disc degeneration, and remolding of the posterior articulations. That is, a hypermobile subluxation indicates laxity of the holding elements—a positional relationship of two vertebrae in which their bodies or apophyseal joint surfaces or both are in a position that they would never occupy during any phase of a normal physiologic movement. The immediate cause can be trauma, disease, or iatrogenic from misapplied surgery or manipulation.

Such hypermobility may be primary (ie, localized trauma or pathology limited to one or more motion units) or secondary. The most common secondary cause is that found in compensation above and below an area of spinal hypomobility (fixation). This subluxation is a dysfunction clinically discernible through motion palpation. Secondary factors also include those resulting from a primary problem often far removed from the spine such as lower-limb asymmetries, eccentric weight bearing, misuse or overuse of spinal tissues associated with postural-occupational stresses, and system-oriented disorders such as hypoglycemia that may increase the degree of spinal curvatures through chronic fatigue.

As severe segmental instability requires stabilization, the primary question in diagnosis is locating and determining the primary problem or maladaption that is overloading and chronically stretching the involved motion unit. A hypermobile unit is not tightened by spinal adjustment; however, it is often self-correcting once its cause is removed.

Implications

Several authorities feel that the first sign of disc disease is that of abnormal motion on flexion. Macnab attributes most pains associated with disc lesions to be from repetitive ligamentous strain due to chronic hyperextension of the posterior vertebral joints and the resulting arthritis. Farfan believes the more advanced changes found in disc disease (eg, marginal osteophytes, degenerated facets, pseudospondylolisthesis) are also due to mechanical stresses. Both Macnab and Farfan consider these changes to be the re-

Table 6.13. Common Causes of Segmental Hypomobility in the Spine

Adhesive capsulitis	IVD anular protrusions
Ankylosis	IVD degeneration
Apophyseal asymmetry	IVD nuclear displacement
Articular adhesions	Ligamentous shortening
Biomechanical dysequilibrium (eg, short leg, hemivertebra)	Meniscoid fragments
Bony encroachment (eg, jammed facet)	Phasic muscular spasm (splinting)
Capsular thickening	Pseudoankylosis
Hypertonic postural reflexes	Somatospinal reflexes
	Synovial tabs
	Viscerospinal reflexes

sult of segmental instability.

Hypermobility is the variant of subluxation that is most apparent in roentgenography. The overt signs include traction spurs, interruption of Hadley's S curve, excessive A-P body shift at extremes of flexion and extension, abnormal opening and closing of disc space during lateral bending, appearance of segmental hyperextension on neutral lateral films, change in articular relations to the joint-body line, reactive spondylosis and arthrosis, etc.

Segmental hypermobility is particularly obvious in spondylolisthesis, laterolisthesis, and retrolisthesis, and in excessive disc-space gapping in the sagittal or frontal plane. Instability in these cases becomes even more obvious at the extremes of movement, hence the value of carefully conducted stress films if they are not contraindicated.

All chronic subluxations appear to follow a progression. For example, a spondylolisthetic vertebra may start with fairly normal mechanics, then slowly become hypermobile with middle age. An evident subluxation must be viewed in the context of the entire clinical picture, and this functional classification is clinically oriented.

SEGMENTAL HYPOMOBILITY

Most pioneer chiropractors viewed a subluxation as a static misalignment. Contemporary research, however, has shown that a spinal articulation may become fixed, totally or partially, in its neutral position, or it may be fixed anywhere within its range of flexion, extension, lateral bending, or rotational motion. Thus, a fixation is not synonymous with a subluxation but a state superimposed upon or independent of a subluxation. If an "off-centered" articular subluxation is not fixed, it undoubtedly would reduce itself automatically during normal spinal motions if the part is not immobilized.

Basic Considerations

According to the *fixation hypothesis*, static anatomical relationships may be normal but dynamic relationships may be far from normal. Because of this, the subluxation complex must be studied *in vivo* and the reason postmortem studies have failed to validate the chiropractic approach is explained.

Various factors that can cause or contribute to one or more vertebrae to be held in a state of fixation (immobility, hypomobility) are shown in Table 6.13.

In compensation to a local area of fixation, adjacent joints are forced to assume roles of increased mobility (hyperkinesia), leading to clinical instability. Also, when a unilateral articulation is partially fixated, its contralateral partner is forced to assume the role of both via pivotal hypermobility about an abnormal axis. Invariably, it will be at the site of excessive mobility that is symptomatic rather than the site of the cause of the abnormal movement. Gillet believes that one exception to this is the suboccipital area, which he feels is often involved in a state of muscular fixation.

Total fixation is most frequently found at the occipitoatlantal, lower thoracic, and sacroiliac articulations. In most instances, however, mobility is not restricted in all directions. The earlier a fixation is corrected, the less chance there is for chronic degenerative changes to occur and the greatest change in mobility can be noted after adjustment.

Clinical Studies

Many clinical studies have been conducted to validate partial or complete segmental fixation. Gillet and Liekens, in Europe, have done much to develop a system of dynamic motion palpation. Much of their findings have been collaborated by Faye, Wiles, and several others in North America.

Stress-view roentgenograpy has also been used extensively to evaluate the existence of segmental fixation in the spine. The first system found in our literature search was developed by Vladef in Detroit during the 1940s and expanded upon by Rich at Lincoln Chiropractic College in the 1950s through cineroentgenology. In more recent years, studies by Illi, Carrick, Giles, Good, Banks, Grice, and Henderson have been highly helpful. Likewise, the work of Vernon, Burnarski, Cox, and Mannen have shed much light on this subject (see chapter bibliography).

Electromyographic studies have also been used to note the somatic changes that occur following adjustive correction of fixations. In this context, the studies of Rebechini-Zasadny, Lewit, and Thabe have greatly added to our knowledge of this concept and its implications.

Implications

When involving one or more vertebrae, a state of decreased mobility of the motion unit encourages neural alterations that can lead to pathologic processes in the areas supplied by the affected nerve root complex, depending upon the degree of fixation and the chronicity of involvement.

An Etiologic Hypothesis

Giles hypothesizes that the main stages evolve as follows:

1. Decreased mobility or vertebral fixation of a motion unit within its normal physiologic range of movement causes sluggish circulatory flow. Keep in mind that the motion unit is normally dynamic and that the following structures may be found in the IVF: the anterior or motor nerve root, posterior or sensory root, part of the posterior nerve root ganglion, recurrent meningeal nerve, spinal ramus artery, intervertebral vein, lymphatic vessels, nervi nervorum, nervi vasorum, vaso vasorum, and vaso nervorum.

2. Sluggish circulatory flow in the vertebral veins and arteries causes venous stagnation. Venous stagnation from arterial backup in turn produces a local toxicity. Toxicity, due to the buildup of metabolic waste products in the area of the IVF, alters the normal pH of the local fluids that causes a breakdown of the Krebs cycle.

3. A breakdown of the Krebs cycle, due to decreased oxygen and toxicity, causes a partial breakdown of the sodium pump mechanism, resulting in an ionic imbalance. Ionic imbalance, as the sodium pump can no longer maintain normal ionic equilibrium, results in some degree of erratic nerve conduction and edema in the tissues of the immediate area. The erratic nerve conduction may be exhibited in all nerves passing through the involved IVF and immediate area. CSF stagnation possibly occurs in association because of the intimate relationship between spinal fluid and venoid blood, contributing to toxicity in the nerve root area.

It should be noted that the hypotheses of several others differ from that of Giles in varying degrees.

Therapeutic Considerations

Segmental hypermobility appears to be the frequent effect of adjacent articular fixation as the result of soft-tissue (muscular and/or ligamentous) contractures. Buerger has shown that there appears to be a lack of stimulation of joint mechanoreceptors that normally inhibit nociceptive afferents. Lack of articular mobility prevents the normal input into the neuronal pool that blocks pain-conducting afferents from conducting impulses to higher CNS levels.

Although nociceptive impulses cannot be measured directly, an accompanying reflex (spontaneous activity of segmental muscles) can be measured by EMG recordings. It has been demonstrated by Thabe that local joint restriction induces abnormal EMG changes and that adjustive therapy normalizes this response concurrently with the correction of joint malfunction.

Adjustive mobilization of spinal fixations has been demonstrated by an EMG study by Rebechini-Zasadny/Tasharski to show a positive gain in muscle strength, and Vernon has shown a significant but short-term increase in serum beta-endorphins (resembling that following acupuncture) immediately after adjustive therapy. Besides the control of pain, the endorphins have far-reaching effects in multiple body systems that are currently undergoing extensive study.

In support of the supposition that fixation is primarily articular in nature, Thabe reports that adjustive techniques could accomplish this correction where local anesthetic injections and mobilization could not. In addition, Mayer and associates found that oral anti-inflammatories do not improve symptoms associated with segmental cervical hypomobility.

STRUCTURAL ADJUSTMENT RATIONALES

For many years, it has been realized that the basis of chiropractic therapy cannot rest on empirical results alone. Controlled research studies have been encouraged through such organizations as the Foundation for Chiropractic Education and Research and various chiropractic colleges. The osteopathic profession and more recently the allopathic profession, as well as the scientific community in general, have also increased their investigation of why corrective manipulative therapy, especially that of the spine, exerts its influence on somatic and visceral functions.

Bergmann states that the most specialized and significant therapy employed by the chiropractor involves the adjustment of the articulations of the human body, especially of the spinal column, manually or mechanically, actively or passively, for restoring normal articular relationship and function, restoring neurologic integrity, and influencing physiologic processes.

Terminology

The objective of any therapy must be based upon a rational hypothesis. According to its founder, the objective of chiropractic therapy is to restore normal "tone" to the nervous system. This goal has never varied, while the primary and secondary methods (technics and techniques) used to achieve this goal have undergone and will continue to undergo constant refinement. This is true for the procedures used within all health-care professions. Although it is recognized that many chiropractic practitioners achieve this by "nonthrust" means (eg, the application of somatosomatic reflexes), objectives are generally achieved by manual articular mobilization unless such a technic is contraindicated in a specific situation.

The terms *technique* and *technic* are generally considered synonymous outside the profession of chiropractic. In chiropractic, however, the term *technic* has been historically restricted to the application of a manually applied adjustive force, while the term *technique* is used concerning the application of any other procedure (therapeutic or diagnostic).

Chiropractic *treatment* should be differentiated from chiropractic *technic*. Case-management treatment includes the application of a primary technique plus all the ancillary procedures incorporated to achieve the clinical objective (eg, physiotherapeutic modalities, nutritional supplementation, diet control, therapeutic exercise, meridian therapy, biofeedback, and psychotherapy or other counseling) in the most efficient manner.

The Uniqueness of the Chiropractic Adjustment

Although the chiropractic "adjustment" is at the foundation of chiropractic therapeutics, few have tried to define it. Sandoz states that it is a passive manual maneuver during which the three-joint complex (IVD and apophyseal joints) is suddenly carried beyond the normal physiologic range of movement without exceeding the boundaries of anatomical integrity. Swezey, an allopath, refers to a dynamic chiropractic adjustment as the high-velocity short-arc-inducing passive movement of one articulating surface over another. Few would strongly object to either of these attempts to define the purely structural effect induced; ie, if the objective is solely to mobilize a fixation or realign a subluxation. Unfortunately, such purely mechanical concepts are limited; eg, they fail to consider the induced neurologic stimulation upon the cord, root, axoplasmic flow, and mechanoreceptors of the area and the local and remote "spillover" effects of such stimuli.

There is a recent trend by some authors and editors to lump what a chiropractor does during an "adjustment" under the general category of *spinal manipulative therapy* (SMT). This appears to be a term originated by the allied health professions for it was rarely seen in chiropractic literature prior to the late 1970s. This author is often uncomfortable with such a generalization because what a chiropractor attempts to do is far removed from the general "mobilization" and gross "manipulation" procedures commonly conducted by physiotherapists and many osteopaths, which typically are passive attempts to increase a restricted range of movement of a joint by stretching contractures. While the term SMT may be appropriate for a large variety of low-velocity extraspinal adjustive techniques or the application of a stretching maneuver to improve a joint's range of motion, it can be argued that its use is a clear misnomer in most instances when applied to the application of scientific chiropractic during spinal therapy.

More than 20 years ago, Levine had the foresight to warn those who defined the chiropractic adjustment *solely in structural terms* without considering the *neurologic overtones* involved:

> "In discussing chiropractic techniques, it is only proper to note that chiropractic holds no monopoly on manipulation. Manipulation for the purpose of setting and replacing displaced bones and joints, including spinal articulations, is one of the oldest therapeutic methods known. It has been and still is an integral part of the armamentarium of healers of all times and cultures.
>
> "What differentiates chiropractic adjusting from orthopedic manipulations, osteopathic maneuvers, massage, zone therapy, etc? In one sentence, it is *the dynamic thrust!* The use of the dynamic thrust is singularly chiropractic. And it is the identifying feature of chiropractic techniques.
>
> "However, chiropractic's rationale is hardly based on the fact that its adjustive techniques are applied with a sudden impulse of force. It is the reasons why these techniques are applied, and why they are applied in a certain manner, that distinguish chiropractic from other healing disciplines, manipulative or not. In fact, some chiropractic techniques of recent vintage are *not* characterized by sudden application. We are thinking of those techniques which have been named 'non-force,' though strictly speaking, the term is a misnomer. What makes them also part of chiropractic is that they are designed to serve the same purpose as the dynamic thrust, though whether they are equally efficient is a moot question."

Motion Barriers During Structural Therapy

Both articular adjustments and manipulation impose static and dynamic forces across joint surfaces. Within its anatomical range of motion, a normal vertebra exhibits (1) a voluntary active range, (2) an involuntary passive range, and a (3) slight quasi-physiologic motion at the end of the passive range that is determined by ligamentous plasticity and elasticity. The comparative ranges of vertebral movement occurring during exercise, mobilization, and dynamic adjustments are shown in Figure 6.18. To recognize the clinical implications of this, an understanding of the barrier concept is necessary.

When a joint is passively tested for range of motion, the examiner will note increasing resistance to motion referred to as a "bind" or the physiologic motion barrier. When the joint is carried past this point, the added motion becomes painful to the patient. This point is called the anatomical motion barrier (AMB). In evaluating the degrees of passive motion, joints should be moved near but not fully to the AMB. Thus, joint motion evaluation is accomplished by passively carrying the joint(s) through a range of motion until the AMB is encountered, and then recording

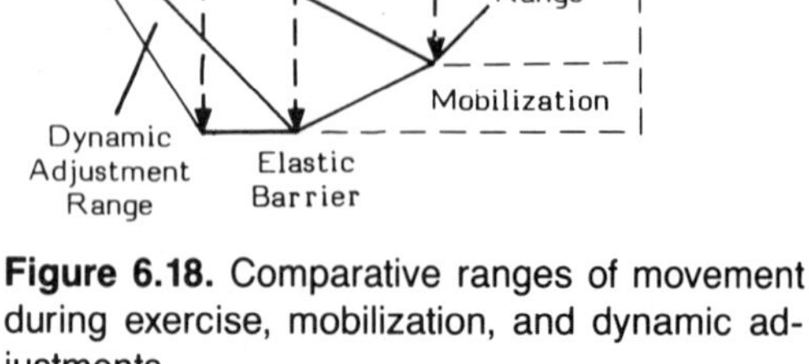

Figure 6.18. Comparative ranges of movement during exercise, mobilization, and dynamic adjustments.

the degrees of movement allowed. Active motion usually exists from the neutral position to the point of tissue resistance, while passive motion extends past this to near the elastic barrier.

Grice points out that the usual objective of mobilization techniques is to restore the normal range of passive joint motion from the neutral position to the normal elastic barrier. Thus, it is longer in range than that of active motion and to the maximum point of passive motion. The objective of mobilization (stretching) techniques is to restore motion from the neutral position to the elastic barrier. Most osteopathic "leverage" techniques are conducted within this range, as are many chiropractic extremity techniques. In contrast, dynamic specific chiropractic spinal adjustments are usually carried a step further into the quasi-physiologic range, often to the anatomical limit, but the duration of the application of force is only a fraction of a second.

Specific Chiropractic Adjustments

It can be generally stated that joints and nerves become painful only when nociceptors are stretched, compressed, or chemically irritated. Analysis consists to a great extent in determining which of these conditions exist to produce the nociceptive input experienced by the patient in pain.

The biomechanical objective in specific chiropractic adjustments is to restore motion throughout the active, passive, and paraphysiologic range of motion (refer to Fig. 6.18). Because of the dynamic forces involved, such techniques should carefully consider the exact geometric plane of articulation (normal or abnormal), asymmetry, the force magnitude to be applied, the direction of force, torque, coupling mechanisms, the state of the holding elements (eg, spastic muscles, articular fixations, stiffness and damping factors), the integrity of the check ligaments (eg, stretched, shortened), and any underlying pathologic processes (eg, infectious, neoplastic, sclerotic, arthrotic, osteoporotic) of the structures directly or indirectly involved. As local temperature, trabeculae arrangement, density, elasticity, plasticity, flexibility, nutrition, etc, are variables that affect the material properties of tissues, these factors also must be considered. The application of any clinical procedure without consideration of the cause-and-effect forces anticipated is not scientific chiropractic.

The Articular Snap

Skilled spinal adjustments often involve the breaking of the synovial seal of the apophyseal joints, which results in an audible "snap." While some feel that this is insignificant, most authorities believe that breaking the joint seal permits an increase in mobility (particularly that not under voluntary control) from 15 to 20 minutes—allowing the segment to normalize its position. Unsuccessful manipulations resulting in increased pain rarely produce an audible joint release, while successful adjustments usually result in an immediate sense of relief even if some pain and spasm remain, a reduction in palpable hypertonicity, and an improvement in joint motion, and are followed by a gradual reduction in symptoms.

Thrust Technics

Thrust technics applied at an articulation can be divided into two general categories: low-velocity and high-velocity adjustments, and each has various subdivisions depending on the joint being treated, its structural-functional state, and the primary and secondary objectives to be obtained. The term *adjustment velocity* refers to the speed at which the adjustment is delivered.

In either low-velocity or high-velocity technics:

- The force applied may be low, medium, or high.
- The duration of the force may be short or sustained.
- The amplitude (distance of articular motion) may be short, medium, or long.
- The direction of the force may be straight or curving and/or perpendicular, parallel, or oblique to the articular plane.

• Overlying soft-tissue tension may be mild, medium, or strong.

• Primary or secondary leverage may be applied early, synchronized, or late.

• Contralateral stabilization may or may not be necessary.

• Thrust onset may be slow, medium, or abrupt.

Fixation (mobility limitations) may be produced by such non-IVF conditions as paravertebral fascial adhesions, ligamentous contractures, IVD dehydration, fibrosed muscle tissue, spondylosis, meningeal sclerosis, or adhesions. A dynamic thrust to these conditions may result in increased mobility by stretching shortened tissues and breaking adhesions, but there is always danger of osseous avulsion or tearing of meninges as scar tissue has a much higher tensile strength than osseous or nerve tissue. In addition, as such states usually involve multiple segments, broadly applied LVTs would be more appropriate.

Low-Velocity Technics (LVTs)

Within the category of low-velocity adjustments fall the many applications that apply slow stretching, pulling, compression, or pushing forces. Sustained or rhythmic manual traction or compression and procedures to obtain proprioceptive neuromuscular facilitation are typical examples. A more specific example would be the application of Spear's double-transverse contact, which is applied to the spine in a deep, low-velocity, alternating, rhythmic fashion to obtain patient relaxation and to stretch paraspinal and intersegmental adhesions and tightened tissues prior to more specific spinal therapy. Many leverage techniques advocated by Cox, Markey-Steffensmeier, and others to reduce IVD protrusions and functional spondylolisthesis can be placed in this category.

High-Velocity Technics (HVTs)

Within the category of high-velocity adjustments fall the many applications of classic *dynamic-thrust* (direct, rotary, or leverage) chiropractic adjustment technics that are applied to a vertebra's transverse or spinous process or a lamina, with various degrees of counterleverage and/or contralateral stabilization. Contact pressure is usually firm, if the underlying tissues are not acutely painful, when the contact is to be maintained at a specific point and the thrust delivered in a precise direction.

The objective of almost all HVTs is to reposition a subluxated joint and/or release a fixated articulation (increase joint mobility). *How* this is achieved has not been specifically determined because more is involved than the application of a mechanical force against a resistance. The most common theories are briefly described below:

• *The mobilization of subluxated articular surfaces.* The apophyseal joints can become fixated because of the effects of joint locking (eg, traumatic), muscle spasm, degeneration, an entrapped meniscoid or other loose body, capsular fibrosis, intra-articular "gluing" or adhesions (eg, postsynovitis, chronic rheumatoid conditions), bony ankylosis, facet tropism, etc.

• *The relaxation of the paravertebral musculature.* While a high-velocity force that suddenly stretches muscles spindles in primary muscle spasm *increases* the spasm, the same force applied to a segment at which its related muscles are in secondary or protective spasm tends to produce relaxation if the thrust succeeds in removing the focal stimulus for the reflex.

• *The shock-like effect on the CNS.* Shock-like forces (1) are known to frequently have a normalizing effect on self-sustaining CNS reflexes; (2) are stimulative to the neurons involved, resulting in increased short-term neural and related endocrine activity; and (3) set up postural and muscle-tone-normalizing cerebellar influences.

Indirect (Functional) Approaches

Manual mobilization and thrust techniques are direct approaches to relieving articular fixations. Indirect functional approaches are often utilized when the cause for fixation has been determined to be primarily muscular in origin or when any form of manipulation would be contraindicated. Within this category fall many manual light-touch cutaneous reflex techniques, trigger-point therapy, galvanism, transverse massage, therapeutic vibration, isometric and isotonic contraction, etc. It is theorized that these procedures produce their effects because of their influence on the gamma-loop system and/or by the superiority of mechanoreceptor input upon nociceptive input.

Bibliography

American Chiropractic Association: *Chiropractic State of the Art.* Arlington, VA, American Chiropractic Association, 1984, pp 4, 8.

Anderson RT, Winkler M: The gravity stress analyzer for measuring spinal posture. *Journal of the Canadian Chiropractic Association,* 27(2):55-58, 1983.

Arkuszewski Z: The efficacy of manual treatment in low back pain: A clinical trial. *Manual Medicine,* 2:68-71, 1986.

Balduc HA: Overview of contemporary chiropractic science for the Chiropractic Association of Oklahoma. Northwestern College of Chiropractic, Convention notes, April 24, 1983.

Baltzell LG, Mackey RH (eds): Firth's Technic Notes. Publishing data not shown, 1967, pp 2-6, 12-23. Distributed by National College of Chiropractic.

Banks SD: Lumbar facet syndrome: Spinographic assessment of treatment by spinal manipulation. *Journal of Manipulative and Physiological Therapeutics,* 6:175-180, 1983.

Benner B, Ehni G: Degenerative lumbar scoliosis. *Spine,* 4:548-552, 1979.

Berger PA, et al: Behavioral acology of the endorphins. *Annual Review of Medicine,* 33:397-415, 1982.

Bergmann T: Integrated chiropractic methods. Compilation of notes presented to the convention of the Oklahoma Chiropractic Association; April 23, 1983; in cooperation with Northwestern College of Chiropractic.

Berthold CH: Morphology of normal peripheral axons. In Waxman SG (ed): *Physiology and Pathobiology of Axons.* New York, Raven Press, 1978.

Bishop B: Pain: Its physiology and rationale for management. Part I, neuroanatomical substrate of pain. *Physical Therapy,* 60:13-23, 1980; Part II, analgesia systems of the CNS, 60:21-23, 1980.

Black RG: The chronic pain syndrome. *Surgical Clinics of North America,* 55:999-1011, 1975.

Bonica JJ: Neurophysiologic and pathologic aspects of acute and chronic pain. *Archives of Surgery,* 112: 750-761, 1977.

Boyd WA: *A Textbook of Pathology.* Philadelphia, Lea & Febiger, 1961.

Bradley KC: The posterior ramsegmental nerves. In Glasgow EF, Twomey LT, Scull ER, Kleynhans AM, Idczak RM: *Aspects of Manipulative Therapy,* ed 2. New York, Churchill Livingstone, 1985, pp 59-63.

Brena SF, Chapman SL: Chronic pain: Physiology, diagnosis, management. In Leek JC, Gershwin ME, Fowler WM Jr: *Principles of Physical Medicine and Rehabilitation in the Musculoskeletal Diseases.* Orlando, FL, Grune & Stratton, 1986, pp 189-216.

Brodin H: Cervical pain and mobilization. *Manual Medicine,* 2:18-22, 1985.

Browde AL: The effect of prolonged pressure on peripheral abdominal nerves. *American Review of Soviet Medicine,* 2:213-217, 1944.

Buerger AA: Experimental neuromuscular models of spinal manual techniques. *Manual Medicine,* 1:10-17, 1983.

Burnarski DJ: Chiropractic biomechanical evaluations: Validity in myofascial low back pain. *Journal of Manipulative and Physiological Therapeutics,* 5: 155-161, 1982.

Burns L, Chandler LC, Rice RW: *Pathogenesis of Visceral Disease Following Vertebral Lesions.* Chicago, American Osteopathic Association, 1948, pp 3-20.

Burt HA: Effects of faulty posture. *Proceedings of the Royal Society of Medicine,* 43:187, 1950.

Cailliet R: Disuse syndrome: fibrositic and degenerative changes. In Brena SF, Chapman SL (eds): *Management of Patients with Chronic Pain.* New York, Spectrum Publications, 1983, pp 63-71.

Canadian Memorial Chiropractic College: *Segmental Neuropathy.* Toronto, Canadian Memorial Chiropractic College, date of publication not shown. Monograph, pp 6-7, 29-32.

Carrick FR: Cervical radiculopathy: The diagnosis and treatment of pathomechanics in the cervical spine. *Journal of Manipulative and Physiological Therapeutics,* 6:129-137, 1983.

Carrick FR: Treatment of pathomechanics of the lumbar spine by manipulation. *Journal of Manipulative and Physiological Therapeutics,* 4:173-178, 1981.

Cassidy JD, Kirkaldy-Willis WH, McGregor M: Spinal manipulation for the treatment of chronic low back and leg pain: an observational study. In Buerger AA, Greenman PE (eds): *Empirical Approaches to the Validation of Spinal Manipulation.* Springfield, MO, Charles C. Thomas, 1985.

Cervero F: Deep and visceral pain. In Kosterlitz HW, Terenius LY (eds): *Pain and Society.* Weinheim, Verlag Chemic, 1980, pp 263-282.

Coggins WN: *Basic Technique: A System of Body Mechanics.* Creve Coeur, MO, published by author, 1983.

Coote JH, et al: Reflex discharges into thoracic white rami elicited by somatic and visceral afferent excitation. *Journal of Physiology,* 202:141-159, 1969.

Council on Chiropractic Education: Position/policy paper, adopted January 21, 1978.

Cox JM: *Low Back Pain: Mechanism, Diagnosis and Treatment.* Baltimore, Williams and Wilkins, 1985.

Crue BB, et al: Neurophysiology of pain—peripheral aspects. *Bulletin of the Los Angeles Neurological Society,* 41(1):13-42, 1976.

Curtis DR, Eccles JC: Synaptic action during and after repetitive stimulation. *Journal of Physiology* (British), 150:374, 1960.

Cyriax E: Some common postural deformities and their treatment by exercise and manipulation. *British Journal of Physical Medicine,* June 1938.

Cyriax J, Schiotz EH: *Manipulation: Past and Present.* London, Wm. Heineman, 1975.
Cyriax J: *Textbook of Orthopaedic Medicine: Vol One, Diagnosis of Soft Tissue Lesions,* ed 8. London, Bailliere Tindall, 1982, pp 22-42, 65-66.
DeBoer KF, Harmon R, Tuttle CD, Wallace H: Reliability study of detection of somatic dysfunctions in the cervical spine. *Journal of Manipulative and Physiological Therapeutics,* 8:9-15; 1985.
Dee R: Articular neurology. In Sokoloff L (ed): *The Joints and Synovial Fluid.* New York, Academic Press, 1978, p 177.
Denslow JS: An analysis of the variability of spinal reflex thresholds. *Journal of Neurophysiology,* 7:207-215, 1944.
Denslow JS, Hassett CC: The central excitatory state associated with postural abnormalities. *Journal of Neurophysiology,* 5:393-402, 1942.
de Reuck AVS, Knight J (eds): *Myotactic, Kinesthetic, and Vestibular Mechanisms.* Ciba Foundation Symposium. Boston, Little, Brown, 1967.
De Rusha JL: Upper cervical technic correlated with neurodiagnosis. *ACA Journal of Chiropractic,* September 1961.
Dowling JJ: *Musculoskeletal Disease: Staged for Rapid Comprehension.* Chicago, Year Book Medical, pp 78-79.
Downing C: *Osteopathic Principles in Disease.* San Francisco, R.J. Orozco, 1923.
Elton D, Burrows GD, Stanley GV: Clinical measurement of pain. *Medical Journal of Australia,* 1:109-111, 1979.
Epstein JA, Epstein BS, Jones MD. Symptomatic lumbar scoliosis with degenerative changes in the elderly. *Spine,* 4:542-547, 1979.
Farfan HF, et al: The effects of torsion on the lumbar intervertebral joints: The role of torsion in the production of disc degeneration. *Journal of Bone and Joint Surgery,* 52A:468, 1970.
Farfan HF: *Mechanical Disorders of the Low Back.* Philadelphia, Lea & Febiger, 1973.
Farfan HF: The scientific basis of manipulative procedures. In Graham R (ed): *Rheumatic Diseases: Low Back Clinics.* London, W.B. Saunders, April 1980.
Farfan HF: Symptomatology in terms of the pathomechanics of low-back pain and sciatica. In Haldeman S (ed): *Modern Developments in the Principles and Practice of Chiropractic.* New York, Appleton-Century-Crofts, 1980.
Farfan HF, Sullivan JD: The relation of facet orientation to intervertebral disc failure. *Canadian Journal of Surgery,* 10:179, 1967.
Foundation for Chiropractic Education and Research: Spinal manipulation—current findings on its therapeutic effects and role in treatment. *Spinal Manipulation,* 2(3):1-3, October 1986. Anonymous.
Freedman BG: The biodynamical aspect of cerebrospinal fluid in disease and health. *Journal of Manipulative and Physiological Therapeutics,* 2:79-84, 1979.
Frogley R: Neurological observations of a subluxation. *The Journal of Clinical Chiropractic,* 1(3), 1973.
Gainsbury JM: High-velocity thrust and pathophysiology of segmental dysfunction. In Glasgow EF, Twomey LT, Scull ER, Kleynhans AM, Idczak RM: *Aspects of Manipulative Therapy,* ed 2. New York, Churchill Livingstone, 1985, pp 87-92.
Giles LG: Spinal fixation and viscera. *Journal of Clinical Chiropractic,* 1(3):144-145, 1973.
Gillet H: The anatomy and physiology of spinal fixation. *Journal of the National Chiropractic Association,* December 1963.
Gillet H: A definition of the subluxation. *The Texas Chiropractor,* February 1974.
Gillet H, Liekens M: *Belgian Chiropractic Research Notes.* Huntington Beach, CA, Motion Palpation Institute, 1981.
Gillet H, Liekens M: A further study of spinal fixations. *Annals of the Swiss Chiropractic Association,* Geneva, IV:41, 1967.
Goldthwait JE, et al: *The Essentials of Body Mechanics in Health and Disease,* ed 5. Philadelphia, J.B. Lippincott, 1952.
Good AB: Spinal joint blocking. *Journal of Manipulative and Physiological Therapeutics,* 6(1):1-7, March 1985.
Goodman CE: Pathophysiology of pain. *Archives of Internal Medicine,* 143:527, 1983.
Greenman PE: Manipulative therapy in relation to total health care. In Korr IM (ed): *The Neurobiologic Mechanisms in Manipulative Therapy.* New York, Plenum Press, 1978.
Grice AS: A biomechanical approach to cervical and dorsal adjusting. In Haldeman S (ed): *Modern Developments in the Principles and Practice of Chiropractic.* New York, Appleton-Century-Crofts, 1980, pp 338-339.
Grice AS, Fligg, DB: Class notes. Department of Biomechanics/Kinesiology, BK101 (Joint Movement and Muscle Testing). Toronto, Canadian Memorial Chiropractic College, date not shown.
Grice AS, Fligg, DB: Class notes. Department of Biomechanics/Kinesiology, BK202 (Spinal Dynamics). Toronto, Canadian Memorial Chiropractic College, date not shown.
Grice AS: Muscle tonus changes following manipulation. *Journal of the Canadian Chiropractic Association,* 19:29-31, 1974.
Grice AS: Radiographic, biomechanical and clinical factors in lumbar lateral flexion: Part I. *Journal of Manipulative and Physiological Therapeutics,* 2: 26-34, 1979.
Grieve GP: *Common Vertebral Joint Problems.* London, Churchill Livingstone, 1981, pp 69-73, 161-196.
Grundfest H: Discussion of excitation and conduction in traumatized nerves. In Korr IM (ed): *The Neurobiologic Mechanisms in Manipulative Therapy.* New York, Plenum Press, 1978.
Gucker T: Changes in vital capacity in scoliosis: Preliminary report on the effects of treatment. *Journal of Bone and Joint Surgery,* 44:469, 1962.
Guillemin R, et al: The endorphins, novel peptides of brain and hypophyseal origin, with opiate like activity: biochemical and biologic studies. *Annals of the New York Academy of Science,* 197:131-157, 1979.
Hadden GR: The development of a static posture analysis instrument with direct application as an objective pre x-ray screening procedure. *Journal of*

the Canadian Chiropractic Association, 27(4): 139-149, 1983.

Haldeman S: Referred pain: Extra spinal symptoms of spinal origin. *The Texas Chiropractor*, July 1974.

Hartman L: Classification and application of osteopathic manipulative techniques. In Glasgow EF, Twomey LT, Scull ER, Kleynhans AM, Idczak RM: *Aspects of Manipulative Therapy*, ed 2. New York, Churchill Livingstone, 1985, pp 82-86.

Henderson DJ, Dorman TM: Functional roentgenometric evaluation of the cervical spine in the sagittal plane. *Journal of Manipulative and Physiological Therapeutics*, 8:219-226, 1985.

Henderson DJ: Significance of vertebral dyskinesia in relation to the cervical syndrome. *Journal of Manipulative and Physiological Therapeutics*, 2(1): 3-13, March 1979.

Hickey RF, Tregonning GD: Denervation of spinal facet joints for treatment of chronic low back pain. *New Zealand Journal of Medicine*, 86:96-99, 1977.

Hildebrandt RW, Howe JW: Spinal biomechanics and subluxation classification. Lombard, IL, National College of Chiropractic, 1974.

Hoag JM, Cole MV, Bradford SG (eds): *Osteopathic Medicine*. New York, McGraw-Hill, 1969.

Homewood AE: A posturometer survey. *Journal of the Canadian Chiropractic Association*, 9(1):9-10, 1965.

Homewood AE: *The Neurodynamics of the Vertebral Subluxation*, ed 3. Place of publication not shown, published by author, 1981, pp 47-66, 69-87, 103-111 162-167, 265-266.

Illi FW: *The Vertebral Column: Life-Line of the Body*. Chicago, National College of Chiropractic, 1951.

Inman VT, Saunders JB: Referred pain from skeletal structures. *Journal of Nervous and Mental Disease*, 99:660-667, 1944.

Janse J: A concept: The neurological element as it relates to clinical chiropractic. *The Chirogram*, December 1975.

Janse J: The integrative purpose and function of the nervous system: A review of classical literature. *Journal of Manipulative and Physiological Therapeutics*, 1(3), September 1978.

Janse J: *Principles and Practice of Chiropractic*. Lombard, IL, National College of Chiropractic, 1976, pp 43-44, 48-50, 161, 205-221, 243-250.

Jaskoviak PA, Schafer RC: Chapter 2: Pain suppression in the twentieth century. In Jaskoviak PA, Schafer RC: *Applied Physiotherapy: Practical Applications Within Clinical Chiropractic*. Arlington, VA, American Chiropractic Association, 1986.

Johnson AC: *Postural Correction*. Los Angeles, Chiropractic Educational Extension Bureau, date not listed.

Johnson J: Manipulative body mechanics therapy. *Journal of the American Osteopathic Association*, vol 60, June 1961.

Judovitch B, Bates W: *Segmental Neuralgia in Painful Syndromes*. Philadelphia, F.A. Davis, 1946.

Kellgren JH: Observations on referred pain arising from muscle. *Clinical Science*, 3:175, 1938.

Kellgren JH, Samuel EP: The sensitivity and innervation of the articular capsule. *Journal of Bone & Joint Surgery*, 32(B):84-92, 1950.

Kendall HO, et al: *Posture and Pain*. Baltimore, Williams & Wilkins, 1952.

Kessler RM, Hertling D (eds): *Management of Common Musculoskeletal Disorders*. Philadelphia, Harper & Row, 1983, pp 27-30, 91-98.

Kfoury PW (ed): *Catalog of Chiropractic Techniques*. Chesterfield, MO, Logan College of Chiropractic, 1977.

Kirkaldy-Willis WH: Manipulation. In Kirkaldy-Willis WH (ed): *Managing Low Back Pain*. New York, Churchill Livingstone, 1983, pp 175-177.

Kirkaldy-Willis WH: The three phases of the spectrum of degenerative disease. In Kirkaldy-Willis WH (ed): *Managing Low Back Pain*. New York, Churchill Livingstone, 1983, pp 24-25, 73-89.

Klausen K: The shape of the spine in young males with and without back complaints. *Clinical Biomechanics*, 1:81-84, 1986.

Korr IM (ed): *The Neurobiologic Mechanisms in Manipulative Therapy*. New York, Plenum Press, 1978, pp 45-47, 137-177.

Korr IM: Proprioceptors and the behavior of lesioned segments. In Stark EH (ed): *Osteopathic Medicine*, Acton, MA, Publication Services Group, 1975, pp 183-199.

Korr IM: The spinal cord as organizer of disease processes: Some preliminary perspectives. *Journal of the American Osteopathic Association*, September 1976.

Kostuik JP, Bentivoglio J: The incidence of low-back pain in adult scoliosis. *Spine*, 6:268-273, 1981.

Kunert W: Functional disorders of internal organs due to vertebral lesions. *Ciba Symposium*, 13(3), 1965.

Lamb DW: The neurology of spinal pain. *Physical Therapy*, 59:971-973, 1979.

Leach RA: *The Chiropractic Theories*, ed 2. Baltimore, Williams & Wilkins, 1986, pp 15-22,28-29, 38-45, 86-105.

Leavitt F, Garron DC, Whisler WW, Sheinkop MB: Affective and sensory dimensions of back pain. *Pain*, 4:273-281, 1978.

Levine M: *The Structural Approach to Chiropractic*. New York, Comet Press, 1964, p 85.

Lewis T: Suggestions relating to the study of somatic pain. *British Medical Journal*, 1:321-327, 1938.

Lewit K: The contribution of clinical observation to neurobiological mechanisms in manipulative therapy. In Korr IM (ed): *The Neurobiologic Mechanisms in Manipulative Therapy*. New York, Plenum, 1978, pp 43-52.

Loomis RC, Steinbach LJ: *Examination of the Spinal Column for Defects of Balance and Subluxation*. Pittsburgh, Universal Chiropractic College, 1930.

Lynch MK, Kessler RM: Pain. In Kessler RM, Hertling D (eds): *Management of Common Musculoskeletal Disorders*. Philadelphia, Harper & Row, 1983, pp 51-72.

Macnab I: *Backache*. Baltimore, Williams & Wilkins, 1977.

Mannen EM: The use of cervical radiographic overlays to assess response to manipulation: A case report. *Journal of the Canadian Chiropractic Association*, 24:108-110, 1980.

Markey LP, Steffensmeier LA: The Markey-Steffensmeier spondylolisthesis maneuver. *The Markey-*

Lloyd Newsletter, 2(2), February 1987.

Mayer ET, Herrmann G, Pfaffenrath V, Pollmann W, Auberger T: Functional radiographs of the cervicocranial region and the cervical spine: A new computer-aided technique. *Cephalgia*, 5:237-243, 1985.

McAlpine JE: A discussion of the dentate ligament neural traction mechanism. *International Review of Chiropractic*, pp 35-39, October-December 1980.

McDowall DA: The subluxation specific, the adjustment specific: an early theory of muscle imbalance. *ACA Journal of Chiropractic*, 13(1):37-39, 1983.

McKenzie RA: *The Lumbar Spine*. Upper Hutt, New Zealand, Spinal Publications Ltd, 1981, pp 9-14.

Mellin G: Physical therapy for chronic low back pain: Correlations between spinal mobility and treatment outcome. *Scandinavian Journal of Rehabilitative Medicine*, 17:163-166, 1985.

Melzack R, et al: Neurophysiological foundations of pain. In Sternbach RA (ed): *The Psychology of Pain*. New York, Raven Press, 1978, pp 1-26.

Nachemson A: Adult scoliosis and back pain. *Spine*, 4:513-517, 1979.

Nall SK: The role of specific manipulation towards alleviating abnormalities in body mechanics and restoration. *Journal of Manipulative and Physiological Therapeutics*, 5(1):11-15, 1982.

Neff SD: The neuroanatomy of vertebral subluxations. *ACA Journal of Chiropractic*, 17(4):S55-57, 1980.

Ochs S: Axoplasmic flow in neurons. In Gaito J (ed): *Macromolecules and Behavior*. New York, Appleton-Century-Crofts, 1966.

Ochs S: Axoplasmic transport. In Tower DB (ed): *The Basic Neurosciences*. New York, Raven Press, vol 1, 1975, pp 137-146.

Ochs S: A brief review of material transport in nerve fibers. In Goldstein M (ed): *The Research Status of Spinal Manipulative Therapy*, NINCDS Monograph No. 15, DHEW Publication No. (NIH) 76-998, Stock No. 017-049-00060-7, Washington, DC, U.S. Government Printing Office, 1975, pp 189-194.

Okubo J: The review of posturography in Japan. *Agressologie*, 21D:3-24, 1980.

Palmer DD: *The Science, Art, and Philosophy of Chiropractic*. Portland, OR, Portland Printing House, 1910.

Parke WW: Applied anatomy of the spine. In Rothman RH, Simeone FA (eds): *The Spine*. Philadelphia, W.B. Saunders, 1975, vol I, pp 33-35.

Perl ER: Mode of action of nociceptors. In Hirsch C, et al (eds): *Cervical Pain*. Oxford, England, Pergamon, 1972, pp 157-163.

Phillips RB: The irritable reflex mechanism. *ACA Journal of Chiropractic*, January 1974.

Pointon R: A possible cause of acute osteopathic lesions. *British Osteopathic Journal*, 8:10-19, 1976.

Poole PB: Considerations of neurogenic pain. *Ortho-Briefs*, Council on Chiropractic Orthopedics of the American Chiropractic Association, Fall 1982.

Raphael R: personal correspondence. Portland, Oregon, 1987.

Rebechini-Zasadny H, Tasharski CC, Heinze WJ: Electromyographic analysis following chiropractic manipulation of the cervical spine: A model to study manipulation-induced peripheral muscle changes. *Journal of Manipulative and Physiological Therapeutics*, 4:61-63, 1984.

Reiter L: Apophyseal joint functional anatomy and experimental findings: A literature review. *PCC Research Form*, 1(2):49-52, Winter 1985.

Roaf R: The basic anatomy of scoliosis. *Journal of Bone and Joint Surgery*, 480: 786, 1966.

Sahlstrand T, Ortengren R, Nachemson A: Postural equilibrium in adolescent idiopathic scoliosis. *Acta Orthopaedica Scandinavica*, 49:354-365, 1978.

Sandoz R: New trends in the pathogenesis of spinal disorders. *Annals of the Swiss Chiropractic Association*, V:93, 1971.

Sandoz R: Some physical mechanisms and effects of spinal adjustments. *Annals of the Swiss Chiropractors Association*, 6:91, 1976.

Sandoz R: Some reflex phenomena associated with spinal derangements and adjustments. *Annals of the Swiss Chiropractic Association*, VII:45, 1981.

Schafer RC: *Symptomatology and Differential Diagnosis*. Arlington, VA, American Chiropractic Association, 1986, pp 226, 290-293, 326-335, 337, 339-340, 841.

Schafer RC: *Clinical Biomechanics: Musculoskeletal Actions and Reactions*. Baltimore, Williams & Wilkins, 1983, pp 121-127, 174-175, 185-187, 194, 199-202, 208-209, 212-215.

Schafer RC (ed): *Basic Chiropractic Procedural Manual*, ed 4. Arlington, VA, American Chiropractic Association, 1984, pp 1-2, 4-9, 15-16.

Schaumberg HH, Spencer PS: Pathology of spinal root compression. In Goldstein M (ed): *The Research Status of Spinal Manipulative Therapy*. NINCDS Monograph No. 15, DHEW Publication No. (NIH) 76-998, Stock No. 017-049-00060-7. Washington, DC, U.S. Government Printing Office, 1975.

Sharpless SK: Susceptibility of spinal roots to compression block. In Goldstein M (ed): *The Research Status of Spinal Manipulative Therapy*. NINCDS Monograph No. 15, DHEW Publication No. (NIH) 76-998, Stock No. 017-049-00060-7. Washington, DC, U.S. Government Printing Office, 1975.

Simmons EH, Jackson RP: The management of nerve root entrapment syndromes associated with the collapsing scoliosis of idiopathic lumbar and thoracolumbar curves. *Spine*, 4:533-541, 1979.

Sinclair DC, Weddell G, Feindel WH: Referred pain and associated phenomena. *Brain*, 7:184-211, 1948.

Spector B, Eilbert L, Finando S, Fukuda F: Video integrated measurement system. *Journal of Manipulative and Physiological Therapeutics*, 5(2):55-61, 1982.

Speransky AD: *A Basis for the Theory of Medicine;* translated by C.P. Dutt. New York, International Publishers, 1943.

Stephenson RW: *Chiropractic Textbook*. Davenport, IA, published by author, 1927.

Strang VV: *Essential Principles of Chiropractic*. Davenport, IA, Palmer College of Chiropractic, 1984.

Sunderland S: Anatomical perivertebral influences on the intervertebral foramen. In Goldstein M (ed): *The Research Status of Spinal Manipulative Therapy*. NINCDS Monograph No. 15, DHEW Publication No. (NIH) 76-998, Stock No. 017-049-00060 -7. Washington, DC, U.S. Government Printing Office, 1975.

Sunderland S: Traumatized nerves, roots and ganglia:

Musculoskeletal factors and neuropathological consequences. In Korr IM (ed): *The Neurobiologic Mechanisms in Manipulative Therapy.* New York, Plenum Press, 1978.

Swezey RL: The modern thrust of manipulation and traction therapy. *Seminars in Arthritis and Rheumatism*, 12(3):326, 1983.

Tehan PJ: Functional technique: A different perspective in manipulative therapy. In Glasgow EF, Twomey LT, Scull ER, Kleynhans AM, Idczak RM: *Aspects of Manipulative Therapy*, ed 2. New York, Churchill Livingstone, 1985, pp 94-96.

Terrett ACJ, Vernon H: Manipulation and pain tolerance: A controlled study of the effect of spinal manipulation on paraspinal cutaneous pain tolerance levels. *American Journal of Physical Medicine*, 63(5):217-224.

Thabe H: Electromyography as a tool to document diagnostic findings and therapeutic results associated with somatic dysfunctions in the upper cervical spinal joints and sacroiliac joints. *Manual Medicine*, 2:53-58, 1986.

Travell JG, Rinzler SH: The myofascial genesis of pain. *Postgraduate Medicine*, 11:425-434, 1952.

Verner JR: *The Science and Logic of Chiropractic.* Englewood, NJ, published by author, 1941.

Vernon H: An assessment of the intra- and inter-reliability of the posturometer. *Journal of Manipulative and Physiological Therapeutics*, 6(2):57-60, 1983.

Vernon HT, Dhami MSI, Howley TP, Annett R: Spinal manipulation and beta-endorphin: A controlled study of the effect of a spinal manipulation on plasma beta-endorphin levels in normal males. *Journal of Manipulative and Physiological Therapeutics*, 9:115-122, 1986.

Vernon HT, Grice AS: The four-quadrant weight scale: A technical and procedural review. *Journal of Manipulative and Physiological Therapeutics*, 7(3): 165-169, 1984.

Vernon HT: Static and dynamic roentgenography in the diagnosis of degenerative disc disease: A review and comparative assessment. *Journal of Manipulative and Physiological Therapeutics*, 5:163-169, 1982.

Vladef T, Hardy M: The theory of fixation points, *National Chiropractic Journal*, June 1945.

Watkins RJ: Subluxation terminology since 1964. *ACA Journal of Chiropractic*, 2(9):S65-70, 1968.

White AA, Hirsch C: The significance of the vertebral posterior elements in the mechanics of the thoracic spine. *Clinical Orthopaedics*, 81:2-41, 1971.

Wiles P: Postural deformities of the antero-posterior curves of the spine. *The Lancet*, April 17, 1937.

Wiles MR: Reproducibility and interexaminer correlation of motion palpation findings of the sacroiliac joints. *Journal of the Canadian Chiropractic Association*, 24:59-68, 1980.

Will TE: The biochemical basis of manipulative therapeutics: hypothetical considerations. *Journal of Manipulative and Physiological Therapeutics*, 1(3): 153-156, September 1978.

Will TE: Hypothetical considerations with regard to the biochemical basis of manipulative therapy. *ACA Journal of Chiropractic*, 13:119-123, December 1979.

Wood KW: Myospasm, myosprain and myalgia. *The Digest of Chiropractic Economics*, pp 126-127, May/June 1985.

Wyke BD: Articular neurology and manipulative therapy. In *Aspects of Manipulative Therapy.* Proceedings of Multidisciplinary International Conference on Manipulative Therapy. Melbourne, Lincoln Institute of Health Sciences, Carlton, Victoria, Australia, August 1979, pp 67-72.

Wyke B: Neurological mechanisms in the experience of pain. *Acupuncture and Electro-Therapeutical Research International Journal*, 4:27-35, 1979.

Yamada K: The dynamics of experimental posture. *Clinical Orthopaedics*, 25:20-31, 1962.

Yamada K, et al: A neurological approach to the etiology and treatment of scoliosis. *Journal of Bone and Joint Surgery*, 53A:197, 1971.

Chapter 7

Specific Potentialities of the Subluxation Complex

This chapter describes the primary neurologic implications of subluxation syndromes, either as a primary factor or secondary to trauma or pathology, within the cervical spine, thoracic spine, lumbar spine, and pelvic articulations.

GENERAL CONSIDERATIONS

Studies reported by Drum, Hargrave-Wilson, Kunert, Burke, Gayral/Neuwirth, and many others have shown that a subluxation complex, often leading to spondylosis, can effect a wide variety of disturbances that may appear to be disrelated on the surface. Most of the remote effects can be grouped under the general classifications of nerve root neuropathy, basilar venous congestion, cervical autonomic disturbances, CSF pressure and flow disturbances, axoplasmic flow blocks, irritation of the recurrent meningeal nerve, the Barré-Lieou syndrome, and/or the vertebral artery syndrome.

This chapter describes many individual causes for and effects of a spinal subluxation complex. In clinical practice, however, causes and effects are rarely found as isolated entities. Several factors will usually be involved and superimposed on each other.

Innervation of the Spinal Dura

It has long been known that the spinal dura mater has an intrinsic nerve supply. Spinal meningeal rami are derived from gray communicating rami and spinal nerves. The spinal nerves contribute sensory fibers to the meningeal rami. Several meningeal rami enter each IVF, and most are located anteriorly to the sensory ganglia within the IVF.

Bridge found that these intrinsic nerve fibers reach the anterior surface of the dura by three main courses. Here the nerves divide into ascending and usually longer descending filaments that run longitudinally and parallel on the dural surface, and a considerable amount of nerve overlaps from adjacent segments. Finer filaments penetrate the dural substance where they subdivide.

Kimmel reported that most of these fibers penetrate the dura near the midline, while others enter laterally near the exiting spinal nerve roots. At each segment level, two or three nerves enter the spinal dura mater and contain only small nerve fibers. In contrast, Edgar/Nundy could determine no definitive nerve endings, but the nerves could be traced to the posterior aspect of the spinal dura. These observations help to clarify the wide distribution of back pain that is often found following protrusion of a single IVD.

Cervical Dura Attachments

Sunderland states that the nerve sheaths in the cervical region are not firmly attached to their respective foramina (Fig. 7.1). Only the C4—C6 cervical nerves have a strong attachment to the vertebral column, and this is to the gutter of the vertebral transverse process. He believes that these observations have relevance to any local lesion that may fix, deform, or otherwise affect the nerve and its roots to the point of interfering with their function, and they also may be important to traction injuries of nerve roots.

Painful Irritations

The sympathetic nervous system, in conjunction with a sensory root compression or independently, plays a role in the interpretation of pain. Compression of the recurrent meningeal branch of the spinal nerves, for example, results in a wider distribution of pain and muscle spasm than the local pathology may indicate.

Many authorities attribute most lumbosciatic pains to IVD faults (Fig. 7.2). The typical disc lesion is thought to produce restrictions in the dura mater during straight-leg-raising or neck flexion tests.

Cyriax believes that lumbago does not arise from tissue that has undergone degeneration (eg, myofibrosis) because the incidence of backache falls by two-thirds between the ages of 60 and 70 and has almost ceased by the age of 80. He attributes the pain to the impingement of discoid material on the dura mater or its root sleeve. He feels that the syndrome is initiated by an attack of internal derangement at a low lumbar IVD as the result of a momentary posterior displacement of a movable piece of intra-articular fibrocartilage. The prolonged subsequent pain is believed to be caused entirely by bruising of the dura mater.

In describing the relationship of structural pathology to the nerve root, Kirkaldy-Willis takes a broader view. He states that the nerves of the lumbar spine may be entrapped (1) at the back of the IVD, (2) laterally in the central canal, (3) in the cauda equina, (4) more laterally in the nerve canal,

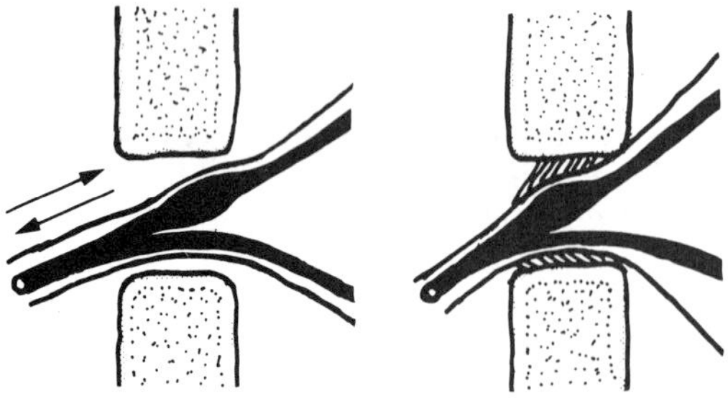

Figure 7.1. *Left,* a normal nerve root within the IVF is quite free to shift in and out of the foramen. *Right,* intraforaminal dural adhesions place considerable traction on the root complex during normal movements that stretch the sensitive tissues of the complex.

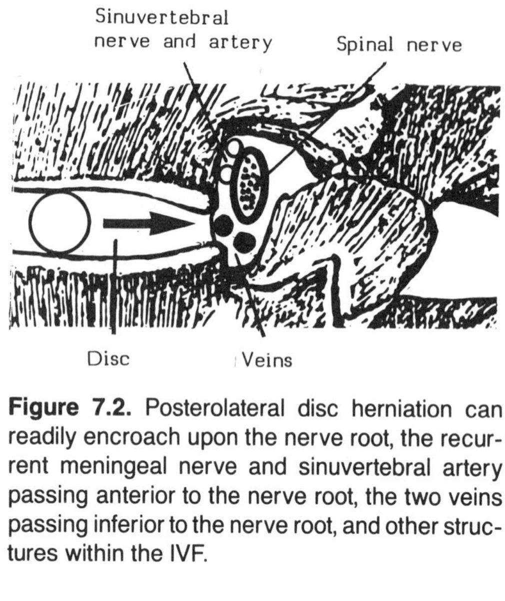

Figure 7.2. Posterolateral disc herniation can readily encroach upon the nerve root, the recurrent meningeal nerve and sinuvertebral artery passing anterior to the nerve root, the two veins passing inferior to the nerve root, and other structures within the IVF.

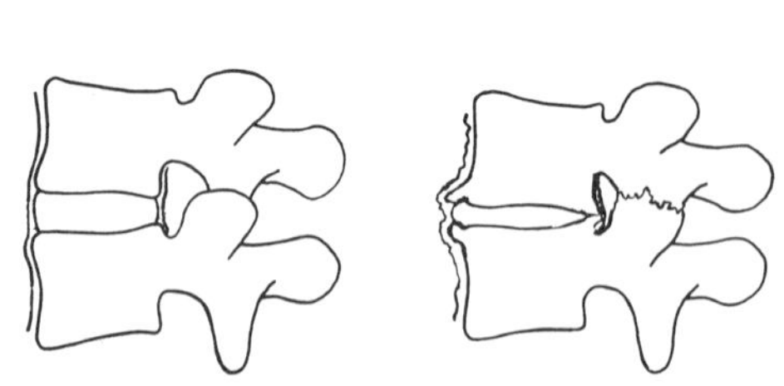

Figure 7.3. *Left,* normal relationships. *Right,* the main products of degenerative spondylosis, including disc degeneration, slackening of the anterior and posterior longitudinal ligaments, osteophyte formation, facet degeneration, apophyseal stenosis, all of which contribute to IVF narrowing.

and (5) posteriorly in the zygapophyseal joints (Fig. 7.3). Changes at these sites can produce dysfunction, disc herniation, instability, lateral entrapment, central stenosis. However, he does state that the pain from a disc lesion or stenosis may come from irritation and inflammation of the dura. The motor loss in these lesions may be attributable a reflex inhibition and vascular insufficiency rather than from nerve compression.

Nerve Root Compression/Irritation

It has long been held within chiropractic that many effects of a subluxation syndrome can be attributed to nerve root compression. Sharpless, Luttges, Sunderland, Pleasure, Schaumber/Spencer, and several others in recent years have contributed greatly to our understanding of the phenomena involved.

Foraminal Encroachment

During their exit from the IVFs, the nerve roots course close to the inner edge of the superior facet. In subluxation, the superior process can override the surface of the inferior process and produce direct irritation of the root by the inferior process, with or without compression (Fig. 7.4). Direct compression also can result by the root being caught between the inferior process and the body of the superior vertebra or caught between a hypertrophied inferior process and the superior body. Olsson and coworkers, however, reported that mechanical pressure on a root is more often from the formation of edema within the nerve sheaths and epineurium, regardless of cause.

Many years ago, Oppenheimer, Hadley, and others noted that a large number of patients suffering from pain and discomfort suggestive of rheumatism or arthritis were the result of nerve root compression arising from narrowing of the IVF. They explained that the primary causes were discogenic disease, inflammatory swelling, and penetration by an articular process.

Sunderland points out that IVF narrowing results from normal extension or any number of pathologic changes in and about the foramen that would reduce its dimensions or lead to nerve compression. Thus, the same effect would be achieved in a subluxation fixed in extension or in some other manner causing IVF narrowing.

Subarticular Entrapment

This type of compression usually occurs from arthritic hypertrophy of an articular facet (Fig. 7.5). It is an occurrence often associated with advanced spondylosis. The bony mass often compresses the nerve root lying beneath the medial border of the superior articular facet. The root is caught between the posterior aspect of the vertebral body and the facet. Besides somatic sensory and

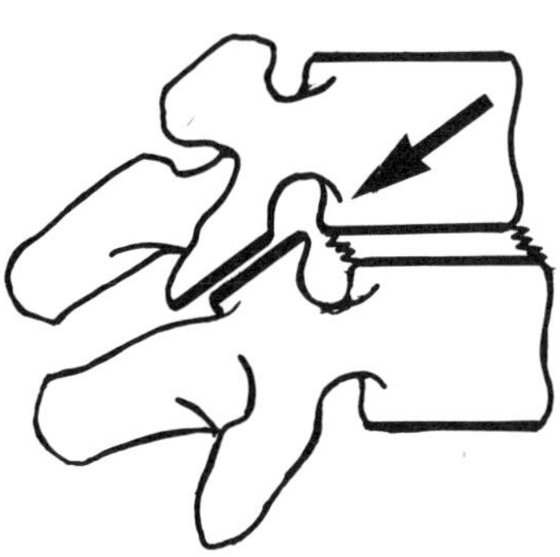

Figure 7.4. Anterosuperior subluxation of a superior process into the intervertebral foramen as the result of weakened or stretched intervertebral disc fibers.

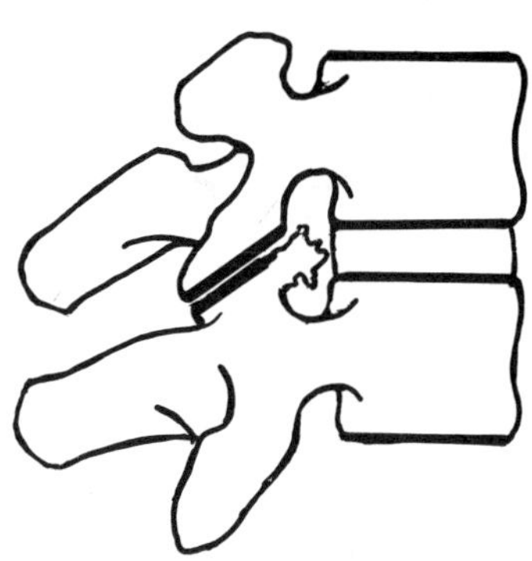

Figure 7.5. Arthritis on an inferior process resulting in an irritative encroachment of the contents of the intervertebral foramen.

motor manifestations, hearing, visual, and equilibrium disturbances may be associated, according to Pang, Chrisman/Gervais, Davis, and others.

Pedicular Kinking

This condition is associated with chronic IVD degeneration where the disc space is quite thin and the vertebral bodies approximate each other asymmetrically because of lateral disc collapse or a laterally tilted vertebral body (eg, scoliosis). As the superior vertebral body descends, it may impose its pedicle on the exiting nerve root (Fig. 7.6). Macnab feels that the most common mechanism is that the nerve root becomes entrapped in the gutter formed by a wide lateral protrusion of the disc and the superior pedicle (Fig. 7.7).

Axial Compression

Axial compression from the upright position is never a problem with a healthy, well-hydrated disc. If the disc space narrows considerably, the spinal canal can be narrowed in the midline by several mechanisms. Typically, these include posterior subluxation of the superior vertebra, anterior subluxation of the inferior vertebra, a diffuse posterior anular protrusion or rupture, kinking of the ligamentum flavum, thickened capsules from laminae shingling, arthritic hypertrophy of the superior processes, or a combination of these factors.

It should be kept in mind, however, that the IVF is usually quite roomy (Fig. 7.8). There can be complete disc collapse without any degree of compression. Also, there can be considerable compression on a root without any overt signs of malfunction if the pressure develops slowly and adaptation is sufficient. Entrapment, from whatever cause, can be encouraged by a transforaminal ligament, an adhesion, or an overgrowth restricting the normal mobility of the root in the IVF.

Spinal Canal Stenosis

Spinal stenosis often produces a bony root entrapment syndrome. Narrowing of the spinal canal can occur either laterally or in the midline of the canal. If it occurs laterally, compression of the nerve roots can result from foraminal impingement (ie, subluxation), pedicular kinking, or subarticular entrapment. If it occurs in the midline, compression of the cord or cauda equina may result (Fig. 7.9).

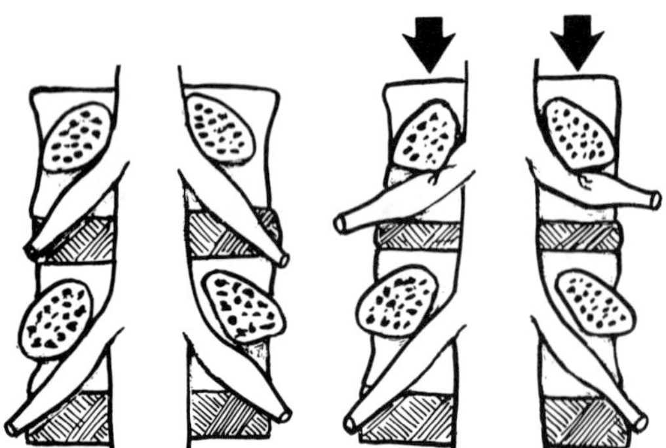

Figure 7.6. *Left,* normal relationship of the pedicle and nerve root. *Right,* caudad migration of the pedicles of the upper segment of the motion unit during IVD thinning producing nerve root compression.

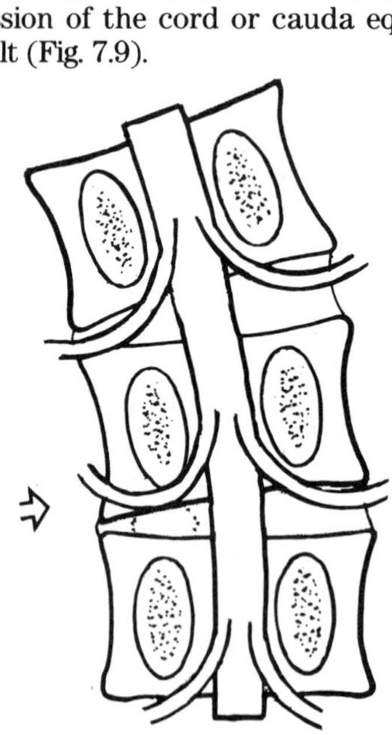

Figure 7.7. During lateral bending under load or in asymmetrical collapse of the disc laterally, the tilt leads to the nerve root being kinked between the adjacent pedicle and a bulging disc, giving rise to root irritation or compression symptoms.

Major Effects of Spinal-Level Nerve Compression

Spinal nerve pressure or irritation may manifest as sensory, motor, autonomic, or combined signs and symptoms. Initial results are often interacting. In studying the effects at injured and compressed nerves, Granit and associates found that nerve impulses set up in a motor root are transmitted to the sensory fibers in a cut or compressed region of the nerve and can be picked up in the sensory root of the same segment.

Causey/Palmer concluded that, in acute experiments, the failure to conduct an impulse after local pressure is applied to a nerve was caused by local anoxia. Rydevik found that this was true but also found that biomechanical nerve root deformation was also a factor in inducing motor weakness and altered sensibilities.

Axoplasmic Flow Disturbances

Most pathologists agree that it takes much more than an invasion of a pathogenic or-

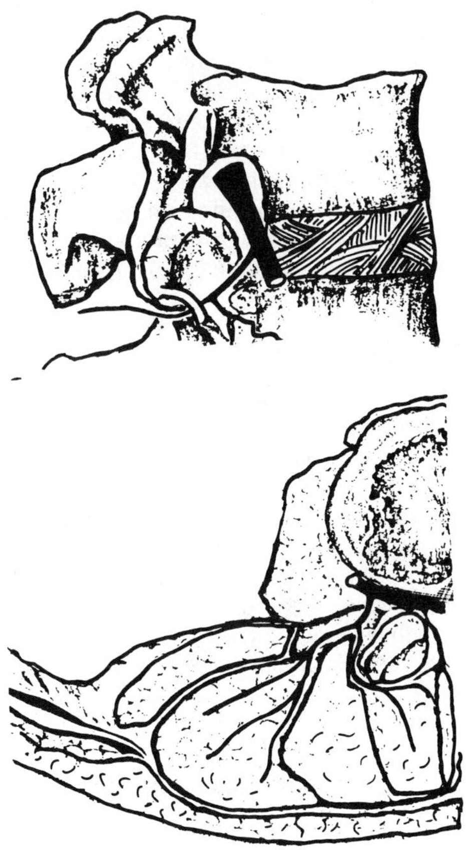

Figure 7.8. *Top,* the lumbar nerve root descends obliquely through the upper IVF, posterior to the vertebral body. The dorsal ramus runs laterally across the superior articular process and through a ligamentous tunnel. Only a small portion of this ligamentous channel is shown in the diagram. *Bottom,* the posterior division of the nerve root as viewed from above. Only the main branches are shown.

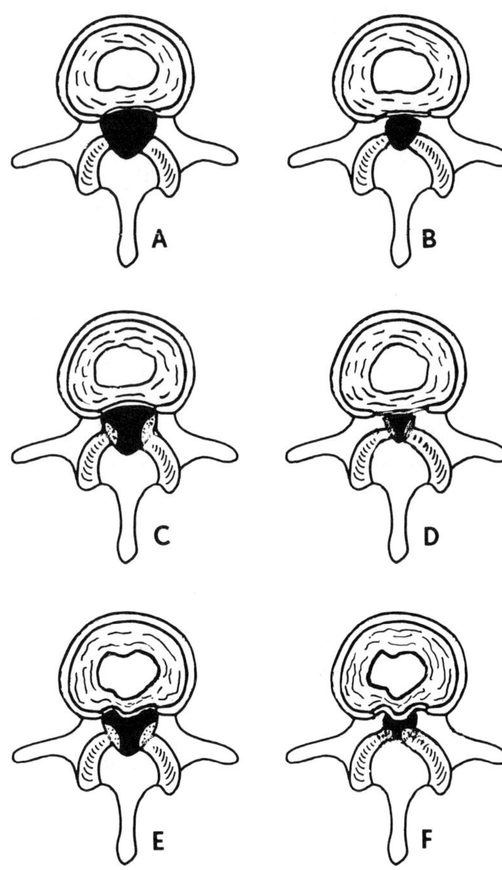

Figure 7.9. Various types of central spinal stenosis as viewed from above. *A,* normal canal (in black). *B,* congenitally small canal. *C,* degenerated canal. *D,* combined congenital and degenerated canal. *E,* combined degenerated canal with disc protrusion. *F,* combined congenital and degenerated canal with disc protrusion.

ganism to cause an infectious disease: an inadequate tissue resistance is also necessary for the invading organism to survive and multiply. The idea of "improving natural resistance to disease" was at the foundation of many pioneer chiropractic concepts. Whereas allopathy has traditionally emphasized the virulence of the invader, chiropractic has emphasized the resistance of the host. During pioneer chiropractic, this hypothesis was based primarily on empiric findings, which were later substantiated considerably by the studies of Zhigalina, Gondienko, Selye, and Speransky that were described in Chapter 2. Studies on the effects of axoplasmic flow interruption have added even greater validity to the chiropractic approach.

The Neuronal Transport System

It has been known for several years that much of the protein synthesized within a nerve cell body moves, along with other materials such as neurotransmitters, from the cell body and along the nerve fiber (anterograde material transport system). Two mechanisms have been isolated, and they are characterized by their fast (410 ±50 mm/day) and slow (1—3 mm/day) rates, regardless of their fiber size. Guth initially recognized this total system for transporting the "trophic" substances normally carried by efferent nerves. It is also recognized that there is a retrograde flow of materials; ie, from terminals toward the nerve cell body.

In recent years, Ochs, Korr, Fernandez, Rainer, Sjostrand, and several other researchers have found that any type of neuronal constriction, compression, or ischemia will cause a local transport block and an accumulation (damming) of the fluid proximal to the restriction. Weiss had earlier described this as a form of persistent endoneurial edema found just proximal to a compressed area.

Pressures successful in blocking axoplasmic flow are far below those necessary to block nerve conduction. It has been hypothesized that some effects previously attributed to nerve root compression (eg, from vertebral subluxation) may be effects from interference with normal axoplasmic flow.

Current Research Findings

Current research supports three important facts: (1) nerve roots are highly susceptible to compression, spinal nerves are not; (2) nerve roots become highly vulnerable to IVF compression when the roots are subjected to traction and the IVF is narrowed; (3) spinal nerves, while not highly susceptible to compression, are highly susceptible to axoplasmic transport block.

Cerebrospinal Fluid Flow Alterations

Stagnant or altered CSF flow has an adverse influence on the CNS. Freedman states that biomechanical aberrations of the spinal column may adversely affect CSF flow and CNS function. It is thought that this factor may be a common physiologic denominator within various (although seemingly different but often equally effective) chiropractic adjustment techniques.

Spinal Nerve Flow

In 1968, Steer/Horney answered the question whether CSF passes peripherally from the spinal cord to spinal nerves. To test the possibility, blue powder suspended in CSF was introduced into the lumbar subarachnoid space of pigs and sheep. Nerves and other tissues were examined 4—21 days later. Particles were found widely distributed; eg, in the brachial and lumbosacral plexuses, thoracic nerves and muscles, skin, and the jugular vein.

Occipital Subluxation Effects

Almost any situation that would cause constriction in the connecting area between the cerebral subarachnoid space and the vertebral canal can limit the escape of CSF into the inferior vertebral canal. This results in a degree of increased intracranial pressure. An atlanto-occipital subluxation may cause the dura mater of the cisterna cerebellaris to be pressed against the posterior medullary velum and partially occlude the foramina of Luschka and Magendie and interfere with the flow from the 4th ventricle. The resulting increase of intraventricular fluid accumulation may create a large variety of symptoms such as deep-seated, stubborn, "internal pressure" headaches; nausea; a tendency toward projectile vomiting; bizarre and unusual visual disturbances; and protopathic ataxias.

Lower Spinal Subluxation Effects

Disorders classified under the category of *CSF flow alterations* refer to the mechanical effect upon the flow of CSF within the CNS and perhaps within the peripheral nerves themselves. Stagnation possibly occurs in association because of the intimate relationship between spinal fluid and venoid blood, contributing to toxicity in the nerve root area. According to some researchers, minute pressure on meninges can alter the flow of CSF and interfere with the system's ability to remove wastes and provide nutritional substances to the cord and related nerves. This may be either the result of direct mechanical pressure or impairment of motion necessary for proper inflow and outflow of this nutrient material.

Cord Compression

Most spinal cord injuries are caused by extreme flexion in which subluxation, fracture, and/or dislocation are co-associated. It is not unusual for what appears initially to be a severe posttraumatic subluxation syndrome to be complicated by a spinal fracture/dislocation. Initial signs are often misleading. Hemorrhage may occur at the site with the same reaction as brain injury (liquefaction, softening, disintegration). Congenital fusions and stenosis may predispose to spinal cord trauma during strenuous activity.

Primary Types

There are direct and indirect classes of spinal cord injuries:

• *Indirect injury* to the cord may be caused by the rupture of tissues of the spine by violent forces such as falls, crushes, or blows. This type of injury, which is normally closed with respect to the spinal column and cord, is of a lesser degree than direct injury. It takes the form of concussion, hemorrhage, or edema of the cord. The cord may cease to function below the site at which the force was applied even if the cord itself received no direct injury. Such dysfunction may be temporary or long standing, thus the prognosis must be guarded. Injuries to the spinal column in which the cerebrospinal fluid is rapidly depleted may be fatal.

If the cervical cord is injured, there is loss of sensation and flaccid paralysis. The lower limbs exhibit a spastic paralysis. If the space in which the spinal fluid flows between the spinal cord and the surrounding vertebral column is either compressed or enlarged, severe headache occurs. Posttraumatic penile erection strongly suggests either cervical or thoracic cord injury.

• *Direct injury* to the cord, the nerve roots, or both may be caused by impact forces or shattered bone fragments. The cord may be bruised, compressed, crushed, pierced, or cut. An open wound is often involved.

Nontraumatic Types

Cord compression also may be the result of chronic subluxation, spondylosis, osteophytes, longitudinal ligament thickening or buckling, or tumor development.

SELECTED CERVICAL CONSIDERATIONS

The tissues of the posterior neck normally provide stability and support for the cranium, a flexible and protective spine for movement, balance adaptation, and housing for the spinal cord and vertebral artery. From a broad viewpoint, primary cervical subluxation syndromes may reflect themselves in the total habitus; from a neurologic viewpoint, insults may manifest throughout the motor, sensory, and autonomic nervous systems. Unlike the lumbar region, cervical disc herniations are not frequently associated with severe trauma; however, traumatic nerve root or cord compression has a high incidence in this area.

Valentini, Fitz-Ritson, Cole, Seeman, Mears, and others have shown that nowhere in the spine is the relationship between the osseous structures and the surrounding neurologic and vascular beds as intimate or subject to disturbance as it is in the cervical region. The effects of local subluxation may express themselves upward within the brain stem and downward to the lumbar spine and pelvis. Many peripheral nerve symptoms in the shoulder, arm, and hand will find their origin in the brachial plexus.

Table 7.1. Local and Remote Features of Cervical Subluxation

Articular grating	Headaches	Poor concentration
Ataxia	Horner's syndrome	Precordial discomfort
Atypical facial pains	Indigestion	Pseudoangina
Blurred vision	Irritability	Psychiatric disturbances
Cold sweats	Lermoyez's syndrome	Retro-orbital pain
Deafness	Memory faults	Stiffness (neck)
Diplopia	Meniere's syndrome	Tenderness
Drop attacks	Mental confusion	Tension
Dysarthria	Neuralgia	Tinnitus
Dysequilibrium	Nausea	Tonsillitis
Dysphagia	Neck pain	Upper extremity coolness, pain, and/or altered reflexes
Dysphonia	Numbness	Vertigo
Epileptiform attacks	Nystagmus	Vomiting
Fatigue	Pallor	
Giddiness	Paresis	

Note: The above list has been developed from the writings of Henderson, Blumenthal, Kovacs, Ryan, Gayral, and Hanflig.

Table 7.2. Function and Innervation of the Major Muscles of the Neck

Muscle	Major Function	Spinal Segments
Erector spinae, upper	Extension, rotation	C1—T1
Longus capitis	Flexion	C1—C3
Longus colli	Flexion	C2—C6
Rectus capitis anterior	Flexion	C1—C2
Rectus capitis lateral	Flexion	C1—C2
Scalenes	Flexion, rotation	C4—C8
Semispinalis capitis	Extension, rotation	C1—T1
Semispinalis cervicis	Extension, rotation	C1—T1
Splenius capitis	Extension, rotation	C1—C8
Splenius cervicis	Extension, rotation	C1—C8
Sternocleidomastoid	Flexion, rotation	C2, XI
Trapezius, upper	Extension, rotation	C3—C4

Note: Spinal innervation varies somewhat in different people. The spinal nerves listed here are averages and may differ in a particular patient; thus, an allowance of a segment above and below those listed in most text tables should be considered.

General Symptomatology

Local and remote effects of cervical subluxation are shown in Table 7.1.

Structural Considerations

The highly mobile cervical spine is unique in that it must provide flexibility and yet protect highly complex neurologic centers within; ie, the lower portion of the medulla oblongata and that portion of the spinal cord which emits the cervical and brachial plexus. The tips of the cervical spinous processes normally correspond to the level of the succeeding cord segment; eg, the C5 spinous process is on a level with the C6 segment of the cord.

The function and innervation of the major muscles of the neck are shown in Table 7.2.

The Cervical Cord Suspension System

The spinal cord is tethered within the dura by the dentate ligaments. Grieve points out that the upper dentates are the strongest and are attached to the dura inside the posterior cranial fossa, behind the canal for the 12th cranial nerve. Because these intraspinal ligaments, which are under tension, project inferiorly and the nerve roots are angled superiorly, the tensile forces on the cord are balanced during spinal motion (Fig. 7.10). This allows the cord to maintain its central position within the vertebral canal—a position which provides maximum protection (Fig. 7.11). Further protection is provided by cerebrospinal fluid, epidural and extradural fat, and the longitudinal ligaments of the canal.

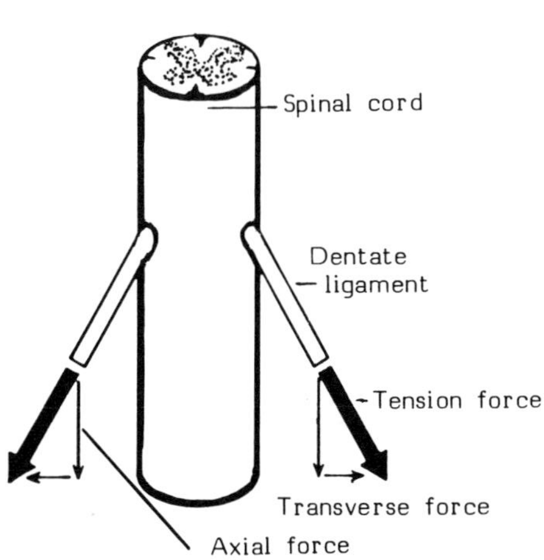

Figure 7.10. A unilateral diagonal dentate ligament would provide the spinal cord with axial and transverse pretension, but the bilateral pair offers the added benefit of resistance against axial tension.

Nerve Root Attachments

It was described earlier that the nerve roots' sleeves of dura and related arachnoid tissue within the cervical canal are *loosely*

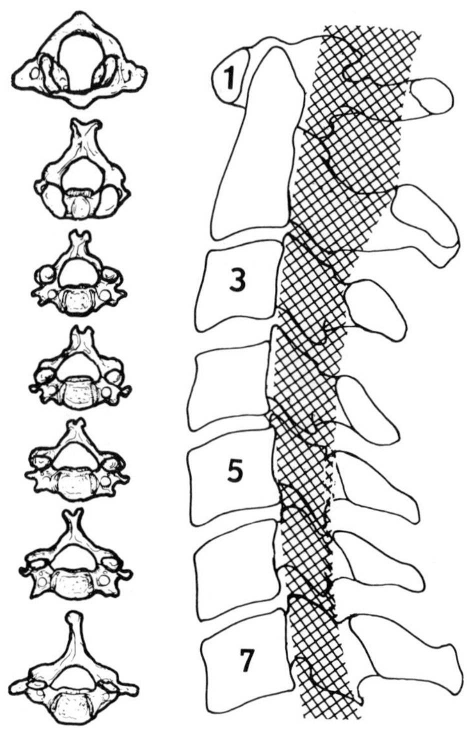

Figure 7.11. *Left,* comparison of cervical vertebrae as viewed from above. Note differences in design of the spinal canal, width of transverse processes, and length of spinous processes. *Right,* sagittal view of the cervical region showing space for the spinal cord within the cervical spine. Dimensions (A-P) are approximately 22 mm at the atlas, 20 mm at the axis, and 12 mm at C4—C7.

attached to the cervical IVFs. These attachments increase in strength during degenerative processes and with advancing age. The lower roots (C4—C7) are *firmly* attached in the gutter of the transverse process by the epineurial sheath, extensions from the prevertebral fascia, and other connective-tissue fibers of the area.

The segmental functions of the cervical nerves are shown in Table 7.3. Subluxation syndromes and traumatic traction involving the cervical and brachial plexuses will be described later in this chapter.

Cervical Spinal Receptors

The abundant proprioceptors of the vertebral column enable the brain to know where each segment is and what it is doing at any given time without visual confirmation. The apophyseal joints of the cervical spine, especially their capsules, are richly innervated with mechanoreceptors and afferent fibers—endowed more than any other spinal region. Activity from the cervical articular receptors exerts significant facilitatory and

Table 7.3. Segmental Functions of Cervical Nerves

Segment	Function
	CERVICAL PLEXUS (C1—C4)
C1	Motor to head and neck extensors, infrahyoid, rectus capitis anterior and lateral, and longus capitis.
C2	Sensory to lateral occiput and submandibular area; motor, same as C1 plus longus colli.
C3	Sensory to lateral occiput and lateral neck, overlapping C2 area; motor to head and neck extensors, infrahyoid, longus capitus, longus colli, levator scapulae, scaleni, and trapezius.
C4	Sensory to lower lateral neck and medial shoulder area; motor to head and neck extensors, longus coli, levator scapulae, scaleni, trapezius, and diaphragm.
	BRACHIAL PLEXUS (C5—T1)
C5	Sensory to clavicle level and lateral arm (axillary nerve); motor to deltoid, biceps; biceps tendon reflex. Primary root in shoulder abduction, exits between C4 and C5 discs.
C6	Sensory to lateral forearm, thumb, index and half of 2nd finger (sensory branches of musculocutaneous nerve); motor to biceps, wrist extensors; brachioradialis tendon reflex. Primary root in wrist extension, exits between C5 and C6 discs.
C7	Sensory to second finger; motor to wrist flexors, finger extensors, triceps; triceps tendon reflex. Primary root in finger extension, exits between C6 and C7 discs.
C8	Sensory to medial forearm (medial antebrachial nerve), ring and little fingers (ulnar nerve); motor to finger flexors, interossei; no reflex applicable. Primary root in finger flexion, exits between C7 and T1 discs.
T1	Sensory to medial arm (medial brachial cutaneous nerve); motor to interossei; no reflex applicable. Primary root in finger abduction, exits between T1 and T2 discs.

inhibitory reflex effects on the muscles of the neck and both the upper and lower extremities.

Wyke believes that the patterns of "normal cervical articular mechanoreceptor reflexes are profoundly distorted when cervical articular nociceptive afferent activity is added to that derived from the normally functioning cervical mechanoreceptors." To underscore this point, he states that (1) manipulation of the head on the neck can produce coordinated flexion and extension movements on the paralyzed arm and leg of a hemiplegic patient, (2) arm movement control without visual aid is considerably affected by rotation of the head, and (3) induced unilateral local anesthesia of the cervical joints in healthy subjects produces severe postural instability, dizziness, nystagmus, and muscular incoordination. These signs and symptoms are similar to those experienced by some patients who suffer from cervical spondylosis, ankylosing spondylitis, and gross fixations, and some while wearing an orthopedic cervical collar.

Lieb shows several full-spine radiographs of severe spinal distortions that have been greatly improved through correction of dental occlusion. If the temporomandibular joint has such a proprioceptive influence upon spinal posture, it is no wonder that chiropractors who specialize in upper-cervical or sacral correction can exhibit an abundance of such before-and-after films because each spinal segment is richly endowed with an equal or greater number of receptors than those of the joint of the jaw.

Cervical Righting Mechanisms

Several extensors of the neck arise from the lower cervical and upper thoracic vertebrae and exert an oblique posteroinferior pull on the occiput. If this line of pull falls behind the atlanto-occipital joint, a rotary movement results that tilts the occiput posteriorly and lifts the face so that the neck is hyperextended. However, if this posterior rotation of the head is inhibited by the cervical flexors (which is normal), the oblique pull tends to have a posterior translatory component when the head is anterior to the midline. This serves to bring the head back toward the vertical gravity line and into better alignment.

The longus group, in addition, exerts a bowstring action on the anterior cervical segments, which assists in axial extension of the neck. Thus, the extensors serve to return the head to the midline following flexion, but axial extension is completed by a straightening of the cervical lordosis produced by segmental *flexion*. If this segmental flexion did not occur during extension, the head would rest in the neutral position facing superiorly. Simultaneously, the thoracic extensors tend to straighten the dorsal curve so that the alignment of the entire cervicothoracic region is improved (Fig. 7.12).

Chronic flexion of the lower cervicals tends to produce elongation of the upper posterior thoracic soft tissues and adaptive shortening of the anterior elements (eg, anterior longitudinal ligament, anterior disc anulus, pectorals, intercostals). This is often seen in aging where it is contributed to by degeneration of the normally elastic ligamentum nuchae, which helps to resist anterior deviation of the head. If this chronic flexion state occurs, cervical extension to the midline following flexion is fairly limited to increasing the cervical lordosis with little axial extension of the neck by segmental flexion. The neck angles forward, and the jaw juts out as the occiput rolls backward.

The Cervical Challenge. Goodheart reports that "challenging" vertebral position during spinal analysis provides a precise method of localizing a subluxation complex

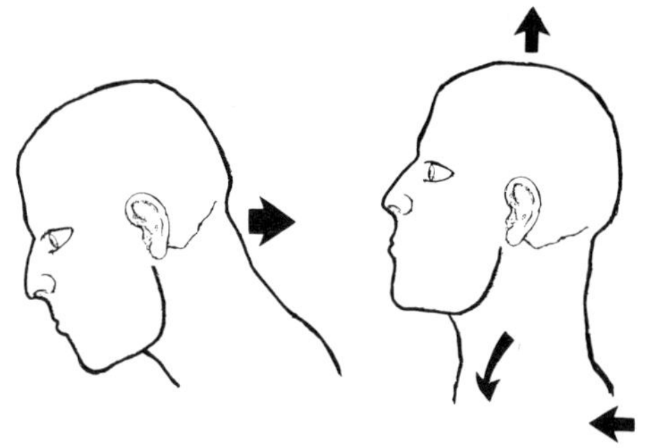

Figure 7.12. *Left,* in axial extension of the cervical spine, the cervical extensors return the neck to the midline. *Right,* the deep cervical flexors straighten the spine, and the thoracic extensors reduce the thoracic kyphosis.

so that a specific adjustment may be made. He has found that light pressure (5—8 lbs) directed into a cervical lesion will cause an increase in strength of a previously weakened muscle and pressure in the opposite direction will produce weakness in the same muscle. It is theorized that when a subluxated facet is pushed farther out of alignment, the righting reflex of the body will temporarily pull this lesion back into position, and vice versa, in an attempt to maintain structural homeostasis. The direction of correction is then said to be toward the side that produces weakness during evaluation.

Dynamics of the Cervical Cord

Breig has shown that the length of the spinal canal shortens during extension and lengthens during flexion (forward and lateral). Thus, the spinal cord must do likewise to avoid injury during flexion. This is accomplished because the cord is pleated in an accordion-like fashion during rest and unfolds during any lengthening process.

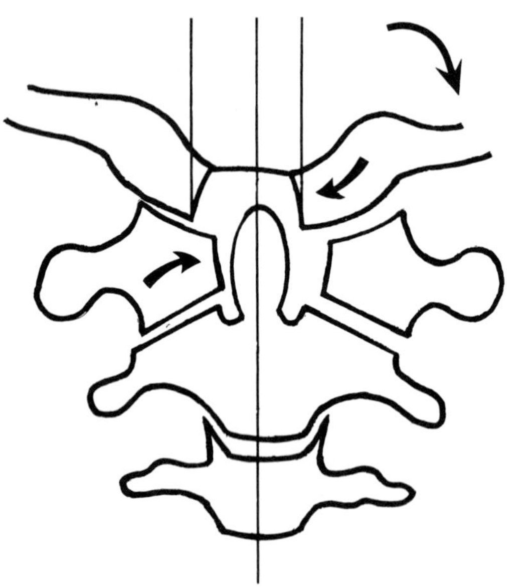

Figure 7.13. Occipitoatlantal and atlantoaxial lateral flexion. During lateral bending, only 5° of motion are exhibited at the occipitoatlantal and 6° at the atlantoaxial articulations. However, the occiput slips towards the convexity and the atlas slips toward the concavity. This creates shear forces at the superior articulations of the atlas and distortion of the odontoid space.

Changes During Rotation and Lateral Flexion. The ipsilateral anterior roots relax and the dorsal roots become taut during rotation. During lateral flexion (Fig. 7.13), the IVFs narrow in height ipsilaterally and elongate contralaterally. Undue tension can be placed on the contralateral dentate bands and IVF contents, and compressive forces can be applied to the contents of the ipsilateral IVF. This is especially true if degenerative changes have occurred.

Changes During Flexion. During flexion, the slack in the cord and its neurons, the dura, and the roots progresses to tension. Because the cord is attached to the coccyx, any tension arising in the cervical area will be transmitted as far caudally as the lower sacral roots. Breig/Turnbull/Hassler report that the cross-section of the cord increases or decreases, as an elastic bar, whenever the cord respectively shortens or lengthens. Although the spinal cord has a high stretch coefficient when tension is applied slowly, Goddard/Reid found that elastic deformation is only necessary at the extremes of spinal motion. Only about 2 or 3 mm of segment-level movement occurs in the cervical spine. The meninges, which have more white fibers than elastic fibers, are not as elastic. They become taut when their length approaches a 5% increase. While the cord and dura are both under tension during spinal motion, according to Penning, that of the dura is from its structural properties and extradural attachments plus root tension, and that of the cord is from the rubber-like dentate bands. This process also mandates that any tension applied to the cord will be rapidly transmitted to the dura and roots, and vice versa.

Changes During Extension. The spinal cord and the roots slacken during extension and slightly gravitate because of gravitational pull, according to Reid. The "free space" of the canal is decreased by three factors during extension: (1) posterior bulging of the IVD, (2) buckling of the relaxed dura, and (3) anterior bulging of the ligamentum flavum.

Selected Clinical Implications

The same tension mechanisms occurring in the cord, dura, and roots during normal physiologic flexion are thought to occur chronically in the relaxed state when the cervical curve or a single motion unit is hypolordotic. In addition, it has been Brodal's experience that normal consequences will be compounded whenever a stretched (bowstring) cord is applied against any space-occupying lesion (spondylotic ridge, IVD protrusion, tumor). In time, this will result in actual flattening of the cord at this point and ischemic degeneration from pressure on the anterior spinal artery, the radicular arteries, and/or their capillary beds. Such findings have been reported by Fried and associates, Hoff, and Brieg. Likewise, it can be projected that the same factors which narrow the canal during normal extension will occur chronically in the relaxed state when the cervical curve or a single motion unit is hyperlordotic.

Nerve function of the cervical and brachial plexuses is shown in Table 7.4.

Cervical Nerve Root Insults

Disturbances of nerve function associated with subluxation syndromes basically manifest as abnormalities in sensory interpretations and/or motor activities. These disturbances may be through one of two primary mechanisms: direct nerve or nerve root disorders, or of a reflex nature.

Sensory Changes. When direct nerve root involvement occurs on the posterior root of a specific neuromere, it manifests as an increase or decrease in sensitivity over the dermatome. A typical example includes foraminal occlusion or irritating factors exhibited clinically as hyperesthesia, particularly on the dorsal and lateral aspects of the thumb and radial side of the hand, when involvement occurs between C5 and C6. Another example is on the dorsum of the hand, the index and middle fingers, and the anteroradial side of the forearm, thumb, index and middle fingers, when involvement occurs between C6 and C7. In other instances, this nerve root involvement may cause hypertonicity and the sensation of deep pain in the musculature supplied by the neuromere. For example, in C6 involvement, there is deep pain in the biceps; or in C7 involvement, there is deep pain in the triceps and supinators of the forearm. Direct pressure near the nerve root or along its distribution may be particularly painful.

Motor Changes. Nerve root insults from subluxations or trauma also may be evident as disturbances in motor reflexes and/or muscular strength. Examples of these reflexes include the tendon reflexes such as seen in the reduced biceps reflex when involvement occurs between C5 and C6; or the reduced triceps reflex when involvement occurs between C6 and C7. These reflexes must also be compared bilaterally to judge whether hyporeflexia is unilateral. Unilateral hyperreflexia is pathognomonic of an upper motor neuron lesion. Prolonged and/or severe nerve root irritation also may produce evidence of trophic changes in the tissues supplied.

Underlying Factors. The common subluxation picture is rarely pure. It is often superimposed upon other manifest and subclinical processes in the mature patient such as vertebral instability, osteochondrophytic ridges at the uncovertebral joints, apophyseal thickening and exostosis, or canal encroachment by a buckling ligamentum flavum, spinal stenosis, posterior vertebral body spurs, disc protrusions, dura and dentate thickening, arachnoid cysts, dura and arachnoid adhesions, and ossification of the posterior longitudinal ligament.

Loss of disc space, especially in the lower cervical area, may contribute as a source of chronic irritation to an already inflamed root by altering the angulation of the IVF tunnel. The sequence of inflammation, granulation, fibrosis, adhesion formation, and nerve root stricture may follow, along with a loss in root mobility and elasticity. These degenerative changes are not as pronounced during youth.

Upper Cervical Trauma

A severely stressful movement of the cervical spine may result in unconsciousness and possible death if the spinal cord is damaged. The cause may be fracture or dislocation that injures the spinal cord, often fatally if it occurs within the upper cervical area. Even mild spinal cord trauma may result in sensory and motor paralysis. Neck hyperextension injuries may cause compression injury to the vertebral arteries causing a temporary oxygen loss to the brain that may result in unconsciousness, if not greater damage through rupture. See Figure 7.14. Less severe disturbances in this area often arise from muscular spasm of one or more of the six muscle bundles that have attachments on the occiput, atlas, or axis. Unequal tension and ultimate fibrotic changes within the paravertebral structures can readily involve the delicate nerve fibers and vascular flow.

A study of most clinical subluxations will reveal that they are infrequently "unusual"

Table 7.4. Nerve Function of the Cervical Nerves

Nerve	Function
Nerve Function of the Cervical Plexus (C1—C4)	
Lesser occipital	Sensory to skin behind ear and mastoid process.
Greater auricular	Sensory to skin over parotid, jaw angle, ear lobe, and front of mastoid process.
Cervical cutaneous	Sensory to skin over anterolateral portion of neck.
Supraclaviculars	Sensory to skin over medial infraclavicular area, pectoralis major and deltoid.
Muscular branches	Motor to capitus anterior and lateralis, longus capitus, longus colli, hyoid muscles, sternocleidomastoideus, trapezius, levator scapulae, scalenus medius.
Phrenic	Sensory to costal and mediastinal pleura and pericardium. Motor to diaphragm.
Nerve Function of the Brachial Plexus (C5—T1)	
Nerve	Function
Radial	Motor for wrist and thumb extension; sensory to dorsalweb space between thumb and index finger.
Ulnar	Motor for little finger abduction; sensory to distal ulnar aspect of little finger.
Median	Motor for thumb opposition and abduction; sensory todistal radial aspect of index finger.
Axillary	Motor to deltoid muscle; sensory to lateral arm and deltoid patch on upper arm.
Musculocutaneous	Motor to biceps muscle; sensory to lateral forearm.

positions. They are often *normal positions in a state of fixation.* In the neutral position, for example, an inferior atlas subluxation-fixation exhibits the posterior arch of the atlas approximating the spinous process of the axis—the *normal* position of the atlas during extension. The same is true of superior, posterior, and lateral listings: all are normal positions if found in flexion, rotation, or lateral bending, but abnormal if found in other positions.

In a discussion of spinal motion of any region or segment complex, it should be kept in mind that minor pathologic changes and individual variances from the "norm" considerably alter the biodynamics that lead to the neurologic insults involved. Neither static position on roentgenography and/or dynamic palpation alone can be used as the basis to determine the need or the results of adjustive therapy. Static palpation is often grossly in error because of the many anomalies in asymmetry found in the typical spine. The whole clinical picture must be utilized.

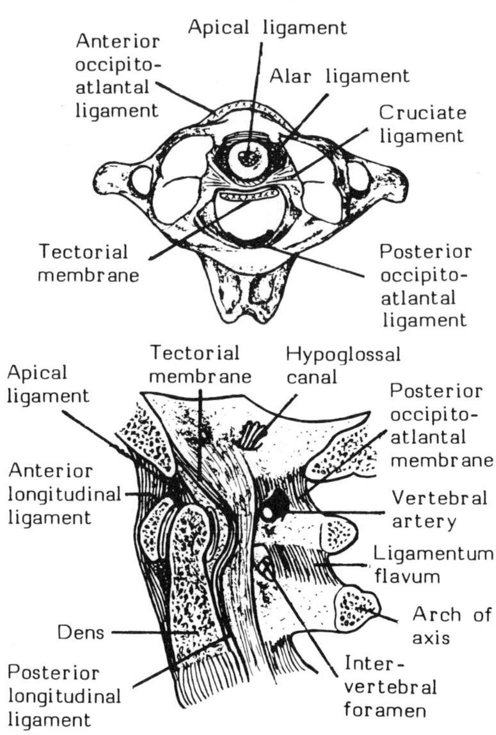

Figure 7.14. The major upper cervical ligaments: *top,* as viewed from above; *bottom,* sagittal section.

Lower Cervical Trauma

The nerve root is anterior and inferior to the facets in the cervical spine. If subluxation of a vertebra occurs in a superior direction, the contents of the IVF become stretched because elongating and narrowing the vertical diameter of the IVF will cause traction upon the nerve trunk plus compression against the anterior portion of the foramen. If there is subluxation in an inferior direction, shortening and widening of the foramen occurs.

Because the nerve sheath is often firmly anchored by tissues connecting it to the borders of the foramen in the adult, an overstretch is exerted on the nerve sheath whenever its shape is altered. It thus can be recognized that enlarging the IVF can cause as much trouble as a reduction in the size of the IVF. Also, it is impossible to subluxate a vertebra between C2 and L5 without changing the shape of its IVD in compensation.

Cervical fractures and dislocations concomitant with a subluxation syndrome are not common except in the elderly where a degree of osteoporosis is evident. In the young, they are usually the result of severe trauma. Signs of paravertebral tenderness, limitation in movement, muscle spasm, and neurologic deficit should be sought. As in upper-cervical damage, emergency management is necessary to avoid paralysis and death. Fracture and/or dislocation of any cervical vertebra require hospitalization for reduction, bone traction, and casting. Keep in mind that overdiagnosing instability of the C2—C3 interface is a common pitfall.

Effects of Pathologic Changes on the Cord

Several factors may produce cord compression (static or dynamic) or reduce cord flexibility (increasing cord tension) besides fracture and dislocation. Some common examples are space-occupying lesions (eg, tumor, hemorrhage, edema), central stenosis, IVD protrusion, end-plate fracture, ligamentous hypertrophy, soft-tissue sclerosis, CSF disorders, root-sleeve fibrosis or swelling, ischemia consequences, glial scars from demyelinating disease, and postinflammatory adhesions. But, according to Kapandji, the most common cause is osteophytes extending from the uncovertebral joints.

Breig feels that it is *increased cord tension* (regardless of cause) and its histologic and microcirculatory effects that produce conductivity and circulatory impairment. He states that these disorders account for most motor, sensory, and autonomic dysfunctions associated with cervical cord syndromes.

Cervical Curve Alterations

Cervical Scoliosis

Cervical scoliosis is often mechanically predisposed by flattening rather than exaggeration of the cervical lordosis. This is especially common during youth. The posterior joints become lax during flattening of the cervical spine, and this encourages retropositioning and posterior subluxations that are frequently the first step toward cervical scoliosis.

In typical rotary cervical scoliosis, the spinous processes tend to rotate toward the convex side of the lateral curve, the vertebral bodies rotate toward the concave side, and the discs and articular facets become subjected to abnormal stretching forces as they open on the side of convexity and to compressive forces on the side of concavity. This type of cervical scoliosis is usually compensatory to a lower scoliosis to the other side and a common cause of recurring episodes of nontraumatic torticollis.

When a cervical disc is loaded unilaterally, the disc initially becomes wedge-shaped. This vertically stretches the anular fibers that are opposite the weight-bearing side, but this action is quickly counteracted by forces transmitted laterally from the resilient nucleus to help the disc return to its normal shape. This self-stabilization factor is the product of a healthy nucleus and anulus working as a mechanical couple.

Cervical scoliotic rotation is also associated with a lateral tilt that increases the distance between the lateral margins of the vertebral bodies on the convex side of the curve. This stretches the lateral anulus, which produces a contraction of that part of the disc and a compensatory bulging of its contralateral (thinned) aspect. If the anular filaments become stretched and weakened, losing some of their stiffness property, the nucleus may shift from its central position so that the vertebral segment is unable to return to its normal position. A firmly locked rotational subluxation can result.

When uninterrupted compression is applied to any active and mobile joint, cartilaginous erosion followed by arthritis can be expected. When continuous stretching is applied to any active and mobile synovial joint, capsulitis and a barrage of nociceptive CNS input can be anticipated. This can produce systemic effects.

Cervical Curve Reversal

Compared with the primary thoracic kyphosis, which is a structural curve, the cervical and lumbar anterior curves are functional arcs produced by their slightly wedge-shaped IVDs. They normally flatten in the nonweight-bearing supine position and quickly adapt to changes involving the direction of force. Although the cervical curve is the first secondary curve to develop in the infant, its maintenance in the erect posture is determined by the integrity of the lumbar curve.

A flattened cervical spine that is not compensatory to a flattened lumbar spine may be the result of a local disorder such as a subluxation syndrome caused by posterior shifting of one or more disc nuclei, hypertonicity of anterior musculature, or anterior ligamentous shortening as the result of local overstress, inflammation, occupational posture, or congenital anomaly. The clinical picture is often the result of trauma-producing whiplash injury, herniated disc, subluxation, dislocation, fracture, or ligamentous injury. Torticollis, arthritis, malignancy, tuberculosis, osteomyelitis, or other pathologies also may be involved. The condition occurs more frequently after the age of 40, and the sexes appear equally affected.

Cervical flattening is often the result of paraspinal spasm secondary to an underlying injury, irritation, or inflammatory process. The acute clinical picture is one of torticollis. Other manifestations include headaches (occipital, occipital-frontal, supraorbital), vertigo, tenderness elicited on lateral C4—C6 nerve roots, neuritis involving branches of the brachial plexus due to nerve-root pressure, hyperesthesia of one or more fingers, and loss or lessening of the biceps reflex on the same or contralateral side. Infrequently, the triceps reflex may be involved. One or more symptoms are often aggravated by an abnormal position of the head such as during reading in bed, an awkward sleeping position, or long-distance driving.

Cervical Subluxation/ Fixation Syndromes

Occipitoatlantal Subluxation/ Fixation Syndromes

Because all freely movable articulations are subject to subluxation, the atlanto-occipital diarthrosis is no exception (Fig. 7.15). The stress at this point is unusual when one considers that the total weight of the cranium is supported by the ring of the atlas, about 1/20th the circumference of the skull, and several spinal muscles, subject to spasm and hypertonicity, have their attachments on the occiput.

In relation to the atlas, the condyles may slip right or left with attended inferiority or superiority and may or may not present with a degree of rotation. In some instances, pure suboccipital jamming may be found as the result of muscle contraction or a blow to the vertex of the skull (Fig. 7.16).

Neurologic disturbances may result from muscular and fibrotic changes along the cranial nerve pathways that emit from the skull and pass intimately between and under suboccipital fasciculi. Five of the cranial nerves are thus vulnerable: the facial, glossopharyngeal, vagus, spinal accessory, and hypoglossal. In addition, circulatory impairment of major and minor nerves of the neck may alter the function of those cranial nerves that do not exit from the skull proper such as the olfactory, optic, oculomotor, trochlear, trigeminal, abducens, and auditory, but which are contained within the cranium and remote from direct vertebral subluxation encroachment effects.

In studying tonic reflexes of the neck during cervical rotation, Deering and associates determined that the reflex is ipsilateral and that the receiver field lies in the region of the upper joints of the neck, especially the atlanto-occipital, C1, and C2 joints.

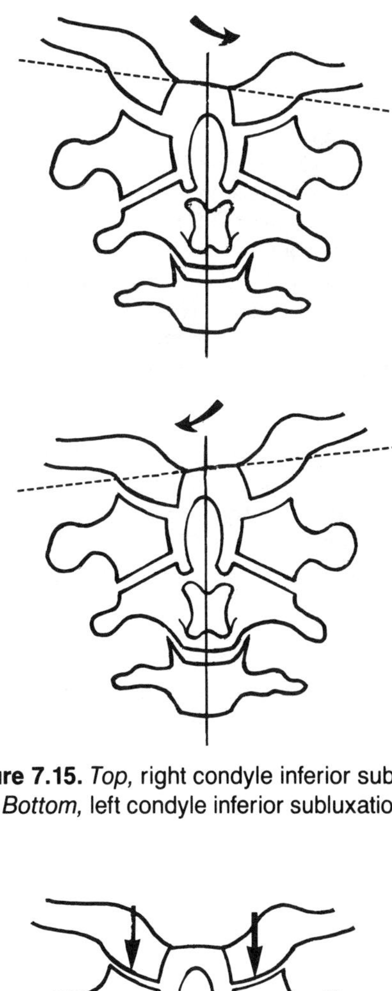

Figure 7.15. *Top,* right condyle inferior subluxation. *Bottom,* left condyle inferior subluxation.

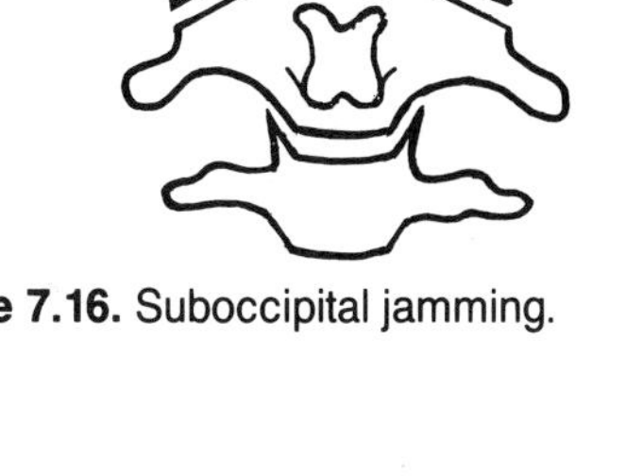

Figure 7.16. Suboccipital jamming.

Atlas Subluxations

Being near the end of a kinematic chain, the atlanto-occipital joints are subject to numerable degrees of subluxation in flexion, extension, rotation, and laterality. Rotary subluxation is not uncommon, especially if the atlantal cups are shallow. Excessive rotation is allowed by the lax check ligaments and capsules. Head weight, the angle of force, the planes of articulation, and the integrity of the para-articular tissues determine the stability present.

The atlas may be found to have side-slipped to the right or left, tipped bilaterally superior or inferior, or rotated, relative to the axis. There are no true bony IVFs for passage of the C1 and C2 spinal nerves, thus avoidance of the type of IVF encroachments produced in the lower spine.

The dura mater of the spinal cord is firmly fixed to the margin of the foramen magnum and to the C2 and C3 vertebrae. In other spinal areas, it is separated from the vertebral canal by the epidural space. Since both the C1 nerve and the vertebral artery pass through this membrane close to the superior pillar of the atlas and beneath the overhanging occiput, atlanto-occipital distortion may cause traction of the dura to produce irritation of the artery and nerve unilaterally and compressional occlusion contralaterally.

There is also a neurosynapse between the upper cervical nerves and the trigeminal that also supplies the dura mater, which helps to explain why irritation of C1 results in a neuralgia not only confined to a small area at the base of the skull but is also referred to the forehead or eye via the supraorbital branch of the trigeminal. The greater occipital nerve does not tend to do this. It exits between the posterior arch of the atlas and above the lamina of the axis, referring pain to the vertex of the head.

Axis Subluxations

With the possible exception of L5, no other vertebra is probably subluxated more frequently than C2. The most common symptom is a unilateral suboccipital neuralgia on the side of posteriority. Sometimes called *cervical migraine*, the neuralgia typically begins in the upper neck and extends over the skull into the temporal and possibly the orbital areas. On the side of posteriority, palpation discloses a tender prominence over the articulating process and a contralateral deviation of the spinous process away from the midline. Posterior axis (or occipital) subluxations are sometimes misdiagnosed as anterior atlantal subluxations.

Rotary subluxations of one or more of the upper three vertebrae (particularly the axis) may cause pressure upon the superior cervical ganglion (Fig. 7.17). The syndrome produced may incorporate excessive facial and forehead perspiration, dry mouth and nasal mucous membranes, dryness and tightness of the throat, dilated pupils, tendency toward exophthalmos, migrainous attacks due to unilateral angioneurotic edema, facial vasomotor disturbances with possible angioneurotic swelling, and moderate tachycardia with functional arrythmias.

De Rusha points out that dysphagia and dysarthria may sometimes be attributed to upper-cervical involvement rather than a CNS situation. The C1 joins the hypoglossal nerve, which supplies the intrinsic muscles of the tongue. It then joins the descending cervical which is derived from C2 and C3. A loop of nerves, the ansi hypoglossi, which supplies muscles necessary for deglutition and speaking, is derived from C1—C3.

The superficial sensory cutaneous set of the cervical plexus (C1—C4) is frequently involved in subluxations of the upper four

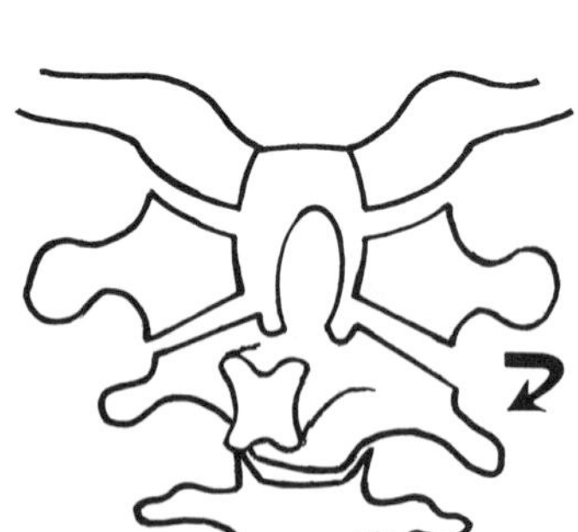

Figure 7.17. Rotary subluxation of the axis, right transverse posterior. The axis slips posteroinferior on the right and anterosuperior on the left, in accordance with the planes of articulation.

segments, particularly when there are predisposing spondylotic degenerative changes. The greater occipital (C2) nerve does not tend to do this. It exits between the posterior arch of the atlas and above the lamina of the axis (Fig. 7.18).

Neurovascular Effects of Upper Cervical Subluxations

Medulla Oblongata. The medulla oblongata extends well into the lower reaches of the foramen magnum and the ligamentous ring that connects it with the atlas, thus any type of occipital or atlantal subluxation may produce abnormal pressure on this portion of the brain stem. Bilateral posterior shifting of the occiput or atlas may cause pressure upon the pyramids or adjacent olivary bodies, producing a syndrome of upper motor neuron involvement characterized by a degree of spastic paralysis or ataxia. A lateral shifting of the occiput may cause pressure upon the tubercle of Rolando producing pain in the area of trigeminal nerve distribution, headache, sinus discomforts, ocular neuralgias, and aches in the jaw.

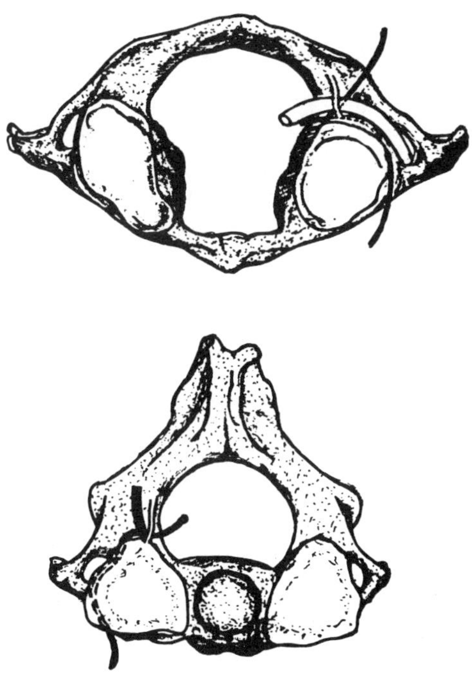

Figure 7.18. The C1 and C2 nerves leave the spinal cord behind their superior articular facets. *Top,* C1 follows a groove on the upper surface of the posterior arch of the atlas, posteroinferior to the occipitoatlantal capsule and beneath the vertebral artery as it crosses the atlas. *Bottom,* C2 traverses the arch of the axis behind the facet and in contact with the capsule. It exits the spinal canal through a small opening in the ligamentum flavum.

Vagus Nerve. As the vagus lies almost in immediate contact with the transverse process of the atlas, rotary subluxation of the atlas may cause pressure which can produce a wide range of symptoms. The syndrome produced may exhibit as nasal and sinus congestion, swallowing and speech difficulties, cardiac arrythmias, coronary artery spasm, gastric and intestinal colic, and other symptoms of vagal disturbance.

Vertebral Arteries. Janse states that any cervical subluxation (particularly atlantal, axial, or occipital) provoking muscle spasm may produce unilateral or bilateral constriction of the vertebral arteries, resulting in circulatory impairment. A large number of equilibrium, cardiac, respiratory, cranial nerve, extrapyramidal, visual, epileptoid, and auditory symptoms may follow. West points out that the vertebral artery can be completely occluded by just turning the head backward and to the opposite side during postmortem studies. Even without a degree of arteriosclerosis, the vertebral artery can be considered a fairly firm tube in the adult that responds poorly to twisting and pressure.

Vertebral Veins and Deep Cervical Veins. Spasm of the suboccipital muscles may cause a decided impediment of venous drainage from the suboccipital area via the vertebral and deep cervical veins, resulting in a passive congestion with consequent pressure upon the sensory nerve endings in the area. This is sensed by the patient as unilateral or bilateral pain and a throbbing discomfort, and may be palpated as knotty lumps within suboccipital muscles.

Sympathetic Disturbances

The vertebral nerve (sympathetic) runs along the vertebral artery within the arterial foramen of the cervical transverse processes.

Neuritis is considered to occur from mechanical irritation to the vertebral artery anywhere along its course, producing symptoms of a vasomotor nature; eg, headache, vertigo, tinnitus, nasal disturbances, facial pain, facial flushing, and pharyngeal paresthesias.

Neuwirth and Kobayshi and associates report that stimulation of the cervical sympathetic trunk can cause alterations of the cerebral circulation and its regulatory mechanism. Thus, irritative lesions involving the cervical region and its articulations may in turn irritate the sympathetic nerve plexuses ascending into the head via the vertebral and carotid arteries. Baklavadzhyan's group found that the cervical sympathetic nerves had a strong influence on the vagus nerve and hypothalamus, as well as on cortical recruiting responses (Fig. 7.19).

Many cases of visual and aural symptoms occur with upper-cervical distortion where the arch of the atlas snugly hugs the occiput, thus possibly irritating the sympathetic plexus of nerves on the vertebral arteries as well as partial compression of the vessels. To appreciate this, we must remember that the visual cortical area of the occipital lobe (cuneate lobe and calcarine fissure area) requires an ideal blood supply dependent on the sympathetics ascending the great vessels of the neck, and this holds true for the inner ear as well.

DeRusha's Maneuver. To test this syndrome, De Rusha suggests having the supine patient read some printed matter while the examiner places gentle traction on the skull cephalad, separating the occipital and atlantal articulations. A positive sign occurs when the patient, often to his or her surprise, experiences momentarily enhanced visual acuity or a reduction in tinnitus.

Cailliet points out that although sympathetic fibers have not been found along the cervical roots, surgical decompression of an entrapped nerve root relieves symptoms attributed to the sympathetics. The mechanism for this effect is not clear.

Lower Cervical Subluxations

A subluxation of one or more of the lower cervical vertebrae often involves the brachial plexus (refer to Table 7.4). Because the distribution of the brachial plexus is so extensive, a multitude of abnormal reflections may be seen in its areas of distribution that must be discerned by knowledge of the pathophysiology involved. A few of the more common disturbances caused by lower cervical subluxations and trauma would include shoulder neuralgias, neuralgias along the medial arm and forearm or elbow, unclassified wrist drop and hand dystrophies, acroparesthe-

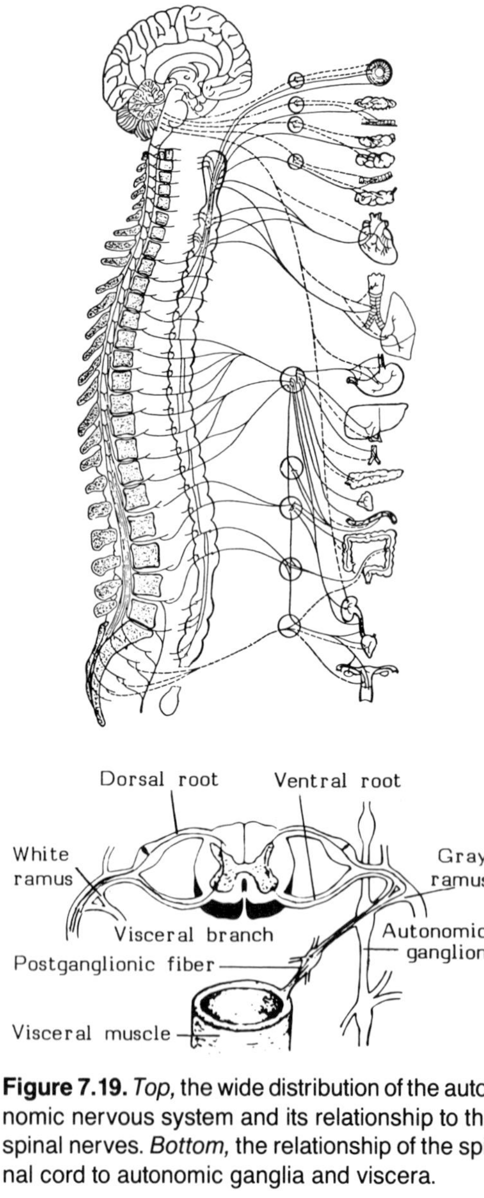

Figure 7.19. *Top,* the wide distribution of the autonomic nervous system and its relationship to the spinal nerves. *Bottom,* the relationship of the spinal cord to autonomic ganglia and viscera.

sia, weak grip strength, and vague "rheumatic" wrist or hand complaints. A subluxation of one or more of the C3, C4, or C5 segments may involve the phrenic nerve and produce symptoms of severe chronic hiccup and other diaphragmatic disorders.

Subluxation-Induced Reflex Syndromes

Various spinosomatic and spinovisceral syndromes may result from cervical subluxations. For example, the involvement may be in the area of C1—C4. This area includes the cervical portion of the sympathetic gangliated chain and the IX—XII cranial nerves as they exit from the base of the skull and pass into their compartments within the deep cervical fascia. The syndrome may include (1) suboccipital or postocular migraine, (2) greater occipital nerve extension neuralgia, (3) mandibular, cervical, auricular, pectoral, or precordial neuralgia, (4) paroxysmal torticollis, (5) congestion of the upper respiratory mucosa, paranasal sinuses, or eustachian tube with hearing loss, (6) cardiorespiratory attacks, (7) ocular muscle malfunction, (8) pathologic hiccups, (9) scalenus anticus syndrome, and (10) painful spasms in the suboccipital area.

Phillips states that if a subluxation produces a stretching of the paravertebral musculature, there will be a continuous barrage of afferent impulses in the Ia fibers. "These afferent impulses monosynaptically bombard the alpha motor neurons causing the paravertebral musculature to go into tetany (spasm). There is a cessation of this afferent barrage when the stretch is released. The muscle stretching also initiates afferent impulses in the Group II afferents from flower spray endings which may reinforce the spastic muscle condition." He goes on to say that trauma to facet joints, disturbed articular relationships, spasms of closely related muscles, and overlying trigger points—all the results of a subluxation—set up a barrage of flexor-reflex afferent impulses via Group II—IV fibers that converge upon the internuncial pool in lamina seven of the spinal cord. "This abundant supply of flexor-reflex afferent impulses excites the alpha motor neurons through multisynaptic connections causing an excess of excitation of paravertebral muscles resulting in spasm."

Neurologic Effects of Whiplash and Similar Cervical Syndromes

Severe sprain (eg, whiplash) can be assumed if cervical pain arises immediately after the accident or shortly thereafter (Fig. 7.20). Difficulty in opening the mouth (when the TMJ is intact) points to severely strained suprahyoid muscles, according to Macnab. If severe muscle splinting of the neck is accompanied by pain in the mastoid-mandible area, the possibility of fracture (probably odontoid or midcervical) must be eliminated immediately. Severe pain and spasm not arising until the following day suggest severe strain of one or more posterior cervical muscle groups. Specific involvement depends on the position of the head and neck during impact.

Pain, spasm, and related neurologic focal signs generally suggest either cord damage or root injury from associated lateral hyperflexion or dislocation that may have been spontaneously reduced. Besides neck pain, a wide variety of usually overlapping features may be exhibited after an extension injury.

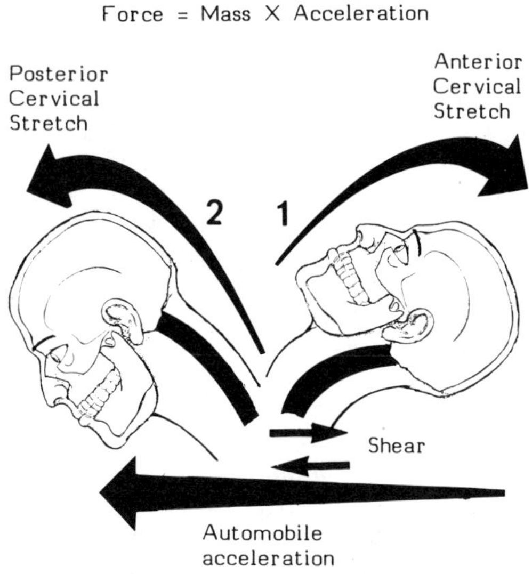

Figure 7.20. Basic kinematic mechanisms involved in a rear-end collision, showing initial and following movement sequences.

For example, expressions may be seen in:

1. Neuropathy (radiculitis, cerebral concussion, IVF fault, hoarseness, dysphagia, headache, visual disturbances, nystagmus).
2. Vasomotor disturbances (vertebral artery injury, tinnitus).
3. Musculoskeletal impairment (overt hypermobility and hypomobility at different segments, and extensive trigger point development).
4. Audiovestibular faults (deafness, vertigo).
5. Deficits of memory (cerebral concussion amnesia).

In discussing the greater occipital-trigeminal syndrome, Palmateer states that whiplash injury can cause trauma of both cervical and upper thoracic areas of the spine. The signs and symptoms may be from altered function of the cervical autonomic spinal accessory nerve, various cervical and upper thoracic nerve roots, and compression of the vertebral artery. Traction on the C2 root may cause pain to radiate through the greater occipital nerve supply to the occipital scalp and into the eye via connections with the ophthalmic division of the trigeminal nerve.

Disturbances of Hearing and Vision of Cervical Origin

In studying cervical syndromes, Chrisman/Gervais associate deafness, tinnitus, blurred vision, pain behind the eye, pupillary dilation, vertigo, and headache (unilateral or bilateral). Pang states that the audiologic symptoms, in most cases, consist of a high-frequency hearing loss and tinnitus. The tinnitus usually varies in intensity and duration, and tends to diminish with time. According to Roca and Dionne, cervical syndromes often result in such visual disturbances as decreased accommodation, nystagmus, decreased prism vergence power, aniscoria, diplopia, blurred vision, photophobia, hyperphoria, hypertropia, exotropia, ptosis, tearing, and the inability to focus. Figure 7.21 illustrates how a cervical nerve is forced against the medial aspect of the transverse process by the much larger vertebral artery.

Disturbances of Equilibrium of Cervical Origin

It has long been recognized that dizziness and/or vertigo can be caused by injury to or a disturbance in the neck muscles. The theories of the mechanism are reported by Pang, Hülse, Baloh, and Jepson to be (1) *neuromuscular*, whereby an alteration in the proprioceptive impulses from deep muscles and tissues causes the dysequilibrium; (2) *neurovascular*, in which the injury produces a disorder of the sympathetic vertebral plexus leading to changes in the blood circulation in the inner ear; and (3) *obstructive-vascular*, by which injury or degenerative processes cause physical obstruction in the vertebral artery.

Headaches of Cervical Origin

Kraus, Markovich, Bogduk, Keith, Gitelman/Fitz-Ritson, and others have noted the significance of upper-cervical disturbances in relation to headaches, occipital neuralgia,

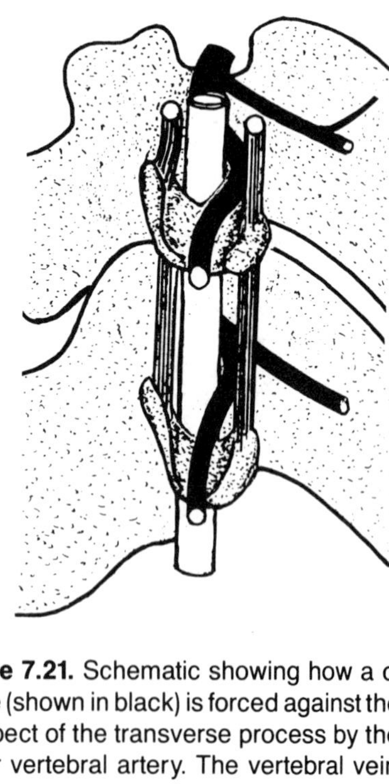

Figure 7.21. Schematic showing how a cervical nerve (shown in black) is forced against the medial aspect of the transverse process by the much larger vertebral artery. The vertebral vein is not shown.

and neck pain. Boake, an allopath, reports that at least 70% of the headache cases he sees in family practice arise from the cervical spine and associated structures, and Mayer and associates relate cervicogenic headaches with upper-cervical hypomobility.

In offering a neurologic appraisal of pain in the head, Kraus states: "It has been my experience that the most common cause of headaches originates in the 'vicious circle' generated by the abnormal and painful contraction of the cervical-nuchal muscles, mainly the trapezius muscle. These contractions generate a type of 'ischemic irritation' that includes the entrapment of the second cervical nerves (greater occipital and lesser occipital) as they travel through the bulk of the muscle, ascending into the back of the head to innervate the posterior scalp region, the temporal areas, and the lobes of the ears, sending terminal branches into the angle of the jaw, the back of the eye, and the vertex of the head." This process can create a distinct clinical syndrome that is easily confused with atypical "vascular migraine" because of the unilaterality of the symptoms and frequent complaints of pain in the back of the eye with or without visual disturbance.

Kraus also states that the second most common entity is the TMJ pain dysfunction syndrome, which has been proven to be more common than many expect and has many protean manifestations to the extent it has become known as *The Great Imposter*. "The fact that a cervical nerve irritation can create a painful condition in the angle of the jaw or in the temple explains the possible common 'irritative' source of both syndromes."

Markovich reports that the most common headache is the type caused by neuromuscular skeletal imbalance. Frykholm and Khurana/Nirankari more specifically emphasize irritation of the posterior cervical sympathetic plexus. Markovich points out that "the head in the human species has changed its position from the quadruped to the erect, thereby changing the basic relationship between the cervical spine and the head, with its important functional structures, and the rest of the body." For reference, he calls attention to the quite delicate interaction and

Table 7.5. Differentiation of Common Types of Headaches

Symptom/Sign	Occipito-cervical Neuralgia	Trigeminal Neuralgia	Vascular Migraine	Temporo-mandibular Traction
Pain	Throbbing, paroxysmal	Excruciating, paroxysmal	Severe, paroxysmal	Severe, dull
Quality	Muscle spasms	Stabbing	Throbbing	Dull ache
Location	Occipital	Facial	Unilateral	Facial
Aura	None	None	Visual	None
Duration	Days	Brief	Hours	Chronic
Associated symptoms and signs	Earache Eye pain Neck pain Paresthesias Anxiety Tinnitus Nausea	Trigger zones	Vomiting Photophobia Irritability	Bruxism Malocclusion Earache Joint clicks

highly sensitive biofeedback or servo-mechanisms that continually make adjustments in body balance, vision, pressure, and hearing with head and neck posture. "These regulatory, homeostatic mechanisms can be disturbed by a variety of conditions, originating at any level, including the inflammation and/or irritation of the cephalic projection of the upper cervical nerves (cervico-occipital neuralgias)."

Abnormal contraction of the muscles at the occipitocervical area appears to generate a type of "ischemic irritation" that includes the entrapment of the C2 nerves (greater and lesser occipital) as they pierce the thick muscle and ascend to the back of the head to supply the back of the scalp, the temples, and the ear lobes, sending branches to the top of the head, the back of the eye, and the angle of the jaw. Differentiation of various types of headaches is shown in Table 7.5, adapted from Markovich's data. However, keep in mind that a patient may not exhibit such a clear-cut picture. For example, vascular migraine may be superimposed on occipitocervical neuralgia or episodes may be interposed, depending upon the causes involved.

Neck and Arm Pain of Cervical Origin

Intervertebral Disc Syndromes

The two most common disorders of cervical IVDs are degenerative disease processes and disc protrusion (Fig. 7.22). These disorders may manifest singularly or be combined. The neurologic signs in the cervical radiculopathies are shown in Table 7.6. These features vary depending upon the direction of the disc bulge; eg, upon the nerve root, IVF vessels, spinal cord, or combinations of involvement. In some acute and many chronic cases, numbness may manifest without pain. In acute disorders, the cervical signs may be confused with those of shoulder or elbow bursitis, epicondylitis, or facet subluxation, especially when no local cervical symptoms exist.

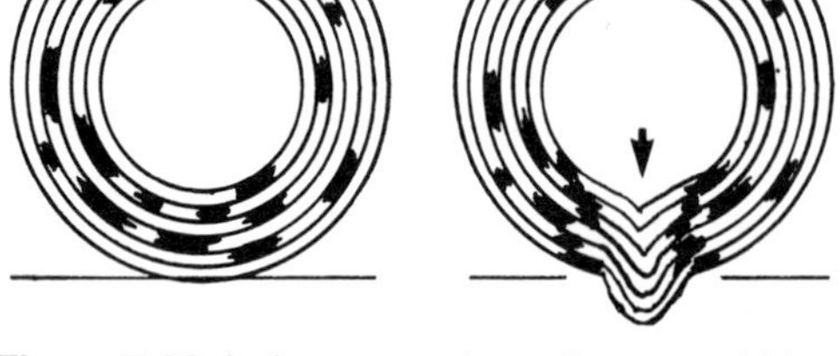

Figure 7.22. *Left,* concentric anular tears within a degenerating disc. *Right,* later progression to anular protrusion.

The clinical picture of cervical disc disorders, states Grieve, is typically a combination of "a hard osseocartilaginous spur, produced by the disc together with the adjacent margins of the vertebral bodies." Furthermore, "the mechanism by which pain and disability originate in the neck region," contends Cailliet, "can be considered broadly to result from encroachment of space or faulty movement in the region of the neck through which the nerves or blood vessels pass." This *encroachment of space* or *faulty movement* commonly comprises apophyseal subluxation with osteophyte formation, contributing to, or superimposed upon disc degeneration and/or protrusion. This occurs most frequently in the C4—C6 area.

Degenerative Disc Disease. Cervical stiffness, muscle spasm, spinous process tenderness, and restricted motion are common features. When pain is present, it is usually poorly localized and often referred to the occiput, shoulder, between the scapulae, arm or forearm (lower cervical lesion), and may be accompanied with paresthesias. Radicular symptoms rarely manifest unless a herniation is present.

Disc Protrusion or Herniation. Generally, central herniation produces local neck pain while lateral herniation produces upper extremity pain. If the protrusion is central, cord signs and symptoms exhibit as lower extremity spasticity and hyperactive reflexes. Sensory changes are rarely evident, but the gait may be ataxic. If the protrusion is posterolateral, the nerve root will be involved rather than the cord. Posterior osteophytes form at the disc attachment peripherally, often compromising the IVFs and vertebral canal. This may be noted by narrowing of the A-P dimension of the spinal canal in lateral films and foraminal encroachment on oblique films. See Figure 7.23. These signs most frequently occur at the C6—C7 level. Anterior osteophytes are considered the result of abnormal ligamentous stress rather than part of the disc degeneration process. They occur most frequently below the C4 level, as do alterations of the covertebral joints.

Spondylosis

Spondylosis is a chronic condition (that may become rapidly symptomatic) in which there is progressive degeneration of the IVDs leading to secondary changes in the surrounding vertebral structures, including the posterior apophyseal joints. It can be the result of direct trauma (eg, disc injury), occupational stress, aging degeneration, or found in association with and adjacent to congenitally defective vertebrae.

The classic picture is one of a middle-aged person with greatly restricted cervical motion, marked muscle spasm, positive cervical compression signs, insidious neck and arm

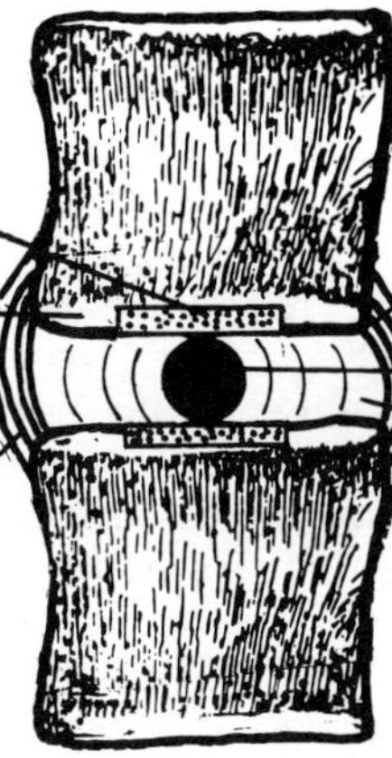

Figure 7.23. Relation of end plates to the intervertebral disc and longitudinal ligaments.

Table 7.6. Neurologic Signs in the Cervical Radiculopathies

Disc Protrusion	Nerve Root Level	Features
C2	*C3*	Posterior neck numbness and pain radiating to the mastoid and ear. The reflexes test normal.
C3	*C4*	Posterior neck numbness and pain radiating along the levator scapulae muscle and sometimes to the pectorals. The reflexes are normal.
C4	*C5*	Lateral neck, shoulder, and arm pain and paresthesia, deltoid weakness and possible atrophy, hypesthesia of C5 root distribution over middle deltoid area (axillary nerve distribution). The reflexes test normal.
C5	*C6*	Pain radiating down the lateral arm and forearm into the thumb and index finger; hypesthesia of the lateral forearm and thumb; decreased brachioradialis reflex; brachioradialis, biceps, and supinator weakness.
C6	*C7*	Pain radiating down the middle forearm to the middle and index fingers, hypesthesia of the middle fingers, decreased triceps and radial reflexes, triceps and grip weakness.
C7	*C8*	Possible pain radiating down the medial forearm and hand to the little finger, ulnar hypesthesia, intrinsic muscle weakness of the triceps and grip. However, these symptoms are uncommon. The reflexes are normal.

pain aggravated by sneezing or coughing, acute radiculopathy from disc herniation, and some muscle weakness and fasciculations. Whiting also includes neck crepitus; local neck tenderness; headaches; neck pain radiating to the scapulae, trapezius, upper extremities, occiput, or anterior thorax; paresthesia of the upper and/or lower extremities; dizziness and fainting; impaired vibration sense at the ankle; hyperactive patellar and Achilles reflexes; and positive Babinski responses.

Spondylosis may produce compression of either the nerve root or spinal cord. During the degenerative process, intradisc pressure decreases, the anulus protrudes, and the end plates approximate through reduction of disc thickness. As the disc protrudes, it loosens the attachment of the posterior longitudinal ligament. This allows the anulus to extrude into the cavity formed between the posterior vertebral body and the ligament, and this portion of the anulus, in time, becomes fibrous and then calcifies. Because of this process, posterior osteophytes prevail in the cervical and lumbar regions, while anterior spurs are more common to the dorsal spine.

Torticollis

Acquired torticollis (wry neck) is a severe stiff-neck syndrome produced by contraction of the neck muscles, causing the head to be drawn to one side with the chin pointing contralaterally. It may have a traumatic, an inflammatory, or a neuropathic origin, or be of various superimposed factors. The condition may be either continuous (tonic) or spasmodic (clonic). The tonic type is frequently seen in cervical Pott's disease of bone and psychoneurotic states. Considerable care must be taken to determine the etiology and differentiate its many possible causes.

The pain associated with acute torticollis is often thought to be attributed to zygapophyseal capsulitis and covertebral joint inflammation. This can generally be confirmed by palpation and should not be confused with the pain aroused from stretching the rigid muscles on the side of the concavity.

Cervical Subluxation. The most common direct cause of torticollis is that from irritating cervical subluxation (eg, trauma, rotational overstress, unilateral chilling, unilateral lifting, instability). Subluxation also may be an asymptomatic complicating factor to various etiologic factors. Barge believes that the structural cause of torticollis is often a rotatory vertebral malposition and abnormal disc wedging, where the nucleus of an involved disc has been forced to shift away from compressive forces. The patient's symptoms are often self-limiting with time and rest that allows the disc to expand in its nonweightbearing (decompressed) state and the vertebral facets to be relieved of their jammed position. It can be theorized that, if the neck does not achieve this subluxation correction through disc imbibition, a rotatory scoliosis will be produced in adaptation so that the patient may at least have a straight eye level. But, as the now chronic subluxation has not been fully corrected, it can serve as a focus for morbid neurologic and degenerative processes, especially at the zygapophyses, covertebral joints, and IVFs.

Inflammation. "Wry neck" spasm (tonic, rarely clonic) of the sternocleidomastoideus and trapezius may be the result of irritation of the spinal accessory nerve or other cervical nerves by swollen glands, abscess, acute upper respiratory infections, scar, or tumor. A spontaneous subluxation of the atlas may follow severe throat infection (eg, bacterial pharyngitis). Neck rigidity also may be the result of a sterile meningitis from blood in the cerebrospinal fluid. Thus, if a patient has slight fever, rapid pulse, and rigid neck muscles, subarachnoid hemorrhage should be suspected. Lateralizing signs are often inconclusive.

Neuropathic and Idiopathic Forms. Focal neuropathic causes include ocular dysfunctions, syringomyelia, and tumors of the spinal cord or brain. Idiopathic forms are seen in acute calcification of a cervical disc, rheumatic arthritis, tuberculosis, or "nervous" individuals. Nelson feels that wry neck also may be the result of a subphrenic or subclinical visceral irritation being mediated reflexly into the trapezius and cervical muscles.

Severe Trauma. Traumatic dislocations of upper cervical vertebrae cause a distortion of the neck much like that of torticollis. A rotary fracture-dislocation of a cervical vertebra, especially of the atlas on the axis or the axis on C3, will produce neck rigidity and a fast pulse, but fever is absent. Local and remote trigger points are frequently involved. Even in mildly suspicious cases, the posttraumatic neck should always be x-rayed in two or more planes before it is physically examined.

Nuchal Rigidity

The term *nuchal rigidity* refers to a spasmotic contraction of the posterior muscles of the cervical spine, but it is not identical to a stiff-neck syndrome or the various types of true torticollis. The most common cause of nuchal rigidity, by far, is meningitis. However, the sign is not pathognomonic. A number of inflammatory conditions may be involved. See Table 7.7.

Traumatic Brachial Plexus Traction

In brachial plexus trauma, the entire plexus or any of its fibers may be injured. The lateral branches of the brachial plexus lie just anterior to the glenohumeral joint. The axillary nerve lies just below the joint. As the roots of the plexus are fixed at their origin in the spinal cord, any sudden or severe traction of the upper extremity may avulse roots from the cord or stretch the plexus to the point of tearing. Attending subluxations are common.

Stretching injuries are common; tearing injuries are rare. Such injuries may be divided into three general types: total arm palsies, upper arm palsies (most common), and lower arm palsies.

Several studies have shown that peripheral nerves have considerable tensile strength

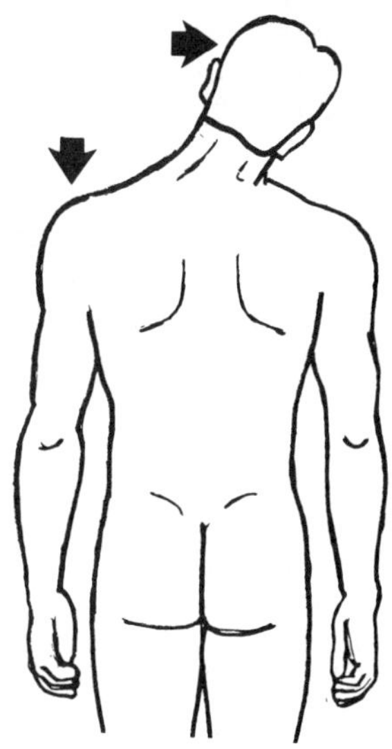

Figure 7.24. Typical forces involved in brachial plexus traction.

Table 7.7. Nuchal Rigidity and Associated Symptoms

Syndrome: Nuchal Rigidity +	Primary Suspect Disorder(s)	
Focal neurologic signs	Cerebral hemorrhage Cerebral abscess Encephalitis Meningitis	Osteomyelitis Spondylosis Subluxation (acute)
Pyrexia	Cervical pyogenic infection Meningitis	Osteomyelitis Retropharyngeal abscess Subarachnoid hemorrhage
Retinal hemorrhage and pyrexia	Collagen disease Stroke	Subarachnoid hemorrhage
Tremor and diffuse spasm	Parkinsonism	

against stretch, but nerve roots do not. Thus, excessive traction forces can create considerable stress, dural leaks, etc. Traction (tension) on the root can pull the IVF contents outward, subjecting the thicker intracanal portion of the root complex to adverse pressure and irritation.

Trauma to the brachial plexus is often seen following severe cervical lateroflexion (Fig. 7.24). The effects vary from mild to severe depending on the extent of nerve contusion, crush, or laceration. Nerve "pinch" or "stretch" syndromes also may be involved. The specific symptomatology, physical findings, roentgenography, and electromyography offer clues to the extent of damage, indicated therapy, and prognosis. Detailed examination is required because multiple nerve injury, related tendon or other soft-tissue damage, and fractured bones may complicate the picture.

Damage to an individual peripheral nerve is characterized by (1) flaccid, atrophic paralysis of the muscles supplied by the involved nerve and (2) loss of all sensation, including proprioception, in the skin areas distal to the lesion. Refer to Table 7.3. When partial destruction to various peripheral nerves occurs, the effects are usually more prominent in the distal extremities. The condition is characterized by weakness, atrophy, and poorly demarcated areas of sensory changes. Trophic lesions of the joints, muscles (atrophy), skin, and nails are common in the late stage.

Ipsilateral vs Contralateral Symptoms. If symptoms appear on the opposite side of forceful bending of the cervical spine, undoubtedly a nerve has been "pinched" within the powerful muscles dorsal to the sternocleidomastoid. If this is the case, the symptoms usually subside in a few minutes with only slight residual tenderness and paresthesia that disappears within a few hours. On the other hand, if symptoms appear on the same side as the direction of the forceful bending, deep skeletal injury such as severe rotary subluxation, fracture, dislocation, or nerve compression can usually be anticipated.

Mild or Moderate Brachial Traction. After lateroflexion injuries of the neck, a sharp burning pain may radiate along the course of one or more cervical nerves—the result of nerve hypertraction from overstretch. Scalenus anticus syndrome may be exhibited. This nerve stretch is often called a "hot shot" by athletes, and recurring injury is common, especially in contact sports. It is not limited to sports, however, for any severe cervical lateral flexion can produce the syndrome. Immediate pain may radiate to the back of the head, behind the ear, around the neck, or down toward the clavicle, shoulder, arm or hand. Frequently, there are arm paresthesias, severe arm weakness, diminished active motion, decreased biceps and triceps reflexes, forearm numbness, and cervical movement restriction. These signs and symptoms may disappear and reappear with greater severity.

Root Avulsion. A similar but more severe nerve injury is that to the proximal brachial plexus or its roots that is usually caused by a fall on the shoulder, a blow to the side of the neck, forceful arm traction, or a combination of these mechanisms. The injury is produced by forceful shoulder depression that stretches the brachial plexus especially in the supraclavicular area. The result may be root tear near the vertebral foramen, spinal cord damage, dural cuff leaks of cerebrospinal fluid, and/or vertebral subluxation, fracture, or dislocation. During avulsion, the spinal cord itself is infrequently damaged and contralateral cord symptoms are found. Such severe manifestations are rarely seen in the well-conditioned patient where the picture is usually limited to pain radiating into the arm and/or hand.

Cervical Rib and Related Syndromes

A cervical rib rising from C7 and ending free or attached to the T1 rib appears in the neck as an angular fullness that may pulsate because of the presence of the subclavian artery above it. It rarely produces symptoms, and it is usually first noticed when percussing the apex of the lung. The bone can be felt behind the artery in the supraclavicular fossa and readily demonstrated in a radiograph. Pain or wasting in the arm and occasionally thrombosis may occur from the impaired circulation.

Grieve points out that some clinicians are far too anxious to blame upper limb paresthesias on the presence of a cervical rib just because it is there. Many patients with a cervical rib have no complaints, many without a cervical rib have similar complaints, and many with complaints have symptoms on the contralateral side of a unilateral cervical rib. However, when any anomaly such as a cervical rib is seen radiographically, the examiner should be suspicious that other anomalies not as evident may be associated.

Symptoms usually occur after the age of 11: after the ribs have ossified. Two groups of symptoms are seen, those from scalenus anticus syndrome and those from cervical-rib pressure. When symptoms are exhibited, they are usually from compression of the lower cord of the brachial plexus and subclavian vessels; eg, numbness and pain of varying intensity in the ulnar nerve distribution. The pain is worse at night because of pressure from the recumbent position. Tiredness and weakness of the extremity, finger cramps, numbness, tingling, coldness of the hand, areas of hyperesthesia, muscle degeneration in the hand, a lump at the base of the neck, tremor, and discoloration of the fingers are also characteristic. Work and exercise generally accentuate these symptoms, while rest and elevation of the extremity relieve them.

Thoracic Outlet Syndromes

The cervicothoracic junction area is a unique spinal area that receives far less attention than it deserves in both medicine and chiropractic. It is a common site of developmental anomalies; it is a major site of arterial, lymphatic, and neurologic traffic; and it presents the juncture of the highly mobile cervical spine with the very limited thoracic spine. This latter point is biomechanically significant.

Etiology. The generally accepted causes of cervicobrachial syndromes are compression of the nerve trunks, trauma to nerve trunks, injuries to the sympathetic and vasomotor nerves, trauma to the scalenus anterior muscle, embryologic defects, postural or functional defects, narrowing of the upper thoracic cap as a result of adjacent infections or anatomical defects, acute infection producing myositis, intermittent trauma to the subclavian artery, or a cervical rib.

There are several defined syndromes to consider under the classification of *neurovascular compression syndromes* (also termed thoracic outlet or inlet syndromes), each of which may produce the symptom complex of radiating pain in the shoulders and down the arms, atrophic disturbance, paresthesias, and vasomotor disturbances. These syndromes, however, do not necessarily indicate the specific cause of the problem; they only define the clinical picture.

Differentiation. Two groups of symptoms are seen, those from scalenus anticus syndrome and those from cervical rib pressure. The symptoms of cervical rib and scalenus syndrome are similar, but the scalenus anticus muscle is the primary factor in the production of neurocirculatory compression whether a cervical rib is present or not. Adson's and similar compression tests will usually be positive.

Compression of nerve tissue results in numbness, pain, paralysis, and loss of function. Compression of vascular structures results in moderate pain and swelling. The obstruction of circulation can result in clotting within the vessels with possible consequent infarction in the tissues supplied. These unilateral phenomena are usually limited to the cervicobrachial distribution.

Craniovertebral Malformations

Varied anomalies arise from upper-cervical malformations. They are usually characterized by an abnormal shift upward of the atlas and axis with the odontoid protruding above Chamberlain's line. Such anomalies are frequently associated with congenital neural malformations and with other osseous deformities (eg, Klippel-Feil syndrome). Aplasia of the arch of the atlas, basilar impression, platybasia, congenital atlantoaxial instability, occipitalization, and odontoid anomalies are important considerations. As they may remain asymptomatic unless precipitated by the forces of trauma or of degeneration, a concern is that these anomalies may easily be confused with the root/

cord signs and symptoms of lower cervical spondylosis. Headache, sensory loss, limb pain, and/or ataxia are often the presenting complaints.

Cervical Ankylosing Spondylitis

Ankylosing spondylitis is characterized by spinal pain, rigidity, spasm, joint deformity, ankylosis, and loss of chest expansion. There may be loose ligaments above a rigid axis leading to atlantoaxial dislocation. Disc spaces are rarely narrowed as the ligaments and discs ossify. The patient moves as if the spine was a metal rod, with head and shoulders moving as a unit. A related fracture (usually lower cervical) through an ossified disc produces a characteristic chin-on-chest deformity, with or without paralysis from an associated epidural hemorrhage. The first signs are not often cervical but found in the dorsal spine (reduced chest expansion), lumbar spine (vertebral body "squaring"), and sacroiliac joints (erosion). The first cervical sign is usually that of reduced lateral flexion, followed by increasing gross neck flexion at rest and upper cervical subluxation. Deformity is usually greatest at the lumbar spine and hips, but spinal motion is first lost in the lower cervical area.

Cervical Pott's Disease

Cervical tuberculosis has the characteristics of joint tuberculosis elsewhere; viz, joint pain and tenderness, malposition of the bones and of the head, abscess formation, and wry neck with stiffness of the muscles of the back and neck and pain in the occiput. The patient is very protective of neck motion, and the chin is often supported by the hand if an abscess is present. Tenderness is present posteriorly on percussion and anteriorly on palpation where an abscess may be felt. Neck pain exists both day and night; it is often relieved somewhat when recumbent and frequently radiates to the occiput and shoulders. Rheumatic or traumatic torticollis, however, may present all these symptoms, and diagnosis may be impossible without the aid of other tests and diagnostic imaging. If in Pott's disease of bone the abscess causes pressure on the anterior spinal cord, a usually spastic paralysis occurs that is characterized by hyperactive reflexes, a positive Babinski, sustained clonus, and difficulty or inability to void.

Pyogenic Infection

Nontubercular pyogenic infection, most common in middle age, produces an exudative inflammation with hyperemia leading to osteoporosis and osteomyelitis. It may predispose a subluxation syndrome or be the effect of or concomitant with a subluxation syndrome. Early diagnosis is vital. The first clues are neck pain (possibly referred to the scapula or shoulder), fever, muscle spasm, and sometimes dysphagia due to a prevertebral abscess that may be palpable. In time, the end plate becomes involved and the infection enters the disc space. Bone destruction leads to collapse. The abscess may enter the cord or a paravertebral abscess may extend into the thorax, or vice versa.

Cervical Rheumatic Disease

The length of the cervical cord and cervical discs is greatest during flexion and least during extension in the normal spine. The opposite is true in the rheumatic spine because of the loss of vertebral disc and centrum height from destruction and absorption.

Neurologic Injury. Nerve roots may become entrapped within one or more IVFs from a combination of subluxation, perivascular adhesions, dural adhesions, rheumatoid nodules, granulation tissue, and sequestrated disc tissue. Neck pain, with or without radiation to the arms, weakness, feelings of instability, ataxia, and paresthesias are common symptoms. However, these cervical symptoms are difficult to differentiate if the disease initiates in the peripheral joints where signs of peripheral entrapment, myositis, tenosynovitis, and subluxated joints from tendon rupture exist. Related giddiness and fainting spells suggest an associated vertebral artery ischemia that is usually linked with an upward migration of the dens which produces a kinking of the vertebral artery at the atlantal level.

Rheumatic Atlantoaxial Subluxation. Orthopedic subluxation is always a danger, proceeding from the synovitis, apophyseal erosion, and erosion of the vertebral bodies involved that lead to instability from joint destruction and ligamentous laxity. As apophyseal erosion progresses, the dens migrates into the foramen magnum and the atlas becomes fixed to the axis to reduce the possibility of dislocation. These signs determine the severity and prognosis of the general disease. The characteristic anterior subluxation of the atlas on the axis is generally considered an adaptation change to help increase the capacity of the spinal canal as rheumatoid tissue accumulates.

Neoplasms

Malignant tumors are more common in adulthood than youth. In metastatic lesions, pain is constant, day and night, and not relieved with rest. The pain is increased by palpation, percussion, and movement. Cord tumors usually present pain with an insidious onset, but other early neurologic symptoms and signs are not always present during the early stages. Most cancerous tumors are associated with some degree of bone destruction, and a mass may or may not be palpable. Osseous tumors, benign or malignant, intramedullary or extramedullary, infrequently occur in youth. Neck pain is typical, and paralysis may or may not be present. Diagnostic imaging (x-ray, ultrasound, magnetic) is necessary to rule out such suspicions.

Vertebral Artery Syndromes

The vertebral arteries are the major source of blood supply to the cervical spinal cord and brain stem, including the medulla oblongata, pons, and midbrain. They also supply the visual cortex of the cerebrum and cerebellum via the basilar artery. For an unexplained reason, one artery is usually smaller than its mate, reports Sweat/Sievert.

Vertebral Artery Deflection

The vertebral artery is a captive vessel from C6 upward (Fig. 7.25). Extremes of rotation and flexion occur at the upper cervical region, but the four normal curves in the vertebral artery help to compensate during neck motion. Deflection may be caused by any stretching or elongation of the artery during neck injury. In later years, it is commonly associated with bony spurs from the covertebral joints or grossly hyperplastic posterior vertebral articulations from arthrosis.

Extension of the cervical spine allows the tip of the superior articular process of the posterior joint to glide forward and upward. If sufficiently mobile, the motion may cause encroachment on the vertebral artery and/or the IVF. Thus, deflection of the artery and any resulting symptoms are exaggerated by rotation and/or extension of the neck. As a result of pressure against the artery, there may be temporary lessening in the volume of blood flow. Atheromatous changes may occur later within the vascular wall. Symptoms include headache, giddiness, vertigo, nausea, vomiting, nystagmus, and suboccipital tenderness—all which may be aggravated by neck motion.

Vertebrobasilar System Patency

The vertebral arteries are unique in their course through several bony foramina, and

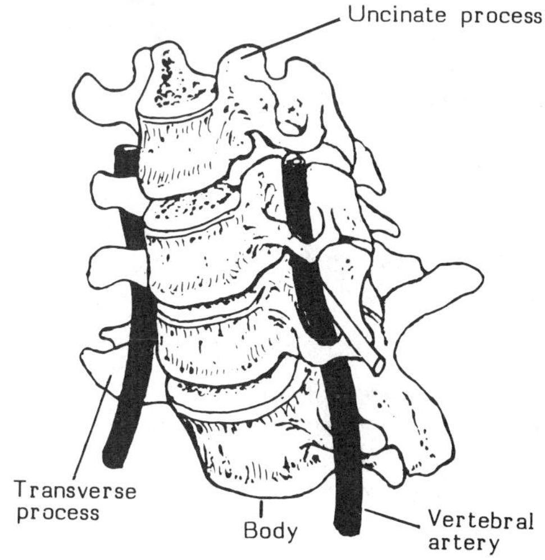

Figure 7.25. Oblique view of the lower cervical vertebrae, with the vertebral artery shown in black.

in this intermittently channeled course from C6 upward they must make four nearly right-angle turns (forming a half square) in just 20—30 mm between entering the C2 transverse and entering the foramen magnum. Adding to this tortuous course is the fact that anomalous loops occur in about one in every 5 people and the C2 area is a common site for aneurysm—allowing additional vulnerability to compressive forces.

The vertebral arteries also exhibit special features for particular sites of predilection for degeneration by the change of fixed and unfixed vessel parts, increased vulnerability to bone and muscle movements, and the occlusion of peripheral arteries in their circulation area by difficult to diagnose pathologic changes of the vascular walls. These factors mandate that the probability of advanced degenerative or inflammatory process involving these arteries be eliminated prior to cervical manipulation or adjustments. Trauma to the vertebral artery has even been reported after emergency resuscitation procedures where passive extension of the neck is usually necessary to insert an airtube.

According to Jepson, Milne, and others, any minor compromise (eg, compression, atherosclerosis, thrombosis, vasospasm, kinking, longus colli and scalenus anticus spasm) producing an insufficiency of blood flow can lead to a singular symptom or a large number of seemingly unrelated cranial manifestations such as occipital headaches, memory lapses, dizziness, tinnitus, nausea and vomiting, lightheadedness or syncope, intermittent blurred vision, suboccipital tenderness, and, sometimes, retro-occular pain (episodic), speech impairment, extremity paresthesia and weakness, drop attacks, and gait defects—all which can be generally grouped under the title of *Barré-Lieou syndrome*, especially when cervical trauma and an underlying spondylosis are involved. These signs and symptoms, which sometimes fluctuate from side to side, can mimic a post-

Table 7.8. Major Muscles of the Trunk

Muscle	Major Functions	Spinal Segment
Diaphragm	Inspiration	C4
Erector spinae	Extension	T1—S3
External oblique	Rotation, flexion, forced respiration	T1—T11
Intercostals, external	Inspiration, extension	T1—T11
Intercostals, internal	Expiration, extension	T1—T11
Interspinalis	Extension, lateral flexion, rotation	T1—S3
Intertransversarii	Lateral flexion, rotation	T1—T8
Internal oblique	Rotation, flexion, forced respiration	T7—T11
Longissimus dorsi	Extension	T1—L5
Multifidus	Extension, lateral flexion, rotation	T1—S3
Quadratus lumborum	Extension	T12—L3
Rectus abdominis	Flexion, forced respiration	T7—T11
Rotators	Extension, lateral flexion, rotation	T1—S3
Semispinalis	Extension, lateral flexion, rotation	T1—S3
Serratus posterior inferior	Expiration	T9—T11
Serratus posterior superior	Inspiration	T1—T4
Spinalis thoracis	Extension	T1—S3
Transverse abdominis	Forced respiration	T7—L1

Note: Spinal innervation varies somewhat among people. The spinal nerves listed here are averages and may differ in a particular patient; thus, an allowance of a segment above and below those listed in most text tables should be considered.

traumatic cervical syndrome, multiple sclerosis, amyotrophic lateral sclerosis, or a tumor within the posterior fossa.

Severe interference (eg, thrombosis, osteophytic kinking, spondylotic foraminal impingement, extension effects of IVD degeneration) leads to involvement of the nucleus ambiguous of the vagus (eg, dysphagia, ipsilateral palatal weakness), descending root and nucleus of cranial V (ipsilateral facial hypesthesia, especially around the lips), descending sympathetic fibers (Horner's syndrome), vestibular nuclei (rotary nystagmus), midbrain and cerebellum (ipsilateral arm/leg malcoordination, intention tremor, ataxia), spinothalamic tract (contralateral hypesthesia), and the effects of impaired venous drainage and CSF flow *(Wallenberg's syndrome)*.

Effects from Cervical Manipulation

It can be readily projected that the many cranial-oriented symptoms that have been relieved by chiropractic adjustments to the cervical region can be attributed to normalization of vertebral artery blood flow. Here we have a clinical paradox in that the same treatment may cause possible distress if precautions are not taken.

Reports of adverse effects (eg, paraplegia) from brainstem ischemia due to mechanical compression of the vertebral artery, dislodgment of a plaque, or a reflex spasm following forced rotation and extension of the head are rare. A Swiss study reported by Dvorak/Orelli states that slight neurologic complications are observed in only 1 out of 400,000 manipulations.

SELECTED THORACIC CONSIDERATIONS

The major muscles of the trunk and their source of innervation are shown in Table 7.8.

Structural Considerations

Several unique factors should be considered regarding the stability of the thoracic spine. The major points are that it: (1) is stiffer, (2) is less mobile, (3) has a smaller vertebral canal, (4) has a high incidence of cord damage associated with structural damage, (5) exhibits less vascularity for the cord, (6) has restricting costal articulations, (7) has an increased moment of inertia because of the added thoracic cage, (8) has an anatomic curvature directed posteriorly, (9) tends to be clinically unstable during flexion, (10) has thin discs, (11) is a common site for bursting anterior centrum fractures (lower region only), (12) has the nuclei more centered within the anuli, (13) has thicker yellow ligaments, (14) has thinner and looser apophyseal capsules, (15) has thinner and weaker interspinous ligaments, (16) has a great resistance to extension, (17) possesses coupling variants from top to bottom, and (18) is the major source of supply of sympathetic fibers. See Figure 7.26.

Thoracic Subluxation/Fixation Syndromes

The entire thoracic region is prone to a large number of various muscular, ligamen-

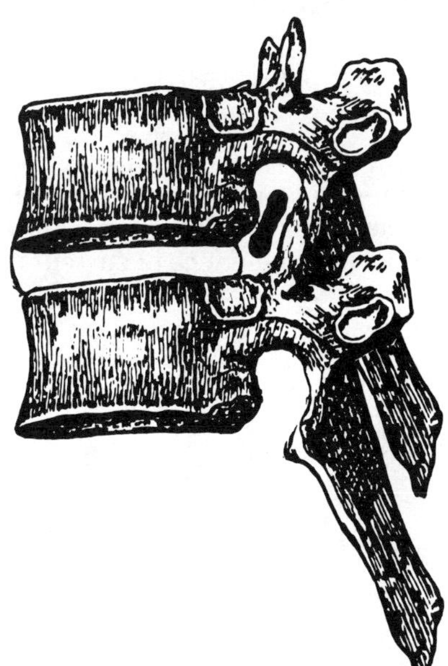

Figure 7.26. The position of the nerve root within the thoracic region is directly anterior to the facets. Most nerve roots occupy about 50% of the ovoid foraminal space.

tous, and costovertebral subluxation/fixations. In addition, primary thoracic fixations tend to produce secondary areas of fixation in the cervical spine, according to the studies of Gillet. In addition, it is a rare thoracic spine that does not exhibit some areas of tenderness upon careful palpation, and there are undoubtedly more trigger points and reflex fasciculations located upon the thoracic walls than any other area of the body.

The lower thoracic region (T9—T12) is predisposed to fixation development more than any other area of the spine. This is likely from the abrupt change in facet planes between the superior and inferior processes of the transitional vertebra, the altered stiffness between thoracic and lumbar vertebrae, the lack of strong supporting muscles enjoyed by the lumbar region, the lack of firm anterior support of the floating ribs, and the large compressive forces concentrated at this area. A sudden change in the stiffness properties of a structure at a given point will subject the structure to stress concentration at that point. This can lead to eventual mechanical failure with resulting neurologic implications. Intercostal neuralgia of the abdominal wall, states Carnett, often simulates gallbladder disease.

Vertebral Subluxations

Probably more than any other region, the thoracic region can be considered a critical zone neurologically and biomechanically, though the predominance of current literature emphasizes the importance of its neighboring regions—the cervical and lumbar spine. Vertebral facet subluxation syndromes, with or without severe fixation, are commonly found in general practice and frequently associated with visceral autonomic symptoms (Fig. 7.27). With the well-developed muscular person subluxation is more commonly associated with acute symptoms of paravertebral strain and sprain.

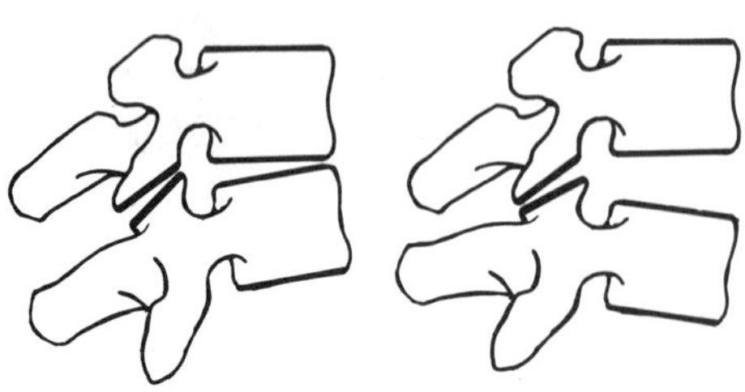

Figure 7.27. Mechanical instability of the intervertebral disc allows considerable abnormal flexion and extension at the posterior joints rather than the normal gliding movements. This state, exaggerated in the drawings, can readily lead to acute subluxation and degenerative changes.

Costovertebral and Costotransverse Fixations

These conditions are usually the result of hypertonic muscles or ligament shortening (eg, the anterior or posterior longitudinal ligaments). Unilateral pain, either stabbing or dull and usually episodic, may be expressed centrally and/or intercostally. The onset is usually rapid following a fall, push, misstep, stretch, sneeze, or cough. Transient but sharp neuralgia, angina, or dyspnea may be reported. Site tenderness, intercostal spasm, and tissue resistance are found at the rib angle and/or near the vertebral or sternal attachments. A midthoracic rib subluxation frequently presents pain radiating down the lateral arm, mimicking a scapulocostal syndrome.

Symptoms are frequently aggravated during deep inspiration when the trunk is flexed. Compressing the rib cage increases pain in fracture and sprain but not in intercostal strain. Springing the ribs P-A of the prone and relaxed patient to create stress at the vertebral connections aggravates symptoms and causes an immediate apprehensive muscle-guarding response in sprain and subluxation. Overreaction should make an examiner suspicious of a hidden fracture.

Thoracic Disc Lesions

The position of the protrusion determines the clinical picture. A midline protrusion usually produces intermittent pain, sensory impairment, pyramidal signs, and possibly bowel and bladder symptoms. Blits states that protrusion laterally causes more pain, is radicular in distribution, and is associated with fewer cord signs. The position of the normal anulus is shown in Figure 7.28.

Thoracic cord signs probably arise because there is less vertebral canal space here for the spinal cord than in other regions of the spine. Thus, a slight posterior disc or end-plate protrusion may manifest cord and cerebrospinal flow symptoms and referred neurovascular signs and symptoms in the thoracic region that would never manifest in the cervical or lumbar spine (Fig. 7.29). Added to this fact is the poor vascularity of the thoracic cord as compared to the cervical cord or even the cauda equina. Although the thoracic cord is comparatively small, its free space is extremely limited.

In moderate cases, the clinical picture is one of relative pain, usually unilateral in chronic cases or bilateral in acute cases, with girdle-like distribution. Baker emphasizes the associated intense girdle pain to be characteristic of a thoracic disc lesion. The pain may radiate to the abdomen, flank, or groin. Spastic paraparesis with sensory complaints may be involved. Motion restriction and tenderness on percussion may be the only local physical signs. Hyperactive tendon reflexes in the lower extremity and a positive Babinski reflex are sometimes seen. If disc protrusion interferes with spinal fluid flow, symptoms may mimic multiple sclerosis, arteriosclerotic myelopathy, etc.

In the *upper thoracic spine*, the pain of a herniated disc usually radiates anteriorly along the involved intercostal nerve. If the T1 root is involved, pain usually radiates down the medial aspect of the arm to the little finger. Sensory loss may be found on the medial side of the forearm, hand, little finger, and half the ring finger. Weakness is exhibited in the intrinsic muscles of the hand. If the T2 root is involved, pain will be referred to the axilla and the medial aspect of the arm. In the *midthoracic spine*, the pain and sensory impairment are intercostal (dermatomal) in nature. In the *lower thoracic spine*, the pain is referred anteriorly to the abdomen, pelvic organs, or groin, depending on the level of involvement. Segmental sensory impairment will help to isolate the lesion.

The associated symptoms of common posterior thoracic pain syndromes are differentiated in Table 7.9.

Spinal Tumors

Naffziger's test gives credence to a suspicion of an abnormal space-occupying mass such as a spinal tumor or disc protrusion. It is performed by having the patient sit or recline while the examiner holds digital pressure over the jugular veins for 30—45 seconds. The patient is then instructed to cough deeply. Pain following the distribution of a nerve may indicate nerve root compression. Though more commonly used for low back involvements, signs of thoracic and cervical root compression also may be aggravated.

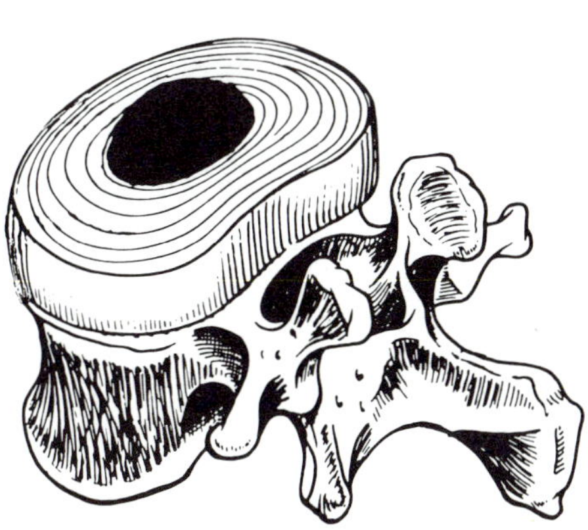

Figure 7.28. Drawing of a vertebra showing its superior disc. The nucleus pulposus is depicted in black, surrounded by the rings of the anulus.

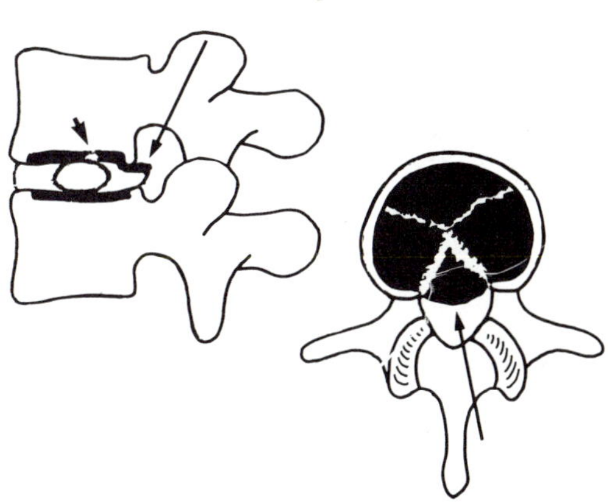

Figure 7.29. Slipped end plate (in black) mimicking nuclear protrusion, as viewed from the lateral and superior. Arrows point to IVF encroachment.

Local pain in the spine does not positively indicate nerve compression; it may indicate the site of a strain, sprain, or another lesion. The sign is invariably positive in the presence of cord tumors, particularly spinal meningiomas. The resulting increased intrathecal pressure above the tumor or disc protrusion causes the mass to compress or pull upon sensory structures to produce radicular pain. The test is contraindicated in geriatrics and extreme care should be taken with any person suspected of having atherosclerosis. In all cases, the patient should be alerted that jugular pressure may result in vertigo.

Thoracic Scoliosis

Scoliosis is a mechanical disorder, but there are always many biologic influences operating as well as purely mechanical forces. The disease processes that are commonly involved with thoracic biomechanical defects are subluxations, disc protrusions and diseases, infections, epiphyseal disorders, tumors, chronic pulmonary disorders, and adverse metabolic manifestations.

Effect of Sensory Input Deficit

Experiments on animals by MacEwen in England have shown that transection of the dorsal root causes a defect in sensory input that produces scoliosis. In each case, the resulting curve was to the side of the disrupted neural elements. Alexander and associates have demonstrated that such a transection also produces a related spinal cord motor impairment.

Involvement of the Righting Reflexes

Separate studies by Michelsson and Ponsetti have shown that unilateral labyrinthine

Table 7.9. Posterior Thoracic Pain and Associated Symptoms

Syndrome: Posterior Thoracic Pain +	Primary Suspect Disorders	
Hematuria	Kidney stone	Pyelonephritis
Neurologic focal signs	Multiple myeloma Spinal cord tumor Spinal tuberculosis	Subluxation complex Vertebral fracture
Pain, local	Aortic aneurysm Carcinoma Multiple myeloma Osteoarthritis	Scoliosis Spinal tuberculosis Spondylitis Sprain/strain
Pain, radiating	Costovertebral subluxation IVD syndrome Pyelonephritis	Radiculitis Rib fracture Spinal cord tumor Trigger point
Pain, upper abdominal	Cholecystitis Duodenal ulcer Gastric ulcer	Hiatal hernia Pancreatic carcinoma Pancreatitis
Pyrexia	Epidural abscess Hodgkin's disease Meningitis Osteomyelitis	Perinephric abscess Poliomyelitis Retrocecal appendicitis Tuberculosis

stimulation or removal have resulted in scoliosis. This points to the delicate relationship between righting reflexes and spinal balance and offers an explanation to how cervical disrelationships with vertebral artery or autonomic effects can produce scoliosis. Yamada found that 99 out of 100 scoliotic patients studied had an associated equilibrium defect and that the greater the spinal distortion, the greater the dysfunction in the proprioceptive and optic reflex systems. These observations, however, have not been confirmed by research in this country.

Pulmonary Impairment

Maximum breathing capacity is usually reduced in proportion to the degree of thoracic scoliosis present. According to Gucker's studies, gross rotary deformity appears to affect cardiopulmonary function to a greater extent than gross lateral deformity. Mechanical pulmonary impairment is not usually a priority concern unless the deformed rigid thoracic cage reaches a point that restricts the pulmonary volume and vital capacity adequate for the demand. This is not to say that restriction far below this threshold will not predispose the patient to numerous cardiorespiratory disorders though there are no signs of obstructive pulmonary disease.

In spinal deformity, the reduced vital capacity may not be due solely to mechanical restriction because weakened thoracic and possibly abdominal muscles, costal fixations, thoracic venous and lymph flow restrictions, and portal pooling are also invariably involved in severe scoliosis. Most of these nonmechanical influences can be attributed to subtle secondary sympathicotonia.

As the spinal deformity increases, the heart is forced downward and traction is placed on its superior nerves and vessels. Arterial restriction in the lung fields leads to right ventricular hypertrophy. While the effects may be perceived by cardiac auscultation, its cause is almost impossible to detect on roentgenography. Cardiorespiratory failure is so slow in these cases that the distortion and its neuromuscular and neurovascular causes are rarely given the credit they deserve.

SELECTED LUMBAR CONSIDERATIONS

The segmental innervation of the lumbosacral spine is shown in Table 7.10, and nerve functions of the lumbosacral plexus are shown in Table 7.11.

The Lumbar Nociceptive Receptor System

Wyke, Gunn, and Lamb report that the lumbar ligaments and fascia are richly innervated by nociceptors. When the lumbar spine is in a relaxed neutral position, its nociceptive receptor system is somewhat inactive. However, any mechanical force that will stress or deform receptors, with or without overt damage, or any irritating chemical of sufficient concentration will depolarize unmyelinated fibers and enhance afferent activity.

Static postural support of the lumbar spine in the prolonged relaxed erect or seated postures is provided primarily by the passive elastic tension of the involved capsules, ligaments, and fascia rather than the spinal muscles whose roles can be considered insignificant during a state of relaxation. This shifting of support from the muscles to the ligaments, however, occurs slowly over a period of several minutes before significant EMG activity can be considered absent.

Mechanical and Chemical Factors of Low Back Pain

According to Calin, Waddell and associates, Kelsey, Frymoyer/Pope, and others, low-back pain experienced after trauma can be the result of mechanical factors, chemical factors, or both.

Features of Mechanical Pain

Normal mechanical force applied to normal tissue does not produce pain. However, abnormal mechanical deformation occurs whenever (1) abnormal stress is applied to normal tissues (eg, postural pain), (2) abnormal stress is applied to abnormal tissues, or (3) normal stress is applied to abnormal tissues (eg, soft-tissue shortening). Pain from mechanical causes is sharp, acute, and occurs immediately. If mechanical pain does not occur until several minutes or hours after an activity, it is most likely that the position assumed following the activity is the cause of the pain rather than the activity itself.

Mechanical pain may be intermittent, appearing and disappearing, or vary in intensity according to aggravating and beneficial circumstances. It is usually intermittent because of increased and decreased mechanical deformation forces. *In cases of pain of mechanical origin, the examiner should be able to reproduce the patient's symptoms by test movements.* Continuous pain from constant mechanical deformation (eg,

Table 7.10. Segmental Innervation of the Lumbosacral Spine

Segment	Major Muscles Supplied
L1—2	Cremaster
L1—5	Iliopsoas
L2—3	Sartorius, pectineus, abductor longus
L2—4	Quadriceps, gracilis, adductor brevis
L3—4	Obturator externus, adductor magnus and minimus
L4—5	Tibialis anticus
L4—S1	Semimembranosus, semitendinosus, extensor hallucis longus, popliteus, plantaris, extensor digitorum longus, extensor hallucis brevis, gluteus medius and minimus, quadratus
L5—S1	Peroneus longus and brevis, tibialis posticus, flexor digiti brevis, abductor hallucis
L5—S2	Gluteus maximus, obturator internus, biceps femoris, soleus, gastrocnemius, flexor hallucis longus
S1—2	Lumbricales, piriformis, abductor digiti, flexor digiti, opponens, quadratus plantae, interossei
S2—4	Levator ani, bulbocavernosus, ischiocavernosus
S4—5	Sphincter vesicae
S5—Cx1	Sphincter ani, coccygeus

Skin Reflexes		Tendon Reflexes	
L1—2	— Cremasteric	*L2—4*	— Patellar
L4—S1	— Gluteal	*L5—S2*	— Achilles
S1—2	— Plantar		
S5—Cx1	— Anal		

Table 7.11. Nerve Functions of the Lumbosacral Plexus

Nerve	Function
Iliohypogastric	Sensory to skin over hypogastric and lateral gluteal areas.
Ilioinguinal	Sensory to skin over genitalia and upper medial thigh area.
Genitofemoral	Sensory to skin over scrotum, upper anterior thigh area; motor to cremaster.
Lateral femoral cutaneous	Sensory to skin over lateral thigh
Obturator	Motor to adductor longus, brevis, magnus; obturator externis; gracilis.
Muscular branches	Motor to major and minor psoas, quadratus femoris, gemellus inferior and superior, piriformis, obturator internus.
Femoral	Sensory to skin over anterior and medial thigh, knee, leg, dorsum of foot to base of 1st metatarsal. Motor to iliacus, pectineus, sartorius, quadriceps femoris.
Superior gluteal	Motor to gluteus minimus and medius, tensor fascia lata.
Inferior gluteal	Motor to gluteus maximus.
Posterior femoral	Sensory to skin over inferior buttock, posterior thigh, cutaneous popliteal space, perineum, external genitalia.
Sciatic	Sensory to skin over posterolateral aspect of leg and lateral foot; heel; over upper third of lateral aspect of leg below knee; over anterolateral aspect of leg and dorsum of foot and toes; medial aspect of sole, great toe, 2nd to 4th toes; lateral aspect of sole, 4th and 5th toes; on dorsum of foot between great toe and 2nd toe. Motor to hamstrings, adductor magnus, gastrocnemius, plan taris, soleus, popliteus, tibialis anterior and posterior, flexor and extensor digitorum longus and brevis; peroneus longus, brevis, and tertius; abductor and adductor hallucis, flexor hallucis brevis, extensor hallucis longus, quadratus plantae, abductor digiti quinti brevis, all interossei, 1st through 4th lumbricales.
Pudendal	Sensory to skin of genitalia, anus, scrotum, labium majorus, penis, clitoris. Motor to levator ani, coccygeus, sphincter ani externus, transversus perinei superficialis, profundus, bulbocaver nosus, ischiocavernosus, sphincter urethrae membranacae.

irreducible disc protrusion) is always possible but not common. The rule to remember is that *pain of mechanical origin is affected by movement*, for better or worse.

Features of Chemical Pain

Chemical irritants accumulate in damaged tissue soon after injury. As soon as the nociceptive receptor activity is enhanced, pain will be experienced. Chemical irritation can be the result of any inflammatory, infectious, or traumatic process of sufficient degree. It also can be the result of any abnormal metabolic by-product, especially that of ischemia when of sufficient concentration to irritate bare nerve endings in the involved tissues.

In contrast to pain of mechanical origin, pain from chemical causes is constant, dull, and aggravated by normal movements as long as the chemical irritants are present in sufficient concentration. It may not occur until several minutes or hours after an injurious event has taken place. Chemical pain subsides during the natural healing process as scar tissue forms. Rarely does chemical pain from trauma extend pass 20 days after the accident.

Considerations in Adjustive Therapy

The specific motion that eases pain the most (reduces mechanical deformation) frequently determines the plane of adjustive therapy. One important exception to this would be the pain produced by motion that stretches shortened tissues. This type of pain subsides immediately when passive stress is removed and the joint returns to its neutral position.

In either subluxation or displaced IVD substance (viz, an end plate, anulus, or nucleus pulposus), a dynamic adjustment is most often given in the direction that *decreases* mechanical deformation and pain. When shortened tissues are involved, slow rhythmic manipulation increasing in force should be given in the direction that stretches the contracted tissues and temporarily *increases* pain. In some instances, an adjustment will be necessary to free adhesions and locked facets. Obviously, this requires careful differentiation prior to therapy.

Lumbar Subluxation/Fixation Syndromes

The articulations of the lower back are located central to the kinematic chain extending from the cranium to the feet. Thus, any alteration in normal dynamics such as a unilateral fixation must manifest biomechanical effects both above and below. Fixation at a link or links of any kinematic chain forces hypermobility and aberrant movements on the nearest possible segments, leading to neurologic and musculoskeletal signs and symptoms.

Rotational malpositions of the lower lumbar vertebrae are frequently found and invariably associated with changes in the related disc and posterior joints. In addition, rotation is coupled with tilting and vice versa. It is usually impossible to tell what is primary and what is secondary as each can cause the other. Periodic recurrence after correction can usually be attributed to congenital asymmetry of the facet planes or acquired asymmetry from the repeated deformation forces of trauma.

Whenever a vertebral motion segment is in a state of prolonged distortion, the involved connective tissues histologically adapt to their biomechanical requirements. Fibers on the side of the concavity shorten, and fibers on the side of the convexity lengthen. This process occurs in all connective tissues but becomes more overt in muscular and ligamentous tissues because motion is no longer symmetrical. Unless corrective action is taken, this state becomes progressively degenerative as the result of the abnormal weight distribution during static and dynamic activity.

Refer to Table 3.12 for the major neurologic signs in the lumbosacral radiculopathies.

Neurogenic Low-Back Pain Syndromes

Because more research has been done on the IVD than any other structure, there is a tendency to attribute almost any type of backache to some type of disc disorder. This leads to tunnel vision on the part of some clinicians because many disorders, both spinal and extraspinal, may simulate disc disease. The most common causes of nondisc functional pain are postural fatigue, spinal strains (acute and chronic), and IVF syndromes. Certain pelvic disorders also may be involved such as chronic abdominal collapse, pelvic infections or neoplasms, sacroiliac sprain, and coccygeal stress.

Acute Lumbosacral Angle Syndromes

An acute lumbosacral angle is frequently associated with low-back pain. The painful status of acute angulation of L5 on S1 is twofold: (1) There is bursal involvement due to an overriding of the facets that stretches the bursa. (2) There is a narrowing of the IVF, causing a telescoping of the facet joints from the superior to the inferior.

Intervertebral Disc Syndromes

Episodic back pain is probably the only consistent symptom in IVD syndromes, and even this may not be present until the late stage (Fig. 7.30). Disc pain is usually intermittent and mechanically aggravated by standing, lifting, coughing, prolonged flexion (eg, while shaving or stooping), or a slight misstep. For some unknown reasons, these episodes often occur early in the day when

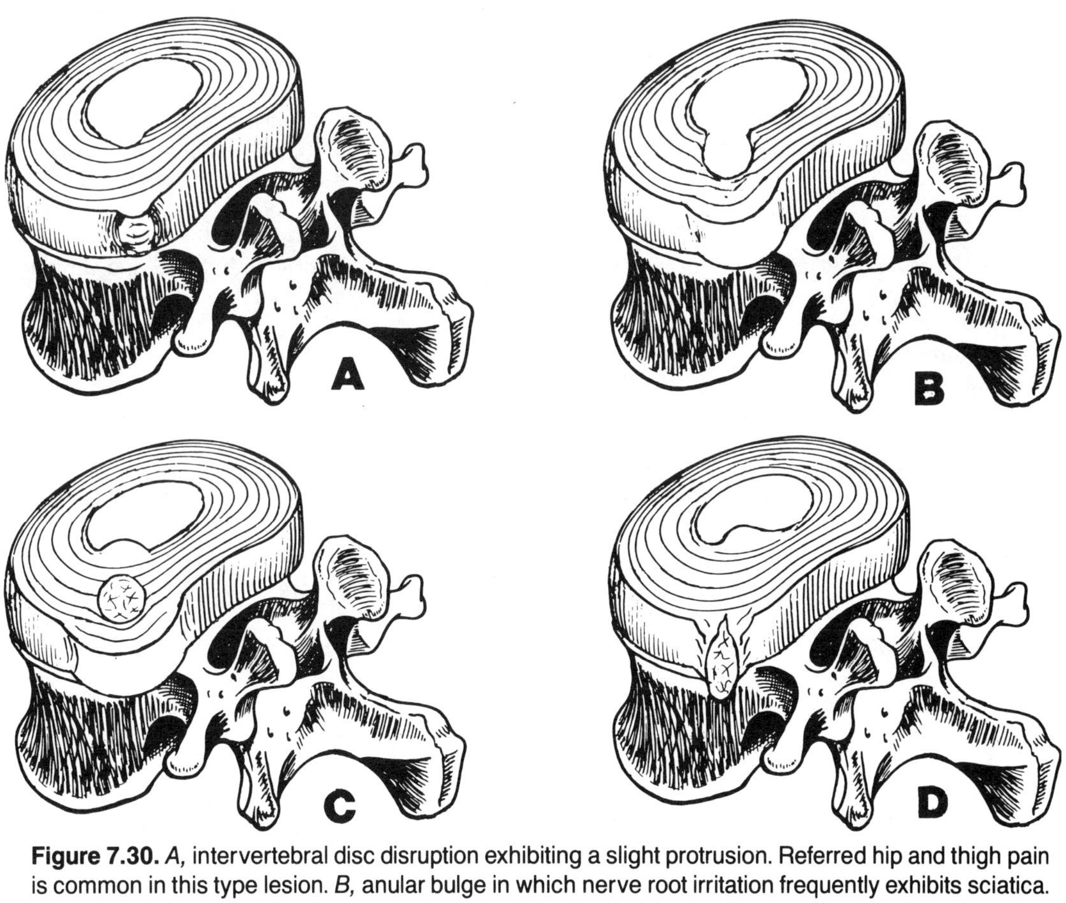

Figure 7.30. *A,* intervertebral disc disruption exhibiting a slight protrusion. Referred hip and thigh pain is common in this type lesion. *B,* anular bulge in which nerve root irritation frequently exhibits sciatica. *C,* disc disruption with a floating, isolated nuclear fragment. Pain usually exacerbates with an increase in intra-abdominal pressure or certain movements. *D,* disc showing a ruptured sequestration. The nuclear fragment may or may not be anchored at some point.

Table 7.12. Differentiation of Nerve, Root, and Cord Lesions

Nerve Lesions	Caudal-Root Lesions	Lumbosacral Cord Lesions
Usually unilateral	Usually bilateral, but not symmetrical	Usually bilateral and symmetrical
Pain on pressure over nerve trunks common	Not present; superficial hyperalgesia or anesthesia dolorosa	Not present
Symptoms present in nerve distribution	Symptoms in segmental distribution	Symptoms in segmental distribution
Pain often aggravated by movement, but spontaneous pain not severe	Spontaneous pain is often severe; movement of limbs not painful; coughing, sneezing are painful	Pain absent unless nerve roots are implicated
Sensory loss involves pain, touch, temperature	Same	Sensory dissociation may be present with unilateral lesions in upper lumbar segments
Reflexes lost in areas affected; others are not increased	Same	Achilles reflex may be absent and patellar increased or vice versa, or all reflexes may be lost
Seldom involve dorsal divisions of peripheral nerves	Involve both dorsal and ventral distributions	Involve both dorsal and ventral distributions
Muscle atrophy and reaction of degeneration may be present	Same	Same
Fibrillation in muscles absent or slight	Same	Fibrillation of muscles active
Trophic sores absent	Trophic sores unusual or mild	Trophic sores common and severe
Sphincters not affected	Sphincters may be affected	Sphincters usually affected
No loss of sexual function	Often some loss of sexual function	Sexual function lost or dissociated
X-ray negative	X-ray may show pathology below L1 (fracture, dislocation, caries)	X-rays may show some pathology in T11, T12, or L1

nuclear turgor is at its maximum. The major points of differentiation for nerve, root, and cord lesions are shown in Table 7.12.

Unilateral sciatic pain following a specific dermatome and not remissive except by a possible position of relief is often manifested. There is usually a C scoliosis away from the side of pain, splinting, and a flattening of the lumbar spine. Lasegue's, Kemp's, and Naffziger's tests are positive. There may be diminished tendon reflexes of the involved segment and possible weakness and/or atrophy of the musculature innervated.

An IVD protrusion initially impinges on the recurrent meningeal nerve in or just medial to the IVF (Fig. 7.31), according to Wyke. At this stage, he feels that the centralized pain produced (without sciatica) is the result of pressure interrupting afferent mechanoreceptor activity and irritating the afferent nociceptive fibers. As the protrusion increases, impingement begins to involve the dorsal nerve roots and their dura sleeves, leading to increased pain extending more peripherally and the development of paresthesias within the distribution of the sciatic nerve. The initially central pain in the midline spreads across the lumbosacral area, into the buttocks and thigh, and possibly as distal as the calf and heel as the lesion becomes worse.

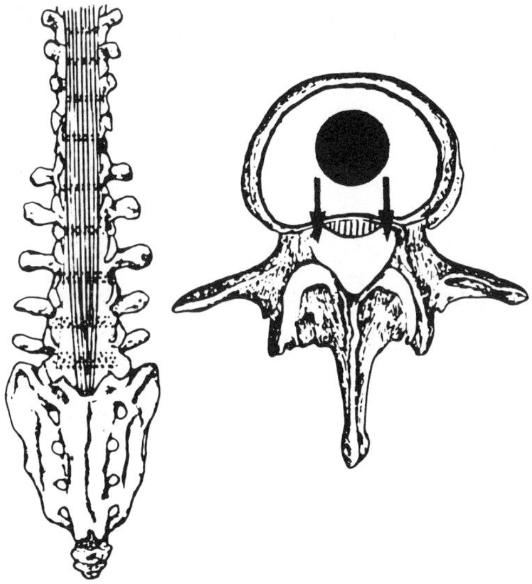

Figure 7.31. *Left,* schematic of the posterior longitudinal ligament. Note how it narrows as it descends the lumbar region, where forces tend to be unrestricted by the strap. The posterior arch of the spine has been removed in the drawing. *Right,* view from above. Arrows show posterolateral areas of disc weakness, where the ligament protects only centrally.

During early disc degeneration, it is impossible to differentiate disc failure from other causes of backache such as instability or postural overstress. Sciatica is frequently absent during the early stage, but it may be elicited by a strong Valsalva maneuver. Many patients with chronic or recurring low back pain exhibit no evidence of a degenerative process, and many patients that display obvious signs of a degenerative process have no low back pain.

A rule of thumb holds that if the protrusion is lateral to the nerve root, the patient will lean laterally away from the side of lesion and the sciatic pain. If the protrusion is medial to the nerve root, the list of the trunk will be toward the side of the lesion and the sciatica.

Facet Syndromes

It has been a popular belief that damage to a facet joint is always secondary to disc failure. However, Farfan, Grieve, and others state that autopsy evidence is clear that varying degrees of facet damage can and frequently do occur that are not secondary to disc failure. Helfet/Lee affirm that lesions of the posterior joints always have an effect on the disc, and disc lesions always have an effect on the posterior joints (Fig. 7.32).

The subluxation of lumbar facet structures, states Howe, is a part of all lumbar dyskinesias and must be present if a motion unit is deranged. In a three-point articular arrangement, such as that present at each vertebral segment, no disrelationship can exist that does not derange two of the three articulations. Thus, determination of the integrity of or subluxation of the facets in any given motion unit is important in assessing that unit's status (Fig. 7.33).

To help differentiate the low back and sciatic neuralgia of a facet syndrome from that of a protruding disc, several physical clues are available. For example, with the patient standing with the feet moderately apart, the

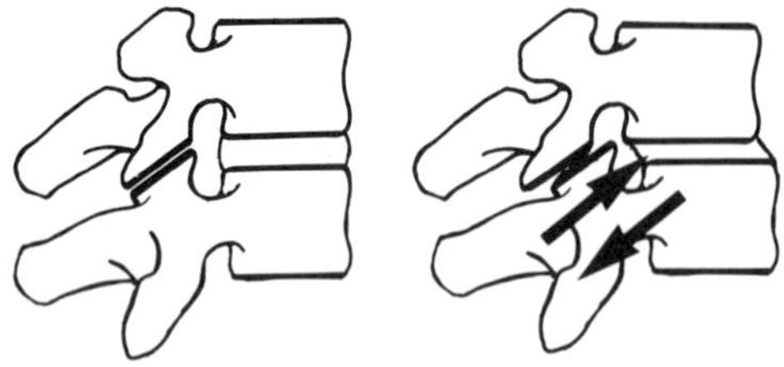

Figure 7.32. *Left,* normal motion unit relationships. *Right,* during abnormal facet motions (eg, thinned disc), a scrubbing action can take place at the posterior facets that sets up the various stages of inflammation, repair, and adhesions that can lead to sites of fixation.

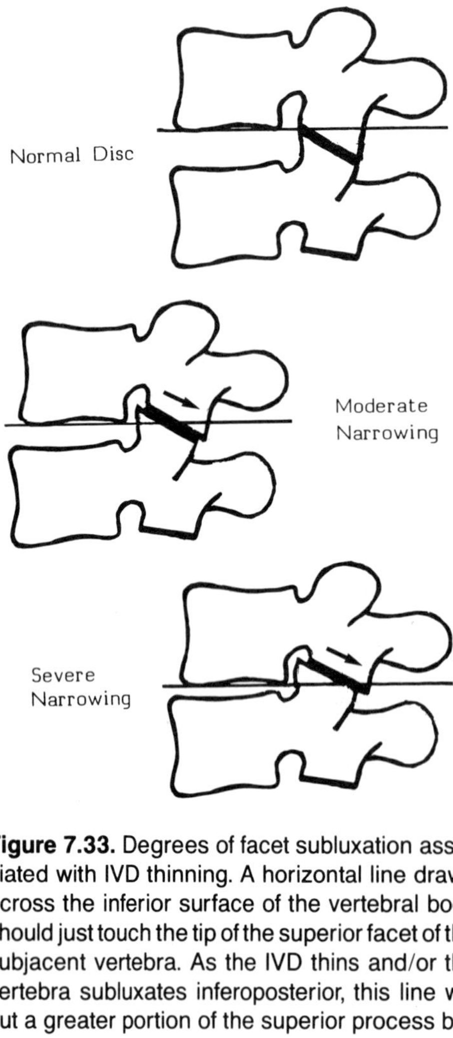

Figure 7.33. Degrees of facet subluxation associated with IVD thinning. A horizontal line drawn across the inferior surface of the vertebral body should just touch the tip of the superior facet of the subjacent vertebra. As the IVD thins and/or the vertebra subluxates inferoposterior, this line will cut a greater portion of the superior process below.

doctor from behind the patient firmly wraps his arms around the patient's pelvis and firms the side of his thigh against the back of the patient's pelvis. The patient is asked to bend forward. If it is a facet involvement, the patient will feel relief. If it is a disc that is stressed, symptoms will be aggravated.

In facet involvement, the patient seeks to find relief by sitting with feet elevated and resting upon a stool, chair, or desk. In disc involvement, the patient keeps the knees flexed, sits sideways in the chair, and moves first to one side and then to the other for relief. If lumbosacral and sacroiliac pain migrates from one to the other side, it is suspected to be associated with arthritic changes.

Sciatica

Although it is the largest nerve of the body and supplies through its branches all the muscles below the knee, the sciatic nerve is rarely injured by sudden trauma. It is often affected, however, by sciatic neuritis (sciatica) that is frequently due to intermittent intrinsic trauma. Sciatic neuralgia or neuritis is characterized by pain of variable intensity to a maximum that is almost unbearable. The pain radiates from the lumbosacral or sacroiliac area down the posterior thigh and even to the sole of the foot. In time, muscular atrophy and a characteristic limp usually occur.

There is a lessening or lack of the patellar tendon reflex in sciatica *(Babinski's sciatica sign)*. When the patient's great toe on the affected side is flexed, pain will often be experienced in the gluteal region *(Turny's sign)*. Also in sciatica, the pelvis tends to maintain a horizontal position despite any induced degree of scoliosis *(Vanzetti's sign)*, unlike other conditions in which scoliosis occurs where the pelvis is tilted.

Sciatic neuropathy must be differentiated from a lumbar impingement radiculopathy, and this is often challenging. The latter can be considered a nerve compression syndrome. As disc herniation rarely involves several segments, neuropathy is first suspected when multiple segments are involved. In contrast to forward flexion in the standing position, flexion in the supine position places little tension on the sciatic nerve. Thus, sciatica aggravated by both standing and supine flexion suggests a disc involvement. Sciatica aggravated in the standing but not the supine position suggests a nerve root involvement.

When Lasegue's straight-leg-raising test is made just short of pain, internal rotation of the femur increases pain and external rotation decreases pain in sciatic neuropathy but has little effect upon lumbar radiculopathies. During Lasegue's supine test, sciatic pain is invariably increased by forced dorsiflexion of the foot and relieved by flexion of the knee. As the point of pain is reached, active flexion of the patient's neck will increase pain in radicular involvement because of the increased tension on the dura. This test is considered a positive Lasegue confirmation, but it does not pinpoint the exact site of the lesion.

Lumbar Stenosis and Claudication

Studies by Porter and associates conclude that the spinal canal is relatively wide in children, reaches a maximum diameter in the late teens, and reduces slightly by late adult life. The size of the canal is particularly significant in patients who have neurogenic claudication and disc symptoms, but size is less significant in root entrapment syndromes.

Intermittent neurogenic claudication is a common manifestation secondary to lumbar spinal stenosis. The syndrome features low back pain and sciatica, which are usually aggravated when the spine is hyperextended or when walking. Gait, bowel, bladder, and sexual dysfunction is commonly associated. Sweere reports that Dejerine's triad is negative, and the femoral, popliteal, and pedal pulses are normal.

Narrowing of the IVD space with sclerosis of the adjacent vertebral bodies may occur as a consequence of infection, neoplasm, trauma, or rheumatic disease. When lumbar disc degeneration reaches the point of rotatory and lateral instability, posterolateral bulging of the anulus fibrosus into the root canal occurs when weight is taken on the ipsilateral lower limb. Symptoms of the spinal stenosis syndrome do not arise until the development of this instability.

Lumbar Nerve Root Entrapment

Entrapment of lumbar nerves may occur (1) at the lateral aspect of the central canal, (2) at the lateral aspect of the IVF, (3) at the posterior aspect of the IVD, (4) at the anterior aspect of the zygapophyseal joints, or (5) in the cauda equina. A wide variety of degenerative changes can occur in both the posterior joints and the disc area, which can produce central stenosis, IVD herniation, lateral entrapment, and/or ligamentous instability.

In addition to the common nerve compression syndrome in the IVF by impingement (eg, subluxation complex), other types of entrapment may occur. After studying the interrelation between lumbosacral nerves and their surrounding tissue, Hasue and associates found several mechanisms leading to sciatica and lower extremity intermittent claudication. Typical mechanisms were the course of nerve roots altered by congenital anomalies or acquired lesions (eg, facet compression) and root compression by ossified ligaments. They also found that the space around the nervous tissue, both in the spinal canal and in the IVF, is narrower in males than in females.

Wiltse and associates describe an entrapment syndrome of L5 by the alar transverse process. They call it the *far-out syndrome.* It appears to be linked with elderly individuals with degenerative scoliosis or younger adults with isthmic spondylolisthesis with at least a 20% slip. Classical symptoms of nerve compression arise, usually at the L5—S1 level.

Lower Extremity Atrophy. Prolonged and/or severe nerve root irritation may show evidence of trophic changes in the tissues supplied. This may be characterized by obvious atrophy. Such a sign is particularly objective when the circumference of an involved limb is measured at the greatest girth in the initial stage and this value is compared to measurements taken in later stages. Chronic L5 root compression exhibits weak dorsiflexion of the foot, featuring a slapping foot-drop during gait. In contrast, chronic L4 root compression manifests weak quadriceps associated with knee pain and buckling during stance. Many knee operations have been unsuccessful because the focal irritation was of the L4 root rather than in the knee.

Referred Pain. Root pain usually has a dermatomal distribution that is aggravated by a Valsalva maneuver. In contrast, abnormal stimuli arising from the lumbar paravertebral soft tissues often refer a dull, diffuse, sclerotomal ache to the sacroiliac joints, buttocks, or posterior thighs. The pain may be solely sclerodermal or be superimposed on dermatomal radicular pain and greatly confuse the clinical picture. It may originate from numerous sources. Poole lists the subcutaneous tissues overlying the motion unit, the posterior aspect of the disc, the dura mater and epidural adipose tissue, the adventitial sheaths of the epidural and paravertebral veins, the walls of the vertebral arteries and arterioles, the articular capsules, the longitudinal ligaments, the ligamentum flavum, the interspinous ligaments, the paravertebral muscles and their tendons, and the periosteum.

Sensory Changes. The posterior sensory root in the lumbar spine is twice the thickness of the anterior motor root. When direct nerve root involvement occurs on the posterior root of a specific neuromere, it manifests as an increase or decrease in sensory awareness over the dermatome. Typical examples might include foraminal occlusion or irritating factors exhibited clinically as hyperesthesia, particularly on the (1) anterolateral aspects of the leg, medial foot, and great toe, when involvement occurs between L4 and L5; and (2) posterolateral aspect of the lower leg and lateral foot and toes when involvement occurs between L5 and S1. In other instances, this nerve root involvement may cause hypertonicity and deep pain in the musculature supplied by the neuromere; for example, L4 and L5 involvement, with deep pain or cramping sensations in the buttock, posterior thigh and calf, or anterior tibial musculature. In addition, direct pressure over the nerve root or distribution may be particularly painful.

Spinosomatic Reflexes. Nerve root insults from subluxations may be evident as disturbances in motor reflexes and/or infrequently as loss of muscular strength. Examples of these reflexes include the deep tendon reflexes such as seen in reduced patella and Achilles tendon reflexes when involvement occurs at L2—L4 or L5—S2, respectively. These reflexes should be compared bilaterally to judge whether the hyporeflexia is unilateral. Unilateral hyperreflexia is highly indicative of an upper motor neuron lesion.

Neurologic-Orthopedic Tests. Such tests as Kemp's, Lasegue's, Naffziger's, Bragard's, Demianoff's, Deyelle-May, and Fajersztajn's are often helpful in differentiating the various etiologies of low-back pain. An examiner should keep in mind that the originators of these maneuvers made specific claims of the significance of these tests, but the projected findings and conclusions are not duplicated consistently in practice. Wyke has shown that because the nociceptive receptor system of the lumbar spine has such an extensive distribution, testing procedures designed to stress selected components and segments by orthopedic stress tests are extremely difficult if not impossible to perform. Only by visualizing the structures being affected by the biomechanical forces being applied will such tests be meaningful to the examiner. See Figure 7.34.

Lumbar Dorsal Ramus Syndrome

This syndrome is described by Bogduk as featuring low-back pain that is referred to the lower extremity. Spasm of the lower back, gluteal area, and hamstring muscles are associated. Careful differentiation must be made to exclude an IVD lesion or nerve root irritation, as only the lumbar dorsal ramus is affected. Recognition of this syndrome may eliminate the need for unnecessary surgical referral.

Meralgia Paresthetica

This syndrome, often called *lateral femoral cutaneous neuropathy,* features a patch of anesthesia, paresthesia, or hyperesthesia, with or without pain, on the anterior surface of one or both thighs in the distribution of the lateral femoral cutaneous nerve. Low-back pain is often associated. The lateral femoral cutaneous nerve arises from the posterior divisions of L1—L3, appears at the lateral border of the psoas, passes obliquely across the iliacus to the anterior superior iliac spine, and then travels under the inguinal ligament to enter the anterolateral aspect of the thigh.

The symptom complex is thought to have its origin in some form of inflammatory process involving the lateral femoral cutaneous nerve or its roots. This focus of irritation may often be found (1) at the L1—L3 IVFs from subluxation encroachment or arthritic hyperplasia or (2) in the pelvis from repetitive trauma as seen in athletic injuries and late pregnancy. Nevertheless, pathology lying anywhere along the course of the nerve may be responsible, whether it be intraspinal, intersegmental, paraspinal, retroperitoneal, pelvic, or, rarely, abdominal.

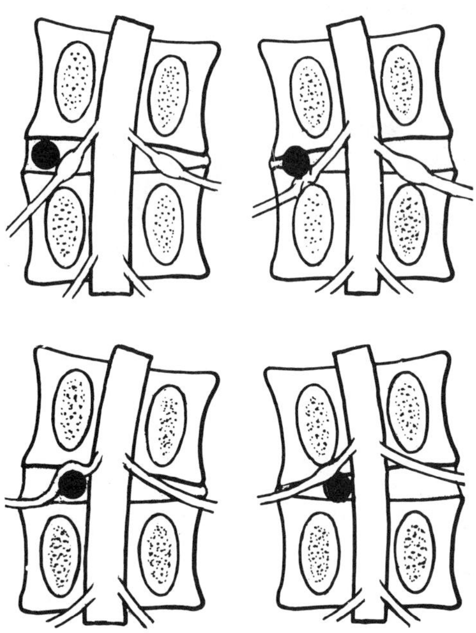

Figure 7.34. Spinal movements in the presence of disc herniation (shown in black) may offer distinct diagnostic clues. *Top,* when protrusion exists lateral to the nerve root, the patient obtains relief by bending *away* from the lesion and pain *(top left).* Pain is increased by bending towards the lesion where the root is caught between the hernia and the inferior pedicle *(top right). Bottom,* on the other hand, when a left protrusion exists medial to the nerve root, pain is increased by bending away from the side of pain because the hernia places an irritative traction on the nerve root *(bottom left).* The patient obtains relief by bending *toward* the side of pain *(bottom right),* which relaxes the tension on the nerve root.

Typically, the patient reports a sense of numbness or burning in the anterolateral aspect of the thigh, which is rarely painful until the late stages. Care must be taken to differentiate this syndrome from trochanteric or iliopectineal (iliopsoas) bursitis, both of which refer pain to the anterolateral thigh. It also should be kept in mind that pronation or supination of the ankle, genu varum, genu valgum, genu recurvatum, flexion contracture, etc, can cause or contribute to anterosuperior thigh pain.

Reiter's Syndrome

The triad of sterile spondylitis, uveitis, and urethritis or prostatitis is called Reiter's Syndrome. The cause is unknown. Backache is usually the presenting symptom, but urinary or conjunctival complaints may manifest first. The weight-bearing joints show the first arthritic changes, and later the proximal joints of the fingers and toes become afflicted.

SELECTED PELVIC CONSIDERATIONS

Serious visceral pathology and hernias often simulate musculoskeletal dysfunction. It is unexplained why leukemia and other systemic diseases may present only backache as the presenting symptom, but it does occur. Back pain often arises early in visceral disease, long before classic physical signs and hematologic changes are noted. A few pathologies may extend from or affect the sacroiliac joints and lumbar spine early that often mimic the symptoms of sprain or chronic subluxation. Confusion may exist when related symptoms are brought out after trauma.

Sacroiliac Subluxation/Fixation Syndromes

For many years, *Gray's Anatomy* classified the sacroiliac joint as an immovable synarthrosis. Throughout the efforts of chiropractic and osteopathic research, however, most anatomists today describe it as a movable diarthrosis, complete with joint cavity, synovial membrane, and synovial fluid.

Sacroiliac subluxations produce (1) irritative microtrauma to the interarticular structures, (2) induction of a vertebral motion unit subluxation and/or contributions to the chronicity of existing subluxations, (3) induction of spinal curvatures and/or contributions to the chronicity of existing curvatures, and (4) biomechanical impropriety of the pelvis in static postural accommodation and locomotion.

The most common errors of analysis stem from misleading visual signs, subjective responses to testing procedures, structural symmetry, and subjective descriptions of pain. Many procedures are helpful in differentiation; eg, the iliac compression test, Piedallu's sign, the belt test, Berry's sign, Erichsen's pelvic rock test, Gaenslen's test, Hibb's test, Mennell's test, and Yeoman's test.

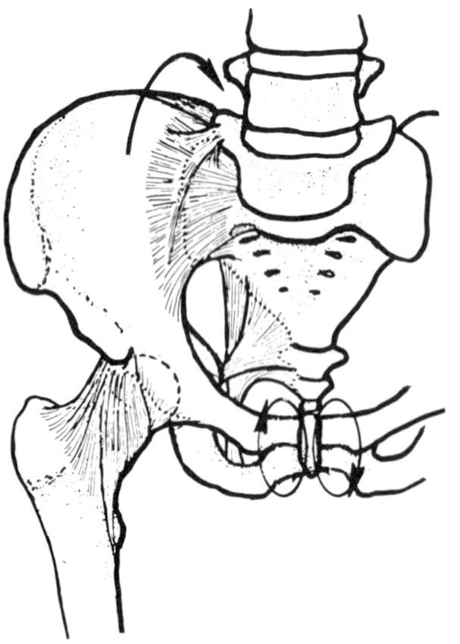

Figure 7.35. Direction of motion in a subluxated posterior right ilium and the torque forces at the symphysis pubis.

Local pain and acute tenderness are rarely seen contralaterally in chronic cases unless the fixated site is irritated by trauma. Old lesions appear to enjoy confusing the examiner by referring signs and symptoms far above or below. Roentgenography is helpful, but rarely is it an end in itself. Thus, signs of immobility, the results of stress tests, and signs of spinal balance are the most reliable clues (Fig. 7.35).

Several authorities say that sacroiliac pain will always be on the side of hypermobility, while others of equal credentials place the pain on the side of fixation. Some say the side of fixation is always the major, while others say that the side of hypermobility is always the major because the joint is normally hypomobile. This confuses everybody except the mentor's disciples. It is this author's opinion that the typical pain of sacroiliac stress is diffuse across the sacroiliac area and most difficult for the patient to isolate with a finger. The palm of the hand is usually used.

It is not uncommon for referred pain to detour from textbook descriptions (eg, gallbladder distress does not always refer to the right scapula, anginal pain does not always refer to the left arm). Even palpable tenderness may be referred. The most reliable clues are the site of consistently increased pain on biomechanical stress tests and, conversely, opposite maneuvers that relieve pain, tenderness, and structural imbalance. When dealing with individual patients, each of which is unique, the doctor is best directed by what is found true in the situation at hand and not on the theories of other doctors that are based upon their patients.

Coccyx Syndromes

The terminal of the spinal cord is attached to the cornua of the coccyx. As the segment moves anteriorly, the apex of the sacrum acts as a fulcrum. As the cornua moves backward and downward, traction is applied to the spinal cord. Thus, symptoms from the resulting cord tension need not be confined to the pelvic region alone (eg, occipital headaches, torticollis).

An irritating coccygeal displacement referring pain to the sacroiliac area is more common among women than men. Coccygodynia may be from mild to severe, and urogenital, rectal, and sciatic-like complaints, along with general nervousness, may be related. The associated pain is usually far greater than the degree of displacement would indicate. In traumatic situations, pain and local levator ani spasm may be pronounced and often episodic. Local tenderness is consistently present, and pain is aggravated by pressure in the direction of displacement.

Pubic Syndromes

Pubic sprain and subluxation are often mistaken for sacroiliac slip, although sacroiliac displacement may have occurred and been spontaneously reduced. The disorder is also associated with lateral hip subluxations. In primary pubic subluxation (essentially torsional), the predominant evidence will be found at the pubic symphysis. The sacroiliac area will not be excessively tender, but acute tenderness will be found over the painful pubis. After severe trauma, pubic and sacroiliac displacement may coexist. Anatomically, they must exist together, but one joint may be more acutely involved than the other.

NEUROLOGIC ASPECTS OF SCOLIOSIS

Kaplan and associates found that a radiculopathic process on the convex side is associated with idiopathic thoracic scoliosis. EMG studies of the erector spinae muscles showed the radiculopathy to be maximal near the apex of the curve. At one time, it was thought that a polyneuropathy or polyneuritis was involved in the development of adolescent idiopathic scoliosis. This theory, however, has been shown by nerve conduction velocity studies conducted by Sahlstrand/Sellden to be false.

The Node Theory

After studying the range of motion from the atlas to the sacrum in 30 cadaveric spines, Kashimoto and associates determined that individual spines had a characteristic level-dependent difference in the capacity for elementary motions at the facet joints. Segments with restricted motion capacity were called *spinal nodes*. The human spine was usually found to have three or four spinal nodes between the skull and the sacrum. Their located was determined at C7—T1, T4—T5, T8—T9, and T11—T12 levels. This intrinsic structural character of the human spine is expressed as "nodal motion structure" by these researchers whom postulated that this state plays an important role in the formation of curve patterns in idiopathic scoliosis and other spinal deformities. It should be noted that Gillet, Illi, King, and Ward have frequently pointed out the high incidence of subluxation-fixation at similar areas.

Spinal Cord Maladaptation

A survey by Lloyd-Roberts and associates has shown that idiopathic structural scoliosis of mild degree is generally not progressive. These researchers report that although the spinal cord is displaced toward the concavity of a scoliotic curve, it does *not* rotate in company with the vertebrae. This exposes the involved nerve roots to traction and possible entrapment. It is suggested that progression occurs when the neuraxis is unable to adjust to the change in the anatomy of the vertebral column: a significant increase in degenerated cells was demonstrated in the posterior root ganglia at the apex of the curve on the convex side.

Equilibrium Sway Effects in Scoliosis

In an analysis by Sahlstrand and associates of sagittal, lateral, and total postural sway when erect, the patterns of scoliotic children were compared to those of healthy children. Scoliotic patients had significantly poorer postural control, especially in tests in which the proprioceptive functions were most important for maintaining postural equilibrium. Patients with a left convex curve had more pronounced reactions quantitatively than patients with a right convex curve, and patients with small curvatures had significantly increased postural sway compared with patients with more severe deformity. It was concluded that these facts together with findings in patients with double primary curves, and the results of studies of brace effects, indirectly indicate the possibility of postural disequilibrium as a contributory cause in adolescent scoliosis. This observation appears to support reports of those who specialize in upper-cervical techniques.

Scoliosis Presenting with Severe Low-Back Pain

The incidence of low-back pain appears to be the same in patients with or without obvious spinal deformity. However, the degree of pain experienced may vary.

Jackson and associates found that patients with major lumbar curves had more pain, and the area of complaint was frequently below the site of the major deformity. The most painful and disabling patterns concerned the compensatory lumbosacral curves. It appeared that the pain originated from the concavity side of the curve and included discogenic, facet joint, and radicular origins. Kostuik/Bentivoglio also found that as the degree of curvature increased, the severity of pain increased, especially for curves of 45° or larger. They also reported that (1) the presence of facet sclerosis correlated with a history of pain in 64% of the cases, and (2) there was a high correlation between radiologic changes to the incidence of pain.

Prophylactic surgery to prevent future back pain in patients having abnormal lumbar curves is generally not justified. Nachemson reports that whether severe low-back pain occurs more often in patients who have distorted lumbar curves than in those whose spines are straight is open to question since calculations show approximately the same incidence of surgery for back pain in scoliotic patients and in those whose spines are straight. Because surgery for scoliosis in the adult carries a high risk and long-term efficacy is unproved, he recommends that all types of conservative measures be tried before considering an operation. However, if unremitting pain from root entrapment occurs (eg, foraminal compression, pedicular kinking) or a painful degenerative scoliosis develops in the elderly, referral for surgical decompression may be the only alternative.

Taylor believes that instances of scoliosis-related pain, especially night pain, are often related to underlying pathology (eg, spinal tumor, osteoblastoma, severe spondylolisthesis).

Bibliography

Abrahams VC: Sensory and motor specialization in some muscles of the neck. *TINS*, 4(1):24-27, 1981.

Aiken P: Meralgia paresthetica. *Orthopedic Brief*, ACA Council on Orthopedics, date not shown.

Albrand OW, Corkill G: Thoracic disc herniation: treatment and prognosis. *Spine*, 4:41-46, 1979.

Bailey RW: *The Cervical Spine*. Philadelphia, Lea & Febiger, 1974, pp 91-97.

Baklavadzhyan OG, Arutyunyan AG, Darbinyan AG: Influence of cervical sympathetic nerve and hypothalamus on direct cortical response. *Neuroscience Translations*, 1:403-410, 1967.

Baloh RW: Dizziness: Matching the symptoms to the source. *Diagnosis*, 5(11):81-98, 1983.

Barge FH: *Scoliosis*. Davenport, IA, Bawden Bros, 1982, pp 119-129, 146, 227-233.

Barge FH: *Tortipelvis*. Davenport, IA, Bawden Bros, 1980, pp 101-102.

Barge FH: *Torticollis*. Davenport, IA, Bawden Bros, 1979.

Barker ME: Manipulation in general medical practice for thoracic pain syndrome. *British Osteopathic Journal*, 15(2):95-97, 1983.

Benner B, Ehni G: Degenerative lumbar scoliosis. *Spine*, 4:548-552, 1979.

Benson DR: The back: thoracic and lumbar spine. In D'Ambrosia RD: *Musculoskeletal Disorders: Regional Examination and Differential Diagnosis*. Philadelphia, J.B. Lippincott, 1977, pp 308-309.

Blits J: Thoracic disk herniation. *Ortho Briefs*, ACA Council on Chiropractic Orthopedics, Spring 1982, pp 8-9.

Blumenthal LS: Injury to the cervical spine as a cause of headache. *Postgraduate Medicine*, 56:147-152, 1974.

Boake HK: Cervical headache. *Canadian Family Physician*, 18:75-76, 1978.

Bogduk N: The clinical anatomy of the cervical dorsal rami. *Spine*, 7(4):19-30, 1982.

Bogduk N: Lumbar dorsal ramus syndrome. *Medical Journal of Australia*, 2:537-541, 1980.

Bohlman HH: The neck. In D'Ambrosia RD (ed): *Musculoskeletal Disorders: Regional Examination and*

Differential Diagnosis. Philadelphia, J.B. Lippincott, 1977, pp 192-193, 203-204.

Bohlman HH: The pathology and current concepts of cervical spine injuries: a critical review of 300 cases. *Journal of Bone & Joint Surgery,* 54A:1363, 1972.

Bradford DS, Moe JH, Winter RB: Scoliosis. In Rothman RH, Simeone FA (eds): *The Spine.* Philadelphia, W.B. Saunders, 1975, vol I, pp 276, 281-283.

Brain, Lord, Wilkinson (eds): *Cervical Spondylosis.* London, Heinemann, 1967.

Breig A: *Adverse Mechanical Tension in the Central Nervous System.* Stockholm, Almquist & Wikell, 1978.

Breig A: *Biomechanics of the Central Nervous System: Some Basic Normal and Pathological Phenomena.* Stockholm, Almquist & Wiksell, 1960.

Breig A: Overstretching of, and circumscribed pathological tension in, the spinal cord—a basic cause of symptoms in cord disorders. *Journal of Biomechanics,* 3:7, 1970.

Breig A, Turnbull I, Hassler O: Effects of mechanical stress on the spinal cord in cervical spondylosis. *Journal of Neurosurgery,* 15:45, 1966.

Bridge CJ: Innervation of spinal meninges and epidural structures. *Anatomical Record,* 133:533-561, 1959.

Brodal A: *Neurological Anatomy in Relation to Clinical Medicine,* ed 2. London, Oxford University Press, 1969.

Brunarski DJ: Functional considerations of spinal manipulative therapy. *ACA Journal of Chiropractic,* May 1980.

Buehler MT: Spinal stenosis. *Journal of Manipulative and Physiological Therapeutics,* 1(2), June 1978.

Burke GL: The etiology and pathogenesis of pain of spinal origin. *Applied Therapeutics,* pp 863-867, October 1966.

Cailliet R: *Low Back Pain Syndrome,* ed 3. Philadelphia, F.A. Davis, 1981, pp 1-21, 25, 44-51.

Cailliet R: *Neck and Arm Pain.* Philadelphia, F.A. Davis, 1974, pp 17-20, 61.

Cailliet R: *Scoliosis.* Philadelphia, F.A. Davis, 1975, pp 1-3, 99-105.

Cailliet R: *Soft Tissue Pain and Disability.* Philadelphia, F.A. Davis, 1980, pp 120-121, 128-130.

Calin A: Back pain: mechanical or inflammatory? *American Family Physician,* 20: 97-100, 1979.

Canadian Memorial Chiropractic College: *Segmental Neuropathy.* Toronto, Canadian Memorial Chiropractic College, date of publication not shown. Monograph.

Carnett JB: The simulation of gallbladder disease by intercostal neuralgia of the abdominal wall. *Annals of Surgery,* 86(5):747-757, 1927.

Causey G: The effect of pressure on nerve fibers. *Journal of Anatomy,* 82:262-270, 1948.

Causey G, Palmer E: The effect of pressure on nerve conduction and nerve fiber size. *Journal of Physiology* (British), 109:220-231, 1949.

Chrisman OD, Gervais RF: Otologic manifestations of the cervical syndrome. *Clinical Orthopedics,* 24:34-38, 1962.

Chusid JG: *Correlative Neuroanatomy & Functional Neurology,* ed 19. Los Altos, CA, Lange Medical, pp 68, 297.

Coggins WN: *Basic Technique: A System of Body Mechanics.* Creve Coeur, MO, published by author, 1983.

Cole WV: The effects of the atlas lesion after 96 hours and after 6 weeks. *Journal of the American Osteopathic Association,* 48(1):7-9, 1948.

Cole WV: The osteopathic lesion syndrome (VIII): the effects of an experimental vertebral lesion on the gross structure of the atlanto-occipital region. *Journal of the American Osteopathic Association,* 49 (9):447-450, 1949.

Cyriax J: Dural pain. *Lancet,* 1(8070):919-921, 1978.

Cyriax J: Lumbago: Mechanism of dural pain. *Lancet,* 249:427-429, 1945.

Cyriax J: *Textbook of Orthopaedic Medicine;* vol one, Diagnosis of Soft Tissue Lesions, ed 8. London, Bailliere Tindall, 1982, pp 297-298.

Davis D: A common type of vertigo relieved by traction of the cervical spine. *Annals of Internal Medicine,* 38:778-786, 1953.

Deering ID, Ling TH, McCouch GP: Location of receptors for tonic neck reflexes. *Journal of Neurophysiology,* 14:191-195, 1951.

De Rusha JL: Upper cervical technic correlated with neurodiagnosis. *ACA Journal of Chiropractic,* September 1961.

De Sterno CV: The pathophysiology of TMJ dysfunction and related pain. In Gelb H (ed): *Clinical Management of Head, Neck and TMJ Pain and Dysfunction.* Philadelphia, W.B. Saunders, 1977.

Dionne J: Neck torsion nystagmus. *Canadian Journal of Otolaryngology,* 3(1):37-41, 1974.

Dittmar E: Cutaneo-visceral neural pathways. *British Journal of Physical Medicine,* 15:208, 1952.

Dove CI: The occipito-atlanto-axial complex. *Manuelle Medizin,* 20:11-15, 1982.

Droz JM: The discoradicular conflict and the radicular involvement in the intervertebral foramen. *Annals of the Swiss Chiropractors' Association,* 2:23-49, 1961.

Drum DC: The vertebral motor unit and intervertebral foramen. In Goldstein M (ed): *The Research Status of Spinal Manipulative Therapy.* Bethesda, MD, National Institutes of Health, 1975, pp 63-70.

Dvorak J, Orelli FV: How dangerous is manipulation of the cervical spine Case report and results of an inquiry. *Manuelle Medizin,* 20:44-48, 1982.

Edgar MA, Nundy S: Innervation of the spinal dura mater. *Journal of Neurology, Neurosurgery, and Psychiatry,* 29:53004, 1966.

Epstein BS: *The Spine: A Radiological Text and Atlas.* Philadelphia, Lea & Febiger, 1962, pp 268-269.

Epstein JA, Epstein BS, Jones MD. Symptomatic lumbar scoliosis with degenerative changes in the elderly. *Spine,* 4:542-547, 1979.

Evans DC: Biomechanics of spinal injury. In Gonzna ER, Harrington IJ: *Biomechanics of Musculoskeletal Injury.* Baltimore, Williams & Wilkins, 1982, pp 165-172, 183-185, 204-212.

Farady JA: Current principles in the nonoperative management of structural adolescent idiopathic scoliosis. *Physical Therapy,* 63:512-523, 1983.

Farfan HF, et al: The effects of torsion on the lumbar intervertebral joints: The role of torsion in the production of disc degeneration. *Journal of Bone and Joint Surgery,* 52A:468, 1970.

Farfan HF: *Mechanical Disorders of the Low Back.* Philadelphia, Lea & Febiger, 1973.

Farfan HF: Symptomatology in terms of the pathomechanics of low-back pain and sciatica. In Haldeman S (ed): *Modern Developments in the Principles and Practice of Chiropractic.* New York, Appleton-Century-Crofts, 1980.

Farkas A: The pathogenesis of idiopathic scoliosis. *Journal of Bone and Joint Surgery,* 36:617, 1954.

Fernandez JL: The transport of protein in nerves. *ACA Journal of Chiropractic,* 10:17-24, 1972.

Fielding JW: Dynamic anatomy and cineradiography of the cervical spine. In Bailey RW (ed): *The Cervical Spine.* Philadelphia, Lea & Febiger, 1974.

Finneson BE: *Low Back Pain.* Philadelphia, J.B. Lippincott, 1973, pp 19-34, 93-132, 332.

Fisk JW: *The Painful Neck and Back.* Springfield, IL, Charles C. Thomas, 1977, pp 28-32, 35-37, 81-84.

Fitz-Ritson DE: The direct connections of the C2 dorsal ganglia in the brain stem of the squirrel. *Journal of the Canadian Chiropractic Association,* 23(4): 131-137, 1979.

Foutz CA: Functional vascular changes affecting the posterior-inferior cerebellar artery. *Journal of the National Chiropractic Association,* 30:13-14, 1960.

Freedman BG: The biodynamical aspect of cerebrospinal fluid in disease and health. *Journal of Manipulative and Physiological Therapeutics,* 2:79-84, 1979.

Fried LC, Doppman JL, Chiro G: Direction of blood flow in the primate cervical spinal cord. *Journal of Neurosurgery,* 33:325, 1970.

Frykholm R: The clinical picture: cervical migraine. In Hirsch C, Zotterman Y (eds): *Cervical Pain.* Oxford, England, Pergamon Press, 1972, pp 5-16.

Frymoyer JW, Pope MH: The role of trauma in low back pain: a review. *Journal of Trauma,* 18:628-633, 1978.

Gayral L, Neuwirth E: Clinical manifestations of the autonomic nervous system sequential to osteoarthritis of the cervical spine. *Lancet,* pp 197-198, May 1958.

Gayral L, Neuwirth E: Oto-neuro-ophthalmologic manifestations of cervical origin. *New York State Journal of Medicine,* 54:1920-1926, 1954.

Gehweiler JA Jr, Osborne RL Jr, Becker RF: *The Radiology of Vertebrae Trauma.* Philadelphia, W.B. Saunders, 1980, pp 76-78.

Gelb H: Patient evaluation. In Gelb H (ed): *Clinical Management of Head, Neck and TMJ Pain and Dysfunction.* Philadelphia, W.B. Saunders, 1977.

Gershon-Cohen J, Budin E, Glauser F: Whiplash fractures of cervicodorsal spinous processes. *Journal of the American Medical Association,* 155:560, 1954.

Giles LGF: Lumbosacral facetal "joint angles" associated with leg length inequality. *Rheumatology and Rehabilitation,* 10:223-238, 1981.

Giles LGF, Taylor JR: The effect of postural scoliosis on lumbar apophyseal joints. *Scandinavian Journal of Rheumatology,* 13:209-220, 1984.

Giles LGF: Vertebral-basilar artery insufficiency. *Journal of the CCA,* 21:112-117, 1977.

Gillet H: The anatomy and physiology of spinal fixation. *Journal of the National Chiropractic Association,* December 1963.

Gillet H: Evolution of a chiropractor. *National Chiropractic Journal,* November 1945, January 1949, December 1949, January 1951.

Gillet H, Liekens M: *Belgian Chiropractic Research Notes.* Huntington Beach, CA, Motion Palpation Institute, 1981, pp 11-39, 61-69, 71, 79-80, 92-100, 104-106.

Gillet H, Liekens, M: A further study of spinal fixations. *Annals of the Swiss Chiropractors' Association,* IV:41, 1967.

Gitelman R, Fitz-Ritson D: Acceleration/deceleration injuries (whiplash). *ACA Journal of Chiropractic,* 17:68, April 1983.

Gitelman R, Fitz-Ritson D: Vertebrogenic headaches. *ACA Journal of Chiropractic,* 20(2):74-75, 1983.

Glasgow EF, Twomey LT, Scull ER, Kleynhans AM, Idczak RM: *Aspects of Manipulative Therapy,* ed 2. New York, Churchill Livingstone, 1985, pp 55-58, 109-122, 128-151.

Glerak RA: Vertebral artery compression and vascular insufficiency of the brain. *Archives of California Chiropractic Association,* 2:28-39, 1972.

Goldthwait JE, et al: *The Essentials of Body Mechanics in Health and Disease,* ed 5. Philadelphia, J.B. Lippincott, 1952.

Goodheart GJ: The cervical challenge. *Digest of Chiropractic Economics,* 15(2): 36-39, 1972.

Granit R, Leksell L, Skoglund CR: Fibre interaction in injured or compressed nerves. *Brain,* 67:125-140, 1944.

Grieve GP: *Common Vertebral Joint Problems.* New York, Churchill Livingstone, 1981, pp 10, 17-33, 24-35, 56-59, 47, 48, 53-55, 60-62, 90-92, 134, 163-170, 176-196, 198.

Gunn CC, Milbrandt WE: Early and subtle signs in low-back pain. *Spine,* 3:267-281, 1978.

Guth L: Degeneration and regeneration of taste buds. In *Handbook of Sensory Physiology: vol 4, Chemical Senses.* Berlin, Springer-Verlag, 1969.

Hadley LA: *Anatomico-Roentgenographic Studies of the Spine.* Springfield, IL, Charles C. Thomas, 1981, pp 69-113, 162.

Hadley LA: Constriction of the intervertebral foramen. *Journal of the American Medical Association,* 140(5):473-476.

Hadley LA: Intervertebral joint subluxation, bony impingement and foramen encroachment with nerve root changes. *American Journal of Roentgenology,* 65(3): 377-402, 1951.

Hanflig SS: Pain in the shoulder girdle, arm and precordium due to foraminal compression of nerve roots. *Archives of Surgery,* 46:652-663, 1963.

Hardy AG, Elson R: *Practical Management of Spinal Injuries,* ed 2. New York, Churchill Livingstone, 1976.

Hargrave-Wilson W: The cervical syndrome. *Australian Journal of Physiotherapy,* 18:144-147, 1972.

Hasue M, Kikuchi S, Sakuyama Y, Ito T: Anatomic study of the interrelation between lumbosacral nerve roots and their surrounding tissues. *Spine,* 8:50-58, 1983.

Helfet AJ, Gruebel Lee DM: *Disorders of the Lumbar Spine.* Philadelphia, J.B. Lippincott, 1978, pp 24-25, 27-30, 145-161, 170-182.

Henderson DJ: Significance of vertebral dyskinesia in

relation to the cervical syndrome. *Journal of Manipulative and Physiological Therapeutics*, 2(1): 3-13, March 1979.

Hewit W: The intervertebral foramen. *Physiotherapy*, 56(8):332-336, 1970.

Hilton RC, Bail J: A systematic pathological study of the dorsolumbar spine. *Journal of Rheumatology*, 9: 95-96, 1983.

Hoff J, et al: The role of ischemia in the pathogenesis of cervical spondylotic myelopathy. *Spine*, 2:100, 1977.

Homewood AE: *The Neurodynamics of the Vertebral Subluxation*, ed 3. Place of publication not shown, published by author, 1981, pp 39, 125-126, 147-161, 167-249.

Hülse M: Disequilibrium caused by a functional disturbance of the upper cervical spine: clinical aspects and differential diagnosis. *Manuelle Medizen*, 1(1): 18-23, 1983.

Howe JW: Determination of lumbo-sacral facet subluxations. *Roentgenological Briefs*, Council on Roentgenology of the American Chiropractic Association, Des Moines, IA, date not shown.

Illi FW: *The Vertebral Column: Life-Line of the Body*. Chicago, National College of Chiropractic, 1951.

Jackson H: Diagnosis of minimal atlanto-axial subluxations. *British Journal of Radiology*, 23:672, 1950.

Jackson RP, Simmons EH, Stripinis D: Incidence and severity of back pain in adult idiopathic scoliosis. *Spine*, 8:749-756, 1983.

Janse J: History of the development of chiropractic concepts; Chiropractic terminology. In Goldstein M (ed): *The Research Status of Spinal Manipulative Therapy*. Bethesda, MD, National Institutes of Health, 1975.

Janse J: *Principles and Practice of Chiropractic*. Lombard, IL, National College of Chiropractic, 1976.

Jeffreys E: *Disorders of the Cervical Spine*. London, Butterworths, 1980.

Jepson O: Dizziness originating in the column cervicallis. *Journal of the Canadian Chiropractic Association*, 11(1):7-8, 1967.

Kale M: The upper cervical specific. *Today's Chiropractic*, part 1, pp 28-29, July-August 1984; part 2, pp 27-30, September-October 1984.

Kapandji IA: *Physiology of the Joints: The Trunk and Vertebral Column*, ed 2. New York, Churchill Livingstone, 1980, vol three.

Kaplan PE, Sahgal V, Hughes R, Kane W, Flanagan N: Neuropathy in thoracic scoliosis. *Acta Orthopaedica Scandinavica*, 51:263-266, 1980.

Kashimoto T, Yamamuro T, Hatakeyama K: Anatomical and biomechanical factors in the curve pattern formation of idiopathic scoliosis. *Acta Orthopaedica Scandinavica*, 53:368-361, 1982.

Keggi, Granger, Southwick: Vertebral artery insufficiency secondary to trauma and osteoarthritis of the cervical spine. *Yale Journal of Biology and Medicine*, 38:471-478, 1966.

Keith WS: "Whiplash"—injury of the 2nd cervical ganglion and nerve. *Canadian Journal of Neurological Services*, 12:133-137, 1986.

Khurana RK, Nirankari VS: Bilateral sympathetic dysfunction in posttraumatic headaches. *Headache*, 26:183-188, 1986.

Kelsey JL, White AA: Epidemiology and impact of low back pain. *Spine*, 5:133-142, 1980.

Kikuchi S, Hasue M, Nishiyama K, Ito T: Anatomic and clinical studies of radicular symptoms. *Spine*, 9(1): 23-30, 1984.

Kimmel DL: Innervation of spinal dura mater and dura mater of the posterior cranial fossa. *Neurology*, 11:800-809, 1961.

King WE: *The King Concept: The Spinal Tetrahedron*, ed 4. Grand Forks, ND, published by author, 1985.

Kirkaldy-Willis WH: Five common back disorders: How to diagnose and treat them. *Geriatrics*, December 1978.

Kirkaldy-Willis WH: Manipulation. In Kirkaldy-Willis WH (ed): *Managing Low Back Pain*. New York, Churchill Livingstone, 1983, pp 175-177.

Kirkaldy-Willis WH: A more precise diagnosis for low back pain. *Spine*, 4(2), March-April 1979.

Kirkaldy-Willis WH: The relationship of structural pathology to the nerve root. *Spine*, 9:49-52, 1984.

Kobayashi S, Waltz AG, Rhoton AL Jr: Effects of stimulation of cervical sympathetic nerves on cortical blood flow and vascular reactivity. *Neurology*, 21 (3):297-302

Korr IM: Discussion: Papers of Sidney Ochs and Davis E. Pleasure. In Goldstein M (ed): *The Research Status of Spinal Manipulative Therapy*. Bethesda, MD, National Institutes of Health, 1975, pp 203-207.

Korr IM (ed): *The Neurobiologic Mechanisms in Manipulative Therapy*. New York, Plenum Press, 1978, pp 8-10, 16-21, 57-58, 291-365.

Kostuik JP, Bentivoglio J: The incidence of low-back pain in adult scoliosis. *Spine*, 6:268-273, 1981.

Kovacs A: Subluxation and deformation of the cervical apophyseal joints. *Acta Radiologica*, 43:1-16, 1955.

Kraus H: Muscular aspects of oral dysfunction. In Gelb H (ed): *Clinical Management of Head, Neck and TMJ Pain and Dysfunction*. Philadelphia, W.B. Saunders, 1977, pp 117-124.

Kunert W: Functional disorders of internal organs due to vertebral lesions. *Ciba Symposium*, 13(3), 1966.

Lamb DW: The neurology of spinal pain. *Physical Therapy*, 59:971-973, 1979.

Lay EM: The osteopathic management of temporomandibular joint dysfunction. In Gelb H (ed): *Clinical Management of Head, Neck and TMJ Pain and Dysfunction*. Philadelphia, W.B. Saunders, 1977.

Leach RA: *The Chiropractic Theories*, ed 2. Baltimore, Williams & Wilkins, 1986, pp 45-46, 49-70, 74-84, 109-119, 121-129.

Lehman JJ: Manual therapy in upper cervical spinal dysfunction: a clinical study. *Physiotherapy Canada*, 30:302-304, 1978.

Levine M: *The Structural Approach to Chiropractic*. New York, Comet Press, 1964, p 85.

Lieb MM: Oral orthopedics. In Gelb H (ed): *Clinical Management of Head, Neck and TMJ Pain and Dysfunction*. Philadelphia, W.B. Saunders, 1977, pp 32-71.

Lloyd-Roberts GC, Pincott JR, McMeniman P, Bayley IJL, and Kendall B: Progression in idiopathic scoliosis: a preliminary report of a possible mechanism. *Journal of Bone & Joint Surgery*, 60B:451-460, 1979.

Logan VF, Murray FM (eds): *Textbook of Logan Basic Methods* (from the original manuscript of Hugh B.

Logan). St. Louis, Logan Chiropractic College, 1950.
Luttges MW, Gerren RA: Compression physiology: Nerves and roots. In Haldeman S (ed): *Modern Developments in the Principles and Practice of Chiropractic.* New York, Appleton-Century-Crofts, 1980, pp 65-89.
MacEwen GD: A look at the diagnosis and management of scoliosis. *Orthopaedic Review,* 3:9, 1974.
MacEwen GD: Experimental scoliosis. In Zorab, PA (ed): *Proceedings of the Second Symposium on Scoliosis: Causation.* Edinburgh, E & S Livingstone, 1969.
Macnab I: Acceleration injuries of the cervical spine. *Journal of Bone & Joint Surgery,* 46A:1797-1799, 1964.
Macnab I: *Backache.* Baltimore, Williams & Wilkins, 1977, pp 19-23, 28-30, 38-63, 69-79, 82-104, 133-207.
Macnab I: Symptoms in cervical disc degeneration. In The Cervical Spine Research Society: *The Cervical Spine.* Philadelphia, Lippincott, 1983, pp 388-394.
Magnaes B, Hauge T: Rheumatoid arthritis contributing to lumbar spinal stenosis. *Scandinavian Journal of Rheumatology,* 7:215-218, 1978.
Markovich SE: Pain in the head. In Gelb H (ed): *Clinical Management of Head, Neck and TMJ Pain and Dysfunction.* Philadelphia, W.B. Saunders, 1977.
Malik DD, et al: Effectiveness of chiropractic adjustment and physical therapy to treat spinal subluxation, *ACA Journal of Chiropractic,* June 1983.
Malik DD, et al: Recovery from radiculalgia by chiropractic adjustment and physical therapy. *ACA Journal of Chiropractic,* June 1984.
Mapstone T, Spetzler RF: Vertebrobasilar insufficiency secondary to vertebral artery occlusion. *Journal of Neurosurgery,* 56:581-583, 1982.
Maurer EL: The thoraco-costal facet syndrome, with an introduction of the marginal line and the rib sign. *ACA Journal of Chiropractic,* December 1976.
Mayer EG, Herrman G, Pfaffenrath V, Pollmann W, Auberger T: Functional radiographs of the craniocervical region and the cervical spine: A new computer-aided technique. *Cephalgia,* 5:237-243, 1985.
Mazzarelli JP (ed): *Chiropractic Interprofessional Research.* Torino, Italy, Edizioni Minerva Medica, 1983. Reprinted in the United States by the International Chiropractors Association, Washington, DC, 1985.
McAlpine JE: A discussion of the dentate ligament neural traction mechanism. *International Review of Chiropractic,* pp 35-39, October-December 1980.
McKenzie JA: The dynamic behavior of the head and cervical spine during "whiplash." *Journal of Biomechanics,* 4:477-490, 1971.
McKenzie RA: *The Lumbar Spine: Mechanical Diagnosis and Therapy.* Waikane, NZ, Spinal Publications, 1981, pp 4-5, 87-90.
Mears DB: Neurological syndrome linking the cervical spine with the dorsallumbar areas. *Digest of Chiropractic Economics,* 14(7):28-29, 1972.
Meyermann R: Possibilities of injury to the artery vertebralis. *Manuelle Medizin,* 20:105-114, 1982.
Michelsson JE: The development of spinal deformity in experimental scoliosis. *Acta Orthopaedia Scandinavia,* Supplement 81, 1965.
Milne E: Giddiness in vertebro-basilar arterial insufficiency. *Medical Journal of Anatomy,* 55:417-418, 1968.
Moe JH, et al: *Scoliosis and Other Spinal Deformities.* Philadelphia, W.B. Saunders, 1978, p 467.
Moe JH, Kettleson DN: Idiopathic scoliosis. *Journal of Bone & Joint Surgery,* 52A:1509, 1970.
Mumenthaler M: *Neurology,* ed 2. Translated by EH Burrows. New York, Thieme-Stratton, 1983, pp 157-158.
Nachemson A: Adult scoliosis and back pain. *Spine,* 4:513-517, 1979.
Nachemson AL: The lumbar spine, an orthopaedic challenge. *Spine,* 1(1):59, 1976.
Naylor A: Factors in the development of the spinal stenosis syndrome. *Journal of Bone & Joint Surgery,* 61B:306-309, 1979.
Nelson WA: personal correspondence. San Francisco, CA, 1980.
Neuwirth E: The vertebral nerve in the posterior cervical syndrome. *New York State Journal of Medicine,* 55:1380, 1955.
Ochs S: Axoplasmic flow in neurons. In Gaito J (ed): *Macromolecules and Behavior.* New York, Appleton-Century-Crofts, 1966.
Ochs S: Axoplasmic transport. In Tower DB (ed): *The Basic Neurosciences.* New York, Raven Press, vol 1, 1975, pp 137-146.
Ochs S: A brief review of material transport in nerve fibers. In Goldstein M (ed): *The Research Status of Spinal Manipulative Therapy.* Bethesda, MD, National Institues of Health, 1975, pp 189-194.
Ochs S: Systems of material transport in nerve fibers (axoplasmic transport) related to nerve function and trophic control. *Annals of the New York Academy of Science,* 228:202-223, 1974.
Olsson Y, Sourander P, Krist K: Neuropathological aspect on root affection in the cervical region. In Hirsch C, Zotterman Y (eds): *Cervical Pain.* Oxford, England, Pergamon Press, 1972, pp 81-88.
Oppenheimer A: Narrowing of the intervertebral foramina as a cause of pseudorheumatic pain. *Annals of Surgery,* 106(3):428-438, 1937.
Palmateer DC: Greater occipital-trigeminal syndrome. *Journal of Clinical Chiropractic,* 2:46-48, 1972.
Pang LQ: The otological aspects of whiplash injuries. *Laryngoscope,* 81:1381-1387, 1971.
Penning L: *Functional Pathology of the Cervical Spine.* Amsterdam, Excerpta Medical Foundation, 1968.
Phillips RB: Upper cervical biomechanics. *ACA Journal of Chiropractic,* X:127-134, October 1976.
Pleasure D: Nerve root compression: Effects on neural chemistry and metabolism. In Goldstein M (ed): *The Research Status of Spinal Manipulative Therapy.* Bethesda, MD, National Institues of Health, 1975, pp 197-200.
Ponsetti IV, et al: Biomechanical analysis of intervertebral discs in idiopathic scoliosis. *Journal of Bone & Joint Surgery,* 54:1993, 1972; 56A, 1973.
Ponsetti IV, Friedman B: Prognosis in idiopathic scoliosis. *Journal of Bone & Joint Surgery,* 32A:381, 1950.
Poole PB: Considerations of neurogenic pain. *Ortho Briefs,* Council on Chiropractic Orthopedics of the American Chiropractic Association, Fall 1982.
Porter RW, Hibbert C, Wellman P: Backache and the lumbar spinal canal. *Spine,* 5:99-105, 1980.
Porter RW, Hibbert CS, Wicks M: The spinal canal in

symptomatic lumbar disc lesions. *Journal of Bone & Joint Surgery*, 60B:485-487, 1978.

Porter RW, Park W: Unilateral spondylolysis. *Journal of Bone & Joint Surgery* (British), 64:344-348, 1982.

Rainer GW, Mayer J, Sadler TR, Dirks D: Effect of graded compression on nerve conduction velocity. *Archives of Surgery*, 107:719-721, 1973.

Reid JD: Effects of flexion-extension movements of the head and spine upon the spinal cord and nerve roots. *Journal of Neurology, Neurosurgery and Psychiatry* (British), 23:214. 1960.

Roaf R: A study of the mechanics of spinal injuries. *Journal of Bone and Joint Surgery*, 42B:810-823, 1960.

Roaf R: Rotation movements of the spine with special reference to scoliosis. *Journal of Bone & Joint Surgery*, 40-B:312-332, 1958.

Roaf R: The basic anatomy of scoliosis. *Journal of Bone & Joint Surgery*, 480:786, 1966.

Roca PD: Ocular manifestations of whiplash injuries. *Annals of Ophthalmology*, 4(1):63-73, 1972.

Rothman RH, Simeone FA: Lumbar disc disease. In Rothman RH, Simeone FA (eds): *The Spine*. Philadelphia, W.B. Saunders, 1975, vol II, pp 476-506.

Ruge D, Wiltse LL (eds): *Spinal Disorders: Diagnosis and Treatment*. Philadelphia, Lea & Febiger, 1977.

Russell AS, Percy JS, Lentle BC: Vertebral sclerosis in adults. *Annals of the Rheumatic Diseases*, 37:18-22, 1978.

Ryan GMS, Cope S: Cervical vertigo. *The Lancet*, pp 1355-1358, December 1955.

Rydevik B, Brown MD, Lundborg G: Pathoanatomy and pathophysiology of nerve root compression. *Spine*, 9(1):7-15, 1984.

Sahlstrand T, Ortengren R, Nachemson A: Postural equilibrium in adolescent idiopathic scoliosis. *Acta Orthopaedica Scandinavica*, 49:354-365, 1978.

Sahlstrand T, Sellden U: Nerve conduction velocity in patients with adolescent idiopathic scoliosis. *Scandinavian Journal of Rehabilitation Medicine*, 12:25-26, 1980.

Sandoz R: Some physical mechanisms and effects of spinal adjustments. *Annals of the Swiss Chiropractors Association*, 6:91, 1976.

Sandoz R: Some reflex phenomena associated with spinal derangements and adjustments. *Annals of the Swiss Chiropractors Association*, 7:45, 1981.

Saternus KS, Fuchs V: Is the artery vertebralis endangered in resuscitation. *Manuelle Medizin*, 20:101-104, 1982.

Schafer RC: *Clinical Biomechanics: Musculoskeletal Actions and Reactions*. Baltimore, Williams & Wilkins, 1983, pp 215-220, 272-273, 289-319, 239-240, 336, 339, 381, 388, 399-401, 406, 427-430.

Schafer RC (ed): *Basic Chiropractic Procedural Manual*, ed 4. Arlington, VA, American Chiropractic Association, 1984, pp 3-5.

Schafer RC: *Symptomatology and Differential Diagnosis*. Arlington, VA, American Chiropractic Association, 1986, pp 335-337, 550-555, 729-732, 829-832, 906, 908.

Schaumberg HH, Spencer PS: Pathology of spinal root compression. In Goldstein M (ed): *The Research Status of Spinal Manipulative Therapy*. Bethesda, MD, National Institues of Health, 1975, pp 141-147.

Seeman DC: C1 subluxation, short leg and pelvic distortion. *Upper Cervical Monograph*, 2(5):1-5, 1978.

Shafar J: The syndrome of the third neuron of the cervical sympathetics. *American Journal of Medicine*, 40:97-109, 1966.

Sharpless SK: Susceptibility of spinal roots to compression block. In Goldstein M (ed): *The Research Status of Spinal Manipulative Therapy*. Bethesda, MD, National Institues of Health, 1975, pp 155-160.

Sheehan S, Bauer RB, Meyer JS: Vertebral artery compression in cervical spondylosis, arteriographic demonstration during life of vertebral artery insufficiency due to rotation and extension of the neck. *Neurology*, 10:968-986, 1960.

Simmons EH, Jackson RP: The management of nerve root entrapment syndromes associated with the collapsing scoliosis of idiopathic lumbar and thoracolumbar curves. *Spine*, 4:533-541, 1979.

Sjostrand J, Rydevik B, Lundborg G, McLean WG: Impairment of intraneural microcirculation, blood nerve barrier and axonal transport in experimental nerve ischemia and compression. In Korr IM (ed): *The Neurobiologic Mechanisms in Manipulative Therapy*. New York, Plenum Press, 1978, pp 337-355,

Smith DM: Vertebral artery. *Roentgenological Briefs*. Council on Roentgenology of the American Chiropractic Association, date and number not shown.

Steer JC, Horney FD: Evidence for passage of cerebrospinal fluid along spinal nerves. *Canadian Medical Association Journal*, 98(2):71-74, 1968.

Steinbach LL: *Spinal Balance and Spinal Hygiene*. Pittsburgh, published by author, 1957.

Strang VV: *Essential Principles of Chiropractic*. Davenport, IA, Palmer College of Chiropractic, 1984, pp 104, 109-110.

Sunderland S: Anatomical perivertebral influences on the intervertebral foramen. In Goldstein M (ed): *The Research Status of Spinal Manipulative Therapy*. Bethesda, MD, National Institues of Health, 1975, pp 129-139.

Sunderland S: The anatomy of the intervertebral foramen and the mechanisms of compression and stretch of nerve roots. In Haldeman S (ed): *Modern Developments in the Principles and Practice of Chiropractic*. New York, Appleton-Century-Crofts, 1980, pp 55-64.

Sunderland S: Mechanisms of cervical nerve root avulsion in injuries of neck and shoulder. *Journal of Neurosurgery*, 41:705-714, 1974.

Sunderland S: Meningeal-neural relations in the intervertebral foramina. *Journal of Neurosurgery*, 40(6):756-763, 1974.

Sweat RW: Scanning palpation: cervical spine. *Today's Chiropractic*, pp 23-24, January-February 1985.

Sweat RW, Sievert T: Chiropractic and the vertebral arteries. *Today's Chiropractic*, part 1, pp 45-48, September-October 1984; part 2, pp 23-24, November-December 1984.

Sweere JJ: Clinical manifestations of lumbar spinal stenosis. *Orthopedic Brief*, ACA Council on Chiropractic Orthopedics, June 1985.

Sweere JJ: A method of physiological testing in the differential diagnosis of acute mechanical low back pain. *Orthopedic Brief*, ACA Council on Chiropractic Orthopedics, September 1984.

Swezey RL: The modern thrust of manipulation and traction therapy. *Seminars in Arthritis and Rheumatism*, 12(3):326, 1983.

Taylor LF: Painful scoliosis: A need for further investigation. *British Medical Journal.* 292:120-122, 1986.

Toole J, Tucker SH: Influence of head position upon cerebral circulation. *Archives of Neurology* (AMA), 2: 616-623, 1960.

Valentini E: The occipito-cervical spine. *Annals of the Swiss Chiropractors' Association*, 4:225-232, 1969.

Verner JR: *The Science and Logic of Chiropractic.* Englewood, NJ, published by author, 1941.

Von Torklus D, Gehle W: *The Upper Cervical Spine.* New York, Grune & Stratton, 1972.

Waddell G, McCulloch JA, Kummel E, Venner RM: Nonorganic physical signs in low back pain. *Spine*, 5:117-125, 1980.

Ward LE: *The Dynamics of Spinal Stress.* Long Beach, CA, SSS Press, 1980.

Watkins RJ: Side effects of subluxation. *Digest of Chiropractic Economics*, 24(4):32-35, 1982.

Weiss P: Endoneurial edema in constricted nerve. *Anatomical Record*, 86:491-522, 1943.

West HG Jr: Physical and spinal examination procedures utilized in the practice of chiropractic. In Haldeman S (ed): *Modern Developments in the Principles and Practice of Chiropractic.* New York, Appleton-Century-Crofts, 1980, p 283.

West HG: Vertebral artery considerations in cervical trauma. *ACA Journal of Chiropractic*, pp 18-19, December 1968.

White AA, Panjabi MM: *Clinical Biomechanics of the Spine.* Philadelphia, J.B. Lippincott, 1978.

Whiting RJ: Cervical spondylosis. *Roentgenological Briefs*, Council on Roentgenology of the American Chiropractic Association, no date or number shown.

Will TE: The biochemical basis of manipulative therapeutics: hypothetical considerations. *Journal of Manipulative and Physiological Therapeutics*, 1(3):153-156, September 1978.

Wiltse LL, Guyer RD, Spencer CW, Glenn WV, Porter IS: Alar transverse process impingement of the L5 spinal nerve: the far-out syndrome. *Spine*, 9:31-41, 1984.

Wyke BD: Articular neurology and manipulative therapy. In *Aspects of Manipulative Therapy.* Proceedings of Multidisciplinary International Conference on Manipulative Therapy, Melbourne, Lincoln Institute of Health Science, Carlton, Victoria, Australia, August 1979, pp 67-72.

Wyke BD: Clinical significance of articular receptor systems. *Annals of the Royal College of Surgeons of England*, 60(2):137, 1978.

Wyke BD: Neural aspects of pain therapy. In Swerdlow IM (ed): *The Therapy of Pain—Current Status of Modern Therapy.* Lancaster, MTP Press, vol 6.

Yamada K: The dynamics of experimental posture. *Clinical Orthopaedics*, 25:20-31, 1962.

Yamada K, et al: A neurological approach to the etiology and treatment of scoliosis. *Journal of Bone & Joint Surgery*, 53A:197, 1971.

Young G: Chiropractic success in epileptic conditions. *ACA Journal of Chiropractic*, 19(4):62-63, 1982.

Chapter 8

Clinical Disorders and the Sensory System

This chapter describes those sensory mechanisms, joint signals, and abnormal sensations (eg, pain, thermal abnormalities) that have particular significance within clinical diagnosis. The basis and differentiation of pain is described, as are the related subjects of trigger points and paresthesia. The chapter concludes with a description of the neurologic basis for the evaluation of the sensory system and the sensory fibers of the cranial nerves.

THE ANALYSIS OF PAIN IN THE CLINICAL SETTING

Although all pain does not have organic causes, there is no such thing as "imagined" pain. Pain that can be purely isolated as a structural, functional, or an emotional effect is rare. More likely, all three are superimposed upon and interlaced with each other in various degrees of status. This is also true for neural, vascular, lymphatic, and hormonal mechanisms.

Common Causes of Pain and Paresthesia

The common causes of pain and paresthesia are: (1) obvious direct trauma or injury; (2) reflex origins in musculoskeletal lesions, which deep pressure often exaggerates, such as trigger areas; (3) peripheral nerve injury (eg, causalgia), which results in an intense burning superficial pain; (4) the presence of nerve inflammations and degenerations of the peripheral or CNS, which frequently cause other changes indicative of such lesions; (5) reflexes from visceral reflexes; (6) vascular disease; and (7) sensory root pressure.

Vascular disease is usually associated with other changes such as swelling, redness, blanching, or other signs of vascular distress —depending upon whether it is an arterial or a venous problem. Certain neurovascular syndromes may be associated with pain and paresthesia. Vasomotor disturbances may be caused or aggravated by vertebral subluxations such as the deep congestive leg aches associated with upper lumbar subluxations or the cranial vasomotor headaches and other symptoms of cervical subluxation.

Sensory root pressure is characterized by pain, paresthesia, and often by abnormal sensitivity to touch along the course of the involved nerve root's segmental skin supply (Fig. 8.1). Thus, this becomes an important consideration and needs to be traced and demarcated with a skin pencil to see if the area corresponds to a specific dermatome.

Pain and other sensory disturbances caused by subluxations may be due to direct nerve root involvement and, therefore, of the nature mentioned above. They also may be due to reflex irritation of the paravertebral ligaments, tendons, or muscles and, like other myofascial trigger areas, refer pain into somatic areas that do not correlate to direct dermatomes or specific nerve roots.

Common disorders that are associated with spinal pain are shown in Table 8.1.

Pain of Mechanical Origin

It was briefly described in the previous chapter that the three major etiologic categories of pain are: (1) mechanical causes, (2) chemical causes, and (3) psychic causes. The mechanical causes of pain include stretching, displacement, and pressure involving various tissues of the body.

When contractions are sustained, the spasm causes pain. Any direct pressure on the supplying nerve will cause pain in the distribution of the nerve. Painful pressure also can arise from hard tissues such as bone or cartilage, but edema, inflammatory exudates, adhesions, gaseous distention, visceroptosis, and muscle tension also will produce mechanical pressure or tension on nociceptors in certain instances. Distention of the venous and lymphatic systems can cause pain if the back pressure is sufficient and prolonged.

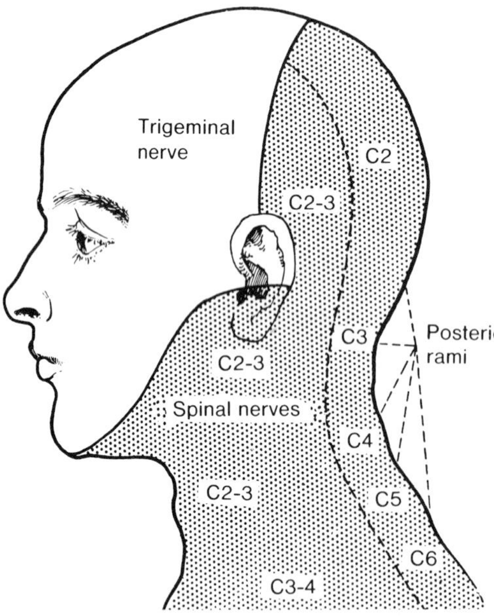

Figure 8.1. Lateral view of the superficial sensory innervation of the head and neck.

Once the difference between the normal and the abnormal is well understood, changes in posture, muscle tone, and movement offer fundamental clinical clues to diagnosis and therapy. When the biomechanical mechanisms involved are acknowledged, painful effects can often be reproduced or relieved at will. Knowing exactly *where*, *when*, and *how* motion increases or decreases pain is the major clue that leads the examiner to find and correct a point of distress whether it is functional or structural.

Pain Induced by Change of Position

Because symptoms often vary with a change in position, this will strongly suggest that the problem has a mechanical origin involving the musculoskeletal system rather than due to some visceral disorder. In fact, positional pain that has existed for years without exacerbation is usually considered to be of mechanical origin.

If pain increases during active or passive compression, it suggests that the tissue being compressed is tender. This compression may be nothing more than normal weight bearing, or it may be from the tissue squeezing that occurs in movement of a joint. Pain that develops when tissues are stretched suggests that the tissues being stretched are hypersensitive. Thus, back pain that develops during side bending is either of compression or tension. If the pain arises on the opposite side of the lateral flexion, then the stretching action is the aggravating factor (eg, torn or tight tissues). If the pain occurs on the side of lateral bending, then, obviously, compression of tender structures is the problem (eg, subluxation, thinned IVD, jammed joint, arthrosis, tissue entrapment).

Observing how the body moves offers the best clues to muscle and joint problems. The patient will invariably assume an antalgic position. In low back spasm, for example, the posteriorly rotated pelvis, the flattened lumbar area, and the slight flexion of the knees and hips, bilateral or unilateral, are unconscious attempts to lessen the tension of the involved sciatic or recurrent nerve and/or to reduce intradisc pressure. Antalgic muscle

Table 8.1. Typical Disorders Associated with Spinal Pain (Acute/Chronic)

Type	Examples	
Degenerative process	Apophyseal osteoarthritis	Nerve root compression
	Cauda equina disorders	Spinal cord disease
	Disc degeneration	Spinal stenosis
	Hyperostosis	Spondylolisthesis
	Joint instability	Spondylosis
Developmental deficit	Bastrup's disease	Short-leg syndrome
	Hypermobility	Spondylolisthesis
	Kyphosis	Various anomalies (eg, hemivertebrae)
	Lordosis	
	Scoliosis	
Iatrogenic origin	Ill-advised manipulation	Poorly fitted support
	Misplaced spinal tap	Postsurgical adhesions
	Myelography	Prolonged support use
Infective arthropathy or neuropathy	Actinomycosis	Smallpox
	Brucellosis	Staphylococcal infection
	Icterohemorrhagica	Subarachnoid hemorrhage
	Influenza	Syphilis
	Leptospirosis	Syringomyelia
	Meningitis	Tetanus
	Osteomyelitis	Tuberculosis
	Paratyphoid fever	Typhoid fever
	Poliomyelitis	
Inflammatory arthropathy	Ankylosing spondylitis	Psoriasis
	Fibrositis	Regional ileitis
	Focal sepsis	Rheumatoid arthritis
	Muscular rheumatism	Reiter's disease
	Osteochondritis	Secondary spondylitis
	Panniculitis	Systemic lupus erythematosus
	Polarteritis nodosa	Ulcerative colitis
	Polymyalgia arteritica	
Metabolic deficit	Gouty rheumatism	Osteoporosis
	Hyperparathyroidism	Paget's disease of the spine
	Osteomalacia	
Spinal tumors	Aneurysmal bone cysts	Neurofibroma
	Hodgkin's sarcoma	Secondary carcinoma
	Myelomatosis	
Trauma	Disc protrusion	Short-leg syndrome
	Dislocation	Spondylolisthesis
	Facet syndrome	Sprain
	Fracture	Strain
	Obesity	Subluxation
	Postural fault	

spasm is extremely common to acute lumbar dysfunction. The greater the pain, the greater will be this "semi-squat" posture in the upright position.

Pain Induced by Chemical Irritation

Several investigators hold that most stimuli that induce pain do so by causing the release of chemical agents such as bradykinin that act upon pain fibers. Shepard states that this is consistent with the observation that the sensation of pain usually outlasts the noxious stimulus which caused it.

Tissue Ischemia

De Sterno reports that an isometric contraction of only 60% of maximum strength results in almost complete occlusion of the blood vessels that supply muscle tissue. This results when the pressure of the contracted muscle exceeds systolic arterial pressure. Such contraction and vascular compression increases nociceptor-irritating lactic acid, reduces oxygen supply, reduces the removal of metabolic ash, lowers muscle pH, and increases the osmotic pressure within the muscle—all of which contribute to pain, fatigue, decreased contractility, and a breakdown in tissue homeostasis.

Naturally Occurring Pain-Producing Substances

Some naturally occurring substances can induce pain at extremely low concentrations. Pain develops if exercise is carried out when local circulation is occluded; but when the circulatory flow is restored, the pain will disappear. Some irritating substance apparently forms in the muscle and this is oxidized by the blood when the circulation to the area is restored. During sustained contraction, relative ischemia develops because, as a rule, blood flows freely only during relaxation. Sustained contraction impedes the blood flow so that P substances (amino-acid peptides) form and pain ensues. This is the probable explanation for the pain of myofibrositis in which some fibers are in a chronic state of contraction. Ischemia, it is postulated, also may give rise to pain because it may allow or aid the release of histamine and bradykinin.

Some other examples of naturally occurring substances that can cause pain are acetylcholine, hydrogen and potassium ions, various peptides, and 5-hydroxytryptamine. This is apparently not true, however, for epinephrine or norepinephrine. Evidence also suggests that prostaglandin E_1 can sensitize bare nerve endings to certain chemical mediators and other stimuli (eg, pressure) though it is not a pain-producing substance except in extremely high concentrations.

Pain of Psychic Origin

Two types of patients commonly frustrate many physicians: (1) the type that complains a great deal of pain and no organic cause can be found and (2) the type that exhibits great damage and makes no complaint. Szasz has pointed out that proper patient care can only result when the two components of pain, *the mechanisms of perception and reaction*, are understood and fully appreciated.

The physician is also confronted with two associated problems: the patient's *complaint of pain* and the *painful person* (homo dolorosus) who has unique experiences, relationships, hopes, and fears. This takes an appreciation of the patient's perspective, not the doctor's. Even monomaniacal hypochondriacs do not choose a "career" of pain unless they see no other alternative.

The physician should be conscious of each action and reaction of the patient during examination. Lynch/Kessier emphasize that pain is not a fixed response to a noxious stimulus. Its perception is modified by a patient's experiences, expectations, and culture. A mental picture should be drawn of how much each patient is suffering. The degree of pain from a fracture may be greater than that of angina; but the overall suffering is greater with angina because the patient is terrorized of what the future might hold, whereas the patient with a fracture knows that the pain will cease in time and that recovery is not in doubt.

Psychic pain can be just as painful as physical distress; if not, it would not drive some people to suicide. People free of physical disease often suffer from the most intractable types of pain. From the standpoint of the patient, there is no such thing as "psychogenic pain"—pain is pain. An unconscious person does not suffer, despite the intensity of noxious stimuli applied, but autonomic manifestations are retained.

Etiologic Factors in Psychogenic Pain

A given stimulus may or may not result in pain, and pain may be experienced in the absence of nociception. In other words, nociception may occur without pain and pain without nociception.

There are two types of pain originated in the psychic: (1) that of *unconscious origin* such as seen in neurotic hysteria, phantom limbs, and conversion syndromes; (2) that of *conscious origin* such as seen in phobias, grief, despair, and umbrage.

Psychogenic pain is located according to body image or appropriate to a fantasy. It may be superficial or deep, well or poorly localized, and may or may not radiate. It is described with vivid, elaborate imagination correlated with ideas of suffering, punishment, and torture that is inconsistent in the retelling. There is a clinical discrepancy between the patient's appearance and the intensity of pain reported. The history may show guilt, a reward from past pain, depression, a recent loss, or other psychic motivations.

When describing pain, picturesque and dramatic phraseology often reflects an underlying neurosis. On the other hand, it should not be assumed that a patient does not suffer because its description is stated in light-hearted terms or the pain appears to be of a nonphysical nature. Sympathy for the patient in pain is never misplaced except, possibly, in conscious malingering.

Some authorities place malingering under the category of psychic pain. A conscious effort by a patient to *pretend* to be in pain, however, is not in the same clinical category as experienced pain whether it be of somatic or psychic origin.

The Reaction Component of Pain and Central Dampening

It was once thought that pain was simply caused by a stimulus sufficient to activate a pain-sensitive structure and send the message to the brain. When this belief prevailed, there was no knowledge of the *reaction component*—central modification of peripherally generated impulses that causes conscious perception which is not necessarily in proportion to the intensity of the stimuli. Thus, it is likely for this reason that pain may express itself differently in different people.

Beecher noticed that some patients with great but painless wounds could feel a clumsy venipuncture. This suggested that the perception mechanism was intact but noxious stimuli were being modified. It was theorized that this was the reason soldiers may not notice their wounds until after battle and why athletes often fail to recognize injuries until after they were out of competition. While people differ in their response to injury and pain, each individual has a more or less predictable pattern that is soon learned by family, friends, physician, and co-workers.

The reaction component can be affected in many ways. Emotional states, placebos, suggestion, and hypnosis are a few examples. Lobotomy can be considered a surgical lesion of the reaction component. Even analgesic narcotics act upon the reaction component, for light touch and temperature stimuli are still preserved. Thus, pain as typically exhibited is a complex process in which the intensity of the focal stimulus plays only a part. Much of the perceived sensation is determined by central processing mechanisms.

Assessing the Origin of Pain

In evaluating pain, it is frequently not possible to determine subjectively how much of a patient's pain is due to pathologic excitation and how much is caused by an emotional factor. In most circumstances, however, some qualified judgments can be made of how large or small a contribution is made by mood and how much is made by the quantity of the stimuli to the overall experience. In this respect, pain differs quantitatively and not qualitatively from other sensory states that may be involved.

The assessment of pain begins with the recognition that it is a subjective experience: a psychic phenomenum. That is, it is something that happens in the mind, although it is described in terms of events that we perceive as originating in the body. This means that our knowledge of pain is subjective; but, we ordinarily attribute it to physical events affecting the body (eg, the forehead, the right arm, the lower back, etc).

There may be times when pain arises from purely physical disorders, but it is made worse by emotional factors. At other times, pain may be primarily of psychic origin. Chronic pain invariably causes emotional disturbances and is strongly colored by it. All measurement of pain has to take into account the fact that people subjected to physical pain are also more than likely to be in a somewhat disturbed emotional state.

The Posterior Lemniscal vs the Anterolateral Spinothalamic Systems

Although both of these systems convey sensory signals, their functions differ. As the types of sensory information that can be transmitted by each is different, knowledge of these differences aids the diagnostic process when a spinal cord deficit is suspected.

The *posterior lemniscal system*, states Guyton, is composed mainly of large myelinated nerve fibers that transmit cephally at a velocity of 30—110 meters per second. It has an extremely high degree of spatial orientation of the fibers with respect to their origin on the surface of the body. Thus, this system conducts signals of fine graduations of intensity that must be transmitted rapidly with temporal fidelity and which are discretely localized to exact points in the body.

The *anterolateral spinothalamic system* is composed of small diameter myelinated nerve fibers that transmit to the brain at a rate of 10—60 meters per second. This system has no or a small degree of spatial orientation of the fibers with respect to their origin on the surface of the body. Thus, this system conducts signals that lack fine gradations of intensity, that need not be transmitted quickly, or in which temporal fidelity or specific localization is not necessary.

The anterolateral spinothalamic system has the advantage of being able to convey a wide spectrum of stimuli (pain, temperature, crude tactile sensations), while the posterior lemniscal system is limited to transmitting mechanoreceptive signals only. A summary of differences of these two sensory systems is shown in Table 8.2.

The Qualities of Pain

The perception of pain may vary from mild discomfort to excruciating, intolerable misery. While the effects of pain can be measured in the office, it is clinically impossible to measure pain accurately by graduated degrees because it is subjective. We must generally rely on the communicative ability of the patient in order to assess the quantity and quality of pain being experienced.

Pain may be referred to in terms of: (1) *time of occurrence* as in posttherapy pain; (2) *duration* or length of time experienced as in acute or chronic pain; (3) *intensity* such as in mild pain or severe pain; (4) *location* as in superficial, deep, or central pain; (5) *mode of transmission* as in referred or projected pain; (6) *ease of transmission* as in inhibited or facilitated pain; (7) *manner experienced* as in sharp, burning, throbbing, or dull pain; (8) *general causative agent* as in self-inflicted pain, spontaneous, organic; (9) *direct source* as in gallbladder or sacroiliac pain; or (10) *autonomic relationship* such as related to sympathetic or parasympathetic origin.

From a purely clinical viewpoint, it seems that differences in the quality of pain are due to: (1) different patterns of stimulation of nociceptors, (2) different locations in the body, and/or (3) simultaneous stimulation of other types of receptors along with pain receptors.

The Intensity of Pain

In studying pain-sensitive tissues, Kellgren/Samuel found that the musculoskeletal structures most sensitive to noxious stimulation were periosteum and joint capsules. Subchondral bone, tendons, and ligaments are moderately pain sensitive, while muscle and cortical bone were slightly less sensitive. The least sensitive tissues were articular cartilage and fibrocartilage. Bone and joint pathology, although appearing well advanced on x-ray films, may be "silent" until the periosteum or joint capsule becomes involved. It is for this reason that IVDs which have become severely degenerated rarely cause discomfort until more sensitive adjacent tissues become involved. A complete muscle rupture is not as painful as a moderate strain/sprain in which the tendinous and ligamentous attachments to periosteum are involved.

There are three commonly held fallacies about pain: (1) persons who are critically ill or gravely injured always experience intense pain; (2) the greater the pain, the greater the amount of tissue damage; and (3) severe chronic pain is symptomatic of incurable illness. Many people who are critically ill (eg, suffering from terminal cancer) or gravely injured do not inevitably experience intense pain. Some do, others do not. The intensity of pain is not directly proportional to the severity or extent of tissue damage; it depends whether pain pathways are intact and activated. In addition, the personality of the neurotic patient may accentuate the pain and the Spartan-like personality may diminish its presence.

The general behavior of a patient in pain can provide a measure of its intensity and the patient's ability to cope with it. If the patient is able to concentrate on something else, or if he completely forgets about the pain when asked something unrelated, then the pain is probably not severe. If the patient is able to continue normal activities (eg, working, sleeping), then the pain may be a nuisance but it would not be considered severe even if the patient may relate it in terms reflecting unbearable agony. Through actions, words, gestures, facial expressions, and voice tones and inflections, the patient slowly, and often indirectly, gives us a picture of how much suffering is occurring.

According to Janse, the acuity of interpreted pain depends greatly on the degree and clarity of consciousness possessed by a particular individual; ie, the greater the degree of mentality, the greater degree of estimating and interpretive capacity of the individual. The more keenly the mind is developed, the more pain sensitive it becomes. People in the sciences and skilled professions appear to show a greater degree of pain symptoms than those in the physical trades where less intellectual development is required.

Pain Threshold

The *threshold of pain* is defined as the smallest intensity of a stimulus at which the subject perceives pain. Some authorities define it as the lowest intensity of stimulus that

Table 8.2. Differences Between the Posterior Lemniscal and Anterolateral Spinonothalamic Systems

Sensations Transmitted by the Posterior Lemniscal System	*Sensations Transmitted by the Anterolateral Spinothalamic System*
Touch signals that require a high degree of intensity graduations or stimulus localization.	Touch and pressure signals capable of only crude localization and discrimination.
Signals of movement against the skin and data concerning fine degrees of pressure intensity.	Pain and thermal (hot and cold) signals.
Positional data and phasic signals (eg, vibration).	Sexual sensations.
	Tickle and itch signals.

will excite the sensation of pain even when the stimulus is applied continuously. Beecher described it as "the first barely perceptible pain to appear in an instructed subject (usually revealed by a verbal statement) under given conditions of noxious stimulation." A literature search will reveal widely diverse definitions of *pain threshold.*

The *threshold* of pain is approximately the same for everyone, but how each individual *grades* pain and *responds* to it can differ greatly from one person to another.

Table 8.3. Factors Known to Affect Pain Tolerance

Factor (+)	Decreased Threshold Level
Anxiety	Lowers with fear of pain, domestic distress, and other anxiety states.
Fatigue	While physical fatigue does not appear to influence pain threshold, mental fatigue often lowers the threshold.
Laterality	Lowers on dominant side for physical pain. Reports differ whether psychic pain is increased on the nondominant side.
Life-style	Lowers in patients confined to bed or home with little to occupy their minds.
Nausea	Lowers, possibly because of autonomic excitement.
Pathology	Lowers if tissue damage is present at the site of measurement, thus such a site should not be used to test general threshold.
Personality	Lower with a history of severe, prolonged childhood pain (eg, beatings).
Race	Lower in Blacks, Jews, and Mediterranean peoples, but higher in East Indian and North European peoples.
Sex	Lower in women with electrical stimuli, but reports differ with heat or mechanical pressure.
Skin temperature	Lowers after skin is warmed.
Factor (-)	Increased Threshold Level
Age	Rises with age.
Distraction	Rises with external distraction (eg, noise).
Pain elsewhere	Hippocrates as well as recent investigators have noted that when pain is produced simultaneously in two places, the lesser tends to be obliterated by the greater.
Placebos and suggestion	Increases.
Miscellaneous conditions	Rises with carbon dioxide retention, impaired judgment, peripheral vasoconstriction, and respiratory depression.

Most people will perceive pain when skin temperature reaches 45°C. It is at this temperature that tissue damage begins to occur because of thermal injury. Almost all subjects perceive pain before the temperature reaches 47°C. Thus, *it is almost never true that some people are unusually sensitive or insensitive to pain.* However, this is not to say that different people do not react differently to the same intensity of pain.

Conditioning impulses entering the sensory areas of the CNS from various parts of the cerebrospinal and peripheral nervous systems can determine whether incoming sensory impulses will be transmitted extensively or weakly to other areas of the brain. See Table 8.3. It has been found that the perception of pain may be strongly modulated according to an individual's experiences and his direction of attention and intention. Since different people have past experiences, expectations, and motivations that cannot be equal, their perceptions are not likely to be the same except in areas where general experiences overlap. Even then, two people will rarely report a simultaneous experience in the same terms or with the same emphasis. Therefore, the same event, as determined by sensory data reaching consciousness, may be experienced as distinctly different events in different people. Some other factors that determine pain responsiveness are an individual's mood, personality, race, sex, age, and health status.

Distribution and Timing

Besides intensity and threshold, two other qualities of pain are its distribution and periodicity. It appears that *distribution* is governed primarily by the myotome, dermatome, or sclerotome area in which the pain may be perceived. Concerning the *periodicity* of pain, various physiologic or psychologic factors may influence whether the pain is worse or better at certain times of the day or night, or following certain activities.

Measuring Sensitivity

A patient's gross sensitivity to a painful stimulus should be measured clinically to (1) determine the integrity of pain pathways, (2) evaluate the level of patient sensibility, and/or (3) determine the patient's pain threshold.

Subjective Methods

The pain threshold and tolerance of a patient is frequently determined in general practice by (1) pricking the skin with a pin or (2) pressing an area of tender tissue (Fig. 8.2). The patient is asked to say "now" when a painful sensation is first felt and say "stop" when the sensation becomes unbearable. This gives the subjective points of (1) threshold and (2) end-point. The span between these points is a measure of tolerance. See Table 8.4.

Pain tolerance can be defined as the greatest intensity of painful stimulation that a subject is able to tolerate. It is common practice, however, to refer to pain tolerance as the quantity of painful stimuli that a subject can bear voluntarily *between* the low and upper pain thresholds. As with pain threshold, an exact definition of pain endpoint and tolerance is controversial. There does not appear to be a definite correlation between the tolerance of pain (reaction interval) and its threshold. During clinical studies, three arbitrary phases are often recorded:

1. When the intensity of a noxious stimulus is slowly increased, there comes a point where pain is experienced by the subject and reported (initial verbal complaint). This can be considered the individual's *low pain threshold.*
2. If the intensity continues to increase, it reaches the degree where it "hurts a lot." This can be considered the individual's *severe pain threshold.*
3. If the intensity is still increased, it reaches a point characterized by a rapid pulse increase and automatic withdrawal. This can be considered the individual's *upper pain threshold.*

Objective Methods

Severe or prolonged pain produces several noticeable signs of which the examiner should be aware. With severe pain, there is an increase in pulse rate, respiratory rate, perspiration, and vasomotor tone. There is also an initial rise in blood pressure and possibly nausea, vomiting, and pallor.

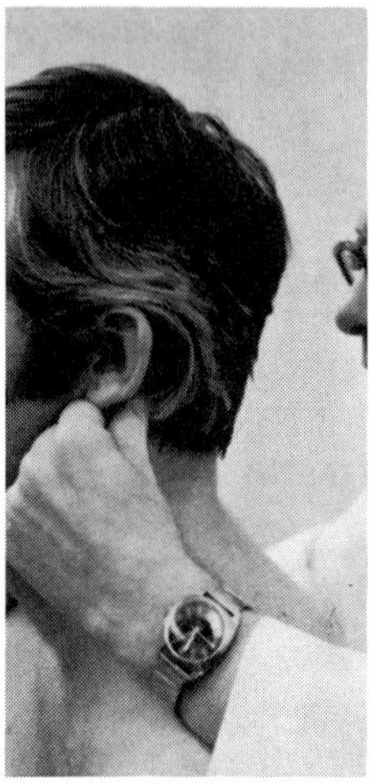

Figure 8.2. Pressing the mastoid processes to evaluate a patient's sensitivity to pressure pain (Libman's test).

Common Patterns of Pain

Determination of the lesion site is often aided by noting the distribution of pain along the course of the involved nerve and the areas of cutaneous sensory disturbance, if any are expressed. The pain may be localized at the site of involvement, below the site of involvement, or be widespread because of referred or projected somatic impulses. It also may be a manifestation of psychic conversion.

Dermatomes, Myotomes, and Sclerotomes

The differentiation of somatic pain reference often rests upon the examiner's knowledge and consideration of dermatomes, myotomes, sclerotomes, and their courses (Fig. 8.3). Grieve points out that the regional distribution and innervation of musculoskeletal and associated tissues evolve from embryonic ectoderm, endoderm, and mesoderm, and these primitive germ layers retain the parenthood of their source connections

Table 8.4. Methods to Measure Patient Sensitivity to Painful Stimuli

Cold	One technique is to immerse a subject's hand in warm water for a measurable time, then quickly transfer it to an ice water bath and record the reaction time.
Heat	A thermal stimulus with various intensities at a constant time or a constant intensity at various exposure times can be used. Changes in environmental temperature and the effects of repeated stimulation, however, are usually difficult to control.
Pressure	A solid object or probe is pressed against a muscle or protruding bone with a measured force. Various procedures have been used by investigators such as applying the pressure of horse hair brushes of varying hardness, pressing the mastoid processes with a thumb (Libman's test) or an object, using a cheese grater concealed within a sphygmomanometer cuff, or using an algesimeter.
Pricking	The simplest method of evaluation is by means of a pin prick. The patient attempts to evaluate different stimuli that the physician applies with a pin.
Ultrasound	A subject's thumb can be kept in contact with an ultrasonic applicator, noting the initial perception of pain and the point of severe pain (ie, withdrawal).
Vascular occlusion	A tourniquet can be applied to the arm while the subject alternately makes a fist at a constant rate. The time taken to produce pain is then recorded.

with mesodermal somites and the ectodermal segments of the spinal cord and the ectodermal nuclei of the cranial nerves. In general, dermatomes overlie myotomes and myotomes overlie sclerotomes. However, areas of the buttock, face, heart, diaphragm, thenar eminence, and upper thorax have a cutaneous innervation that differs from that of the deeper tissues.

Dermatomes. Dermatomes are areas of sensation on the skin (skin segments) that are primarily supplied by the dorsal root of a single spinal segment. Dermatomal pain follows the anatomical course of the involved nerve fibers, and pain limited in distribution to one or more dermatomes is called *radicular pain.* It is typically sharp, sometimes shooting, and well localized. Specific determination of the segmental level of involvement is usually impossible because, in most cases, each dermatome overlaps about 50% or more of adjacent skin segments. For example, the superior aspect of the T5 dermatome is superimposed on the inferior aspect of the T4 dermatome and the inferior aspect of the T5 dermatome is superimposed on the superior aspect of the T6 dermatome.

Myotomes. Myotomes are muscles or groups of small muscles innervated by a single spinal segment. Some authors refer to

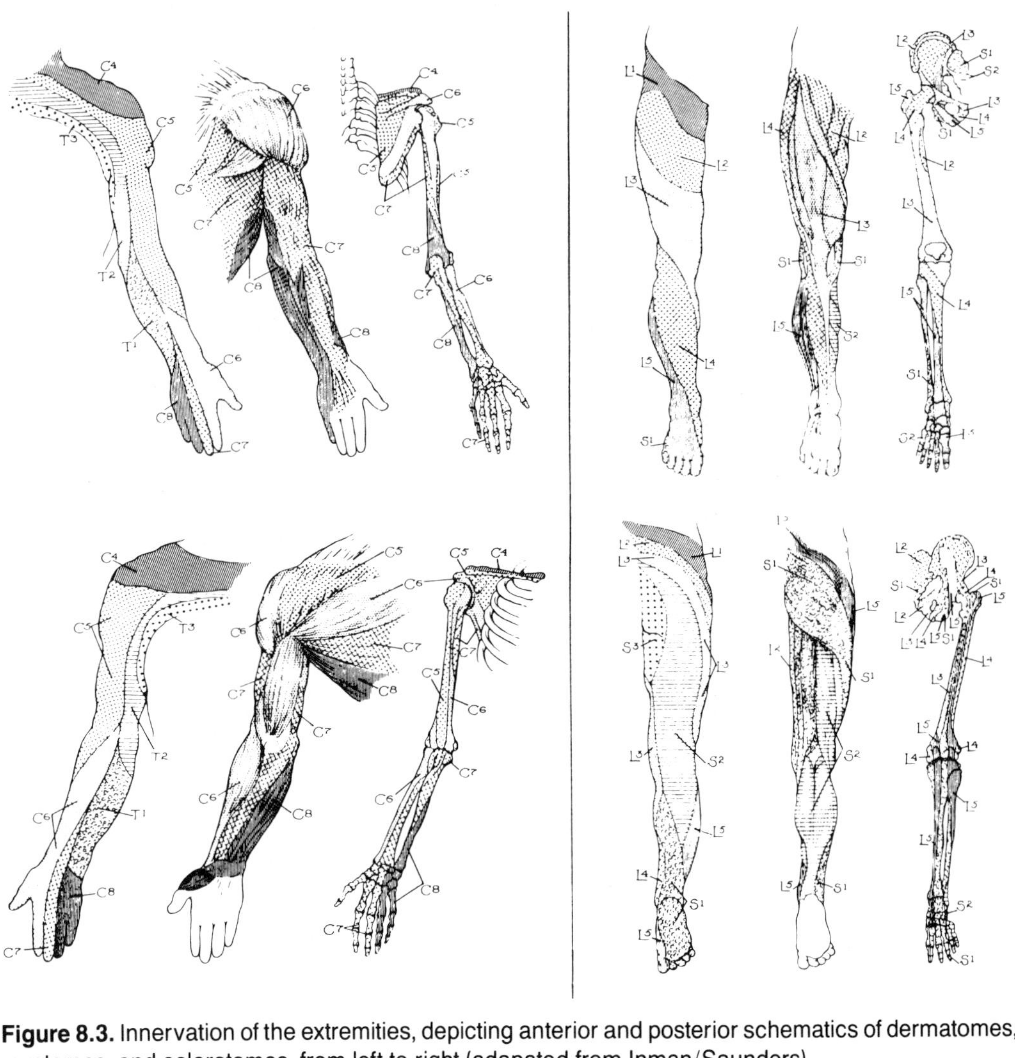

Figure 8.3. Innervation of the extremities, depicting anterior and posterior schematics of dermatomes, myotomes, and sclerotomes, from left to right (adapated from Inman/Saunders).

them as a muscle mass whose total population of motor units is supplied by one nerve root. Because most muscles are supplied by more than one nerve root, most muscles help to form more than one myotome.

Sclerotomes. Sclerotomes are areas of bone, cartilage, and other deep tissues innervated from a single spinal segment. A sclerotome, whose parent is a single mesodermal somite, forms the embryonic tissue that ultimately develops into the skeleton. In contrast to dermatomal pain, sclerotomal pain is typically deep, aching, and poorly localized. An example of its significance is seen with the patient whose pain does not correspond to the site of a known lesion. The pain will be described as traveling down one side of a limb and then abruptly spiral down the other side in a manner that does not correspond to any nerve or muscle. The patient may be describing a sclerotome pattern arising from C6 or L4, for example.

Table 8.5. Typical Syndromes Associated with Pain Referred to the Spine

Origin	Examples	
Psychic focus	Anxiety Camptocormia Compensation neurosis	Depression Hysteria Malingering
Cranial focus	Encephalitis Hematoma Meningitis	Skull fracture (basilar) TMJ dysfunction Tumor
Neck focus	Malignant lymphadenopathy Postpharyngeal abscess	Subarachnoid hemorrhage Vertebral artery deficit
Thoracic focus	Aortic aneurysm Bronchial carcinoma Cardiac enlargement Coronary artery disease Esophageal carcinoma Gallbladder disease	Herpes zoster Hiatus hernia Malignant lymphadenopathy Mediastinal mass Pancoast tumor Pulmonary disease
Abdominal focus	Abdominal sphincter spasm or obstruction Ascites Enteritis (chronic) Malignant lymphadenopathy	Pancreatic carcinoma Pancreatitis (chronic) Peptic ulcer(s) Pyelonephritis Renal carcinoma
Pelvic focus	Aortic obstruction Colon cancer Disseminated sclerosis Ectopic pregnancy Endometriosis Endometritis Ileocecal stenosis	Iliac artery obstruction Malignant lymphadenopathy Ovarian cyst/tumor Prostate carcinoma Prostatitis Rectal carcinoma Uterine carcinoma
Lower extremity focus	Ankle/foot dysfunction Hip disorder	Postural stress (eg, somatosomatic reflexes)

Referred Pain

Pain is said to be *referred* when it originates at one site in the body and is perceived in another such as when it initiates from a deep visceral lesion and is felt to be located in the surface of the body. Common syndromes that are known to refer pain to the spine are listed in Table 8.5.

Distress sensed at the point of injury is called *homotopic* pain. In contrast, *heterotopic* pain and tenderness are distressing sensations that are referred; ie, perceived to arise from an area other than its origin.

Radiating pain may or may not imply intrinsic nerve involvement; ie, it may arise from any structure containing nociceptors. When pain is referred, it is usually expressed in a structure that developed from the same *dermatome* (ie, the same embryonic segment) as the irritated structure. Shepard points out that pain caused by an irritation of the heart is commonly referred to the chest, axilla, and/or inside the left arm; the diaphragm to the neck and shoulder (Fig. 8.4); the stomach to between the scapulae; the appendix to the umbilical area; and the ureter to the groin or testes.

One mechanism widely held responsible for referred pain is *convergence*. This theory assumes that the localization of pain depends on what area or areas of the brain are stimulated. For example, heart pain referred to the arm is explained by the fact that pain fibers from the heart and pain fibers from the arm have an identical final common pathway (refer to Fig. 3.36).

Projected Pain

While most authors treat referred pain and projected pain as synonyms, Lynch/Kessler define *projected pain* as that which is composed of both dermatomal and sclerotomal expression. They believe it shows a direct irritation of nerve pathways projecting afferent input from a particular site (eg, a nerve root). Thus, an IVD lesion or IVF osteophyte may excite fibers in a nerve root servicing sensory or motor functions and thus produce symptoms and signs confined to the relevant dermatome, myotome, and sclerotome. Peripheral entrapment syndromes, however, primarily exhibit as paresthesias long before pain manifests.

The classic courses of referred/projected pain are shown in Table 8.6.

Prolonged Pain

When the normal pattern of adequate activity and rest becomes unbalanced in either direction, malfunction and deterioration are likely to result. Inadequate physical activity can lead to a large number of systemic changes that serve as percursors to chronic pain of somatic origin. The common points of differentiation of pain by duration and intensity are shown in Table 8.7.

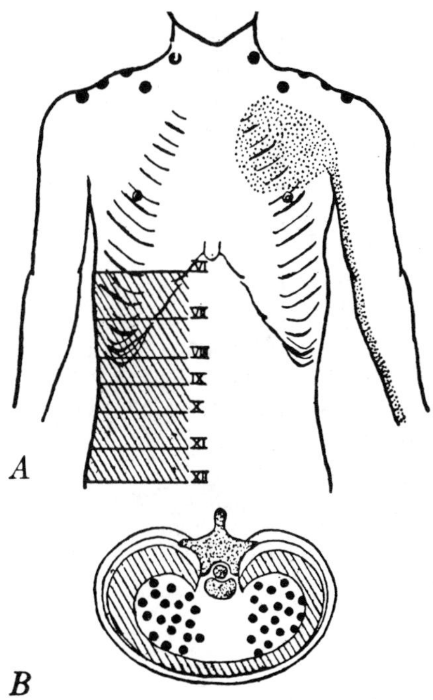

Figure 8.4. Schematic of possible referred pain in diaphragmatic disorders. *A*, cutaneous areas to which pain is referred. *B*, pleural surface of the diaphragm. If the center of the diaphragm (dotted area) is stimulated, pain is felt in the region of the lower neck (black dots) supplied by C3—C4 nerves. If the edge of the diaphragm (striped area) is stimulated, pain is felt in the lower thorax, abdomen, and lumbar region supplied by T6—T12 nerves. Pain of the cardiac region is usually referred to the left side of the chest and down the inside of the left arm (stippled area).

Table 8.6. Classic Courses of Referred/Projected Pain

Priority Suspect Nerve(s)	*Area of Localized Pain*	*Priority Suspect Nerve(s)*	*Area of Localized Pain*
Trigeminal	Anterior head and face	T5—12	Peritoneum
C1—2, T7—12	Occiput	T6—10	Pancreas, spleen
C2—3	Forehead	T7—9	Ascending colon
C3, T1—5	Neck	T8—9	Gallbladder
C3—4, T1—3	Aortic arch	T9—10	Small intestines
C3—4, T1—5	Heart	T9—11	Transverse colon
C3—4, T1—8	Head and face	T10—11	Umbilical area, ovary, testicle
C3—4, T3—5	Lungs		
C3—4, T6—7	Stomach, cardiac aspect	T10—12	Crown of head, scrotum, lower limbs
C3—4, T8—10	Stomach, pyloric aspect		
C3—4, T7—9	Liver	T10—12, S1—3	Prostate
C4	Shoulder girdle, temple area	T10—L1	Kidney, uterine body
		T11—L1	Urethra, epididymis
C5	Deltoid area	T11—L2	Bladder neck, descending colon
C6	Thumb		
C7	First or index finger	T11—L1	Suprarenal area
C8	Fourth finger	T12—L1, S1—4	Uterine neck
T1	Fifth finger	T12—L2	Ureter
T1—4	Thorax	L1	Groin
T2	Nipple area	L1—3, S1—4	Bladder body, rectum, genital organs
T2—4	Bronchi		
T2—5	Upper limbs	L3	Knee, medial aspect
T2—12	Pleura	L5	Great toe
T4—5	Mammae bodies	S1	Fifth toe
T4—7	Thoracic aorta	S2	Thigh (posterior)
T5—8	Esophagus (caudal)	S2—4	Cervix

Note: Authorities differ somewhat as to exact levels, and variances of a segment above or below are commonly stated by different authorities. The above data are a composite of the findings of Pottenger, Firth, Head, and Harvey, et al.

Table 8.7. Differentiation of Pain by Duration and Intensity

Type of Pain	Suggested Etiology
Continuous, dull, spontaneous	Expanding inflammation, muscle strain
Continuous, sharp, with paresthesia	Neuritis
Exacerbative or paroxysmal	Vasospasm (sympathicotonic)
Intermittent, sharp, with paresthesia	Neuritis
Intractable pain	Metastatic invasion, obstructed duct
Remittent pain	Colic, neuralgia

Pain responses initiated through reduced physical activity may become strengthened in time by learning (operant conditioning) processes, according to Fordyce. This process, *the learned pain syndrome*, is similar to any behavior that is modified by positive and negative reinforcements or mimicry (eg, drug tranquility, financial gain, increased attention, reduced responsibilities, relief, sympathy). It is characterized by dependency, disability exaggeration, disuse atrophy, dramatization of complaints, and drug overuse (the "Five Ds").

Persistent pain that is unaffected by activity, rest, or position is likely to have a visceral, obstruction, or neoplastic origin. There are some exceptions to this, of course, such as most headaches, toothaches, earaches, etc. A psychologic origin may be a consideration, but psychogenic pain is unrelieved by analgesic-producing therapies unless the patient is highly receptive to suggestion.

Recurrent Pain

Acute pain or a dull ache recurring at nonspecific intervals is a common characteristic of chronic visceral disease. It is expressed in those dermatomes supplied by neurons whose cell bodies lie adjacent in the cord to the cell bodies of the afferent neurons from a viscus that is or has been the site of distress. This pain may occur when there is no other evidence of pathology, and it is often precipitated at a time of psychic stress or hormonal change (eg, grief, worry, fatigue, menstruation, weather changes, etc).

The cause of recurring pain, states Pottenger, is often a hypersensitive viscerosomatic reflex (ie, a functional cord conditioning lowering the threshold response) established by a previous visceral pathology and initiated by a stimulus that would be insufficient to produce overt malfunction under normal conditions. If this hypothesis is true, then a somatosomatic reflex from an old musculoskeletal injury could produce a similar effect.

Nocturnal Pain

Nocturnal pain that is relieved during the day may have a positional explanation or be the effect of gout or a bone disease. Anxiety states that are worse at night often increase physical pain of other origins during the evening hours. Febrile diseases usually have their crises during the early morning hours.

Effects of Spinal Manipulation in Pain Control

The positive benefits of chiropractic adjustments for the relief of back pain have been written of extensively in chiropractic and osteopathic literature for over 90 years. However, except for German journals, it has only been recently that such reports have begun to appear in allopathic literature. Livingston, Paris, Burns, and Tobis/Hoebler, for example, found that a large percentage of injuries or disorders of the spine can be helped by manipulative treatment. Two other examples are described below:

- A study by Terrett/Vernon assessed the response of paraspinal cutaneous pain tolerance measurements to spinal manipulation. They found that a statistically significant elevation of pain tolerance (140%) occurred after manipulation as compared to the control group.
- A syndrome of back pain is described by Glover that consists of skin hyperesthesia associated with tender areas, a dull ache, and limitation of spinal movement by pain. The tender areas followed the distribution of sclerotomes rather than dermatomes. After one successful manipulation, the syndrome usually disappeared within a few minutes. The hyperesthesia was thought to be the skin component of pain arising in deep mesodermal structures such as nipping of the synovial membrane between the apophyseal facets or the sacroiliac joint, or to tension of a joint ligament. In either case, manipulation restored the normal function of the joints and relieved the patient's pain.

MYOFASCIAL TRIGGER POINTS

Trigger points are functional transient entities; ie, like a pea-shaped spasm, there is no overt histologic change. During palpatory examination, a trigger point (myodysneuria) is noted as a small, deep, hypersensitive area within a myofascial structure. From this focus, high-intensity impulses bombard the CNS and give rise to a deep-aching, sharply demarcated area of referred pain—as contrasted with the ischemic compression nerve pain of prickling, tingling, and numbing that follows the segmental distribution of an entrapped peripheral nerve.

A little-recognized cause of spasm and myofascial pain is often an irritable trigger point in or near a muscle. When a trigger point becomes irritated, the pain may manifest at the site or be referred to a remote area. Many cases of torticollis, shoulder pain, tennis elbow, substernal aches, lumbago, sciatica, hip pain, knee pain, and ankle pain can be traced to trigger-point mechanisms. Such conditions are frequently misdiagnosed as myalgia, myofascitis, nonarticular rheumatism, and sometimes as muscle strain or joint sprain. This is especially true when symptoms persist long after precipitating events.

Sola reports that myofascial pain may be the most common pain problem faced by most physicians. It may present as a primary complaint or as a crippling adjunct to any number of other problems (eg, unequal leg lengths, disuse, immobilization, chronic strains, poor posture, gait disturbances, connective-tissue diseases, arthritides).

Kraus states that visceral or somatic trigger-point irritation can produce a degree of spasm of the paravertebral muscles ipsilaterally in 2—3 segments on the same side as the entering afferent. If the irritation is severe, this effect can spread up, down, and contralateral (eg, as in renal colic). In this regard, Stoddard reminds us that the sharp "textbook" demarcation made between the somatic and autonomic nervous systems is erroneous.

Common Locations

Although one or more trigger points may occur in any muscle, they usually form in clusters. Certain muscles and muscle groups (eg, the antigravity muscles) appear to be more liable than others. The major trigger points producing posterior thoracic pain (low, middle, upper areas) are related to the most common muscles involved in Table 8.8.

One or more trigger points may be localized in one muscle or group, or it also may involve remote muscles or groups. Primary trigger points in the gluteus medius, for example, are commonly related to secondary trigger points in the neck and shoulder girdle. Thus, while trigger points in the neck and upper thoracic muscles may be found to be responsible for or contributing to tension headaches, a group of "mother" trigger points should be sought on the dorsal aspect of the ilia. See Figures 8.5 and 8.6.

Table 8.8. Major Trigger Points Causing Posterior Thoracic Pain

Area of Perceived Pain	Primary Suspect Muscles	
Low thoracic area	Iliocostalis thoracis Longissimus thoracis Multifidi	Rectus abdominis Serratus posterior inferior
Middle thoracic area	Iliocostalis thoracis Infraspinatus Latissimus dorsi Levator scapulae Multifidi	Rhomboids Scaleni Serratus posterior superior Serratus anterior Trapezius
Upper thoracic area	Levator scapulae Multifidi Rhomboids	Scaleni Supraspinatus Trapezius

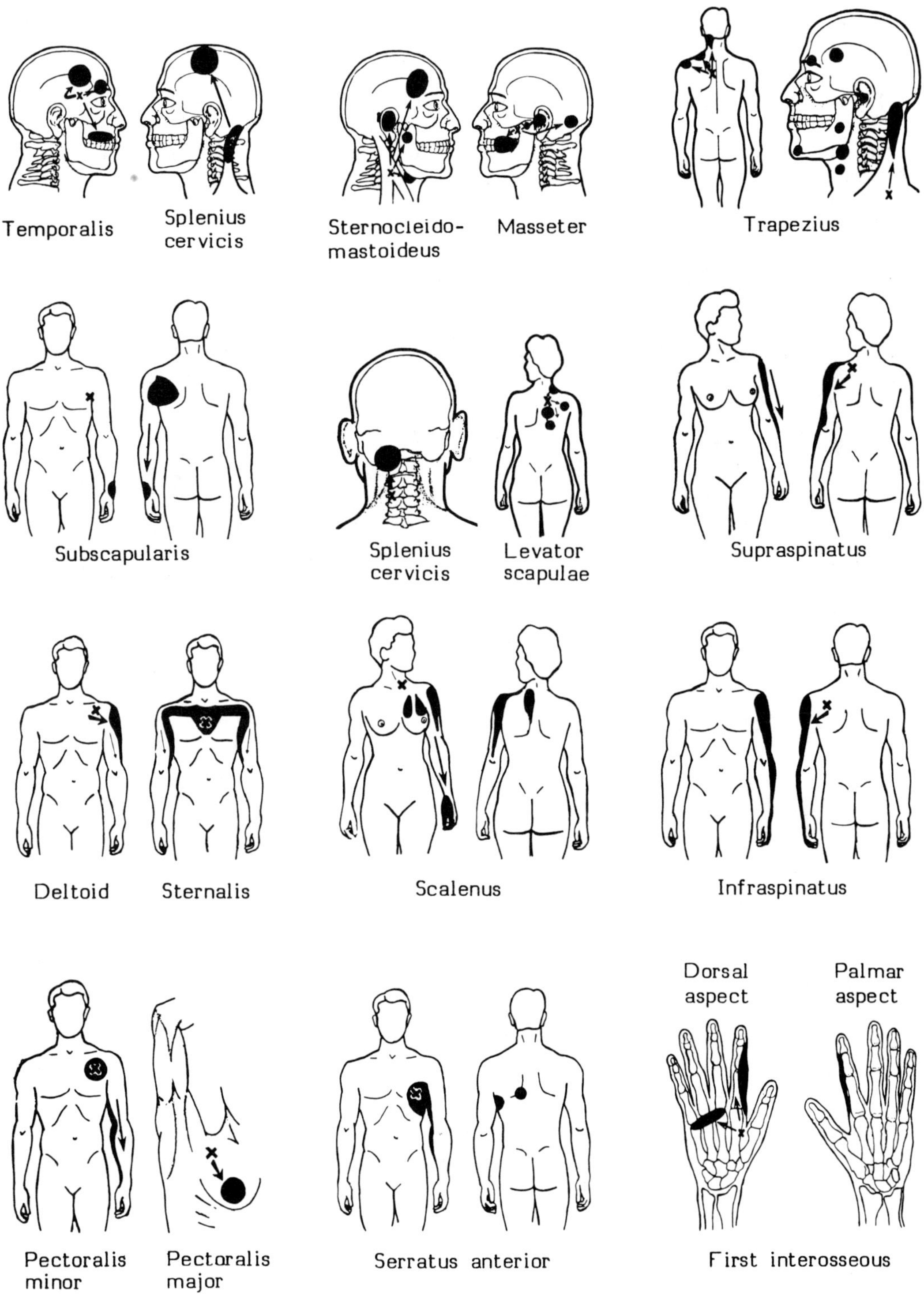

Figure 8.5. Some examples of common trigger points; where X, indicates the common site of the trigger point, and the blackened areas indicate typical areas of referred pain.

Predisposing Conditions

Trigger point syndromes often appear related to a lack of appropriate (but not excessive) exercise; thus, they are less common (but not absent) in athletes and laborers than they are in sedentary workers.

The major conditions that appear to predispose myofascial trigger mechanisms near the spine are chronic strain as the result of prolonged repetitive movement, subluxation, fatigue, tension, infection, neural lesions, nutritional deficiencies, syndromes of the menopause or male climacteric, and hypometabolic states exhibiting creatinuria.

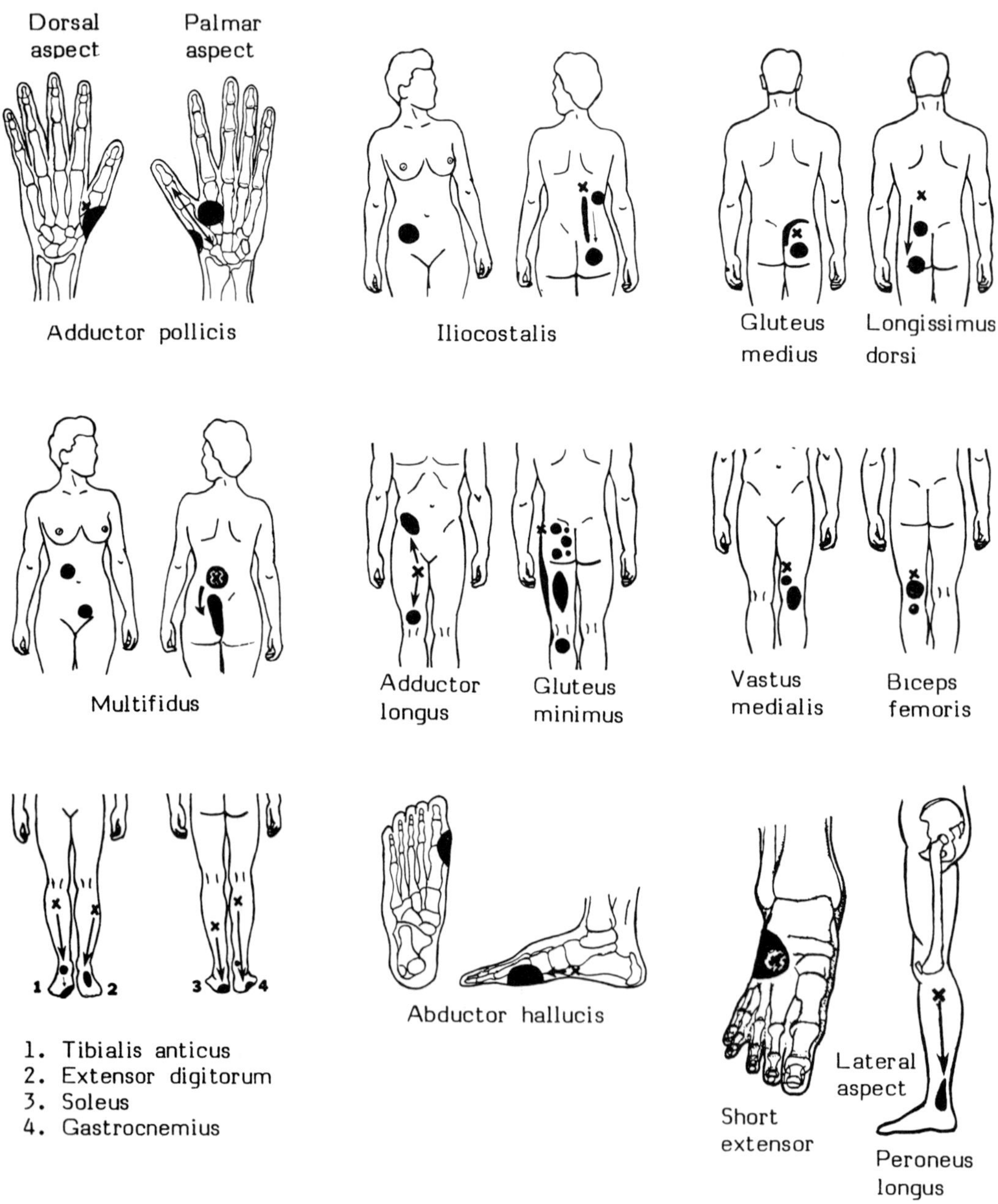

Figure 8.6. Other common trigger points.

Precipitating Factors

Clinicians for many years have found highly localized, exquisitely sensitive areas within or near a painful region. When pressure is placed on the sensitive spot (trigger point), local pain, referred pain, or both may be initiated. Besides deep pressure, an application of heat, cold, electrical stimulation, needling, or some other stimulus may evoke a painful trigger-point reaction. The force of such a reaction appears to be moderated by several factors (eg, conditioning, genetic predisposition, hormonal balance, scar tissue from previous injury, and prolonged emotional stress).

It is generally considered that trigger points are "weak" points within myofascial tissue which are particularly sensitive to stress-induced change. That is, they may remain quiescent until a certain stress (mechanical or metabolic) triggers a syndrome that involves some positive feedback cycles such as sensory and motor reflexes, sympathicotonia, vascular responses, and, possibly, extracellular fluid changes. These can eventually lead to hypertonia, fatigue, and endogenous pain or the intensification of traumatic pain.

According to Travell, the most common precipitating factor is thought to be motion that produces stretching of the tissue containing the focal spot. This ignites a self-perpetuating cycle of pain—spasm—pain that may persist even after the precipitating cause has been removed (eg, subluxation). Other precipitating factors include acute trauma, an inflammatory process, unusual or excessive exercise, chills, IVD herniation producing nerve root pressure, immobilization, and severe anxiety.

The cycles of physiologic responses arising from trigger points involve (1) well-defined pathways (eg, motor reflexes, sensory changes), (2) anticipated autonomic feedback reflexes, and (3) hypothesized microscopic tissue changes. Motor and sensory reactions usually manifest as local and general muscle fatigue, hypertonia, weakness, possibly a fine tremor, hyperirritability, pain, and hypoesthesia.

The autonomic concomitants are similar to those seen with Meridian acupoints. Travell believes that these are frequently expressed as decreased skin resistance, increased pilomotor reaction in the reference area, vasodilation (possibly with dermatographia), and skin temperature changes (coolness). In the typical myofascial syndrome, laboratory analyses and roentgenography fail to show significant bone, joint, or metabolic changes.

Etiologic Hypotheses

Kraus states that the frequent result of chronic muscle tension and spasm is trigger-point development. The effect can be referred pain on pressure over the trigger area, hyperalgesia, joint stiffness, movement limitation, weakness, and autonomic dysfunction occurring in the area of reference (target area). Once one muscle has been affected by trigger points, its whole system of related antagonists and synergists is affected. This muscular dysfunction leads to episodes of tension, spasm, radiating pain, and more trigger points unless proper therapy is applied.

The exact etiology of trigger-point development is unknown. Several hypotheses are described below, and it should be noted that many facets of each overlap to some degree.

The Neurophysiologic Theories

Although the exact physiologic mechanisms of trigger point pain are unknown, Sola offers a neurophysiologic explanation. He feels that, because of physiologic defense mechanisms such as splinting and bracing of muscles, vasomotor changes, increased sympathetic discharge, and hormonal and other humoral changes in plasma and extracellular fluids, the spastic muscle or its fascia (which is probably more sensitive than surrounding tissue due to previous injury or a genetic weakness) fatigues and signals its distress to the CNS. Several responses may result. For example, various muscles associated with the trigger point may become more tense and begin to fatigue because of motor reflexes or because sympathetic responses may lead to vasomotor changes within and around the trigger point.

Zimmermann reports that local ischemia following vasoconstriction or increased vascular permeability following vasodilation may lead to changes in the extracellular environment of the cells involved, release of algesic agents (eg, bradykinins, prostaglandins), osmotic changes, and pH changes—all which may increase the sensitivity or activity of nociceptors in the area. The sympathetic hyperactivity also may cause smooth muscle contraction in the vicinity of nociceptors, thus increasing their activity. This increased nociceptor input may then contribute to the cycle by increasing motor and sympathetic activity, which, in turn, leads to increased pain. This pain may be shadowed by growing fatigue that adds an overall mood of distress to the patient's status and feeds back to the cycle.

As tense muscles in the affected area begin to fatigue in an environment of local sympathicotonia and biochemical change, Sola believes that latent trigger points within the involved muscles also may begin to fire—thus adding to the positive feedback cycle and spreading the pain to these muscles or muscle groups. Finally, the stress of pain and fatigue, coupled with both increased muscle tension and sympathicotonia throughout the body (conceivably with ipsilateral emphasis through the sympathetic chain), may lead to focal exacerbations or trigger points in other muscles that are far remote from the initial area of pain. Common sites and reference zones are shown in Table 8.9.

Sandman states that the focus of pain appears to be from exercise of an ischemic muscle and/or chemoreceptor and mecha-

Table 8.9. Common Trigger Point Syndromes*

Upper Body Location	Primary Reference Zone or Symptoms†
Infraspinatus	Posterior and lateral aspects of the shoulder.
Intercostal muscles	Thoracodynia, especially during inspiration.
Levator scapulae	Posterior neck, scalp, around the ear.
Pectoralis major	Anteromedial shoulder, arm.
Pectoralis minor	Muscle origin or insertion.
Quadratus lumborum	Anterior abdominal wall, 12th rib, iliac crest.
Rectus abdominus	Anterior abdominal wall.
Semispinalis capitis	Headache, facial pain, dizziness.
Splenius cervicis	Headache, facial pain, dizziness.
Sternocleidomastoideus	Headache, dizziness, neck pain, ipsilateral ptosis, lacrimation, conjunctival reddening, earache, facial and forehead pain.
Trapezius	Lower neck and upper thoracic pain, headache.
Lower Body Location	**Primary Reference Zone or Symptoms†**
Anterior tibialis	Anterior leg and posterior ankle.
Gastrocnemius/soleus	Posterior leg, from popliteal space to heel. These trigger points may be involved in intermittent claudication.
Gluteus medius	Quadratus lumborum, tensor fasciae latae, gluteus maximus and minimus, sacroiliac joints, hip, groin, posterior thigh and calf, cervical extensors, upper upper thoracic muscles.
Tensor fasciae latae	Lateral aspect of the thigh, from ilium to the knee.

*Adapted from Sola, with slight modifications.

†Reference patterns vary considerably according to the severity and chronicity of the trigger point phenomenon involved.

noreceptor stimulation from pressure by accumulated metabolic debris or irritation by released acetylcholine, blood serum, bradykinin, histamine, inflammatory exudates, substance P, and 5-hydroxytryptamine. He feels that the amount of degeneration or pathologic alteration created may relate directly to the length of time these conditions are allowed to exist within a muscle.

The Neurochemical Theory

Simons offers a neurochemical explanation of trigger point development that also deserves consideration. He feels that a traumatically induced tear in the sarcoplasmic reticulum initially causes the release of calcium that acts in conjunction with adenosine triphosphate (ATP) to stimulate continuously local contractile activity. This uncontrolled contraction shortens and tenses fibers within the involved muscle bundle(s). Such increased physiologic activity can initiate a subsequent increase in sustained, uncontrolled, localized metabolic activity by the muscles that is capable of producing substances that cause a hypersensitivity of involved sensory nerve fibers and, possibly, stimulate localized reflex vasoconstriction to help control what otherwise might be a rapidly increasing metabolic activity. The result is local tenderness, referred pain, and decreased blood flow within the involved muscle area.

Once the local energy and nutrient supply becomes restricted in this manner, ATP stores become depleted. When this occurs, the local physiologic contracture of muscle fibers is converted to an energy-deficient contraction. Thus, the sarcoplasmic reticulum of the muscle must be repaired. If sufficient energy is not available, the calcium pump (which is the most energy-sensitive step in the contractile mechanism) will respond with continued muscle contraction, creating an even greater energy depletion.

It has been found clinically that normal function may be restored by stretching the locked actin and myosin filaments far enough apart to eliminate contraction (eg, deep friction massage). Following stretching, enough ATP will then accumulate to restore a normal sarcoplasmic reticulum, according to Simons, which would allow the inhibited circulation to remove the accumulation of metabolic by-products slowly.

Correlation with Acupoints

Trigger points, associated with myofascial and visceral pains often lie within the areas of referred pain, but many are found far from them. These properties of trigger points, their widespread distribution, and the pain relief produced by stimulating them resemble those of acupuncture. A study by Melzack (coauthor of the "gate theory") and associates determined a correlation between trigger points and acupuncture points for pain on the basis of two criteria: spatial distribution and associated pain pattern. A high degree (71%) of correspondence was found. This correlation suggests that trigger points and acupuncture points for pain, though discovered independently and labeled differently, represent the *same* phenomenon.

VISCERAL PAIN

Pain originating from viscera features a diffuse dull ache that is entirely unrelated to posture. There are, generally, no *articular* signs of muscle guarding (splinting), blocked motion, or sharp pain during movements of the part, unless somatic soft tissues are also involved (eg, peritonitis). The major causes of true visceral pain are chemical irritation, distention, ischemia, and/or visceral spasm.

Viscerally produced pain is often difficult to distinguish from deep somatic pain except for colic. A distended viscus can produce intermittent regular pain, sometimes of an extreme degree, which is characteristic and quite unlike the intermittent pain produced by somatic structures. Nociceptive impulses from viscera travel mainly through C-fiber (unmyelinated) afferents.

Splanchnic Pain

Although research has not been directed to visceral nociceptors to the extent it has to somatic nociceptors, specific visceral nociceptors have been shown to exist by Cervero and others. In general, visceral organs have sensory receptors primarily for pain, especially terminals sensitive to tension and pressure forces such as seen in distension or prolonged isometric muscle contraction of hollow organs. For example, a ruptured, ulcerated, burned, or severed viscus is not painful in itself, but one distended by gas or a space-occupying mass is (eg, tumor, aneurysm, swollen gland or capsule).

Receptors for light touch, compression, heat, and cold are either not found within visceral walls or are very sparsely distributed. It is for this reason that highly localized types of damage to an internal organ rarely give rise to pain. However, any stimulus that causes diffuse stimulation of nociceptors throughout a viscus can cause pain that may be extremely severe. An occlusion of the blood or lymph supply also can do this. Thus, any stimulus that excites pain-sensitive receptors in diffuse areas of a viscus can elicit visceral pain.

Parietal Reflexes

Visceral pain also may have an underlying parietal cause or contribution. Some pain sensations are transmitted from the viscera to nerve fibers that innervate the parietal peritoneum, pleura, and pericardium. These are primarily spinal cord arcs (viscerosomatic reflexes). The parietal surfaces of visceral cavities are supplied mainly by sensory fibers that penetrate centrally from more superficial branches. Thus, parietal pain and tenderness is due to this extension innervation. It is frequently sharp and pricking in quality but may be perceived as a burning sensation or a dull ache (Fig. 8.7).

Visceral Pain Mimicking Musculoskeletal Disorders

Most visceral sensations travel the same pathway as somatic sensations in the spinothalamic tracts and the thalamic radiation. The major exceptions to this are the few (but potent) sensory fibers that travel to the brain along with the vagus nerve.

Pathologic conditions in many organs of the body have been noted to exhibit painful symptoms that are directly related to specific cutaneous zones. These skin areas have been noted to be so characteristic that they have become useful to the physician during diagnosis. Although pain has been known to be referred from one organ to another (viscerovisceral reflex), pain is most often referred from a visceral organ and interpreted as pain in the skin (viscerosomatic). In fact, many splanchnic ailments exhibit no other sign except that of pain referred to the periphery.

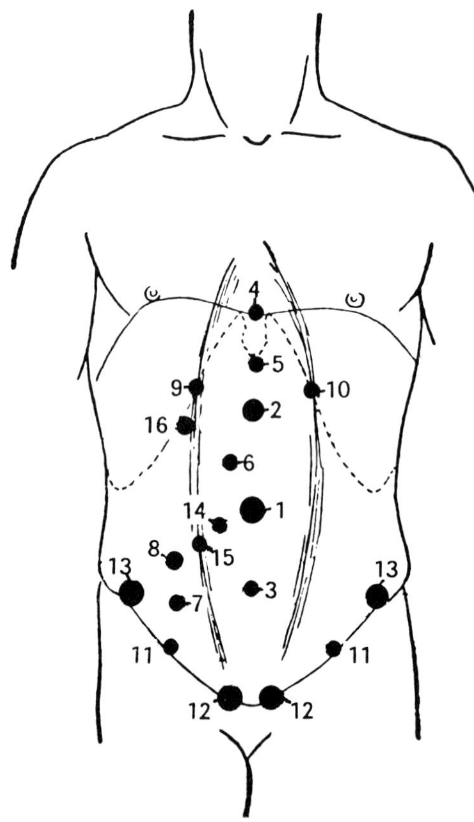

Figure 8.7. Classic abdominal points: *1,* umbilicus; *2,* Addison's or midepigastric point; *3,* mid-hypogastric point; *4,* sternoxiphoid point; *5,* tip of xiphoid process; *6,* Robson's point; *7,* Lanz's point; *8,* McBurney's point; *9,* right costorectal point; *10,* left costorectral point; *11,* mid-Poupart point; *12,* pubic spine; *13,* anterior superior iliac spine; *14,* Morris's point; *15,* Munro's point; *16,* tender point with acute cholelithiasis.

It is hypothesized that when visceral pain fibers are intensely irritated, especially by overdistension or an impaired blood supply, the intense stimulation produces such a bombardment of impulses to the cord that some spill over to affect synapses that connect with cutaneous afferents from the skin and subcutaneous tissues. This can produce referred hyperesthesia and deep tenderness. The patient then has the feeling that the sensations are originating in peripheral tissues. In this context, it should be noted that a paravertebral inflammatory reaction need not be from infection but of irritation from malfunction in a part of the gastrointestinal tract that reflexly produces vasospasm in the para-articular tissues and hence pain.

Many back pains and certain types of headaches appear to be caused by muscular spasm, with the spasm originating reflexly from much weaker pain impulses originating elsewhere in the body. Other examples are the severe cluster-like temporal headaches associated with gastric ulcers or the migraine-type headaches associated with many gynecologic syndromes. Another example is the pain associated with a ureter or prostate, which can result in reflex spasm of the lumbar muscles. Thus, irritation produced by malfunction of an abdominal/pelvic organ or valve may produce many signs and symptoms that can confound the diagnostician.

Some comparative characteristics between splanchnic and somatic pain are shown in Table 8.10.

Musculoskeletal Disorders Mimicking Visceral Disease

In investigating the history of any visceral problem, the sympathetic and parasympathetic innervation to the viscera and the structures related to the viscera must be considered. Next, the somatic and visceral

Table 8.10. Splanchnic vs Somatic Pain

	Splanchnic Disorders	Somatic Disorders
Origin	Diseased organ	Neuromuscular tissue
Location and radiation	Deep, poorly localized, often radiates or is referred to the surface	Same
Distribution	Segmental	Dermatome, myotome, sclerotome
Intensity	Correlates with the intensity of stimulation	Same
Quality	Gripping, cramping, aching, squeezing, crushing, stabbing, or burning	Vague, aching, dull, heavy, boring, or pounding character that is intensified by movement, compression, pulsation
Alleviating-exacerbating factors	Intensified by motor activity or compression of an involved viscus that correlates with secretory or motor rhythms of the involved viscus	Relieved by rest and inactivity
Associated factors	Patient presents a trial-and-error behavior, often based upon past experience, in an attempt to relieve the pain	Patient avoids movement, pressure, and presents awkward motions because of the protective spasm associated

reflexes that affect other tissues must be appraised. Visceral dysfunction frequently refers pain to the spinal segments supplying the involved viscera and also alters the function of other viscera sharing the same nerve supply. In addition, the probability should be considered of somatic dysfunction occurring in segmentally involved areas causing visceral dysfunction or in other somatic structures sharing the same nerve supply.

Just as visceral disease can exhibit solely as signs of a somatic nature, musculoskeletal disorders can mimic visceral disease. Several examples are described below.

Headaches. Headaches, the most frequent symptom in America today, are usually attributed to tension, migraine, abnormal sinus, tumor, vascular disorders, or hysteria. Often neglected causes are overall postural strain and trauma to the cervical spine (Fig. 8.8), and headaches caused by viscerosomatic reflexes from the gallbladder, stomach, and duodenum are much more common than suspected. Nausea or vomiting with headaches is usually considered to have a neurologic basis of a vascular nature; however, a vagal disturbance due to upper cervical malfunction may be the cause.

Vertigo. Vertigo makes basilar insufficiency or Meniere's syndrome suspect, but vertebral artery ischemia due to upper cervical dysfunction or an atlanto-occipital subluxation may be the reason. In blackout spells of an unexplained nature, epilepsy and arterial occlusive disease are suspect, but somatic dysfunction involving the cervical ganglia may be the cause.

Chest Pain. Chest pain usually points to acute or chronic coronary insufficiency, dissecting aneurysm, or it may be of esophageal or pleural origin. It also may be referred from the gallbladder, stomach, duodenum, or pancreas. However, chest pain also may be the result of somatic rib cage dysfunction, costochondral or costovertebral strain, or pseudoangina.

Chest Pains Associated with Cough. In chest pains associated with a cough, acute and chronic pulmonary infections, pneumonia, lung abscess, and chronic bronchitis are usually suspected, along with pleuritis and lung or pleural tumors. Bronchial tumor, pulmonary embolism, broncholith, bronchiectasis, postnasal discharge, or the inhalation of irritants also should be considered. Reflex considerations would include costovertebral dysfunction, costochondral dysfunction or separation, or costal fracture. Reflexes from clavicular strains affecting recurrent laryngeal nerves, cervical subluxation, or cerumen impaction should not be overlooked.

Respiratory Symptoms. Ventilatory impairment is usually suspected in dyspnea or of metabolic origin, but it may be the result of rib cage dysfunction, spondylitis, or paravertebral muscle spasm and pain. Air hunger at rest is a cardinal sign of anxiety, and it is often seen in chronic obstructive pulmonary disease. However, it is also a reflex sign of rib cage dysfunction.

Upper Extremity Symptoms. Several diseases may refer pain to the shoulder or arm. This is seen often in disorders other than those of the gallbladder such as coronary artery disease, empyema, pneumothorax, pericarditis, mediastinal lesions, peptic ulcer, diaphragmatic hernia, perisplenitis,

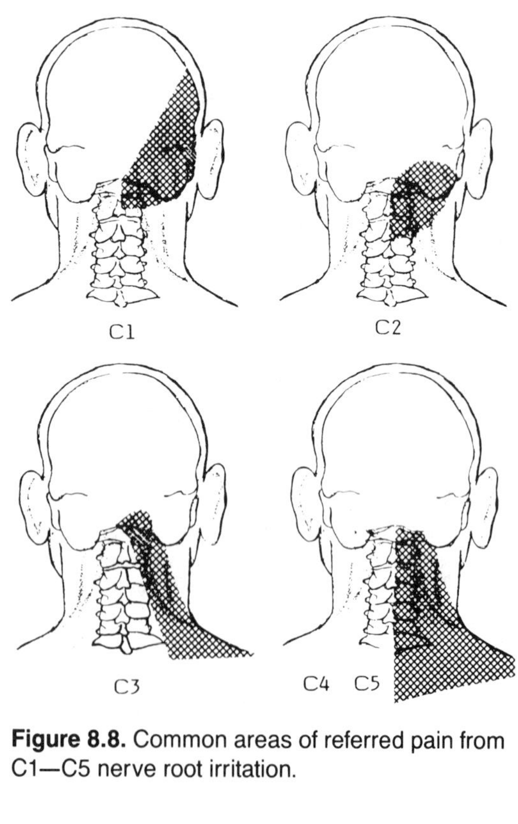

Figure 8.8. Common areas of referred pain from C1—C5 nerve root irritation.

and subphrenic abscess. Pain radiating to the arm may be referred from coronary disease. It also may be a reflex from brachial neuropathy caused by dysfunction or degenerative disease of the cervical spine. The referred scapular pain of gallbladder disease and other visceral disorders have been mentioned. Frequently overlooked is the gallbladder reflex causing cardiac arrhythmia. Pain, numbness, or tingling in the hands is seen in many neuropathies. However, the cause may be musculoskeletal in origin such as degenerative disease or somatic dysfunction of the cervical spine, brachial plexus entrapment due to clavicular and upper rib dysfunction, carpal tunnel syndrome, or cervical cord compression.

PARESTHESIA

The term *paresthesia* refers to a perverted sensation or uncomfortable sensation not amounting to pain—but it may be concomitant with pain. The most common paresthesias are sensations of numbness, tingling, formication or itching, weight or bearing down, coldness, faintness, fullness, girdle sensation, precordial constriction, and weakness or debility.

Paresthesia is commonly witnessed in the form of the familiar prickling and tingling felt when one's arm or leg has "gone to sleep." Sensations as of crawling insects are not uncommon; the "hot feet" of many elderly persons with arteriosclerosis and the "burning hands" of people who work in hot water are other familiar examples. Local paresthesia is common in lesions of the cerebral cortex and constitutes the preliminary aura with which many attacks of epilepsy are ushered in. Well-developed tabes dorsalis shows many curious or distressing varieties of paresthesia, as do many other varieties of peripheral neuritis.

Common Types

Numbness. Numbness and tingling may occur in the feet during the initial stages of locomotor ataxia, apoplexy, tumor of the brain, spinal meningitis, neuritis, myelitis, and neurasthenia to name a few associated disorders. It indicates the loss of sensory function.

Itching. Formication is a sensation of insects crawling upon the skin. It occurs in diabetes, jaundice, and skin diseases. General formication is more common in cases of hysteria, neuresthesia, and drug intoxication.

Precordial Constriction. Precordial constriction is a feeling of tightness in the chest that is near the point of suffocation. It is encountered in those diseases accompanied by intense dyspnea such as bronchial asthma, emphysema, angina pectoris, meteorism, and heart trouble.

Girdle Sensation. A girdle sensation is an important and common paresthesia found in disease of the nervous system. It is a subjective sensation of a tight band drawn around the waist and often associated with locomotor ataxia, myelitis, and tumor of the spinal cord.

Bearing Down. The sensation of weight is most commonly found in the pelvis and is more frequently found in women than in men. It is symptomatic of prolapse of the uterus, pelvic tumors, or falling of the abdominal viscera.

Fullness. The sensation of fullness is usually perceived when the abdomen is distended by gas or fluid as in gastritis and ascites, or it may be present when there is pressure by an enlarged or prolapsed organ.

Coldness. The sensation of coldness is present at the beginning of a fever or during the chill stage but also occurs in a few cases in which the body temperature is normal. These latter instances are usually diseases of the nervous system in which the sensation is only mentally initiated. Such sensations of coldness are found in neurasthenia, hysteria, and chorea.

Faintness. Faintness is a feeling of extreme bodily weakness with a cloudiness of the intellect and occurs from cerebral anemia. Early chiropractors often attributed this to a subluxation in the region of T2 in which the heart is affected to such an extent that the brain is not receiving sufficient oxygen to maintain consciousness. It was also felt it may be caused by an atlas subluxation in which the vasomotor nerves of the vessels of the brain are impinged, thus causing a spasm of these muscles and rendering a part or whole of the cerebrum anemic to some extent. It occurs in diseases of the heart and hydrothorax, pleurisy with effusion, or sometimes as a result of great emotion, fatigue, or excessive heat.

Vertigo. This is a subjective sensation of a loss of equilibrium. When it appears that the patient himself is falling, rising, or whirling, it is called *subjective vertigo.* When the objects around the patient appear to be in a state of motion, it is called *objective vertigo.* Both subjective and objective vertigo may be classed as horizontal if present when the patient is lying down. Horizontal vertigo always disappears when the patient assumes an erect position. Vertigo itself is a symptom and not a disease. It is often found in disorders of the heart, liver, stomach, disease of the semicircular canals of the internal ear, and in acute alcohol intoxication.

Weakness. Weakness or debility attends the onset of all febrile diseases and appears toward the close of wasting diseases. It may be especially marked in diseases such as diabetes mellitus, cancer, anemia, influenza, tuberculosis, and neurasthenia.

Meralgia Paresthetica

This syndrome, often referred to as *lateral femoral cutaneous neuropathy,* features a patch of anesthesia, paresthesia, or hyperesthesia, with or without pain, on the anterior surface of one or both thighs in the distribution of the lateral femoral cutaneous nerve. Sites defines the condition simply as a sensory disturbance affecting the lateral cutaneous nerve.

The lateral femoral cutaneous nerve arises from the posterior divisions of L1—L3, appears at the lateral border of the psoas, passes obliquely across the iliacus to the ASIS, and then travels under the inguinal ligament to enter the anterolateral aspect of the thigh. The focus of irritation is often found (1) at the L1—L3 IVFs from subluxation encroachment or arthritic hyperplasia or (2) in the pelvis from repetitive trauma as seen in athletic injuries and late pregnancy. Nevertheless, pathology or impingement anywhere along the course of the nerve may be responsible, whether it be intraspinal, intersegmental, paraspinal, retroperitoneal, pelvic, or, rarely, abdominal.

The typical patient inflicted reports a sense of numbness or burning in the anterolateral aspect of the thigh, which is rarely painful until the late stages. Care must be taken to differentiate this syndrome from trochanteric or iliopectineal (iliopsoas) bursitis because both refer pain to the anterolateral thigh. It also should be kept in mind that pronation or supination of the ankle, genu varum, genu valgum, genu recurvatum, flexion contracture, etc, can cause or contribute to anterosuperior thigh pain.

Notalgia Paresthetica

Pleet/Massey describe this disorder of unknown etiology as a sensory neuritis that affects the posterior rami of several thoracic spinal nerves (T2—T6), producing itching, burning, dysesthesia, and hyperesthesia. They point out that the posterior rami of these spinal roots traverse at a 90° course through the multifidus spinae muscles, making them unique among the posterior rami.

DIAGNOSTIC CONSIDERATIONS

Testing sensory perception helps to determine the condition of the peripheral receptors, their afferent fibers, the sensory columns of the spinal cord, and the higher sensory areas of the nervous system. If not conducted on a regional basis, some examiners leave this portion of the neurologic examination to the last because it is the most tedious and challenging part of the investigation.

General somatic sensations are divided into two major classes: *exteroception* and *proprioception.* Exteroception includes the sensations of pain, temperature, and light touch from the surfaces of the body. Proprioception includes the sensations of muscle, tendon, ligament, and joint activities, along with vibratory awareness, deep pain, and deep pressure perceptions. In evaluating *exteroceptive qualities,* tactile, pain, and temperature tests should be conducted. In judging *proprioceptive qualities*, position, motion, vibration, deep pain, stereognosis, and two-point discrimination tests should be conducted.

Daube/Sandok recommend that the examination of sensation should consist of three portions: (1) *qualitative*, to determine the elements of sensation that are affected; (2) *quantitative*, to determine the degree of involvement when sensation is impaired; and (3) *anatomical*, to map out the areas of sensory impairment.

The Clinical Differentiation of Pain

One of the first steps in the differential analysis of pain is to determine whether the patient's pain is being expressed superficially or deeply within the body part and then to determine whether the pain is of somatic, splanchnic, or psychic origin. If this can be determined, the physician is then in an advantageous position to locate the specific tissues involved.

Significance of Localization

The localization of pain usually depends on whether the source of the pain is superficial or deep. Kellgren has shown that, in general, the closer the involved tissue is to the surface of the body, the better the site of pain corresponds to the site of noxious stimulation. His research team also found that pain of deep musculoskeletal origin was usually delocalized; ie, the site at which the pain is perceived rarely corresponds exactly to the site of its origin.

Pain can be localized only because most of the stimuli that excite nociceptors also excite touch, pressure, or stretch receptors at the same time. Thus, localized pain arises only because more than one type of receptor is activated. If it were not for this important fact, pain would be practically impossible, if not completely impossible, to localize.

Superficial vs Deep Pain

Pain perceived to be on or near the skin (superficial) is usually sharp, localized, of short duration with a sudden onset. In contrast, deep pain is dull, diffuse, of long duration with a gradual onset.

Deep pain of a physical nature can arise from either a splanchnic or a somatic disorder. It can rarely be distinguished easily from pain that is derived from the viscera if the sources are linked with the same segment. Deep pain may give rise to variations in sudomotor, visceromotor, and myotomic activity; but, it is not associated with a loss of muscle strength, a loss of normal reflexes, or a loss of sensory perception (eg, light touch, pressure, temperature, position, two-point discrimination).

Pain of deep somatic origin often radiates into a characteristic pattern that tends to follow dermatome or sclerotome pathways. The extent of this radiation, which almost always radiates distally rather than proximally, depends on the intensity of the noxious stimulation.

When a tissue of a particular sclerotome is irritated, the pain will be perceived to arise from any or all tissues innervated by the same segmental nerve even when they are healthy. Inman/Saunders attribute this to a lack of precision in the central neural connections rather than being related to impulse overflow down a nerve. They feel that the problem is central, not peripheral. This effect has been seen in many chiropractic offices whensevere knee pain, which failed to be corrected by repeated surgery, was relieved when adjustments corrected a lumbar lesion. Similar experiences with chronic elbow pain are commonplace after a lower cervical (C5—C7) subluxation has been corrected. When pain expresses over a sclerotome, state Inman/Saunders, there need not be anything wrong with the area in which the pain seems to arise.

Painful Muscles

Pain originating from muscle tissue has peculiar characteristics. It can arise from an injury to muscle tissue elicited by making the muscle contract against resistance without allowing it to shorten; ie, preventing movement of adjacent joints. This test, although it may be of help in differentiating myalgia from the pain of other etiologies, is not absolute because it is not always possible, even with great care, to avoid some indirect pressure or tension on adjacent structures. An additional feature is that the pain which arises from a chronic contraction of the involved muscle is not increased by contracting the muscle further.

Any type of excessive motor fiber stimulation results in pathologic, involuntary, and painful muscle spasm. Severe spasm places considerable tension on highly sensitive periosteum via tendinous attachments. The spasm itself may be the result of toxic irritation of the anterior horn cells; encroachment irritation of the nerve root; irritation, stretching, or pressure upon a nerve trunk or plexus; irritation or pressure upon peripheral nerve branches; muscle spasm secondary to trauma of an adjacent structure; primary muscle spasm from direct irritation or trauma; or psychogenic muscle spasm.

Tendon Pain. Pain in damaged tendons usually arises when the attached muscle is contracted. The tendon fibers that are torn will usually not cause pain when the muscle is relaxed; but, with the least muscle shortening, pain ensues. The pain of true tendinitis is often superficial, resulting from a tenosynovitis. It is evoked by passively moving the tendon to and fro within its sheath.

Lymph Stasis. Although skeletal muscle tissue lacks an intrinsic lymph supply, a muscle's connective-tissue sheath and tendons are richly endowed with lymphatic vessels. During the normal physiologic exchange of fluids through capillary walls, the quantity of fluid leaving the capillary is usually greater than that entering the venule. The related lymphatic network takes up the excess and eventually delivers it to the venous system. It is this process that allows a continuous exchange of tissue fluids and maintains a constant pressure of interstitial fluid. The flow of lymph is increased during activity as is capillary circulation, but this flow can be restricted by excessive pressure exerted by a constantly hypertonic or phasic contracted muscle. De Sterno explains that inhibited lymph drainage contributes to muscular pain during prolonged activity by (1) causing a buildup of interstitial fluids that increase hydrostatic pressure and (2) encouraging the accumulation of metabolic waste products that would normally be drained by the lymphatics and venules.

Painful Joints

Pain may arise from any joint tissue containing nociceptors such as ligaments, tendon insertions, periosteum, fibrocartilages (slightly), capsules, and vascular walls. Authorities disagree whether the synovial lining contains nociceptors.

Ligamentous Pain. Pain is elicited from irritable ligaments by stretching and deep pressure. Joint ligaments can be stretched by passive movements of the related joint to the limit of the range of motion. When accessible to palpation, an irritated ligament will be tender; and if it can be squeezed, pain will be evoked. Ligamentous pain is the type that develops when a joint is under extremely prolonged stretch (tension). A hypomobile joint should be the first suspicion in such cases. Generally, chronic ligamentous pain comes on slowly after assuming some posture in which the involved joint(s) is held at a limit of motion. The ache arises from the irritation of the intraligamentous and periosteal receptors.

Painful Adhesions. Adhesions do not in themselves contain nociceptors. During movement, however, pain arises when they stretch or occlude adhering, connecting, or congruent pain-sensitive tissues (eg, periosteum, vascular walls, joint or visceral capsules). The cause may be from direct compression or tensile forces or be the product of ensuing stasis, ischemia, or distention. The pain is immediate in onset and not delayed as when the ligaments are relaxed. Another diagnostic clue is the fact that there is a pronounced structural hypomobility when adhesions are present. The most common situation encountered is the painful adhesions that develop after surgery or major trauma. However, adhesions may develop as the result of adhesive capsulitis, rheumatoid arthritis, and septic arthritis. The pain originating in capsules tightened by adhesions occurs at once when the capsule is stretched. If the adhesions are stretched further, a sharp pain may ensue, leaving the surrounding muscles flaccid. The intensity of such a pain varies with the site and size of the adhesions. For the most part, pain arising from adhesions is only momentary because motion is quickly halted as soon as the sharp pain is felt.

Cartilaginous Pain. As with adhesions, pain arises from most cartilaginous tissues only when they are displaced or swollen and stretch or pressure is applied upon adjacent pain-sensitive receptors. The periphery of intervertebral fibrocartilage and the menisci of the knee and jaw contain a few nociceptors, but the degree that they are involved in a patient's report of pain is difficult to determine. A cartilaginous loose body (eg, in the knee) will certainly produce pain if it is caught between two apposing articular surfaces (joint block). If adjacent tissues are inflamed, then both compression and tensile forces will give rise to pain.

Evaluating the Sensory System

Testing should be conducted in a warm room when the patient is relaxed. Examination begins with the face and scalp, then proceeds anteriorly and posteriorly to the soles of the feet. Reactions in both the right and left sides of the body and the upper and lower extremities should be compared.

According to Cabot, the most important types of sensations evaluated during the examination are anesthesia, hyperesthesia, paresthesias, pain, and disorders of the special senses. These disturbances may all be seen in different stages or types of lesions of the spinal cord or peripheral nerves. They are less common in brain lesions. Brain stem lesions can usually be determined through the pupillary reaction to light, corneal reflex, gag reflex, jaw reflex, and ciliospinal reflex.

Mechanoreceptive Sensations

The mechanoreceptive somatic senses are stimulated by mechanical displacement of some tissue of the body. These senses include touch, pressure, vibration, and tickle senses (all which are called the *tactile* senses) and the position sense, which determines the relative positions and rates of movement of different segments of the body.

The Tactile Senses

The perception of light touch is called *esthesia;* increased sensation, *hyperesthesia.* The term *graphesthesia* refers to the sense by which figures or numbers written on the skin are recognized by the patient without being seen (Fig. 8.9).

The patient should close the eyes and be instructed to answer "Yes" when the touch is felt. The examiner frequently outlines with a skin pencil any area that shows a tactile alteration. Lighter and heavier touches may be attempted for comparison, and a graphic record is prepared when appropriate. Some examiners prefer to use a wisp of cotton (Fig. 8.10) for the very light touch and their finger or a blunt instrument (Fig. 8.11) is used to evaluate moderate touch. Light stroking stimulates only the receptors of the skin, thus normal responses are lost in pyramidal tract disease.

Decreased sensation is called *hypesthesia;* loss of sensation, *anesthesia.* Sensory loss may be the result of the same factors that produce pain; however, upper motor neuron lesions also may exist. In such cases, abnormal reflexes and other signs are associated such as loss of superficial reflexes, exaggerated deep tendon reflexes, and paralysis (spastic or rigid).

Superficial Pain Perception

During examination, the patient's eyes should be closed. The patient is touched lightly with the point of a pin and directed to

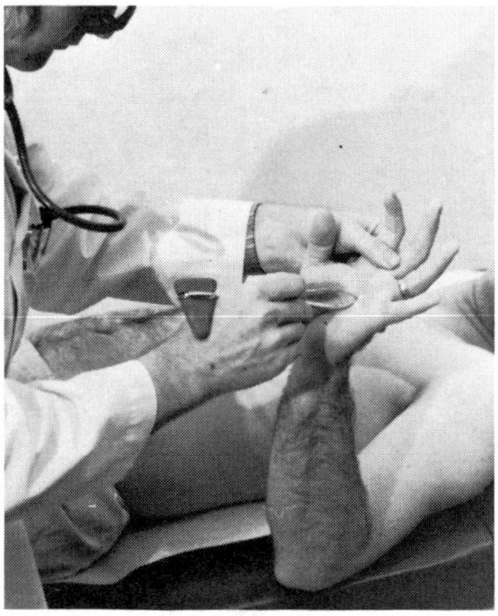

Figure 8.9. Testing graphesthesia on the left palm (American Chiropractic Association).

say "Yes" when the pressure is detected as being "sharp." The procedure then proceeds as in the tactile test. Reactions are then compared using the point and head of the pin or a bent pin, noting the patient's ability to appreciate the difference quickly (Figs. 8.12 and 8.13). If known beforehand, the unaffected side should be tested first—taking care to use the same degree of stimulation over unaffected and affected areas.

Pain is technically called *algesia;* a decrease in pain sensation, *hypalgesia (hypoalgesia);* an absence of pain sensation, *analgesia;* increased pain sensation, *hyperalgesia*—as seen in irritative lesions.

Hypalgesia and Analgesia. Diminished or lack of superficial pain sensation commonly occurs in peripheral neuritis, disorders of the spinothalamic tract, and hysteria. The distribution of anesthesia depends, like the distribution of paralysis, on the lesion. Hemianesthesia is seen most often in hysteria and organic brain lesions. Cord lesions such as transverse myelitis or compression of the cord usually produce anesthesia in the area supplied by the spinal nerves below the lesion. Peripheral nerve lesions may produce anesthesia of the skin supplied by the nerve in question. Areas of hysterical anesthesia (with hyperesthesia and paresthesia) usually do not correspond to the distribution of any set of nerves or centers and are distinguished by this fact.

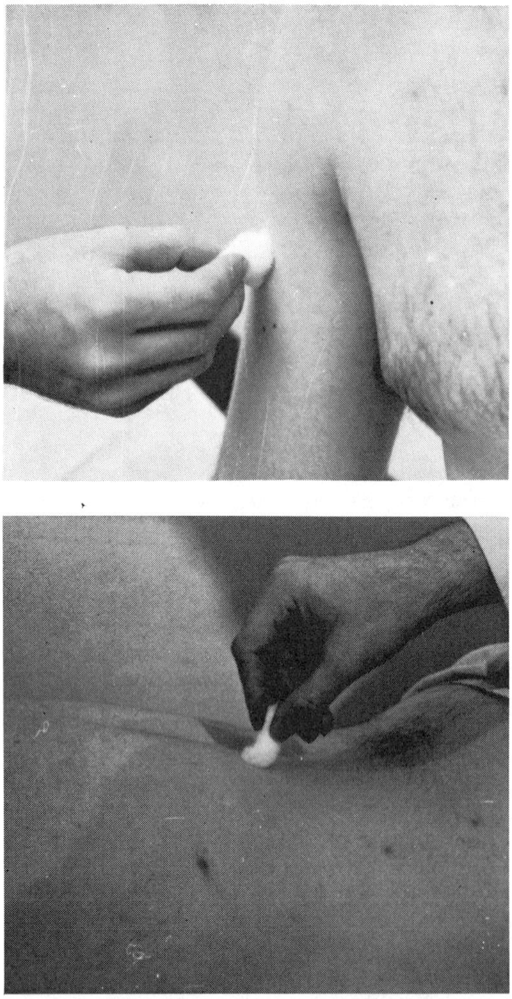

Figure 8.10. *Top,* testing light tactile sense on the right arm with a cotton ball. *Bottom,* testing thoracolumbar light tactile sense (American Chiropractic Association).

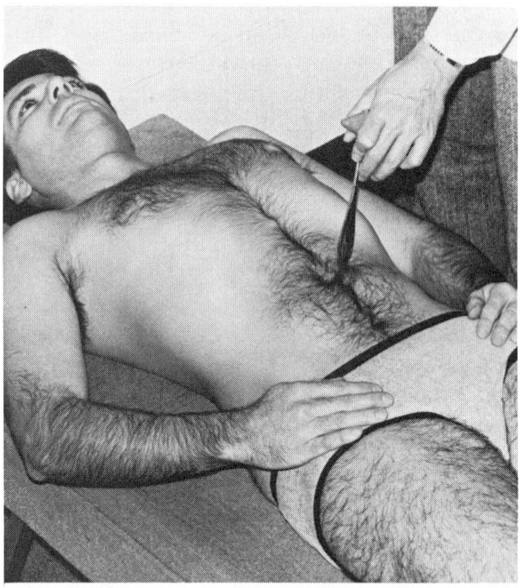

Figure 8.11. Testing the abdominal reflex. Contractions above the navel on sharp downward friction of the abdominal wall indicate normal activity of the spinal cord from the 5th to the 12th thoracic nerves. An absent reflex could indicate the following defective arc: upper quadrant reflex absent, T5—T8; midquadrant reflex absent, T9—T11; lower quadrant reflex absent, T11—T12; all sites diminished or absent, suspect upper motor neuron involvement. Abdominal reflexes are normally diminished or absent in the obese and the elderly.

Hyperesthesia. An increase in pain sensation is most often recognized as hypersensitivity to light tough, abnormal tenderness, or, in the special senses such as hypersensitivity to light or noise. It is most common in peripheral nerve lesions and in hysteria. Increased superficial pain sensation is seen in cases of posterior root irritations caused by local inflammatory processes. A ticklish person is one whose superficial reflexes (skin and muscles) are normally very lively.

Deep Pain Perception

Tenderness on pressure along the various nerves should be tested. Tendons and muscles should be squeezed firmly. The patient *should* be able to detect a painful sensation. Certain areas are more important than others such as squeezing the Achilles tendon, where upon absence of pain is called *Abadie's sign.* In tabes dorsalis, the patient will not feel pain upon normally painful pressure.

Thermal Perception

Decreased temperature sensation is called *thermhypesthesia;* increased sensation, *thermhyperesthesia.*

In evaluating temperature perception *(thermesthesia)*, metal tubes (eg, 5 cc steritube containers) are commonly used: one

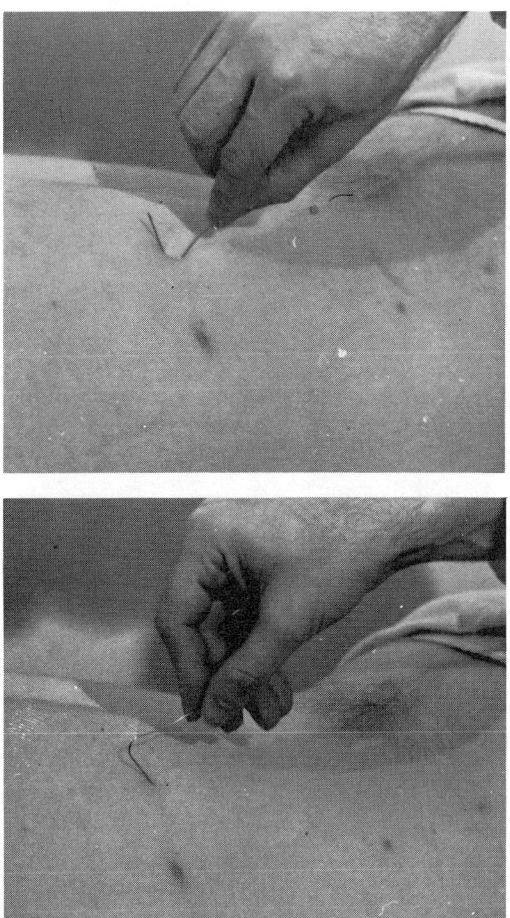

Figure 8.12. *Top,* testing dull superficial pain sense; *bottom,* testing sharp superficial pain sense (American Chiropractic Association).

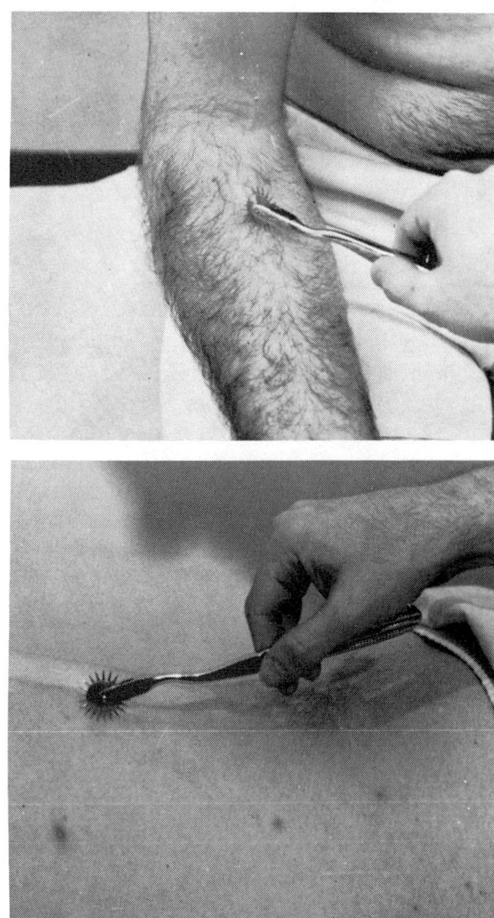

Figure 8.13. Testing a patient's superficial pain sense with a pinwheel (American Chiropractic Association).

containing hot water and the other containing cold water (Figs. 8.14 and 8.15). The patient's eyes should be closed, and the patient should be asked to name the temperature as it is applied to the skin. The patient should be able to perceive which is hot and which is cold, and the examiner should note the quickness of response, mistakes, etc. The procedure then proceeds in a manner similar to that used for the tactile and pain tests.

Areas of impaired temperature sensation usually follow a pattern similar to the areas of impaired pain sensations. The receptors in the skin for the sense of cold and heat are thought to consist of both naked and encapsulated endings, and the neurons serving the sensory path for temperature perception follow the same course as those of the pain pathway. The two systems are so closely associated in the CNS that they can scarcely be distinguished anatomically, and an injury to one usually affects the other to a similar degree. Thus, for most practical clinical purposes, testing either pain or temperature sensibility accomplishes the same result.

Local Temperature Changes

During health, bilateral skin temperature readings are about equal unless an ipsilateral inflammatory reaction exists. For example, a painful joint with overlying hyperemia or a local sympathetic block may alter this pattern. Upon this fact, many instruments have been developed to measure skin temperature differentials. The conclusions drawn from the interpretation of these recordings, however, have been controversial for many years.

In recent years, the study of skin temperature differentials has advanced considerably, with the introduction of liquid crystal thermography, thermal cameras, infrared detector instruments, and improved thermograms. Rask concluded that thermography of the spine was more accurate in evaluating and differentiating IVD syndromes than myelography, and Hendler and associates found current techniques valuable in differentiating somatic from psychogenic causes of pain.

There is little doubt that there is a correlation between sympathetic activity and skin temperature. Normell/Wallin demonstrated concomitant changes in evoked skin sympathetic activity in a peripheral nerve and in skin temperature in the corresponding skin area that strongly supports the concept that the cutaneous thermoregulatory response is a consequence of changes in efferent sympathetic nerve activity.

Effects of Chiropractic Adjustments on Peripheral Temperature. In studying the effects of spinal adjustments on distal skin temperature, McCullough, Haldeman,

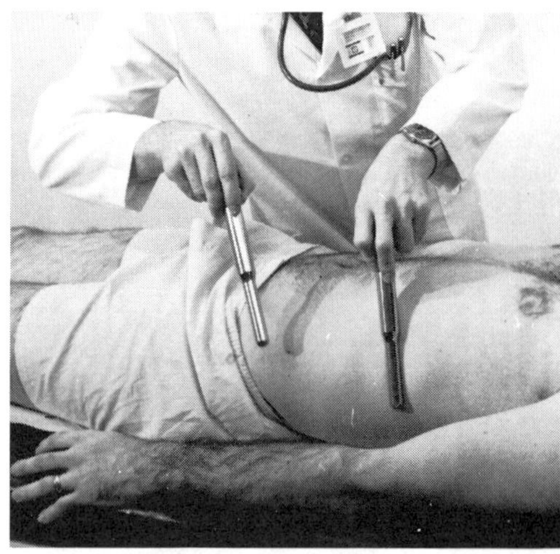

Figure 8.14. Testing thermesthesia sense of the left lateral thorax (American Chiropractic Association).

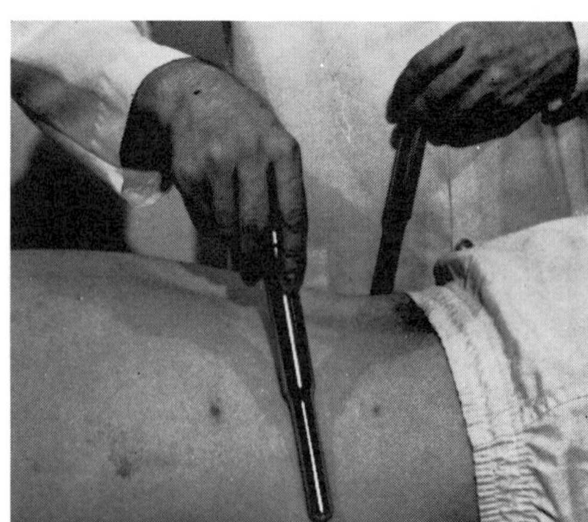

Figure 8.15. Thermesthesia test (Courtesy of the American Chiropractic Association).

Pierce/Stillwagon, and Kelso and associates have noted before and after changes following chiropractic adjustments. In a recent study, Harris/Wagnon concluded that (1) adjustments to the spine can significantly affect temperature (probably through changes in blood flow) in tissues distant from the spine; (2) changes in fingertip temperature varied, depending upon which region of the spine was adjusted; (3) adjustments within the classic sympathetic outflow caused activation of the sympathetic nervous system; and (4) adjustments outside this region caused apparent sympathetic inhibition. The changes in temperature recorded in this study were quite small, but their presence strengthens the contention that manual adjustments of the spine can cause measurable changes in the physiology of distal tissues.

Interpretation of current localized skin temperature methodology remains controversial. The American Chiropractic Association has not adopted a specific policy on this procedure.

Vibration Perception

A decreased perception of vibratory sensation is recorded as *pallhypesthesia;* loss of sensation, *pallanesthesia.* Pallesthesia refers to the normal perception of vibration from the fork when placed against any subcutaneous bony prominence.

During typical evaluation, a vibrating tuning fork is placed over bony prominences (eg, the lower ends of the radius and ulna, the ASIS, the patellae, and the external and internal malleoli), then the patient is asked to state when he feels a vibration or humming sensation. When the vibratory sense is lost, the patient cannot differentiate between a vibrating fork and a silent one. See Figures 8.16 and 8.17.

Testing begins at the head and proceeds to the feet, and compared with the examiner's own hand or other bony prominences. The nonvibrating fork is alternately placed over a point to determine if the patient is guessing. If the patient fails to feel the vibration, it suggests an impairment of the posterior columns of the spinal cord; ie, those tracts that convey the vibratory impulses. Normal vibratory perception is commonly impaired in tabes dorsalis, subacute sclerosis of the cord following pernicious anemia, and in generalized arteriosclerosis. It is first detected with a C256 fork and later by a C128.

Position and Motion Senses

Joint sensation is called *arthresthesia;* decreased sensation, *arthrhypesthesia;* loss of sensation, *anthranesthesia;* increased sensation, *arthrhyperesthesia.*

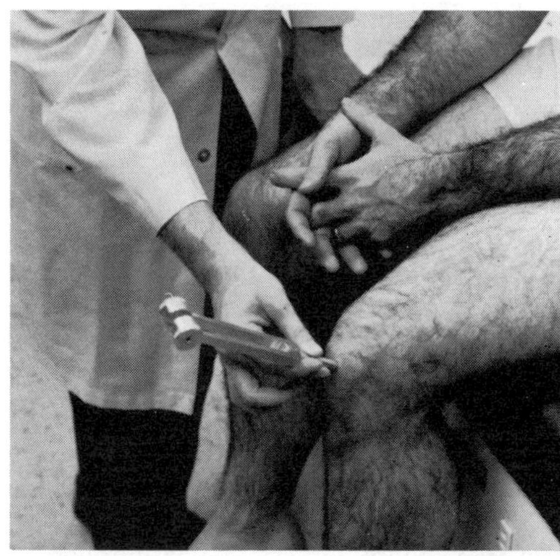

Figure 8.16. Testing pallesthesia sense of the right patella (American Chiropractic Association).

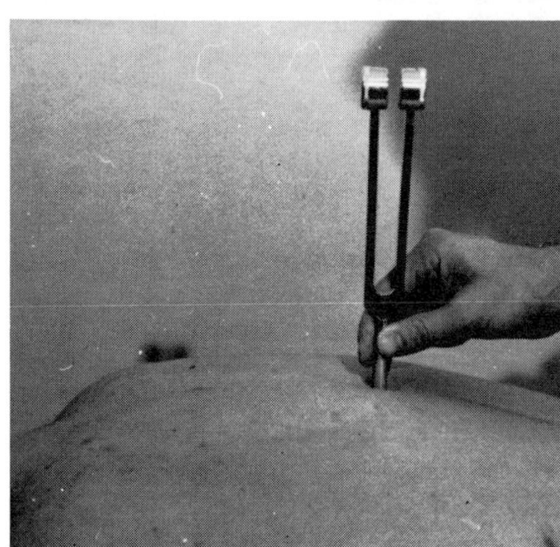

Figure 8.17. Spinal pallesthesia test (Courtesy of the American Chiropractic Association).

With the eyes closed and extremities relaxed, the patient is asked to tell what position a particular joint has been placed or what joint is being moved (Fig. 8.18). Each part should be tested several times. The patient should be able to perceive joint motion with the eyes closed. The examiner should be cautious that the patient completely relaxes the joints being manipulated. The best joints to test appear to be those of the great toe and thumb.

Stereognotic Perception

Stereognosis refers to the ability to sense the form, nature, and solidity of objects through the sense of touch. Familiar objects as keys, coins, marbles, pencils, etc, are commonly used. Different objects are placed in either hand of the patient when the patient's eyes are closed. The patient is asked to handle them and to name them. Loss of the ability to recognize familiar objects occurs in contralateral brain lesions in the parietal area.

Two-Point Discrimination

There is loss of the normal ability to recognize two points simultaneously applied to the skin as distinct from a single point when there is impairment of the proprioceptive pathway. In testing, it is common to use the two ends of an opened paper clip (Fig. 8.19) or the points of a compass.

Tenderness

The perception of tenderness is a highly subjective symptom influenced by many individual structural, functional, and psychologic factors that often make it an unreliable sign.

Localized Tenderness. Tenderness is a frequently encountered sensory symptom that can be defined as pain upon pressure. *Rebound pain* or *rebound tenderness* refers to the sensation or intensification of discomfort when pressure is released; eg, rebound pain at McBurney's point is a classic symptom of acute appendicitis. It should be remembered whenever muscle tenderness is found that the sensory innervation of muscle follows the *motor* innervation and not that of the cutaneous zones. See Figure 8.20.

Paravertebral Tenderness. Determining the specific location of paravertebral tenderness is often helpful in its differentiation. For example, paravertebral tenderness is frequently found at the apices of spinal curves and rotations and not infrequently where one curve merges with another. Tenderness about spinous or transverse processes is usually of low intensity and suggests articular strain. Tenderness noted at the points of nerve exit from the spine and continuing in the pathway of the peripheral division of the nerves is a valuable aid in spinal analysis; however, the lack of tenderness is not a clear indication of lack of spinal dysfunction.

Nerve Tracing

Nerve tracing is the art of following by palpation a tender nerve from its spinal origin to some inflammatory or pathologic lesion or zone or the act of tracing a tender nerve from an inflammatory zone to its spi-

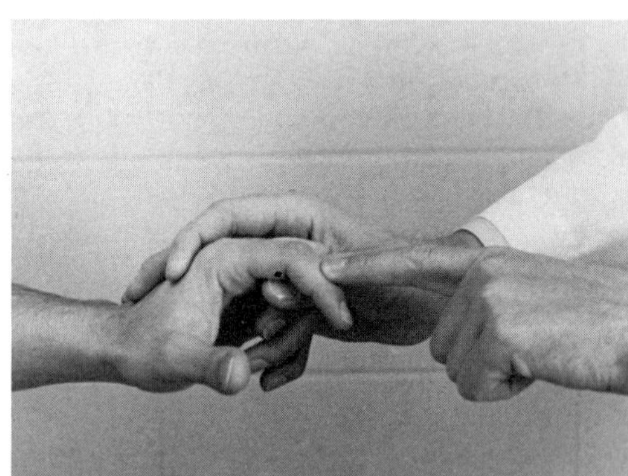

Figure 8.18. Testing position sense in the upper extremity, wherein the patient is asked to indicate (with the eyes closed) the direction in which a finger is being moved. Raphael points out that the patient could interpret the examiner's finger pressure in the position illustrated to give the position change. Thus, it is suggested that it would be better to have the examiner lightly grasp the patient's finger on the medial and lateral sides and move the joint to evaluate position sense.

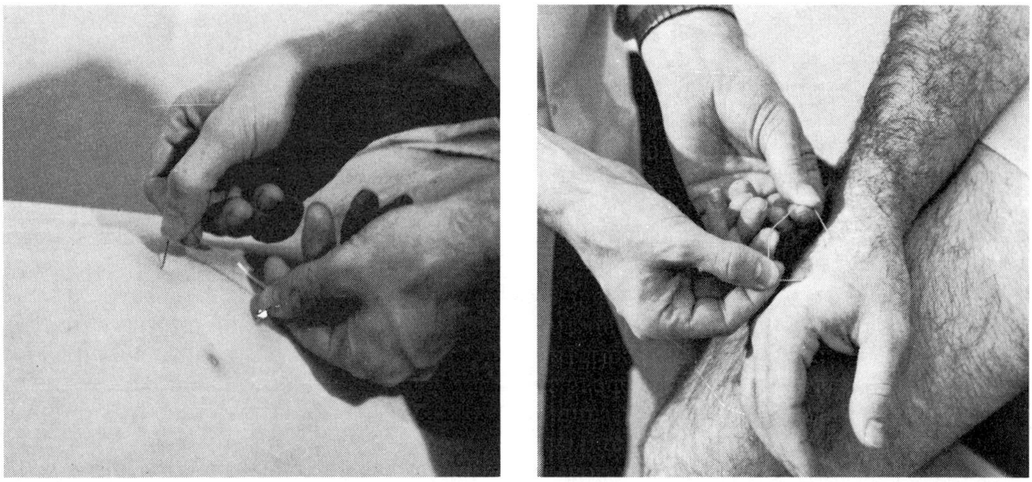

Figure 8.19. *Left,* testing two-point discrimination on the thorax; *right,* on the dorsal surface of the hand (American Chiropractic Association).

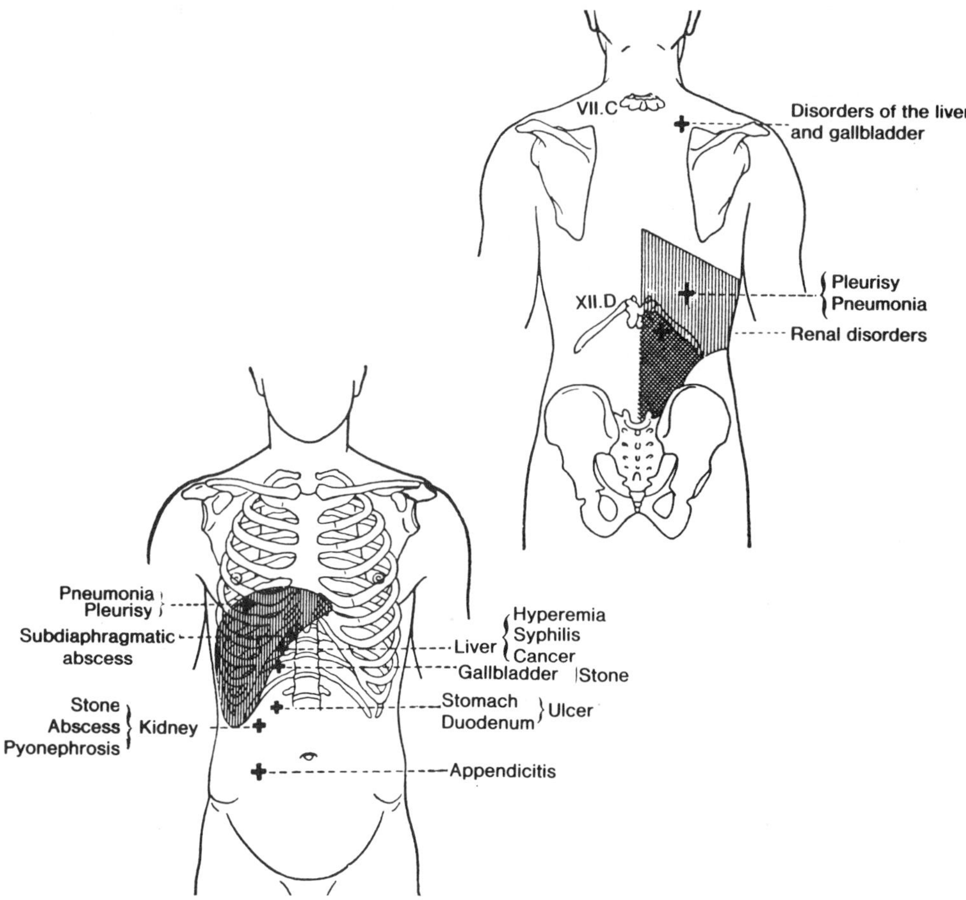

Figure 8.20. *Left,* points of anterior tenderness in right hypochondrium with their respective common causes and modes of radiation. *Right,* points of posterior tenderness associated with right hypochrondriac tenderness with their common causes.

nal exit. A nerve may be traced if it is tender and situated at a point where it may be reached while palpating. To be traced, it is necessary that the nerve be hypersensitive, regardless of cause.

Tenderness is a frequently encountered sensory symptom that may be defined as *pain on pressure.* Pain produced by external pressure results from trigger points, traumatic lesions of sensitive subdermal tissue, or the development of a toxic accumulation or deep-seated inflammatory irritation. There may be a condition that would cause tenderness when pressure is applied, but no abnormal sensation is felt if there is no pressure. It is upon this fact that nerve tracing is based. Nerve tracing is a method of following the course of tenderness over nerves that are irritated or impinged that will usually assist in locating the cause of pain, tenderness, and headache.

Nerve tracing as a diagnostic procedure is a technique once widely practiced by pioneer chiropractors. Although it has fallen into disuse in recent years (like outlining the borders of organs through percussion), the art has considerable merit. Firth, Janse, and Harper mentioned the importance of nerve tracing in their writings on spinal analysis. More recently, Kirby, using the early works of Gregory as reference, offers a concise explanation of the methodology from which the following has been adapted.

Points to be considered in nerve tracing:

1. *Method of holding the palpating finger.* It is necessary to perform deep palpation by considerable pressure to elicit tenderness along the nerve pathway and thus determine its course. To avoid finger fatigue during continuous deep pressure, the index finger is placed on the top surface of the middle finger for support and the thumb is placed against the under surface of the middle finger to support the bottom of the palpating middle finger.

2. *Method of following a nerve.* Once a sensitive point along a nerve pathway is found by digital exploration, palpation is continued along the anticipated course of the nerve. If tenderness is lost, pressure is applied above or below the expected course by palpating in a half-moon direction. The nonactive hand usually holds a skin pencil that can be used to mark the course of tenderness.

3. *Unpalpable nerve pathways.* If a tender nerve passes under a bone or thick muscle where tenderness cannot be elicited, the examiner must try to anticipate its route and pick it up past the obstruction where the nerve will again be elicited by tenderness. This is common when a nerve passes under the scapula or clavicle and the pathway must be reaffirmed.

4. *Method of tracing nerves from the spine.* Standard paraspinal palpation is performed, but then the palpation continues along the nerve pathway step-by-step until the pathologic zone is reached. Sometimes nerve pressure upon a tender nerve tract may relieve the tenderness or numb it to the degree that it cannot be traced further. For that reason, it may be difficult to retrace a nerve from its spinal origin to the periphery.

5. *Method of tracing nerves to the spine.* First, the tender point along the nerve pathway near the inflammatory area should be elicited, but deep palpation is avoided over the actual tender zone of the affected area. Palpation should be made a short distance toward the spinal origin of the nerve supply. If pressure on the nerve numbs its sensitivity, only the distal portion of the nerve will be affected. Deep pressure along the nerve pathway will frequently relieve pain or at least afford temporary relief. This is often a therapeutic aid but a diagnostic obstacle.

6. *Dual routes.* It is often found that the nerve will branch and the tender pathway can be traced to two different points of the spinal column. This is most likely because multiple organs are involved or because a nerve supply from different segments of the spine are given off to the same pathologic zone that has become involved.

7. *Locating tender points along the nerve pathway.* It is important to realize that as the nerve is traced from its spinal origin to the region of some pathologic zone, or vice versa, certain points along the nerve pathway may prove more tender than others. These points, likely trigger points or acupoints, should be marked. Pressure along the nerve may excite a sharp and decisive pain in the pathologic area. This site also should be marked and noted.

8. *Tracing of the peripheral nerve rami.* Nerves and their branches that innervate internal viscera cannot be directly traced because they are too deep to be palpated. How then in such a condition can the examiner elicit information that will help to determine correctly the location of the etiologic spinal lesion The explanation is that if a deep nerve is sensitive or tender, usually its branches are equally sensitive or tender. If we cannot trace a nerve to the end site of a trunk or cavity of the organ, it may be possible to trace a peripheral branch of the same nerve back to its spinal origin. Needless to say, an excellent working knowledge of neurology is essential for this particular work. If the peripheral nerve branches can be traced to the proper point or locality of the spinal lesion, then an excellent tool of analysis is at hand.

Not all nerve pathways follow the course shown in anatomy textbooks. Some deviate and wander somewhat wildly along their classic course. In these cases, by palpating in a fantailed manner, tenderness may be found and nerve tracing may then proceed as normal. Gregory felt that when a nerve is tender at all, it is tender throughout its entire length. Consequently, any tender nerve will be tender near its spinal origin.

Gregory illustrated these wandering nerves by describing a patient with pain over the right hypochondriac region when a full breath was drawn. He expected to locate the tender zone and trace it from this region back to the spine following the intercostal spaces and nerves. For the first 1½ inches, this was true; then suddenly the tender pathway took an upward direction through the axillary region to the front of the shoulder, under the clavicle, and back to the origin at C6 on the same side as the tender zone. If this seems to be a peculiar tracing, then understanding the ramifications of the long posterior thoracic nerve will provide an explanation.

Clinical Reflexes

Testing the superficial, deep, and visceral reflexes evaluates the integrity of the peripheral receptors and the respective motor response. See Table 8.11. Such reflexes evaluate both the sensory afferent and motor efferent portions of the arc. See Figure 8.21.

Skin Resistance

Electrodermograph recordings of skin resistance are sometimes used as an aid during the diagnosis of musculoskeletal and internal disorders, but their interpretation is controversial. Due to cutaneous overlap, segmental localization is imprecise, therefore, neither segment nor organ specific.

General Bilateral Differences. The common asymmetry of the conduction of the skin between the two complete sides of the body has not yet been explained, state Bauch/Hartig, but CNS influences are assumed to be the cause. In studies of bilateral basal skin resistance (BSR), Varni and associates found that the side of the body having the lower BSR corresponded with the side with the lesser vasomotor constriction during experimental stress (eg, breath holding). Their findings suggested that the asymmetry of autonomic activity is typical rather than atypical for the normal individual and that various autonomic variables form patterns of asymmetry. Not all authorities agree with this assumption, however.

Correlation with Pain. Riley/Richter studied electrical skin resistance in patients with neck and upper extremity pain without clinical or radiographic evidence of spinal cord or nerve root irritation but who did exhibit evidence of an abnormality with a cervical IVD or involving a facet joint of the cervical spine. They found that, in general, areas of low skin resistance (assumed to be the result of sympathetic hyperactivity) corresponded well to areas of subjective pain. The skin resistance pattern did not lead to localization of the level of the abnormality within the cervical spine, but it was of value in confirming the clinical impression that a pain-producing mechanical or degenerative lesion existed. It was therefore concluded that the test added some objective measure to a subjective report of pain.

Correlation with Manipulative Therapy. After manipulative treatment of the segment involved in patients with lumbago, Ivanov found that electrosensitivity remained the same as that of the controls and conductivity was near normal values. Further research is necessary to substantiate Ivanov's findings, however, as many clinicians report conflicting findings.

Evaluating Cranial Nerve Sensory Fibers

The cranial nerves have a variety of functions that often become involved in combined lesions because of their proximity to each other. Examination of the cranial nerves is a specialized task that is often referred to the neurologist, but several tests can be performed by the general practitioner that may offer many distinct clues to a cranial nerve lesion. Refer to Table 4.8.

The Olfactory Nerve (Cranial I)

The olfactory nerve is a pure sensory nerve that provides the sense of smell and flavors except for salty, sweet, bitter, and acid.

The patient's sense of smell can be tested with various unlabeled solutions or oils such as cinnamon, peppermint, clove, menthol, vanilla, wintergreen, etc. One of the patient's nares is closed, and the patient is asked to smell a solution held a short distance from the nose. The tube is usually rapidly passed

Table 8.11. Summary of Normal Reflexes

Superficial Reflex	Afferent Nerve	Center	Efferent Nerve
Anal	Pudendal	S4—S5	Pudendal
Consensual	Optic	Midbrain	Oculomotor
Corneal	Trigeminal	Pons	Facial
Cremasteric	Femoral	L1	Genitofemoral
Lower abdominal	T10—T12	Cord level	T10—T12
Nasal (sneeze)	Trigeminal	Brain stem, upper cord	Cranial V, VII, IX, X, and spinal nerves of respiration
Plantar	Tibial	S1—S2	Tibial
Upper abdominal	T7—T10	Cord level	T7—T10
Uvular	Glossopharyngeal	Medulla	Vagus
Visceral Reflex			
Accommodation	Optic	Occipital	Oculomotor
Bulbocavernous	Pudendal	S2—S4	Pudendal
Carotid sinus	Glossopharyngeal	Medulla	Vagus
Ciliospinal	Sensory nerve	T1—T2	Cervical sympathetics
Light	Optic	Midbrain	Oculomotor
Oculocardiac	Trigeminal	Medulla	Vagus
Deep Tendon or Periosteal Reflex			
Achilles	Tibial	S1—S2	Tibial
Biceps	Musculocutaneous	C5—C6	Musculocutaneous
Jaw jerk	Trigeminal	Pons	Trigeminal
Patellar	Femoral	L2—L4	Femoral
Radial	Radial	C6—C8	Radial
Triceps	Radial	C6—C7	Radial

inward from a distance of about a yard. The patient is then requested to tell the examiner what it is. Then the opposite side is tested with a different solution. Some patients smell a substance correctly but are unable to name it.

The least amount of odor necessary for recognition is called the *minimal identifiable odor* (MIO). When this is determined, House and associates recommend that a steady stream of test odor should be passed through the nostril until stimulus fatigue occurs, at which time the patient is no longer aware of the odor. Each nostril is then tested at 30-second intervals with the MIO to determine the duration of fatigue. It should be kept in mind that any nasal disorder (eg, a head cold) will influence the results of such tests.

Ischemia of the nasal mucosa has been shown by Kuntz to provide the milieu for the filterable viruses associated with common upper respiratory infections, which, in turn, are often superimposed by bacterial infection. Homewood points out that an infection at the thin roof of the nasal cavity may easily spread to the olfactory bulb and from there to the meninges to establish meningitis. In this context, it should be noted that the blood vessels of the nasal mucosa are supplied by sympathetic postganglionic fibers originating in the superior cervical ganglion,

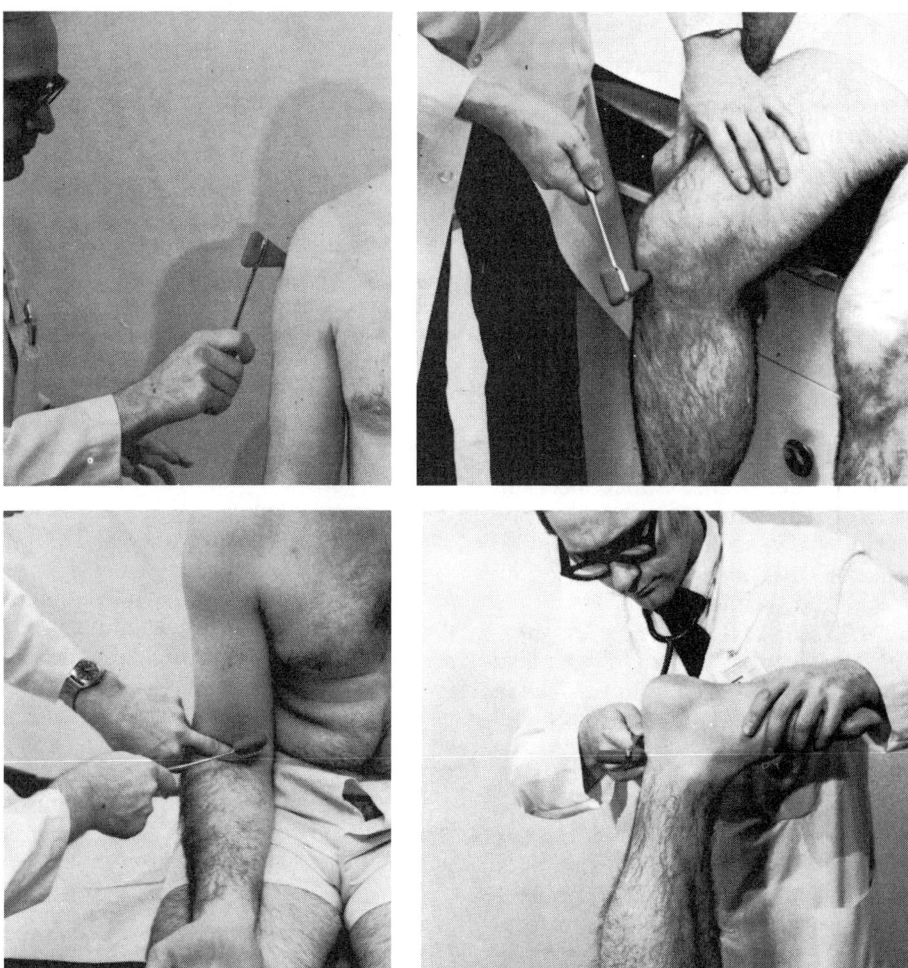

Figure 8.21. Testing some tendon reflexes: *top left,* deltoid reflex; *top right,* patellar reflex; *bottom left,* biceps reflex; *bottom right,* Achilles reflex (American Chiropractic Association).

whose preganglionic fibers stem from T1—T4 segments. Thus, upper cervical and upper thoracic subluxations may cause or encourage such nasal-focus syndromes in their initial stages.

The Optic Nerve (Cranial II)

The optic nerve is a pure sensory nerve that provides the perception of vision. A large number of visual defects, however, may exist that are due to mechanical defects anterior to the optic nerve (eg, lens and accommodation defects).

Injury to the optic nerve is not uncommon. Loss of vision often accompanies a fracture through the sphenoid involving the orbital foramen. Complete blindness of one eye invariably indicates a lesion of the optic nerve. Refer to Figure 4.5. Optic neuritis and tumors compressing the optic nerve are the most common lesions causing loss of the direct light reflex. Lesions of the optic nerve are especially noted with optic atrophy, optic neuritis, papilledema, and visual impairment. Thus, the optic nerves should be tested for visual acuity and fields of vision, and directly inspected by observing the condition of the fundi.

Visual Acuity and Color Perception. The ability to recognize objects and to read the standard Snellen eye charts can be tested. Jaeger or similar test cards can be used at the bedside. If the examiner is not concerned with errors of refraction, the patient can be tested with the glasses on. Color perception also should be determined, and this can be tested by colored yarn or test cards.

Fields of Vision. Visual fields are measured most accurately with a mechanical perimeter or tangent screen by one skilled in its use. A rough estimate of the fields can be obtained in the following manner: With the patient and examiner facing each other about 2 feet apart, the patient is asked to close one eye and fix the open eye on the examiner's eye which is opposite (examiner's right, patient's left). A small object, preferably red, is moved on a line equidistant from the eyes of the two individuals, from the periphery toward the center of the field. This procedure is carried out in the four quadrants, and the patient mentions when he first sees the object enter his field of vision. A comparison is thus made between the extent of the patient's fields and those of the examiner. Obviously, the examiner's fields must be normal; and if so, gross quadrantic or hemianopic defects are often found in this manner.

Some of the gross signs are as follows: *Bitemporal hemianopsia* indicates a lesion at the optic chiasma. *Homonymous contralateral hemianopsia* points toward a lesion at the optic tract or optic radiation. *Homonymous contralateral quadrantopsia* indicates a lesion in the upper or lower area of optic radiation. *Complete blindness* of one eye indicates a lesion of the optic nerve. *Isolated blind spots* (scotomata) surrounded by areas of normal vision may be the result of optic neuritis, optic atrophy, cataracts, detached retina, or lesions of the optic chiasm.

The Fundi. The fundi are examined with an ophthalmoscope, preferably through clinically dilated pupils if legally allowed in the state of practice. Papilledema appears with increased intracranial pressure. Doubtful signs should be confirmed by a specialist. *Papilledema* first appears as a loss of sharpness of the disc margins, which progresses until evidence of the margin disappears. The normal optic disc is glistening white with sharply defined edges. There is a normal minimal indistinctness of the disc margins along the nasal aspect of the disc. *Optic atrophy* appears as a combination of pallor of the lateral aspect and a lack of normal vascularity in the lateral area. The retinal vessels should be inspected for signs of arteriosclerosis, diabetes, retina detachment, pigmentation, hemorrhage, and exudation.

After ruling out local ocular causes of disturbed vision, patterns of visual loss offer one of the best means of locating intracranial lesions when such lesions affect the visual pathway. A sharp disc outline and pulsations of the disc veins are of particular neurologic significance because these findings indicate normal intracranial pressure.

The Trigeminal Nerve (Sensory Fibers of Cranial V)

The trigeminal is a mixed sensory-motor nerve that serves as the chief sensory nerve of the face. The three sensory bundles of the trigeminal nerve (which travel in separate foramina) and their distribution are the: (1) *mandibular branch*—chin, lower lip, cheek, upper ear, and lateral scalp; (2) *maxillary branch*—cheek, upper lip, lateral nose, and lower eyelid; and (3) *ophthalmic branch*—anterolateral nose, eye, forehead, and anterior scalp to the midpoint of the crown. These areas should be tested for touch, pain, and sometimes for temperature. A wisp of cotton is used for touch, a pin for pain, and warm and cool tubes for temperature sensation. Pain perception is tested over the nasal and buccal mucous membrane as well as the face.

The Corneal Reflex. The cornea and conjunctiva are tested for light touch perception with a thin wisp of cotton or a fine hair. The patient should be looking upward, and the cornea should be approached from the side. Each eye should be tested separately, and both eyes should blink quickly with the stimulation. The corneal reflex involves three corneal nerves: III (to open eyelid), V (for sensitivity), and VII (to close eyelid). This reflex is frequently diminished unilaterally from either a central or peripheral lesion. Positive signs will be seen in tic douloureux, herpes zoster, alcoholism, neuritis, and cerebellopontine angle tumors. Irritating lesions result from encephalitis, tabes, and tetanus, and clonic spasm is occasionally seen in petit mal attacks.

The Sneeze Reflex. Sneezing when the nasal membrane is irritated is absent or greatly diminished in lesions of the cranial nerves V to X and the upper cervical nerves.

Visceral Reflexes. Pottenger attributed the tooth decay commonly associated with pulmonary tuberculosis and the unilateral hectic flush associated with pulmonary disorders to vagal afferent impulses mediating in the medulla with sensory efferent fibers of the trigeminus. It also should be noted that most of the dilator fibers contained within the cervical sympathetics unite in their course with the trigeminus, which has some dilator fibers of cerebral origin. Pottenger also felt strongly that the herpes associated with pneumonia, the common cold, and some gastrointestinal disorders are common parasympathetic viscerovisceral reflexes mediated by the vagus and trigeminal nerves.

The Facial Nerve (Sensory Fibers of Cranial VII)

The facial nerve is a mixed sensory-motor nerve. Its sensory fibers supply the taste buds in the anterior two-thirds of the tongue.

Taste perception is tested with solutions of sour (vinegar), sweet (sugar), and salty (salt) substances. Certain signals are arranged with the patient before the test is made. For instance, holding up two fingers may mean that no taste is recognized and three fingers may mean that a taste is recognized. Then the applicator is dipped in the solution, and the patient is asked to protrude the tongue. It is kept protruded with the aid of a sterile pad, and a solution is applied to one side of the tongue. After the patient has signaled that a taste is perceived or not, a request is made to name the flavor. Each side of the tongue should be tested separately. It is best to have the patient rinse the mouth thoroughly with warm water after each solution is used to avoid confusion between the solutions.

The Cochlear Division of the Auditory Nerve (Cranial VIII)

The cochlear division of Cranial VIII is a pure sensory nerve that provides the sense of hearing. To screen hearing, sound perception can be evaluated on both sides by using a watch. During examination, widespread and conversational tones can be compared. Cochlear involvement is commonly seen in otitis media, skull fractures, otosclerosis, and basal tumors.

If an abnormality is noted during a screening procedure, the integrity of the cochlear nerve can accurately be tested by audiometry. However, using a tuning fork is common procedure in general practice. Bone conduction (with the base of the fork held against the vertex or occiput) should be equal in both ears. Covering one ear should shift the sound to the closed ear *(Weber's lateraliza-*

tion test). When sound is no longer heard with bone conduction, bringing the fork near the ear without setting it in vibration again should again be heard by air conduction (*Rinné's test).* Air conduction should be about twice the duration of bone conduction.

Rinné's Test. To test for deafness, a tuning fork is vibrated and placed next to each ear opening (for air conduction) and then against the mastoid bone (for bone conduction) to see which tone is heard longer (Fig. 8.22). Normally, the tone will be heard longer through the otic canal via air conduction.

Weber's Test. To test for deafness and lateralization, the base of a vibrating tuning fork is placed in the center of the forehead at the hairline and the patient is asked if the tone is heard better in one ear than the other. Normally, the tone is heard equally in both ears.

Nerve Deafness vs Conduction Deafness. Deafness resulting from cochlear division impairment is called nerve deafness, as opposed to deafness resulting from middle ear pathology (conduction deafness). Weber's and Rinné's tests differentiate. In *Weber's test,* the sound heard best when the fork is on the vertex is by the unaffected ear if the deafness is due to disease of the auditory apparatus (Fig. 8.23). If the deafness is due to obstruction of the air passages, the vibration will be heard by the affected ear. A positive Rinné's test, if the sound is heard better by bone conduction, points toward a blockage of the middle ear. In nerve deafness, both air and bone conduction will be impaired. Tinnitus is often associated, but it also may be found also in middle ear disease or due to wax in the external meatus. Nerve deafness is the result of cochlear neuropathy; eg, extension of otitis media, skull fracture (especially temporal), otosclerosis, tumors, syphilis, congenital syphilis, and genetic defects.

The Vestibular Division of the Auditory Nerve (Cranial VIII)

The vestibular division of cranial VIII is a pure sensory nerve that serves as the primary mechanism for balance and equilibrium via afferents from the semicircular canals. The complete system provides the nervous system with information concerning gravity, rotation, and acceleration and is located primarily at the posterior fossa level.

Vestibular function is ordinarily not evaluated unless vertigo, nausea, or disturbances of postural coordination on the affected side are reported or observed. These symptoms and signs suggest a lesion of cranial VIII, sensory ataxia, or brain-stem disease.

Stein states that vertigo from whatever cause means a disturbance of the vestibular apparatus and can be analyzed by ear tests.

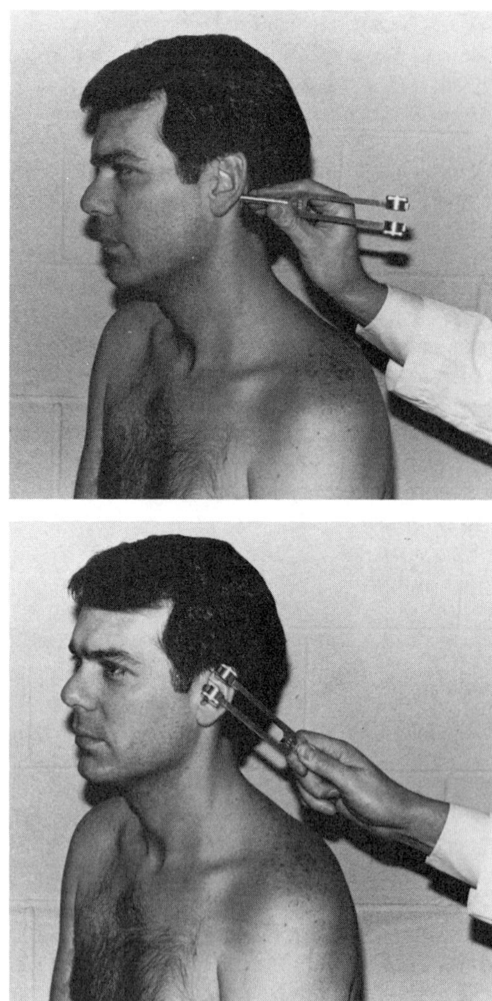

Figure 8.22. Testing bone conduction *(above)* and air conduction *(below)* during Rinne's test.

In vestibular dysfunction, a clinical clue of nystagmus is often a finding of the *caloric test.* This procedure is sometimes called *Barany's test* or the *thermal test.*

Caloric test. Hot and cold water are alternately douched into the patient's ear, after it has been determined that the eardrum is not perforated. The patient should be seated with the head tilted backward about 60° to bring the horizontal semicircular canal into a vertical plane. Normally, hot water (not exceeding 120°F) produces rotary nystagmus, first away and then toward the irrigated ear. Cold water produces an opposite effect—nystagmus first toward and then away from the ear irrigated. The final response normally will appear within 30—40 seconds. Lack of response shows decreased or absent vestibular nerve function; ie, no nystagmus results if the labyrinth is diseased. The test should be discontinued if there is no reaction within 3 minutes.

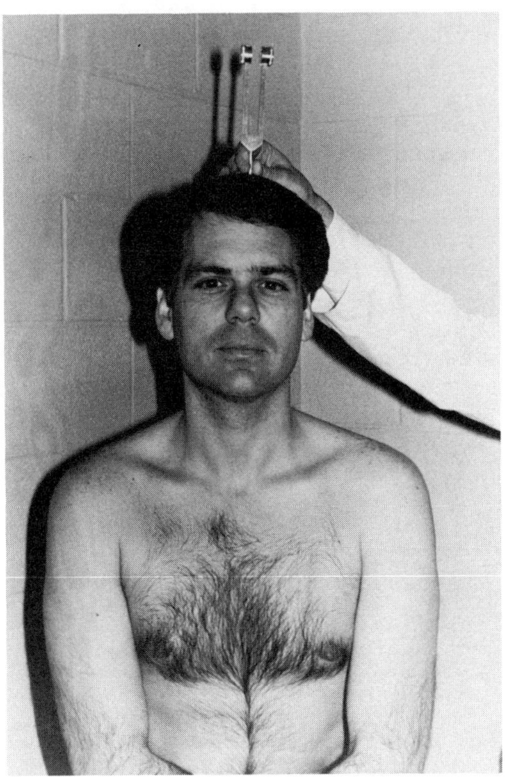

Figure 8.23. In Weber's test, the activated fork is placed on the vertex and the patient states where the sound is heard.

The classic origins of vertigo and imbalance syndromes are seen in Meniere's syndrome and vestibular neuritis. *Meniere's disease* is a syndrome of deafness, tinnitus, and dizziness in association with nonsuppurative disease of the labyrinth. In *vestibular neuritis,* which often occurs in epidemics, there is severe vertigo without a hearing impairment. The dizziness passes off in a few days but may recur at times during sudden movements or quick turns of the head. *Positional vertigo* is usually the result of otolith disease, a lesion of the posterior fossa, a vertebral or basilar artery deficit, or an upper cervical subluxation complex.

Lewit writes of the relationship of the cervical spine to Meniere's disease (Review in *Czechoslovak Medicine,* VII:2, 1961) after 120 cases of Meniere's disease and similar forms of vertigo were sent by leading ear departments of Prague for manipulative treatment. The conclusions reached were: "(1) The results of manipulative treatment in Meniere's disease whether there is any noticeable symptomatology from the cervical spine at the same time or not and in cases of vertigo (Barre-Lieou's syndrome) are practically the same. (2) There are gradual transitions between all the groups of vertigo, sometimes even in one and the same patient. (3) The vertebral origin of Meniere's disease can frequently be directly proved by the aid of tests; ie, experimentally. Thus, cases of cervical origin can be diagnosed from the start. And (4) although Meniere's disease (labyrinthine vertigo) may be provoked by other ways than that of the cervical spine, by labyrinthitis for example, it appears that we have to cope with a syndrome that in the large majority of cases is connected with functional disturbances of the cervical spine; therefore, it should be indicated for manipulative treatment."

Vestibulospinal Postural Reflexes. Molina-Negro and associates report that, through its activation from the utricule in response to displacement of the center of gravity, the vestibular system seems to provoke an increase of the excitability of gamma-static motor neurons of extensor muscles of the trunk and legs and to a lesser degree of the gamma-dynamic and alpha motor neurons. This contributes to the adaptation of muscle tone for the maintenance of the standing static posture and for the alternative change from the extensor to flexor phase during gait. Temporary vestibular hyperfunction provoked by central or peripheral stimulation is manifested clinically by vertigo. The presence of adequate gammastatic innervation on one side seems contradictory to complete suppression of labyrinthine function ipsilaterally. On the other hand, the absence of response to caloric stimulation in one or both labyrinths does not exclude the possibility of vestibular hyperfunction. These researchers conclude that the study of phasic stretch reflexes appears to be a valid method of measurement of the functional state of the static labyrinth and vestibular apparatus.

In describing manipulative treatment based upon a study of postural reflexes, Stejskal states that labyrinthine postural reflexes have relatively little clinical importance. Rather, he emphasizes the importance of the stretch reflex of the axial musculature, of the visual afferentation that is closely connected with the deep neck reflexes, and of the influence of the respiratory phase.

The Glossopharyngeal Nerve (Sensory Fibers of Cranial IX)

The glossopharyngeal is a mixed sensory-motor nerve. Its sensory fibers supply the posterior third taste buds of the tongue, the pharynx, parotid gland, and middle ear.

Taste sensation of the posterior third of the tongue is tested in the same manner described for the VII nerve. In practice, testing the integrity of the sensory fibers of cranial nerves VII and IX is usually conducted at the same time.

The Vagus Nerve (Sensory Fibers of Cranial X)

The vagus is a mixed sensory-motor nerve. Its sensory fibers supply the pharynx, larynx, heart, lungs, and alimentary tract.

Upper vagal integrity is screened by the motor response to the gag reflex, and the oculocardiac reflex *(Aschner's sign)*. Gag reflexes can be tested by irritating the posterior pharyngeal wall. A laryngoscopic examination should be performed if there is any sign of involvement of the pneumogastric nerve. To evaluate the *oculocardiac reflex*, note any irregularities or changes in respiratory rhythm or cardiac action via carotid sinus sensitivity.

Carotid Sinus Syndrome. The carotid sinus syndrome of vasovagal syncope is the result of pressure on a hypersensitive carotid sinus. Pressure causes marked bradycardia, vasodilation, a lowered blood pressure, and associated vertigo, syncope, and convulsive seizures. The associated fainting is called *carotid sinus syncope*. This reflex is especially irritable in hypertension, arteriosclerosis, and vasomotor instability. The response is often absent in lesions of the cranial nerves IX and X. When testing the sensitivity of this reflex, pressure should be put on only one side of the neck, while monitoring pulse and blood pressure. Bilateral testing in the prone position is usually avoided as it may provoke a convulsion.

The Salivary-Taste Phenomenon. Worthy of note here is the *salivary-taste phenomenon*, which is considered a reflex of the *vagus*. When a drop of weak acid such as vinegar is placed on the tongue, the salivary glands will normally increase their output of saliva that can be observed. The sensation is carried by afferent facial nerve fibers with efferent motor action by vagal parasympathetics to the salivary glands.

Tests to determine the possibility of parasympathicotonia (vagotonia) and sympathicotonia will be described in Chapter 10.

Bibliography

American Hospital Association: *Stress*. Chicago, American Hospital Association, 1977.

American Orthopaedic Association: *Manual of Orthopaedic Surgery*. Chicago, American Orthopaedic Association, 1972, pp 27-38.

Anderson KV: Endogenous opioid peptides and the control of pain. In Brena SF, Chapman SL (eds): *Management of Patients with Chronic Pain*. New York, Spectrum, 1983, pp 33-46.

Arbuckle BE: Reflexes. *Journal of the American Osteopathic Association*, 46(7), July 12, 1946.

Balduc HA: Overview of contemporary chiropractic science for the Chiropractic Association of Oklahoma. Northwestern College of Chiropractic, Convention notes, April 24, 1983.

Bauch K, Hartig W: Electrodermatographic examination of segmental sweat secretion in the diagnosis and differential diagnosis of internal diseases. *Acta Neurovegetativa*, 30(4):536-545, 1973.

Beck JW (ed): *The Management of Pain*. Amsterdam, Elsevier, 1979, pp 306-316.

Beecher HK: *Measurement of Subjective Responses*. New York, Oxford University Press, 1959.

Berthold CH: Morphology of normal peripheral axons. In Waxman SG (ed): *Physiology and Pathobiology of Axons*. New York, Raven Press, 1978.

Bishop B: Pain: Its physiology and rationale for management. Part I, neuroanatomical substrate of pain. *Physical Therapy*, 60:13-23, 1980; Part II, analgesia systems of the CNS, 60:21-23, 1980.

Black RG: The chronic pain syndrome. *Surgical Clinics of North America*, 55:999-1011, 1975.

Bonica JJ: Neurophysiologic and pathologic aspects of acute and chronic pain. *Archives of Surgery*, 112: 750-761, 1977.

Brena SF, Chapman SL: Chronic pain: Physiology, diagnosis, management. In Leek JC, Gershwin ME, Fowler WM Jr: *Principles of Physical Medicine and Rehabilitation in the Musculoskeletal Diseases*. Orlando, FL, Grune & Stratton, 1986, pp 189-216.

Brown AG: The termination of cutaneous nerve fibers in the spinal cord of man. *TINS*, 4(3):64-67, 1981.

Burns L, Chandler LC, Rice RW: *Pathogenesis of Visceral Disease Following Vertebral Lesions*. Chicago, American Osteopathic Association, 1948, pp 3-20.

Burns R: The cervical spine in manipulative medicine. *Practitioner*, 222:803-806, 1979.

Cabot RC: *Physical Diagnosis*. New York, William Wood, 1919, p 484.

Canadian Memorial Chiropractic College: *Segmental Neuropathy*. Toronto, Canadian Memorial Chiropractic College, date of publication not shown. Monograph, pp 12-21.

Cervero F: Deep and visceral pain. In Kosterlitz HW, Terenius LY (eds): *Pain and Society*. Weinheim, Verlag Chemic, 1980, pp 263-282.

Chatton MJ: General symptoms. In Krupp MA, Chatton MJ, Werdegar D: *Current Medical Diagnosis & Treatment—1985*. Los Altos, CA, Lange Medical, 1985, p 1.

Chusid JG: *Correlative Neuroanatomy & Functional Neurology*, ed 19. Los Altos, CA, Lange Medical, 1985, pp 222-239, 241-243.

Clark WC, Hunt HF: Pain. In Downey J, Darling R (eds): *Physiological Basis of Rehabilitation Medicine*. Philadelphia, W.B. Saunders, 1971, pp 373-401.

Coote JH, et al: Reflex discharges into thoracic white rami elicited by somatic and visceral afferent excitation. *Journal of Physiology*, 202:141-159, 1969.

Crue BB, et al: Neurophysiology of pain—peripheral aspects. *Bulletin of the Los Angeles Neurological Society*, 41(1):13-42, 1976.

Curtis DR, Eccles JC: Synaptic action during and after repetitive stimulation. *Journal of Physiology* (British), 150:374, 1960.

Cyriax J: *Textbook of Orthopaedic Medicine: Vol One, Diagnosis of Soft Tissue Lesions*, ed 8. London, Bailliere Tindall, 1982, pp 22-42, 65-66.

de Reuck AVS, Knight J (eds): *Myotactic, Kinesthetic, and Vestibular Mechanisms*. Ciba Foundation Symposium. Boston, Little, Brown, 1967.

De Rusha JL: Upper cervical technic correlated with neurodiagnosis. *ACA Journal of Chiropractic*, September 1961.

Dee R: Articular neurology. In Sokoloff L (ed): *The Joints and Synovial Fluid*. New York, Academic Press, 1978, p 177.

De Sterno CV: The pathophysiology of TMJ dysfunction and related pain. In Gelb, H (ed): *Clinical Management of Head, Neck and TMJ Pain and Dysfunction*. Philadelphia, W.B. Saunders, 1977.

Ditmar E: Cutaneo-visceral neural pathways. *Journal of Physical Medicine (British)*, 15:208, 1952.

Elton D, Burrows GD, Stanley GV: Clinical measurement of pain. *Medical Journal of Australia*, 1:109-111. 1979.

Fordyce WE: *Behavioral Methods for Chronic Pain and Illness*. St. Louis, C.V. Mosby, 1976.

Fowler WM Jr, Taylor RG: Differential diagnosis of muscle disease. In D'Ambrosia RD: *Musculoskeletal Disorders: Regional Examination and Differential Diagnosis*. Philadelphia, J.B. Lippincott, 1977, pp 93-95.

Friedman AP (ed): Symposium on headache and related pain syndromes. *Medical Clinics of North America*, 62:427-623, 1978.

Friedman HH: *Problem-Oriented Medical Diagnosis*, ed 2. Boston, Little, Brown, 1979, pp 316-341.

Frogley R: Neurological observations of a subluxation. *The Journal of Clinical Chiropractic*, 1(3), 1973.

Gandhavadi B, et al: Autonomic pain: Features and methods of assessment. *Postgraduate Medicine*, 7(1):85-90, 1982.

Giles LG: Spinal fixation and viscera. *Journal of Clinical Chiropractic*, 1(3): 144-145, 1973.

Glover JR: Back pain and hyperesthesia. *Lancet*, 1(7135):1165-1169, 1960.

Goldstein M (ed): *The Research Status of Spinal Manipulative Therapy*. Bethesda, MD, National Institutes of Health, DHEW Publication No. (NIH) 76-998, 1975, pp 173-180, 185-187.

Goodheart GJ: *Collected Published Articles and Reprints*. Montpellier, OH, Williams County Publishing, 1969, pp 23-24.

Goodman CE: Pathophysiology of pain. *Archives of Internal Medicine*, 143:527, 1983.

Granit R: *Receptors and Sensory Perception*. New Haven, CT, Yale University Press, 1955.

Grieve GP: *Common Vertebral Joint Problems*. London, Churchill Livingstone, 1981, pp 69-73, 161-196.

Guilliam N: Evolution of the nervous system. *ACA Journal of Chiropractic*, May 1970.

Guyton AC: *Textbook of Medical Physiology*, ed 6. Philadelphia, W.B. Saunders, 1981, pp 588-625.

Haldeman S: Observations made under test conditions with synchrotherme. *Journal of the Canadian Chiropractic Association*, 14(1):9-12, 1970.

Hardy JR, et al: *Pain Sensations and Reactions*. Baltimore, Williams & Wilkins, 1952.

Harris W, Wagnon RJ: The effects of chiropractic adjustments on distal skin temperature. *Journal of Manipulative and Physiological Therapeutics*, 10(2):57-60, April 1987.

Hart FD (ed): *The Treatment of Chronic Pain.* Philadelphia, F.A. Davis, 1974, pp 1, 4, 8, 15, 64, 113.

Hendler N, Uematesu S, Long D: Thermographic validation of physical complaints in "psychogenic pain" patients. *Psychosomatics*, 23(3):283-287, 1982.

Hertz AF: On the sensibility of the alimentary canal in health and disease. *Lancet*, 1:1051, 1911.

Homewood AE: *The Neurodynamics of the Vertebral Subluxation*, ed 3. Place of publication not shown, published by author, 1981, pp 112-125, 132-146, 250-260, 267-281.

Hoppenfeld S: *Orthopaedic Neurology.* Philadelphia, J.B. Lippincott, 1977, pp 1-3.

House EL, Pansky B, Siegel A: *A Systematic Approach to Neuroscience*, ed 3. New York, McGraw-Hill, 1979, pp 215-216.

Huskisson EC: Measurement of pain. *Journal of Rheumatology*, 9(5):768-769, 1982.

Igneizi RJ, Atkinson JH: Pain and its modulation: Part I. *Neurosurgery*, 6(5): 577-583, 1980.

Inman VT, Saunders JB: Referred pain from skeletal structures. *Journal of Nervous and Mental Disease*, 99:660-667, 1944.

Ivanov BN: Changes in electrical skin sensitivity and conductivity in the lumbago syndrome after manipulative therapy. In Lewit K, Gutmann G (eds): *Rehabilitácia. Proceedings of the IVth Congress.* Prague, International Federation of Manual Medicine, supplement 10-11:171-176, 1975.

Janse J: A concept: The neurological element as it relates to clinical chiropractic. *The Chirogram*, December 1975.

Janse J: The integrative purpose and function of the nervous system: A review of classical literature. *Journal of Manipulative and Physiological Therapeutics*, 1(3), September 1978.

Janse J: *Principles and Practice of Chiropractic.* Lombard, IL, National College of Chiropractic, 1976, pp 48-50, 73-74, 243-250, 310-312.

Jaskoviak PA, Schafer RC: *Applied Physiotherapy: Practical Applications Within Clinical Chiropractic.* Arlington, VA, American Chiropractic Association, 1986, pp 15-44.

Judge RD, Zuidema GD (eds): *Methods of Clinical Examination: A Physiological Approach*, ed 3. Boston, Little, Brown, 1968, pp 341-366.

Karvinen E, Komi PV: Neuromuscular performance. In Larson LA (ed): *Fitness, Health, and Work Capacity.* New York, Macmillan, 1974, pp 73-78, 81-86.

Keegan JJ, Garrett FD: The segmental distribution of the cutaneous nerves in the limbs of man. *Anatomical Record*, 102:409-439, 1948.

Kellgren JH: Observations on referred pain arising from muscle. *Clinical Science*, 3:175, 1938.

Kellgren JH: On the distribution of pain arising from deep somatic structures with charts of segmental pain areas. *Clinical Science*, 4:35-46, 1939.

Kellgren JH, Samuel EP: The sensitivity and innervation of the articular capsule. *Journal of Bone & Joint Surgery*, 32(B):84-92, 1950.

Kelso AF, Grant RG, Johnston WL: Use of thermograms to support assessment of somatic dysfunction or effects of osteopathic manipulative treatment: Preliminary report. *Journal of the American Osteopathic Association*, 82(3):182-185, 1982.

Kessler RM, Hertling D (eds): *Management of Common Musculoskeletal Disorders.* Philadelphia, Harper & Row, 1983, pp 27-30, 91-98.

Kirby JD: The technique of nerve tracing. *The Chirogram*, June 1976.

Kitzinger E: Vertebrogenic syndromes and nondrug treatment. *International Journal of Chinese Medicine*, 1(3):3-7, September 1984.

Korr IM: The spinal cord as organizer of disease processes: Some preliminary perspectives. *Journal of the American Osteopathic Association*, September 1976.

Kraus H: Muscular aspects of oral dysfunction. In Gelb H (ed): *Clinical Management of Head, Neck and TMJ Pain and Dysfunction.* Philadelphia, W.B. Saunders, 1977.

Krupp MA, Chatton MJ, Werdegar D: *Current Medical Diagnosis & Treatment—1985.* Los Altos, CA, Lange Medical, 1985, 581-630.

Krupp MA, Tierney LM Jr, Jawetz E, Roe RL, Camargo CA: *Physician's Handbook*, ed 21. Los Altos, CA, Lange Medical, 1985, pp 34-53.

Kunert W: Functional disorders of internal organs due to vertebral lesions. *Ciba Symposium*, 13(3), 1965.

Kuntz A: Anatomic and physiologic properties of cutaneo-visceral vasomotor reflex arcs. *Journal of Neurophysiology*, 8:421-429, 1943.

Kuntz A: *The Autonomic Nervous System.* Philadelphia, Lea & Febiger, 1949, pp 22, 486.

Lamb DW: The neurology of spinal pain. *Physical Therapy*, 59:971-973, 1979.

Laufenberg PC: New dimensions in neurologic evaluation. *The Digest of Chiropractic Economics*, pp 10-12, 105-106, May/June 1979.

Livingston MC: Spinal manipulation in medical practice: A century of ignorance. *Medical Journal of Australia*, 1:552-554, 1968.

Lundeberg T: Long-term results of vibratory stimulation as a pain relieving measure for chronic pain. *Pain*, 20(1):13-23, 1984.

Lundeberg T: Naloxone does not reverse the pain-reducing effect of vibratory stimulation. *Acta Anaesthesiologica Scandinavica*, 29:212-216, 1985.

Lundeberg T, Nordemar R, Ottoson D: Pain alleviation by vibratory stimulation. *Pain*, 20(1):25-44, 1984.

Learmouth JR: Neurosurgery in the treatment of diseases of the urinary bladder, II: treatment of visceral pain. *Journal of Urology*, 26:13, 1931.

Leavitt F, Garron DC, Whisler WW, Sheinkop MB: Affective and sensory dimensions of back pain. *Pain*, 4:273-281, 1978.

Lewis T: Suggestions relating to the study of somatic pain. *British Medical Journal*, 1:321-327, 1938.

Lynch MK, Kessler RM: Pain. In Kessler RM, Hertling D (eds): *Management of Common Musculoskeletal Disorders.* Philadelphia, Harper & Row, 1983, pp 51-72.

MacDonald ML, Stanish WD: Neuromuscular system. In Scott WN, Nisonson B, Nicholas JA: *Principles of Sports Medicine.* Baltimore, Williams & Wilkins, 1984, pp 15-24.

Mayer DJ, Price DD: Central nervous system mechanisms of analgesia. *Pain*, 2:379404, 1976.

McCullough JW: An overview of medical thermographic imaging. *ACA Journal of Chiropractic*, 21(4):22-23, 1984.

McKenzie RA: *The Lumbar Spine*. Upper Hutt, New Zealand, Spinal Publications Ltd, 1981, pp 9-14.

McNaught AB, Callander R: *Illustrated Physiology*, ed 4. New York, Churchill Livingstone, 1983, pp 244-245.

Melzack R, et al: Neurophysiological foundations of pain. In Sternbach RA (ed): *The Psychology of Pain*. New York, Raven Press, 1978, pp 1-26.

Melzack R: The gate theory revisited. In LeRoy PL (ed): *Current Concepts in the Management of Chronic Pain*. Miami, Sympopsia Specialists, 1977.

Melzack R, Stillwell DM, Fox EJ: Trigger points and acupuncture points for pain: Correlations and implications. *Pain*, 3:3-23, 1977.

Melzack R, Wall PD: On the nature of cutaneous sensory mechanisms. *Brain*, 85: 331-356, 1962.

Melzack R, Wall PD: Pain mechanisms: A new theory. *Science*, 150:971-979, 1965.

Merskey H, et al: The lateralization of pain. *Pain*, 7:271-280, 1979.

Mitchell GAG: *Cardiovascular Innervation*. London, Livingstone, 1956, p 356.

Molina-Negro P, Bertrand RA, Martin E, Gioani Y: The role of the vestibular system in relation to muscle and postural reflexes in man. *Acta Oto-Laryngologica*, 89:524-533, 1980.

Nathan PW: The gate-control theory of pain—A critical review. *Brain*, 99:123-158, 1976.

Normell LA, Wallin BG: Sympathetic skin nerve activity and skin temperature changes in man. *Acta Physiologica Scandinavica*, 9(3):417-426, 1974.

Olson WH, Brumback RA, Gascon G, Christoferson LA: *Practical Neurology for the Primary Care Physician*. Springfield, IL, Charles C. Thomas, 1981, pp 1-32, 98-114, 157-178, 236-269.

Pastan RS: Diffuse musculoskeletal pain. *Diagnosis*, 5(3):42-46, 1983.

Perl ER: Mode of action of nociceptors. In Hirsch C, et al (eds): *Cervical Pain*. Oxford, England, Pergamon, 1972, pp 157-163.

Phillips RB: The irritable reflex mechanism. *ACA Journal of Chiropractic*, January 1974.

Pierce WV, Stillwagon G: Charting and interpreting skin temperature differential patterns. *Digest of Chiropractic Economics*, 12(5):37-39, 1970.

Pleet AB, Massey EW: Notalgia paresthetica. *Neurology*, 28:1310-1311, 1978.

Poole PB: Considerations of neurogenic pain. *Ortho-Briefs*, Council on Chiropractic Orthopedics of the American Chiropractic Association, Fall 1982.

Pottenger FM: *Symptoms of Visceral Disease*, ed 6. St. Louis, C.V. Mosby, 1944, pp 183, 187, 189, 266.

Prichard JW: Nerve. In Albright JA, Brand RA (eds): *The Scientific Basis of Orthopaedics*. New York, Appleton-Century-Crofts, 1979, pp 396-399, 405-408.

Raphael R: personal correspondence. Portland, Oregon, 1987.

Rask MR: Thermography of the human spine: Study of 150 cases with back pain and sciatica. *Orthopaedic Review*, 8(11):73-82, 1979.

Reiter L: Apophyseal joint functional anatomy and experimental findings: A literature review. *PCC Research Form*, 1(2):49-52, Winter 1985.

Research Group of Acupuncture Anesthesia; Peking Medical College: Effect of acupuncture on pain threshold on human skin. *Chinese Medical Journal*, 3:151-157, 1973.

Riley LH Jr, Richter CP: Uses of the electrical skin resistance method in the study of patients with neck and upper extremity pain. *John Hopkins Medical Journal*, 137(2):69-74, 1975.

Sandman KB: Myofascial pain syndromes: their mechanism, diagnosis and treatment. *Journal of Manipulative and Physiological Therapeutics*, 4(3):135-139, September 1981.

Schafer RC: *Basic Chiropractic Paraprofessional Manual*. Des Moines, IA, American Chiropractic Association, 1978, pp XV:39-42.

Schafer RC: *Chiropractic Physical and Spinal Diagnosis*. Oklahoma City, Associated Chiropractic Academic Press, 1980, pp II:20, 33; III:4-14; V:1-17, 26-27, 34-54.

Schafer RC: *Chiropractic Management of Sports and Recreational Injuries*. Baltimore, Williams & Wilkins, 1982, pp 91, 170-171, 231-252, 262-265, 281.

Schafer RC: *Clinical Biomechanics: Musculoskeletal Actions and Reactions*. Baltimore, Williams & Wilkins, 1983, pp 137, 140-185, 221-223, 240-243, 246-249, 397-401, 405-408, 427-428.

Schafer RC (ed): *Basic Chiropractic Procedural Manual*, ed 4. Arlington, VA, American Chiropractic Association, 1984, pp 39-40, 73-80.

Schafer RC: *Physical Diagnosis: Procedures and Methodology in Chiropractic Practice*. Arlington, VA, American Chiropractic Association. In preparation, to be released in 1989. Chapter 4, The Clinical Interpretation of Pain; Chapter 7, Basic Neurologic Considerations.

Schafer RC: *Symptomatology and Differential Diagnosis*. Arlington, VA, American Chiropractic Association, 1986, pp 8-9, 203-288, 326-340.

Shepard RS: *Human Physiology Examination Review*. New York, Arco, 1975, pp 321-322.

Simons DG: Myofascial triggerpoints: a need for understanding. *Archives of Physical Medicine and Rehabilitation*, vol 62, March 1981.

Sinclair DC, Weddell G, Feindel WH: Referred pain and associated phenomena. *Brain*, 7:184-211, 1948.

Sites JS: Meralgia paresthetica: A case report. *Research Forum*, 2(2):55-58, 1986.

Sola AE: Myofascial trigger point therapy. *Medical Times*, January 1982, pp 70-77.

Stein HI: Diagnosis and treatment of disturbances of the vestibular system. *Journal of the American Medical Association*, 5(8):407-412, 1952.

Stejskal L: Five suggestions for manipulative treatment based upon a study of postural reflexes. In Lewit K, Gutmann G (eds): *Rehabilitácia. Proceedings of the IVth Congress*. Prague, International Federation of Manual Medicine, supplement 10-11:171-176, 1975.

Stoddard A: *Manual of Osteopathic Technique*, ed 2. London, Hutchinson, 1962.

Sutton DC, Lueth HC: Pain. *AMA Archives of Internal Medicine*, 45:827, 1930.

Szasz TS: The psychology of persistent pain. In Soulairac A, et al: *Pain*. London, Academic Press, 1968, pp 93-113.

Terrett ACJ, Vernon H: Manipulation and pain tolerance: A controlled study of the effect of spinal manipulation on paraspinal cutaneous pain tolerance levels. *American Journal of Physical Medicine*, 63(5):217-224.

Thomas AH: The anatomy, physiology, and psychology of pain. *Journal of Occupational Medicine*, 7:526-534, 1965.

Tobis JS, Hoebler FK: Musculoskeletal manipulation in the treatment of low back pain. *Bulletin of the New York Academy of Medicine*, 59(7):600-608, 1983.

Tran TA: Essentials of the neurological examination: Tests for cerebral function. *The Chirogram*, July 1975.

Travell JG, Bigelow NH: Referred somatic pain does not follow a simple segmental pattern. *Federation Proceedings*, 5:106, 1946.

Travell JG: Myofascial trigger points: clinical view. In Bonica JJ, Albe-Fessard D (eds): *Advances in Pain Research and Therapy*. New York, Raven Press, 1976.

Travell JG: Referred pain from skeletal muscle. *New York State Journal of Medicine*, February 1, 1955.

Travell JG, Rinzler SH: The myofascial genesis of pain. *Postgraduate Medicine*, 11:425-434, 1952.

Travell JG, Simons DG: *Myofascial Pain and Dysfunction: The Trigger Point Manual*. Baltimore, Williams & Wilkins, 1983, p 663.

Vallbona C: Bodily responses to immobilization. In Kottke FJ, Stillwell GK, Lehman JF (eds): *Krusen's Handbook of Physical Medicine and Rehabilitation*. London, W.B. Saunders, 1982.

Ufberg SH: Muscular nociception. *ACA Journal of Chiropractic*, 14:93-96, September 1980.

Varni JG, Doerr HO, Franklin JR: Bilateral differences in skin resistance and vasomotor activity. *Psychophysiology*, 8(3):390-400, 1971.

Vazuka FA: *Essentials of the Neurological Examination*. Philadelphia, Smith, Kline, & French Laboratories, 1962.

Wall PD, Sweet WH: Temporary abolition of pain in man. *Science*, 155:108, 1967.

Wall PD: Gate control theory of pain mechanisms: a re-examination and re-statement. *Brain*, 101:1-18, 1978.

White JC, et al: Cardiac innervation: Experimental and clinical studies. *AMA Archives of Surgery*, 26:765, 1933.

Willer JC, Boureau F, Albe-Fessard D: Role of large diameter cutaneous afferents in transmission of nociceptive messages: Electrophysiological study in man. *Brain Research*, 152:358-364, 1978.

Wyke BD: Articular neurology and manipulative therapy. In *Aspects of Manipulative Therapy*. Proceedings of Multidisciplinary International Conference on Manipulative Therapy. Melbourne, Lincoln Institute of Health Sciences, Carlton, Victoria, Australia, August 1979, pp 67-72.

Wyke BD: Neurological aspects of pain therapy: A review of some current concepts. In Swerdlow M (ed): *The Therapy of Pain*. Lancaster, England, MTP Press, 1981.

Wyke BD: Neurological mechanisms in the experience of pain. *Acupuncture and Electro-Therapeutical Research International Journal*, 4:27-35, 1979.

Wyke BD: Neurological mechanisms in spasticity: A brief review of some current concepts. *Physiotherapy*, 62(10):316-319, 1976.

Zimmermann M: Physiological mechanisms in chronic pain. In *Pain and Society*, report of Dahlem Workshop, Berlin, November 1979. Deerfield Park, FL, Basle, 1980, pp 283-298.

Chapter 9

Clinical Disorders and the Motor System

This chapter describes the clinical implications of abnormal muscle mass, tone, and weakness. The primary features of muscle pain, stiffness, cramps, spasms, movement disturbances, and paralysis are described. The chapter concludes with a description of motor reflexes and the neurologic basis for the evaluation of the somatic motor system, including the cerebellar system and the cranial nerves.

OVERVIEW

Such clinical features as fatigue, weakness, nervousness, pain, tenderness, paralysis, sensory loss, paresthesia, and abnormalities of muscle mass or tone are the most common signs and symptoms noted in neural disorders. Fatigue, weakness, and nervousness are frequently presented together. This triune can usually be attributed to a functional disorder or appear as a complication in organic disease.

Abnormal striated muscle function has its origin in diseases of the brain, spinal cord, peripheral nerves, or muscle tissue itself. Dysfunction occurs in a variety of symptoms and signs such as (1) impaired movements, (2) spontaneous movements, (3) coordination defects, (4) abnormal reflexes, (5) distortions of muscle tone, and (6) postural and movement distortions. Weakness, wasting, and sometimes paralysis are represented in these conditions. Common types of motor lesions are shown in Table 9.1.

Basic Neuromuscular Activities

There are two fundamental types of neuromuscular activity. One type consists of reflex *postural contractions*, which are the basis of posture and physical attitudes and maintain muscle tone. The other type consists of *phasic contractions*, which produce movement. Phasic contractions may be either reflex or volitional in origin. While reflex actions are always purposeful, predictable, and involuntary, cortical activity is not.

Neurons carrying phasic and tonic impulses have distinct characteristics. Phasic motor neurons are large, have a rapid conduction velocity, have a high threshold of physiologic excitability, present large impulses of short duration, and are electrically silent during rest. In contrast, tonic motor neurons are smaller in size, have a slower conduction velocity, have a lower threshold of physiologic excitability, present smaller impulses of longer duration, and are electrically active during rest.

Muscle and Joint Correlations

Functional and degenerative lesions of joints are principally the result not only of a pathologic process in a joint but of altered function of the motor system as a *whole*, according to the findings of Janda. Because of their physiologic properties, he believes that the muscles, which represent the most liable link of the motor system, respond early and distinctly in most clinical pictures of functional and degenerative joint disease. However, the muscular reaction is not of the same quality in all muscles: muscles with predominantly postural function tighten and muscles with predominantly phasic function weaken. To understand the fine control of motion, the separate activity of individual muscles is not as important as their coordinated activity within different movement patterns. Understanding this, states Janda, seems to be the best basis for rational treatment and good long-term therapeutic results.

MUSCLE MASS AND ATROPHY

The strength of healthy muscle is generally proportional to its size (bulk). The term *atrophy* refers to the loss of muscle bulk as the result of disease. Atrophy is especially difficult to evaluate in the aged or malnourished individual.

The Determination of Atrophy

Palpation and mensuration are used to determine muscle volume. Upon palpation, there should be a mass that is symmetrical bilaterally. Measurements should be made with a flexible tape from a bony prominence to the belly of a suspected muscle and the point marked with a skin pencil. This dis-

Table 9.1. Common Types of Motor Lesions

UPPER MOTOR NEURON LESIONS

Motor Cortex	*Brain Stem*
Cerebral palsy (birth injuries, etc)	Inflammation
Inflammation	Multiple sclerosis
Neoplasms	Neoplasm
Skull fracture	Trauma
	Vascular lesions
Internal Capsule	*Spinal Cord*
Embolism	Combined sclerosis
Hemorrhage	Inflammation
Inflammation	Lateral sclerosis
Neoplasm	Multiple sclerosis
Stroke	Neoplasm
Thrombosis	Trauma

LOWER MOTOR NEURON LESIONS

Anterior Horn	*Peripheral Nerve*
Amyotrophic and other combined conditions	Demyelination disease
Poliomyelitis	Entrapment
Progressive muscular atrophy	Inflammation
	Trauma
Spinal Root and Nerve	*Muscle*
Inflammation	Amyotonia congenita
IVD protrusion	Muscular dystrophy
Osteophyte	Myasthenia gravis
Subluxation complex	Myotonia congenita

tance should be recorded for future reference, then the circumference at that point is measured. The same procedure is then conducted on the opposite side. The two sides should be approximately the same circumference unless there is a large degree of unilateral occupational activity. A decrease in size (eg, midcalf or thigh) indicates atrophy and is usually associated with some degree of hypotonicity and a decrease in strength (Fig. 9.1).

Local Atrophy

General emaciation should not be confused with local atrophy. Local muscle atrophy occurs as a result of a peripheral nerve lesion, poliomyelitis, neuritis, or trauma to a spinal nerve. The affected muscle becomes shrunken, poor in tone, and weak in strength. Age, sex, occupation, and right- and left-handedness must be considered.

Weakness, flaccidity, and atrophy occur in the face, tongue, and pharyngeal muscles with disease of the lower motor neurons of the brain stem. The result is described by Daube/Sandok as a breathy, imprecise, nasal speech called *flaccid dysarthria*.

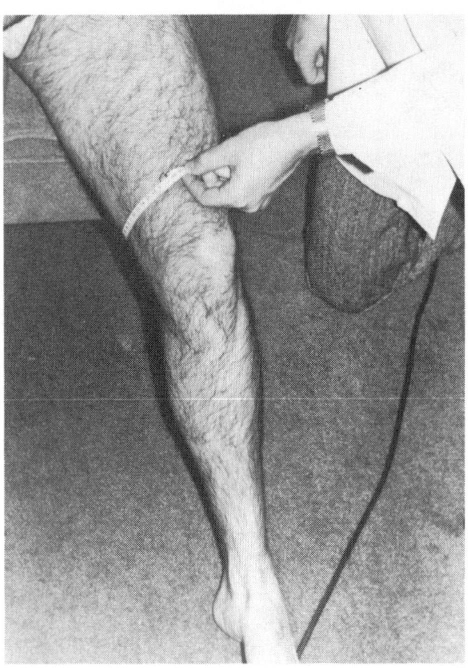

Figure 9.1. Measuring for quadriceps atrophy.

Types of Atrophy and Their Differentiation

When signs of atrophy are found, it is important to keep in mind those features that distinguish *disuse atrophy* from *denervation atrophy*.

Disuse Atrophy

Disuse atrophy occurs with a loss of use. With the possible exception of noxious spinal influences, disuse atrophy is the most common cause of local muscle weakness. It may be the result of immobilization, an occupational lack of use of a particular muscle group, or disuse as a result of painful injury, nerve disease, or muscle disease.

The features of disuse atrophy include moderate reduction in visible muscle size, from mild to moderate diminished muscle strength (with paralysis in upper motor neuron lesions), normal tendon reflexes (hyperactive after initial shock in cases of upper motor neuron lesions), normal response to direct muscle stimulation, and mild slowly progressing atrophy. Pottenger observed that visceral malfunction also can produce these symptoms. In disuse atrophy, the weakness exhibited is *proportional* to the muscle's bulk.

Denervation Atrophy

Neurogenic atrophy occurs with a loss of innervation. Rapid reduction in visible muscle size, zero voluntary muscle strength, absent tendon reflexes, no response to brief direct muscle stimulation, and rapidly progressing atrophy are characteristic of denervation atrophy. The weakness exhibited is *unproportional* to the muscle's bulk.

MUSCLE TONE

A healthy muscle has a small amount of tension even at complete rest. It feels resilient rather than flabby. Palpable muscle firmness is normally the result of a slight sustained flow of low-frequency asynchronous impulses from the spinal cord generating slight contractions of a small fraction of skeletal muscle fibers plus any degree of active tension. If the function of the ventral roots is impaired, a muscle loses its basic tone immediately; and the same is true if the dorsal roots containing sensory fibers from the muscle are damaged. Thus, tone must be considered not a property of muscle itself, but of reflex activity.

Evaluation of Muscle Tone

The typical feeling of a normal muscle upon palpation is one of resilience (Fig. 9.2). An increased perception of tone by the examiner denotes a hypertonic muscle; decreased tone, a hypotonic muscle. Tone, age, sex, body structure, occupation, physical avocations, and nutritional status of the patient must be considered in evaluating muscle health.

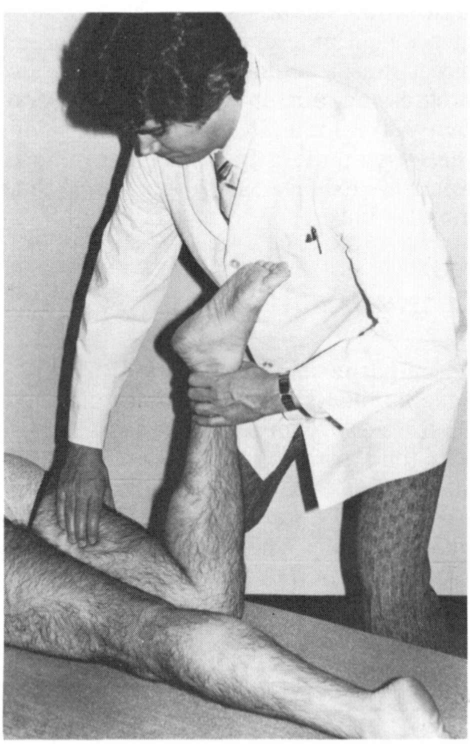

Figure 9.2. Hamstring palpation while testing hamstring strength with the patient prone.

During passive manipulation of a joint, a slight degree of resistance is encountered in the muscle that is not part of conscious effort by the patient. Thus, it can be said that the chief characteristics of normal muscle tone are (1) subdued activity during relaxation and (2) an involuntary reaction opposing mechanical stretch.

Postural Tone and Balance

Postural tonus refers to the sustained contraction of muscles supporting the upright position. The stimuli producing the volley of nerve impulses that continually excite the postural muscles can arise from every sense organ of the body. For example, postural tone is increased by loud noises, bright lights, strong odors, and jarring shocks. When such stimuli are absent, postural tone diminishes.

The stretch reflex is responsible for regulating tension within various muscle groups that provides the basis of postural muscle tone. Stretch (myotatic) reflexes are tested clinically by testing tendon reflexes.

Muscle Tone and the Stretch Reflex

Muscle tone is sustained by the stretch reflex. Gravity pulls on all antigravity muscles, and this stretch elicits muscular tone that reflexively helps maintain the body erect. It is on the foundation of postural muscle tone that all voluntary movements are superimposed.

As explained previously, the stretch reflex is a major component of maintaining muscle tone and is well developed in the antigravity muscles to control body posture. However, although basic muscle tone and postural patterns involve local cord reflexes, they are under brain control (eg, the cerebral cortex, cerebellum, inner-ear proprioceptors). In states of unconsciousness, the body quickly gives in to the force of gravity.

Dystonia

Dystonia means a state of impaired or disordered tonicity. It is a general term that may be applied to either muscular hyperto-

Table 9.2. Types of Dystonia and Typical Causes

FLEXION DYSTONIA	**Degenerative Disorders** Amyotrophic lateral sclerosis Hallevorden-Spatz syndrome Hunt's pallidal degeneration Idiopathic parkinsonism Olivopontocerebellar atrophy Pick's disease Wilson's disease (late) Alzheimer's disease (late) Huntington's chorea (late) **Infectious Disorders** Encephalitis Jakob-Creutzfeldt disease Meningitis Postencephalitic parkinsonism Syphilis Tuberculosis **Metabolic Disorders** Anoxia Fahr's disease Hypoparathyroidism Pseudohypoparathyroidism	**Toxic Disorders** Carbon monoxide Carbon disulfide Cyanide Kernicterus Lead Manganese Nitrous oxide Phenothiazines **Traumatic Disorders** Injury to cortex or globus pallidus connections **Vascular Disorders** Diffuse arterial disorders
HEMIPLEGIC DYSTONIA	**Degenerative Disorders** Dystonia musculorum deformans (mild) Huntington's chorea Olivopontocerebellar atrophy Parkinsonism (some forms) Shy-Drager syndrome Striatonigral degeneration Wilson's disease (juvenile) **Infectious Disorders** Jakob-Creutzfeldt disease Postencephalic parkinsonism	**Metabolic Disorders** Anoxia Hepatic encephalopathy **Toxic Disorders** Manganese Methanol Phenothiazines **Traumatic Disorders** Birth trauma Skull trauma
SPASTIC DYSTONIA	**Degenerative Disorders** Familial spastic paraplegia **Metabolic Disorders** Anoxia Hypoglycemia	**Vascular Disorders** Embolus Stroke Thrombosis Vasculitis
TORSIONAL DYSTONIA	Dystonia musculorum deformans	Tentorial herniation

nicity or hypotonicity, or to an imbalance within the autonomic nervous system. Clinically, the term *dystonia* is often used to describe an abnormal limb position: an alpha-type rigidity from sustained contraction of EMG-normal motor units.

There are four major types of muscular dystonia:

• *Flexion dystonia*, exhibiting a sustained four-limb flexion posture (pallidal syndrome).

• *Hemiplegic dystonia*, characterized by flexed upper extremities and extended lower extremities, without spasticity. Athetosis is often associated.

• *Spastic dystonia*, featuring the same picture as hemiplegic dystonia except the spasticity is overt.

• *Torsion dystonia*, portraying an attitude of decerebrate rigidity.

The differentiation of various types of dystonia is shown in Table 9.2.

Cerebral Palsy Hypotonicity

The general term *cerebral palsy* refers to any upper motor neuron deficit that has its origin in a perinatal insult. The muscle hypotonia exhibited may be temporary or permanent. The various types of cerebral palsy are shown in Table 9.3.

Hypertonicity

With few exceptions, states Chusid, hypertonic and hyperkinetic states are invariably

Table 9.3. Types of Cerebral Palsy

Type	Features
Ataxic palsy	The major features are trunk and extremity ataxia, dysdiadochokinesia, dyssynergia, dysmetria, and mental retardation.
Atonic diplegia	Pronounced hypotonic quadriparesis in the lower extremities with less weakness in the upper extremities. There are also inadequate trunk control, hyperreflexia, and mental retardation. The involved muscles become spastic after a few years.
Dyskinetic palsy	Spontaneous involuntary trunk movements at rest and after effort. There is mental retardation and often deafness.
Spastic diplegia	The lower limbs are weaker and more spastic than the upper limbs. There are also pathologic reflexes, hyperreflexia and mental retardation.
Spastic hemiplegia	Unilateral involvement, usually sparing the face. Other major signs include upper extremity spastic distally, lower extremity weak proximally, pathologic reflexes, and hyperreflexia. Retardation is not present.
Spastic monoplegia	One limb is weaker and more spastic than its partner. Retardation is not present.
Spastic quadriplegia	Four limbs are weak and spastic. There are also inadequate trunk control, pathologic reflexes, hyperreflexia, and profound mental retardation.
Spastic triplegia	Three limbs are weak, spastic, and exhibit increased deep tendon reflexes and pathologic reflexes. Retardation is present.
Mixed forms	Any combination of the above.

the result of involvement of the *extrapyramidal system.* There are three major types of hypertonicity: rigidity, spasticity, and flexor spasms.

Rigidity and spasticity are differentiated in Table 9.4. The characteristics of various types of rigidity are as follows:

• *Cogwheel (ratchet) rigidity:* extrapyramidal rigidity alternating with releases in muscle tension. It is commonly associated with parkinsonism.

• *Decerebrate rigidity:* constant contraction of all antigravity extensors, which is caused by a lesion between the vestibular nuclei and the superior colliculus.

• *Decorticate rigidity:* constant contraction of upper-extremity flexors and lower-extremity extensors, which is the result of a lesion above the superior colliculus.

• *Paratonic rigidity (Gegenhalten):* involuntary stiffening of a limb against the direction of passive movement. *Reverse Gegenhalten* refers to the involuntary movement of a limb toward the direction of passive movement. Both types are commonly associated with frontal-lobe lesions and their related behavioral disturbances.

MUSCLE WEAKNESS

Terminology is often confusing when strength is described. The phrase "isometric strength" (equal in length) refers to muscle activity occurring without muscle shortening. "Isotonic strength" (equal in tone) means muscle activity with shortening of the muscle. Both of these general terms are physiologic misnomers in that there *is* a degree of length change in isometrics due to tendon stretching; and in isotonics, normal tone *is* influenced by the altered mechanical advantage and resistance. Strength is also described in terms of dynamic (isotonic), explosive, and static (isometric) types.

Weakness is characterized by feelings of lassitude, tiredness, weariness, depletion, exhaustion, malaise, loss of energy and motivation. Its cause may be general or local. If local, the weakness may be described in lower or upper extremities, either distal or proximal. It may be localized in the trunk, head, or in respiration. A rule of thumb is that proximal weakness is the result of a myopathy, while a distal weakness is caused by a neuropathy (Fig. 9.3).

It is important to analyze weakness in terms of body segments because weakness almost always follows a neuroanatomical distribution in organic disease.

Psychomotor Responses

Weakness without related symptoms or signs suggests an emotional problem (eg, depression). These responses refer to the reaction of musculature to emotional effects on the nervous system as the body depicts its

Table 9.4. Hypertonicity: Differentiation of Rigidity and Spasticity

Feature	Rigidity	Spasticity
Description	Increased tone in opposing muscles produces steady resistance to passive stretch throughout range of motion.	Increased tension in a muscle dependent on the speed of passive stretch.
Release after shortening response	Slow	Rapid, clasp-knife response
Stretch reflex velocity	Slow	Exaggerated
Typical cause	Lower motor neuron lesion	Upper motor neuron lesion

psychologic stresses. They may be environmentally, socially, or intrinsically initiated.

Pathologic Weakness

Inequality in muscle balance has many causes. It may be initiated by trauma, postural distortion phenomena, biochemical reactions, psychomotor responses, paralytic effects, or somatic and visceral responses. Weakness may be the only symptom of an early systemic disease such as Guillain-Barré syndrome.

Primary disease of the neuromuscular system itself (eg, paralytic diseases) affects musculoskeletal tone and strength, thus affecting position and quality of motion. Typical causes of pathologic muscle weakness and spasm are atrophy, muscle rupture, spastic paralysis, flaccid paralysis, myopathy, myasthenia gravis, periodic paralysis, root or nerve disease, upper and lower motor neuron syndromes, parkinsonism, and cerebellar disease.

In weakness or paralysis due to final common pathway disease, there is an inability to obtain voluntary contraction, a loss of involuntary movements, and a loss of reflex contraction of the involved muscles (Fig. 9.4). This weakness is either the result of failure of the action potential to be transmitted to the muscle because of a neural block (eg, impingement, disease process) or the result of diseased muscle fibers that cannot respond to the action potentials of their lower motor neurons.

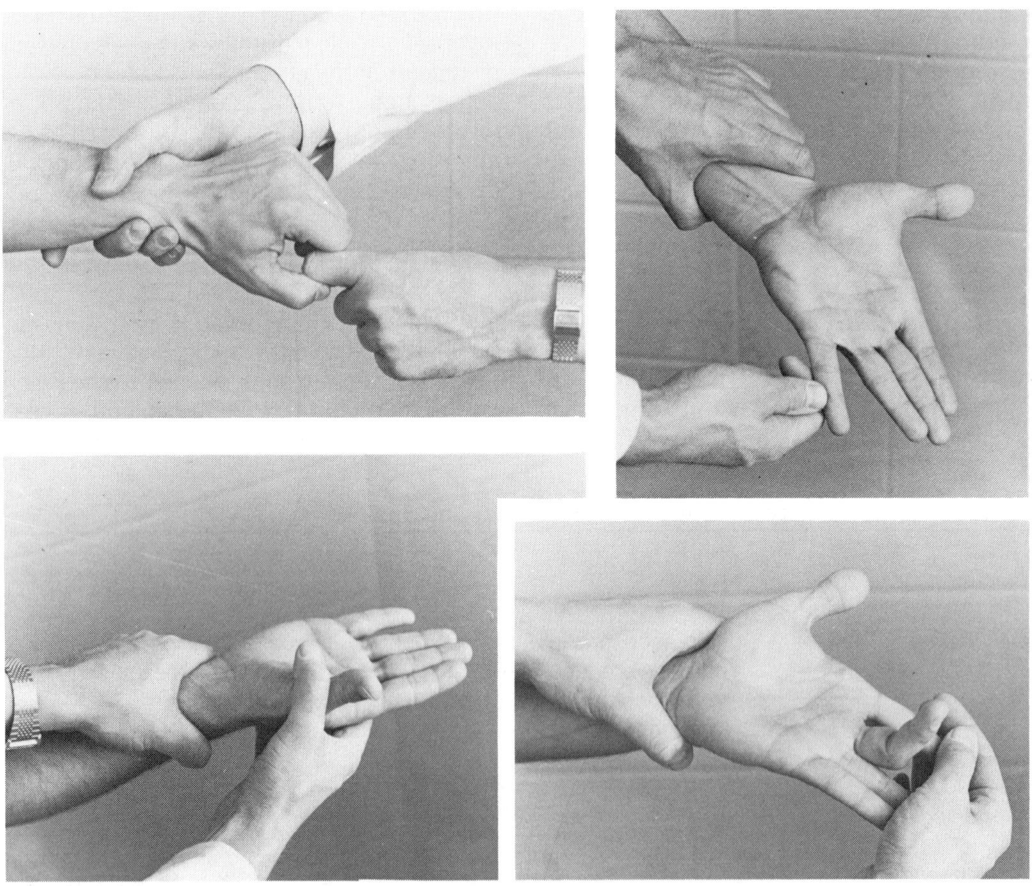

Figure 9.3. Ulnar entrapment tests: evaluation of pinch strength (top left), little finger abduction strength (top right), thumb abduction strength (bottom left), and active flexion of the metacarpophalangeal joints (bottom right).

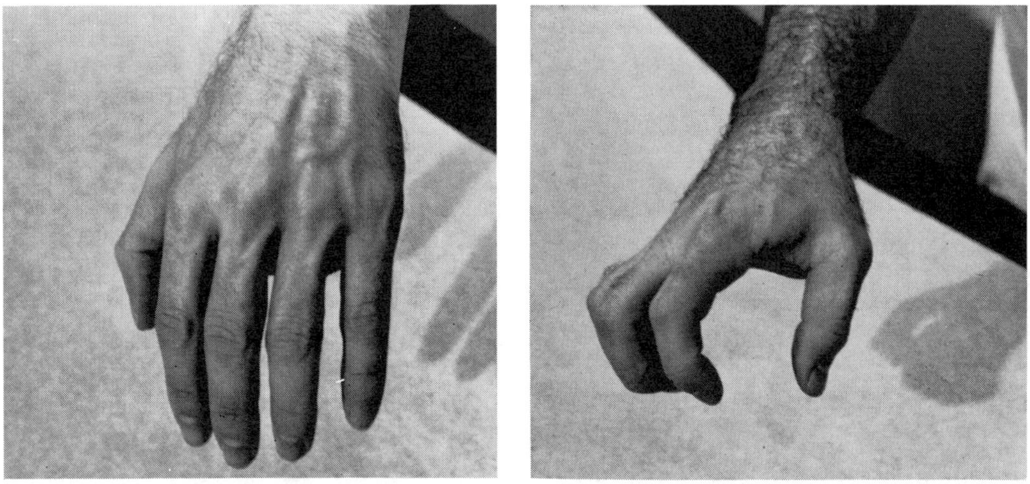

Figure 9.4. *Left,* the inability to separate fingers indicates an ulnar nerve lesion. *Right,* ape (simian) hand is usually the result of injury to the median nerve (Courtesy of the American Chiropractic Association).

A thorough evaluation of weakness should consider its site, anatomical origin, and rate of progression.

Weakness Evaluated by Its Site

The site of weakness may be symmetrical, asymmetrical, distal, proximal, or general in distribution. Regardless, the fault may be sited in the anterior horn cells, myoneural junction, muscles, or be of unknown origin.

In generalized weakness, there is little or no wasting with periodic paralysis, myasthenia gravis, myasthenic syndrome, steroid myopathy, or hyperthyroidism. Wasting will be associated with generalized myositis ossificans, congenital dystrophy with arthrogryposis, and the congenital myopathies.

Weakness Evaluated by Its Anatomical Origin

Weakness originating from a lesion at a particular anatomical location offers characteristic clinical findings.

Involvement of the Corticospinal Pathway. The stretch reflexes are hyperactive, and there is increased resistance to passive motion and abnormal sensory perceptions. Weakness is usually more pronounced than atrophy.

Involvement of the Anterior Horn Cells. The stretch reflexes are absent or hypoactive. The weakness is generalized, but occasionally distal only. Weakness parallels the atrophy present.

Involvement of the Peripheral Nerves. The stretch reflexes are absent or hypoactive. Weakness is usually distal but sometimes generally distributed. Weakness parallels the atrophy present. Muscle fasciculation is sometimes seen, and paresthesia and sensory changes are usually present.

Involvement of the Myoneural Junction. Stretch reflexes are normal. Fatigue is greater than the weakness, and strength returns quickly with rest after exertion. Muscle fasciculation is rarely present. The disorder is usually seen first in the extraocular muscles, progressing in a variable, fluctuating course.

Involvement of the Muscle Fibers. Stretch reflexes are absent or hypoactive, but the distal reflexes are usually normal. Weakness is proximal and parallels the atrophy present. Muscle fasciculation is rarely present.

Involvement of Function. Stretch reflexes are normal, and there is no fasciculation or atrophy. Cogwheel responses and slowness of motion are present. There is a distinct activity overflow and inconsistency in responses.

Weakness or Paralysis Evaluated by Its Rate of Progression

Weakness or paralysis may have a fast, variable, or slow rate of progression and thus point toward specific conditions.

Disorders with a Fast Rate of Progression. Examples include the muscular dystrophies, inflammatory myopathies, toxic myopathies, periodic paralysis, myasthenic syndromes, muscle tumors, a large variety of atrophies and neuropathies, amyotrophic lateral sclerosis, syringomyelia, and poliomyelitis.

Disorders with a Variable Rate of Progression. The myoglobinuric myopathies, amyloid myopathy, sarcoidosis, infantile spinal muscular atrophy, myositis ossificans, and myasthenia gravis are examples.

Disorders with a Slow or Static Rate of Progression. Examples include the congenital myopathies, endocrine myopathies, and glycogen storage diseases.

MUSCLE FATIGUE

When physical activity is conducted under highly warm-humid conditions, precautions must be taken to avoid dehydration fatigue, heat cramps, exhaustion, and stroke. Under such conditions, muscle cramps result from electrolytic depletion and are temporarily disabling.

An excised rested muscle tests alkaline with litmus paper, while a fatigued muscle tests acid because muscle contraction consumes nutrients and oxygen and produces acids as well as the body's major source of heat. Acids accumulating as a result of continued activity apparently tend to contribute to fatigue.

Fatigue may be the only early symptom of myopathy. Either progressing central or local fatigue adversely affects skill: diminished skill is commonly associated with approaching exhaustion. As muscle perfusion is greater in a strong muscle as contrasted with that of a weak muscle, fatigue can be the result of inadequate perfusion. However, the overt signs of pallor and the energy-wasting poor coordination, confusion, and staggering gait are usually blamed on inadequate blood flow to the posture-regulating center. Strength also has an influence on recovery because strength tends to minimize the microtrauma secondary to oxygen lack and local weakness.

TYPES OF PARALYSIS

True paralysis refers to the complete loss of sensation, muscle function, or the inability to control a muscle or group of muscles. It may be either temporary or permanent.

Spastic paralysis is commonly seen in lesions of upper motor neurons. *Flaccid paralysis* occurs in the peripheral type of nerve lesions involving the lower motor neurons of the anterior horn cells. *Peripheral nerve paralyses* are especially apt to be accompanied by sensory symptoms, electrical changes, and wasting. *Brain-originating paralyses* have few sensory symptoms (sometimes paresthesias), and slight wasting, mental changes, coma, or convulsions often precede or follow the attack. *Cord paralyses* may or may not show these associations, but they are often accompanied by disorders of the bladder and rectum.

Flaccid Paralysis

A flaccid type of paralysis exhibits if there is no or extremely poor regeneration after injury. It manifests in the peripheral type of nerve lesions affecting the anterior horn cells, nerve roots, peripheral motor neurons, or myoneural junction. The cause can be anything that will block the flow of peripheral impulses (eg, cord tumor or disease process, root compression, nerve laceration or block, junctional deficit). Muscle tone no longer exists because the nerve is unable to maintain it. The muscles become limp and feel small and flabby. Local reflexes are decreased, strength is diminished, and the muscles involved eventually shrink and possibly become replaced by connective and adipose tissues. Deformity results because normal antagonistic muscles overcome the weakened agonists. Weakness with some paralysis in one longitudinal half of the body is called *hemiparesis*.

Spastic Paralysis

Spastic paralysis is the clinical opposite of flaccid paralysis. It is seen with lesions of upper motor neurons (Table 9.5). A spastic type of paralysis occurs on the opposite side of the body and below the level of the lesion if it is at or above the medullary pyramid. Increased muscle tone is felt as firmness and stiffness, especially in the arm flexors and the leg extensors. Although the muscles involved show weakness on resistance, they palpate tight and tense at rest.

Weakness is especially pronounced in the musculature of the limbs, and there is great difficulty with movements of the hands. However, incoordination is the more common complaint rather than weakness. Besides the neurologic deficit, incoordination results from the varying degrees of strength between the prime movers and antagonists. Deformity by flexion contraction results when the flexors of a part remain strong while the extensors become weak (Fig. 9.5).

In some cases, lesions in the brain stem can involve both upper and lower motor neurons. This results in an *alternating hemiplegia.*

Tran states that the extent of the symptomatology frequently offers the examiner a clue to the location of the disorder. In most chronic pyramidal tract lesions, especially when the trauma has been sudden but not insidious, a partial recovery of control is expected. This occurs mostly in the large proximal muscles of the shoulder and hip. Disorders of the pyramidal tract commonly produce defects that are more conspicuous in

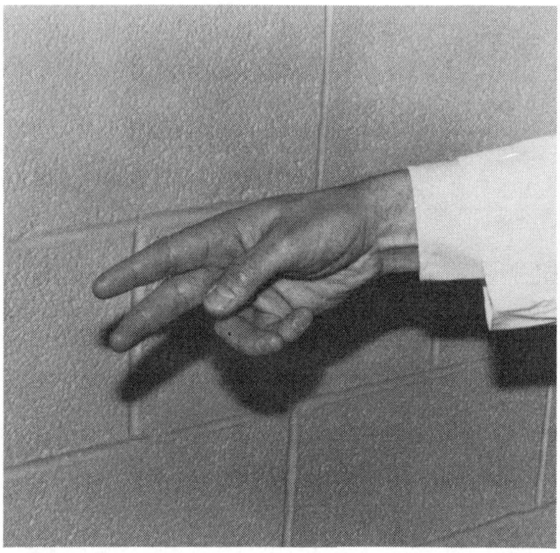

Figure 9.5. Position the hand assumes in carpopedal spasm such as seen in Trousseau's phenomenon.

Table 9.5. Differentiation of Upper and Lower Motor Neuron Lesions

Consideration	Upper Motor Neuron Lesion	Lower Motor Neuron Lesion
Site	Cerebral cortex or pyramidal tract	Anterior horn or peripheral motor neuron
Distribution	Diffuse or patchy	Segmental (number)
Reflexes		
Superficial	Absent	Absent
Deep	Exaggerated	Absent or hypotonic
Atrophy	Disuse, not prominent	Rapid extension, trophic
Trophic lesions	Minimal	Intense and extensive
Pathologic signs and reflexes	Present	Absent
Fasciculations	Not present	Present
Paralysis		
Type	Spastic and rigid	Flaccid
Location	Contralateral hemiparesis	Paresis limited to specific muscles

the upper limb. This is possibly because highly skilled movements are more prevalent there in comparison to necessary mass contractions.

MUSCLE SORENESS AND STIFFNESS

Tender muscles may occur shortly after activity and pass quickly, or they may not appear until up to 48 hours after exercise and persist for several days. Stiffness, a sign of poor physical fitness in the weekend athlete or of unusual stress in the trained athlete, may be confused with minor strain, as both stiffness and strain produce pain due to increased intramuscular pressure. The stiffness syndrome features gradually increasing pain, swelling, and restricted motion.

Most authorities now believe that muscle stiffness is not the result of local accumulation of lactic acid produced by activity. Rather, the stiffness is thought to result from the accumulation of extracellular muscle

Table 9.6. General Interpretation of Resisted Motion Signs

Response	*Probable Cause*
Strong with excessive range of motion	Capsule laxity, ligamentous instability.
Strong and painful in a specific direction	Minor musculotendinous lesion.
Strong and painful in all directions	Neurosis.
Strong with pain on repetitive resisted movements	Arterial flow deficit.
Strong and unchanged pain in all directions	Referred pain syndrome.
Strong, painful, and hypomobile	Guarded joint for some reason.
Strong, painless, and hypomobile	Contracture, adhesion.
Weak and sharply painful	Fracture, dislocation, rupture, gross pathology.
Weak without aggravation of pain (painless or unchanged constant pain)	Neurogenic disorder, muscle or tendon rupture.
Weak and painless in all directions	Nonmusculotendinous lesion, probable neurogenic lesion.
Pain only at specific point of arc	Functional entrapment, lax joint, dislocated tendon.
Pain at one range extreme	Subluxation, tissue entrapment, eroded cartilage.
Painful with gross hypermobility	Severe sprain.
Painless with gross hypermobility	Ruptured tissues with interrupted sensory path.

fluid due to increased capillary filtration pressure in an unconditioned muscle area where the vascular bed is unable to keep up with the necessary vascular return. The dispersal of the accumulating extracellular fluid is also delayed because of the lack of lymphatics within voluntary muscle.

MUSCLE CRAMPS AND SPASMS

It has been estimated that from 50% to 60% of the pains and discomforts that the average ambulatory patient has are the direct or indirect result of involuntary muscle contraction. Thus, the physician is compelled to consider the relationship of muscle contraction to pain symptoms in both diagnosis and therapy.

Musculoskeletal and peripheral vascular disorders are characterized by associated muscle cramps or spasms. These spasms are powerful involuntary muscular contractions shortening the flexor muscles. The result is extreme, often incapacitating, pains initiated by ischemia and hypoxia of muscle tissue. Such spasms are commonly associated with myositic, fibrositic, and articular disorders.

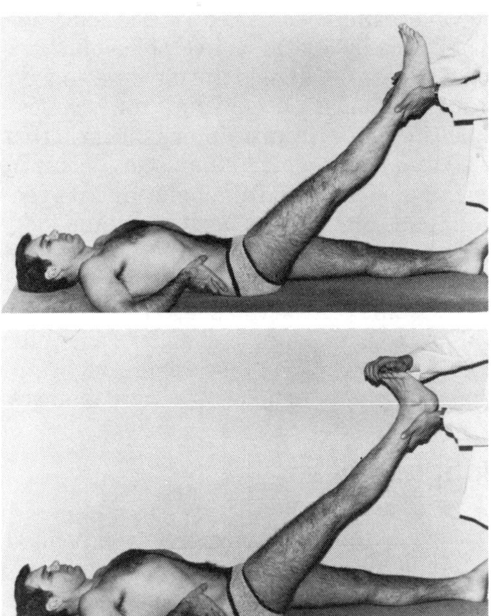

Figure 9.6. *Top,* Lasegue's supine straight-leg-raising test; *bottom,* Bragard's test.

Hypertrophy and spasm must be differentiated from the muscular enlargement that follows exercise. The increase in muscle bulk following exercise is caused by two factors: (1) the opening of capillaries during activity that are closed during rest; and (2) prolonged activity (months), which appears to increase thesize of individual muscle fibers.

The general points of differentiation when restricted motion is found are shown in Table 9.6.

Neuromechanisms

Many motor units normally rest while others are firing; but in the cramp phenomenon, all motor units fire and cause the spasm. Why this happens is not clear, but impaired fluid intake, electrolytic balance, and blood flow are often involved. Cramps are characterized by spontaneous, prolonged, painful muscle contraction, usually occurring in voluntary weight-bearing flexor muscles. They often develop during sleep or soon after violent exertion and may vary from slight contractions to violent spasms.

Muscle spasm is an involuntary and aberrant contraction of a muscle part or whole as a result of some excessive motor fiber stimulation such as irritation of (1) the anterior horn cells by the toxic elements of catabolic débris, accumulations consequent to faulty elimination, and circulatory disturbances; (2) an encroached nerve root from subluxation (Fig. 9.6), paraforaminal congestion, herniated disc, and/or ligamentous thickening; (3) a nerve trunk or plexus; eg, piriformis, psoas major, scalenus anticus contraction; (4) peripheral nerve branches; eg, common peroneus by contracted tensor fascia lata or occipital nerve by suboccipital spasm. Spasm also may occur as splinting secondary to injury as in sprain, avulsion fracture, and compression; within a muscle as the result of direct injury or irritation, often resulting from toxic accumulations; eg, toxic lumbago; or consequent to psychic stress.

Etiology

The primary causes of muscle spasm (from minor to severe) are postural and occupational fatigue, electrolyte imbalance, stress, trauma, emotional tension, psychic conversion syndromes, referred irritation from visceral involvement, and nerve root irritations associated with interosseous derangements.

When a synovial articulation is subjected to excessive stresses or toxic insult, the muscles that move the joint are reflexly provoked into spasm because of the irritation of the articular sensory bed. This spasm, often asymmetrical, will frequently force the joint into greater derangement or compression and thus set up the inimical phenomenon of circulus vitiosus.

In cases of pathologic spasm, the patient's history may show that muscles in painful spasm may be relaxed at times if the muscles are provided a position of physiologic rest and an appropriate therapy is applied.

Heat cramps also can cause muscle soreness and stiffness. These cramps are often caused by excessive salt loss. However, other factors may be involved such as muscle anoxia, a blow or strain, or for some yet unexplained reason. Violent exercise too soon after a meal increases the danger of active-extremity cramps because much of the general circulation is diverted to the abdomen for absorption purposes. Hormonal factors may be involved in the female, especially during the menstrual period. Cramps frequently follow drinking ice water or other cold drinks too quickly or in too large a quantity after exercise.

Abdominal Cramps

Abdominal cramps are common and frequently associated with gastralgia and enteralgia in which there is contraction of the muscles of the stomach, intestines, and sometimes of the abdominal wall. *Windedness* is an acute cause of abdominal pain and is associated with a diaphragmatic cramp.

General Spasms

General myospasm guarding joint motion can be grossly evaluated by watching the body attitude (eg, stiff carriage) and by efforts to bend the joint forward, backward, and to the sides. If the examiner is familiar with the average range of mobility in each direction at different ages and physical condition, this test is usually easy and rapid. Care should be taken to differentiate phasic spasm (usually antalgic) from frequently exhibited reflex hypertonicity.

It is one thing to find muscle spasm present and another to determine if it is protective, compensatory, hysterical, or a causative factor. Careful analysis of the dynamic motion of the involved joint is an important method of gaining differential clues. Limitations of motion due to spasm are seen with special frequency in joint pathology and subluxation-fixations, but they may occur in almost any form of joint trouble, particularly in the larger joints.

Painful Splinting

Striated muscles, especially the erectors, become painfully splinted (intrinsically immobilized) by spasm, active or involuntary, when they are fatigued. If this is prolonged, trophic changes occur and tone is lost. Splinting differs from ordinary spasm in that relaxation of the affected muscles occurs at rest. Prolonged pain from bone, muscle, tendon, and joint lesions with resultant long-term splinting or pseudoparalysis may lead to eventual osteoporosis in the involved bones. Joint contractures also may develop. This is another example, similar to a psychic conversion symptom, where a sensory symptom may lead to definite structural changes.

Fatigue Spasm

More neuromuscular energy is expended in human postural, locomotive, occupational, and recreational efforts than in any other vertebrate. Fatigue therefore intrudes itself upon most clinical profiles. A characteristic of all erector muscles of the axial skeleton is that when they experience postural and stress fatigue, they go into a splinting-type painful spasm. When such a provoked muscle tires and goes into fatigue spasm as a compensatory necessity, the muscle becomes painful because the spasm impinges upon the neurotendinous and neuromuscular receptors, and trigger mechanisms are created. This pain is usually asymmetrical and of a distorting, compressing nature.

If there is a pre-existing defect, the asymmetrical fatigue spasm may be the burden that triggers a subliminal situation into an acute syndrome or may become the provocative factor in a nagging chronic discomfort that is stubborn to relieve. On the other hand, muscles get stronger with use. The only time a used muscle gets weaker is when its nutrition is absent or reduced. This can be the product of noxious neurologic reflexes of inhibition.

MUSCLE TRAUMA

Muscles are often injured by strain, contusion, laceration, indirect trauma, rupture, hernia, and less frequently by disease.

Frank trauma may cause inflammation, degeneration, etc, and particularly the muscular splinting reaction that muscles make when their surrounding tissues are injured. This alters the position and motion of the structural tissues that are related. Sustained microtrauma, although of a less acute nature, may cause a slow continual irritation and eventually create degenerative changes that similarly alter muscular reaction.

The obvious trauma of a fall or blow that surprises a joint with the intrinsic muscles unprepared will cause a joint sprain with ligament injury, and a sudden slip during a lift is equally damaging to the unprepared muscles or a weak joint. However, the slower trauma of occupational strain is not as easy to visualize. Holding a baseball bat at arm's length to the side for 2 minutes will cause the shoulder to ache within 1 minute; but the big "catch" will be at the lumbosacral level in ensuing hours and days.

A muscle in pronounced traumatic or reflex spasm will become inflamed. This is likely to produce some degree of transudation precipitation of fibrin, collagen, and mineral salt deposition, and, if extended, this state can easily result in chronic myositis and myofibrosis. The myofascial planes usually become inflamed at the points of major stress, wherein transudation and fibrin formation produce myofascial plane adhesions. Some authorities feel that this process encourages or is the cause of the development of trigger points.

LOCAL MOVEMENT DISTURBANCES

Extrapyramidal disorders produce abnormal tone, movement disturbances, and there may be decreased associated movements and pauses in motion. Such neuromuscular disorders as fibrillations, tics, tremors, convulsions, and spasms can be generally classified as local movement disorders. The early stage of such disturbances is easy to miss if not observed under good lighting. In the late stages, spontaneous movements can often be noticed while taking the history.

Fibrillation

Fibrillation is a spontaneous, rhythmic episode of irregular twitching contractions of individual muscle fibers or small groups of muscles. The movements are fine, minute, vermicular waves that can rarely be seen or palpated in muscle except possibly under extremely thin skin such as of the tongue and hands. They are best seen on the tongue when the tongue is resting on the floor of the mouth. Fibrillation is usually only discernible by EMG studies. The minute twitching occurs during muscle atrophy or in the presence of a biochemical impairment of the lower motor neurons. The causative lesion may occur at the cord, root, or peripheral nerve level.

Fasciculation

Fasciculation is a spontaneous, isolated contraction (twitch) of individual motor units. The contractions are usually brief, and the quantity of the reactions depends on the size of the muscle involved (extra-ocular vs trapezius). Light percussion of affected muscles usually activates fasciculation.

Fasciculation is a primary sign of anterior horn disease, root disease, or diffuse motor neuron disease (eg, amyotrophic lateral sclerosis), but rarely are the twitches a complaint. The sign is also associated with electrolytic disturbances, myasthenia gravis, and early poliomyelitis (inflammatory stage) or in chronic cord damage (eg, neoplasm, scar, compression).

Fasciculation is more often seen with nerve root compression than it is with more distal peripheral nerve compression. It may be generalized in myokymia, but it usually appears first in the calf muscles. Generalized fasciculation is often described as a "slow shiver." Transient psychomotor benign fasciculation is often seen in normal subjects under stress and offers no clinical significance.

Spontaneous fasciculations persist even during rest. However, contraction fasciculations (nonspontaneous) disappear when the involved muscles are relaxed. Contraction fasciculations may occur during weak muscle contractions and are usually witnessed in the tense patient who has difficulty in relaxing. They are also associated with amyotrophic lateral sclerosis and poliomyelitis.

Tics and Habit Spasms

Tics are brief, recurrent, inappropriate, involuntary twitching movements repeated in the same pattern (stereotyped). The more common tics are twitchings of the eye, side of the face, lips, or arm and shoulder. Tics are commonly the result of habit, encephalitis, or idiopathic extrapyramidal neuropathy. Idiopathic tics usually begin in childhood and diminish in later life. Episodes are frequently precipitated by emotional stress. Tics may be briefly controlled voluntarily, but such control is likely to be followed by an intense episode of contractions.

Gilles de la Tourette syndrome is a childhood disorder characterized by bizarre tics, coprolalia, imitative gestures, and severe behavior changes. Differential diagnosis should give priority consideration to early parkinsonism, chorea, basal ganglia disease, cerebellar lesion, and Wilson's disease.

Myokymia

Myokymia is a benign form of muscle twitching. It is characterized by brief, spontaneous, tetanic contractions of muscles or fiber groups. Sometimes a continual undulation of muscle surface is produced. The muscle movements are slower and more prolonged in myokymia than they are in fasciculation or tics. Myokymia usually occurs without apparent cause but sometimes is associated with metabolic and infectious disorders.

Tremors

Tremors are rapid, oscillating, involuntary movements that usually involve the tongue or hands. There is a state of continuous contraction of individual muscles with a varying pattern of rhythm. A tremor may occur only during rest, only during volitional motion, during postural sustentation (ie, maintaining a specific posture), or during various combinations of these acts.

Tremors may result from fatigue, alcoholism, drug addiction, thyrotoxicosis, anxiety, multiple sclerosis (intention tremor), or Parkinson's disease (rest tremor). The tremor of anxiety, hyperthyroidism, idiopathic dementia, alcoholism, and toxicosis is most evident in the outstretched hands.

To screen for tremor, Olson and associates recommend that the patient be instructed to point closely at (but not touch) the index fingers of each hand. This may bring out a proximal tremor. A patient with essential tremor will show the tremor throughout the range of motion during a finger-to-finger test.

Basic Classes

• *Cerebellar tremor*. When the tremor is not present at rest or during sustentation but only when an act is being performed, it is called an *intention tremor*. The tremor of cerebellar dysfunction is invariably an intention tremor, and it is worse at the end of movement. The tremor is at right angles to the direction of movement (eg, from side to side). The muscles involved are hypotonic and other signs of cerebellar disease will be present. In chronic alcoholism, the intention tremor is slow, irregular, and unsteady.

• *Essential tremor.* An *essential tremor* is present during intention movements and sustentation but not during rest. It is common to a number of senile, benign, and inherited disorders. The tremor appears in the direction of movement. A staggering gait (titubation) is usually associated.

• *Metabolic tremor.* This type of fine tremor is present with intention and sustentation. It may increase or decrease during rest. Mild pyrexia and tachycardia are often associated.

• *Rubral tremor.* This is a constant tremor. It never disappears and may worsen with intentional activity. The involved muscles are hypotonic, and mesencephalic signs will invariably be present.

• *Parkinson's tremor.* A static tremor at rest that is absent during action or sustentation is characteristic of parkinsonism. It is most noticeable in the upper extremities. Plastic or cogwheel rigidity and hypokinesia are often associated. Anxiety and senile tremors and those associated with early Wilson's disease often resemble parkinsonism, but they are coarser in character.

Parkinson's Disease

Parkinson's disease (paralysis agitans) is a primary or secondary degenerative disease process where deep reflexes are normal and muscle tone is increased to rigidity, especially in the upper flexors and lower extensors. It affects 1.5% of the population over the age of 65, and has four cardinal clinical features: bradykinesia, rigidity, tremor, and a characteristic disorder of posture and gait. The syndrome of bradykinesia and rigidity is called *parkinsonism.*

One of the most early signs of Parkinson's disease is that the patient rarely blinks his eyes, and this can occur from 5 to 7 years before all symptoms develop. Later, there is a characteristic resting "pill-rolling" tremor in the fingers and a fixed facial expression (Parkinson's mask). Passive extremity flexion and extension result in increasing resistance that collapses and gives way to alternating, jerky, cogwheel motions. While erect, the head and shoulders are stooped. The gait is short, shuffling, and the arms (held at the side) do not swing in rhythm with the legs. The gait is the progressive type. Hyperthyroidism, Wilson's disease, and drug toxicosis should be ruled out early.

Myoclonus

Myoclonus is a state of involuntary, short, rapid, rhythmic bursts of muscle contractions involving individual muscles, groups of muscles, or entire limbs. It may be either generalized or segmental. A sudden jerk or series of jerks may occur with rates as fast as 50—60 per minute or as slow as 5—10 per minute. The disorder is commonly associated with diffuse neuron disease and childhood convulsions.

Myoclonic jerks are likely to occur in the muscles of the limbs, face, and oral cavity, and disappear during sleep. If large groups of muscles are affected, states Chusid, they produce joint movements that may be of sufficient violence to jar patients or throw them to the ground. Palatial myoclonus usually results from lesions in the pathways connecting the red nucleus, the olivary bodies of the medulla, and the dentate nucleus of the cerebellum.

Chorea and Choreiform Movements

Chorea is a disease that results from basal ganglia damage. It is characterized by sudden, spontaneous, irregular, highly variable, purposeless muscle movements, resembling a dancing part. *Huntington's chorea* is an inherited variety associated with cerebral cortex defects. It is progressive and leads to severe mental deterioration. *Sydenham's chorea* occurs in children as a result of rheumatic fever, frequently presenting rapid recovery without complications. The direct cause of chorea is sequential firing of agonists and antagonists, resulting in quick jerky motions.

With chorea, the muscles are not as rigid as in paralysis agitans. The condition may occur hemilaterally as a result of a vascular lesion. Grimaces may occur on the face or aberrations may be present in other parts of the body, but, like athetosis, chorea has a predilection for distal involvement. The features are most noticeable in the hands, fingers, face, tongue, and lower extremities. In the early stages, slight twitching and digit flicking are noticed. In advanced cases, whole extremities are involved.

Choreiform movements are usually the result of a fault in the basal ganglia, their distribution is highly variable, and they may occur during sleep. They begin suddenly and are without rhythm and are generally purposeless, coarse, rapid, and jerky in character.

Ballismus and Hemiballismus

Ballismus (ballism), resembling Huntington's chorea, is exhibited as violent flinging of the extremities by vigorous involvement of the proximal muscles, often to the point of self-injury. The condition represents an extreme lack of inhibitory control. Between episodes, purposeful movements can be conducted. A pathologic substrate of subthalamic involvement is usually associated (eg, a small infarct). In differential diagnosis, chorea, focal seizures, and drug dyskinesia must be excluded.

Hemiballismus (hemiballism) is a rare sign that involves one side of the body and is usually marked in an upper limb. It is characterized by continual malcoordinated activity of the axial and proximal extremity musculature, sometimes to the extent that the limb thrashes about and resembles hemichorea. The face is often spared. The onset is usually sudden. In most cases, the cause is a lesion (eg, hemorrhagic softening) of the contralateral subthalamic nucleus.

Athetosis

Athetosis is a disease of the corpus striatum that is characterized by involuntary slow, twisting, repetitive, worm-like movements in the extremities, especially prominent in the wrists, fingers, tongue, lips, jaw, neck, or feet. It is the result of simultaneous firing of agonists and antagonists, which produces continuous writhing snake-like movements. While variable, the clinical picture is always the same in the same patient and ceases only when the patient is asleep.

Athetosis is often noted in spastic paralysis of infants with brain damage that occurred before or at delivery. *Pseudoathetosis* is the result of severe proprioception loss from whatever cause.

Dystonic Movements

Dystonia usually refers to mobile spasms of the axial and proximal muscles of the extremities. Dystonic movements tend to involve the large portions of the body and have an undulant, sinuous character that may produce grotesque posturing and bizarre writhing, twisting movements of the trunk and body as a whole, with some of the muscles being hypertonic. Torsion spasm (eg, spasmodic torticollis), with resulting twisting or turning movements, is considered a form of dystonia.

Ataxic Movements

Ataxia means a failure or irregularity of muscular activity or coordination. With few exceptions, it especially manifests when volitional motions are attempted. In gait ataxia, the affected individual staggers while walking on a wide base in a manner similar to a drunken gait (unable to stand with the feet together), and usually sways to the side of the unilateral lesion. The loss of equilibrium is the result of a lack of muscle synergy and not of a defect in the proprioceptive pathway. Closing the eyes in the Romberg station has little worsening effect in cerebellar ataxia. Lesions in the midline of the cerebellum cause a difficulty in maintaining an upright stance.

Convulsions and Seizures

Convulsions and seizures are sudden, violent, involuntary muscular contractions of all muscles or large groups of muscles due to a large variety of intracranial lesions. They may vary in intensity from a momentary lapse in consciousness (petit mal) to prolonged violent convulsions (grand mal).

Tonic vs Clonic Spasms

Convulsions and spasms may be either tonic or clonic. A *tonic spasm* is a continuous contraction of a muscle or muscles as in trismus. A *clonic spasm* is marked by alternating contractions and relaxations of the involved muscles such as seen in spasmodic torticollis. Convulsions are common in epilepsy, hysteria, tetanus, uremia, strychnine poisoning, eclampsia, hydrophobia, and lesions of the brain.

Epileptic Seizures

Epilepsy presents a good example of both tonic and clonic convulsions. The seizure is divided into two parts: the first being brief and of the tonic type, the second of the clonic type. Immediately preceding the attack, the patient may have a premonitory symptom of an aura that may vary in different individuals but usually consists of an imaginary vapor arising from the region of the knees toward the head. When the vapor reaches the level of the head, the patient gives a scream, the head and eyes are turned to one side, and the patient passes into the tonic convulsion. This tonic condition may last about a minute, then there is relaxation, after which contractions and relaxations alternate. In this clonic part of the convulsion, the muscles of the face, eyes, and jaw work convulsively. The head and extremities jerk rhythmically. The action of the jaws may be such as to bite the tongue, causing the foam forming in the mouth to be bloodstained. There may be incontinence of urine and involuntary movements of the bowels. After a duration of 2—3 minutes, the patient passes into the deep epileptic coma. Although tonic and clonic convulsions may occur in other diseases, the mode and manner of onset and the course of the convulsion will differ according to the disease in which it is present.

As described above, grand mal is often preceded by a sensory aura and mild motor disturbances leading to violent convulsions and unconsciousness. The specific pattern of a seizure depends on the specific site of the lesion. A prodromal twitching of a limb or side of the face usually indicates a lesion in the *motor area*. The perception of a peculiar odor points toward a lesion in the *temporal lobe*. Perceptions of flashes of light and other visual phenomena indicates a lesion in the *occipital area*. A *parietal area* lesion usually exhibits numbness, tingling, and odd crawling sensations.

Miscellaneous Types of Movement Disturbances

Other forms of involuntary movements may be witnessed. *Clonic convulsive movements* are focal seizures—sudden, brief, rhythmic or irregular, involuntary—that usually involve the great toe, thumb and fingers, or perioral area. Initial localized clonic jerks may progress to prolonged and generalized tonic contractions. *Oculogyric crises* are involuntary, tonic, upward eye movements that last from a few minutes to several hours and are presumed to be the result of a psychogenic problem, upper brain stem dysfunction, or basal ganglia lesion.

GAIT DISTURBANCES

Muscle Analysis During Gait

In walking, most of these muscles are most active during the beginning and end of the stance and swing phases to accelerate and decelerate the angular moments of the lower extremities (Fig. 9.7). This point is important diagnostically, as it is at these periods of gait that specific muscular disorders will become most apparent. Activity is minimal during midstance and midswing, though this is the period of most obvious movement.

Stance Actions

Immediately after heelstrike, the *gluteus maximus* is first elongated before its maximal contraction to assure the development of considerable tensile force to the hip. Also during early stance at a moderate speed, the *quadriceps* becomes elongated and active when the knee is flexed, to smooth flexion up to the point that the center of mass moves anterior to the knee. During rapid gait, the quadriceps contract to inhibit knee flexion and begin extension after toeoff.

During the stance phase, the *gluteus medius* and *minimus* (hip abductors) are in active lengthening contraction when the pelvis is dropping on the swing side and the femur is being slightly adducted. This helps to stabilize the pelvis. The *tibialis anterior* and *toe extensors* rest during midstance, but just after heelstrike, they elongate and achieve their maximum contraction to dorsiflex the foot. At the end of stance, the *iliacus* is elongated as the hip extends and shortens as the swing phase begins to start hip flexion.

At the time of toeoff, there is slight action by the elongated *hamstrings*, which increases with walking speed, to increase knee flexion. The initially stretched *triceps* surae contract when the ankle is in 0° flexion, just long enough to achieve heel flexion.

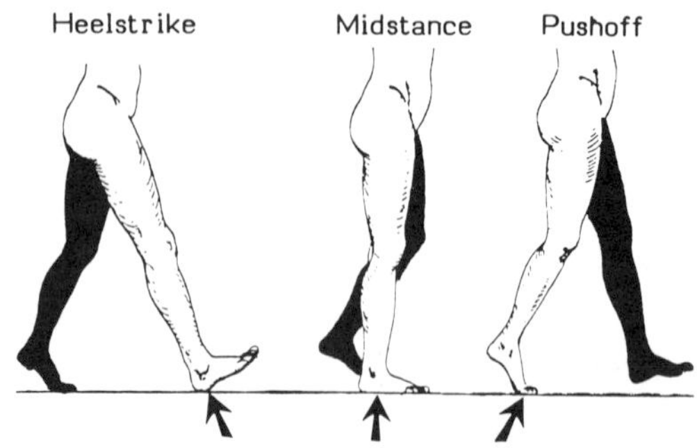

Figure 9.7. During locomotion, the reaction force of the floor is equal in action line and magnitude but counter in direction. Heelstrike force is greater than that of midstance force due to the momentum of the body. Pushoff force is greater than midstance force because of the force produced by calf contraction to plantar flex the foot and propel the body forward.

Swing Actions

The *tensor fascia lata* contracts twice during a single cycle: (1) Its maximum contraction occurs when the swing phase is initiated, simultaneous with iliopsoas contraction, as an aid in hip flexion. At this point in gait, the band is elongated prior to activation. (2) It also contracts at the end of swing and at the start of stance. This is simultaneous with gluteus maximus contraction and resists posterior dislocation of the iliotibial tract where much of the gluteus maximus is inserted.

The *thigh adductors* are in a state of lengthening contraction at the beginning and during the end of the swing phase. See Figure 9.8. At the end of the swing phase, the *hamstrings* become elongated and active into early stance to aid hip extension by the gluteus maximus.

Neurologic Gaits

Neurologic gaits are usually the result of unilateral flexor or extensor spasticity. The

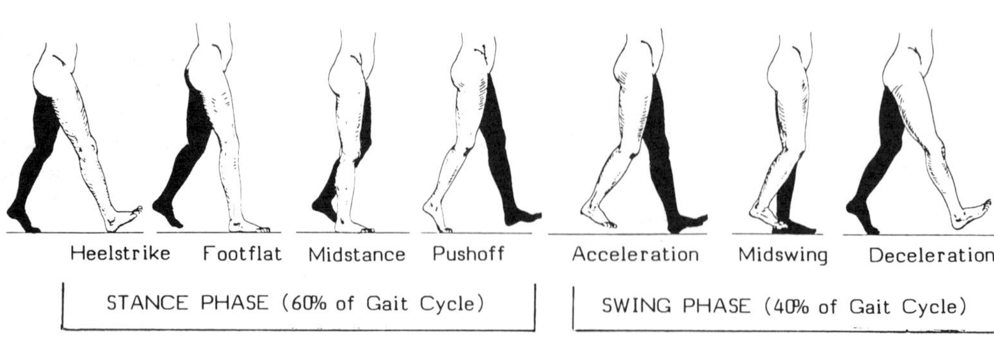

Figure 9.8. The complete gait cycle: stance and swing. Walking is a purposeful disturbance in body equilibrium where alternating leg displacement sustains body weight.

clinical picture is the result of exaggerated stretch reflexes, reflex impairment of the antagonists, and poor flexor-extensor coordination. Most all spastic gaits exhibit a slow cadence and a repetitive pattern during each cycle.

Unilateral Flexor Spasticity

This gait is characterized by a distinct forward lurch of the trunk, a narrow base of support, a decreased stride length, and an absent heelstrike. Adductor tone is usually normal.

Unilateral Extensor Spasticity

A spastic gait is common in upper motor neuron diseases that have a spastic paralysis of the extensor muscles. It is a feature of spinal paralysis, lateral sclerosis, and some other forms of myelitis and anterior tract or brain damage. The upper body is flexed while the lower extremity is extended. The locomotion pattern is characterized by a short stride length, a narrow base of support, and pelvic elevation during swing so that the foot will clear the floor. The legs are firmly extended, the back foot is dragged along in a shuffling manner with the toes scraping on the ground to permit one foot to pass the other. There is little knee flexion during the swing phase if the quadriceps are spastic. Heelstrike is absent and the knee is hyperextended in midstance if the plantar flexors are spastic or if the ankle dorsiflexors are weak. Adductor tone is usually normal.

Adductor Spasticity

In some cases of this condition, the adductors become bilaterally spastic to cause the legs to cross (scissors gait) and the knees often scrape each other in passing (eg, Little's disease). The steps are short and progression is slow. The lower limbs are thrust forward in a stiff, jerky manner, which is often associated by pronounced compensatory motions of the trunk and upper extremities.

Mowing (Hemiplegic) Gait

In spastic hemiplegia, as in unilateral extensor spasticity described above, there is a unilateral spastic gait in which the pelvis is tilted and the affected leg is swung around in a semicircle in front of the other with the toes often scraping the ground. The patient leans to the affected side and the ipsilateral arm is held in a rigid, semiflexed position. The spastic limb is thrown forward with difficulty because of the impaired joint mobility. The hemiplegic limb hangs so that abduction and circumduction of the limb are necessary to move it forward. The most common cause of a *mowing gait* is hemiplegia due to cerebrovascular disease, but any condition that would result in an upper motor neuron lesion can produce such a gait. On first notice, this paralytic gait can be easily confused with any musculoskeletal disorder restricting the action of a hip or knee.

Proprioception Impairment: Ataxic and Tabetic Gaits

This gait is characteristic of posterior column disease and frequently called an *ataxic gait* because it occurs in locomotor ataxia. The patient walks in a clumsy, uncertain manner on a wide base in a stooped posture. Each foot is raised unusually high, thrown forward with force, and brought to the ground flat-footedly with a stamp to increase sensory awareness. While in the air and before being lowered, the foot wavers as if there is a degree of uncertainty in bringing it down. The patient walks with the feet wide apart and is constantly looking at them. This is done to supplement the loss of proprioception. To maintain a large area of foot contact throughout weight bearing, heelstrike is usually eliminated.

An ataxic gait is sometimes called a *tabetic gait* when it is characteristic of a lesion in the dorsal ganglia, dorsal roots, or posterior column of the cord—rarely in higher levels. The ataxia is increased when the eyes are closed or when the patient must walk in a darkened room. This gait is typical of tabes dorsalis but also seen in pernicious anemia and other disorders involving proprioceptive pathways.

Basal Ganglia Dysfunction

This gait is characteristic of paralysis agitans or Parkinson's disease. In these conditions, it is called a *propulsive gait* or *festination* (increasing speed). However, an identical gait is also characteristic of drug poisoning, multiple neuritis or sclerosis, brain tumor, and general paresis.

The hurried walk of parkinsonism is the result of the forward tilt of the trunk (in the attitude of a stoop) and the attempt of the patient to maintain balance. As the center of mass is anterior to the base of support, the patient appears to be chasing his center of gravity (marche à petis pas). Almost all joint motion is restricted, as is arm swing, pelvic tilt, pelvic rotation, and knee flexion. The body and head lean far forward. The trunk, hips, knees, and ankles are flexed to some degree, and the subject walks with short, hurried, shuffling steps, which makes it appear as if the patient is being pushed from the rear and about to fall. Heelstrike is absent, and toes drag during the swing phase. It is difficult for a person with this gait to stop suddenly or to turn a corner. Thus, falls are frequent. Progression is slow at first and then increases rapidly with minimal voluntary control.

Cerebellar Dysfunction

This gait, a sign of cerebellar ataxia, resembles the actions of an intoxicated person. The patient walks with the feet wide apart, takes short steps, and irregularly sways to and fro to such an extent that progression in a straight line is almost impossible. Unsteadiness and a tendency to reel to one side are associated. The lower extremities appear loose. Movement of the advancing limb starts slowly, but the limbs appears to be unexpectantly, erratically, and vigorously flung forward to land with a stamp on the floor. Staggering often occurs on turning. The gait resembles that of a person trying to walk on a rolling ship, constantly trying to maintain equilibrium with little success.

This gait is found with tumor of the cerebellum and diseases of the semicircular canals. Cerebellar lesions are invariably associated with vertigo. It may be indicative of long-term use of alcohol or other drugs (Jake legs) or high CNS neurosyphilis. If the causative factor is unilateral, deviation is to the involved side because of hypotonia.

Paralytic Gaits

Paralytic or paretic gaits with varying patterns are the result of spinal root lesions, brain lesions, nerve compression syndromes, peripheral mononeuritis, abnormal reflexes, and trauma.

General Considerations

If the quadriceps are extremely weak, locomotion is usually impossible as the knee is too unstable during stance. If knee flexion and plantar flexion are weak during swing, compensation is made by hip elevation. The two typical patterns are referred to as the *steppage gait* and the *waddling gait*.

Steppage Gait. This gait is also called the prancing, highstepping, or footdrop gait. It resembles that of a person walking in tall grass, hence its name. The flexor muscles of the foot are subject of a flaccid paralysis so that the toes hang downward when the foot is raised from the floor. To prevent the toes dragging on the floor or catching upon objects, the foot is raised high and brought to the floor forcibly before the toes can drop. Thus, the foot strikes the floor heel first or flat-footed. With bilateral footdrop, the gait often resembles that of a high-stepping horse. This gait, the result of paralysis of the anterior tibialis group of muscles, points to tertiary syphilis, alcoholic neuritis, peroneal nerve injury, poliomyelitis, progressive muscular atrophy, multiple neuritis, and arsenic poisoning.

Waddling Gait. This occurs when there is extreme muscular weakness in the thigh and hip muscles as commonly found in pseudohypertrophic muscular paralysis and muscular atrophy or dystrophy where the trunk muscles must be strongly utilized. The shoulders are thrown back, the lower section of the spine is lordotic, the pelvis is severely tilted, and while in this state, the leg is brought around and placed on the floor. The "waddle" results from difficulty in maintaining the pelvis at an adequate level to the weight-bearing extremity, with slump of the pelvis toward the nonweight-bearing side, which, in turn, produces an exaggerated compensatory trunk sway toward the weight-bearing side.

When walking, the subject swings from side to side in a very noticeable manner, thus it is often called a *goose gait.* Such a "clumsy" gait is also seen in bilateral hip dislocation. In gaits involving muscle weakness, the compensatory pattern is largely the result of the patient's attempt to alter the center of gravity about the base of support.

Hip Weakness

Extension Weakness. During extension paralysis, the gait is grossly altered in weight bearing after heelstrike when the extensors normally contract. Because of the weakness, the trunk is thrown backward to maintain balance by keeping the center of gravity behind the axis of the hip.

Flexion Weakness. Weak hip flexors affect acceleration during swing, the pelvis is usually elevated, the trunk is thrown backward toward the unaffected side in compensation, but stance is rarely involved. The stride is usually short on the involved side.

Abductor Weakness. In upper motor neuron weakness of the hip abductors, the trunk is thrown toward the affected side during weight bearing. If uncompensated, the pelvis distinctly lunges laterally toward the involved side and dips on the side of swing. At midswing, hip and knee flexion is exaggerated on the unaffected side. In less severe cases, there is little sideward lunging because of trunk compensation. Use of a cane on the contralateral side of involvement also eliminates this lateral lurch.

Knee Weakness

Extensor Weakness. This pattern is often difficult to see. In stance, the knee is normally fully extended. The features of the weakness are most prominent after heelstrike when the quadriceps normally contract and the knee flexes. Signs of excessive heel lift during gait and excessive knee flexion during the swing phase should be sought. Knee extension is maintained at heelstrike and throughout stance by hip extension (eg, the gluteus maximus via the iliotibial tract) and plantar flexion. This is helped by throwing the trunk forward at heelstrike to move the center of gravity anterior to the axis of the knee. In pronounced cases, the patient will push the affected thigh backward with the hand to aid extension.

Flexor Weakness. Weak hamstrings allow full knee extension and inhibit deceleration as heelstrike approaches. This produces a hard heelstrike, often called an "overshot." Near the end of the stance phase, the knee fails to flex until pushoff. In prolonged conditions, the result is often the development of distinct knee hyperextension (genu recurvatum).

Ankle Weakness

Plantar Flexion Weakness. If these muscles are weak, propulsion is inhibited because heeloff is impaired. The foot leaves the floor as a unit, the knee is fully extended, and the hip flexes at pushoff to begin the swing phase. Because pushoff is controlled primarily by foot plantar flexion, triceps surae paralysis or Achilles tendon trauma will force some compensation by the gluteus maximus and posterior hamstrings.

Dorsiflexion Weakness. When the ankle dorsiflexors are mildly weak, it is possible to lift the foot from the floor, but during the swing phase, relaxation occurs, which causes the foot to be slapped down during flatfoot. In severe weakness, toestrike replaces heelstrike. This requires a compensatory increase in hip and knee flexion during the swing phase so that the foot clears the floor (steppage gait).

Psychomotor Disorders

Besides the gaits described, locomotion may be restricted by various types of psychomotor disorders. The two major types are those due to hysteria or central apraxia.

Hysteria

A hysterical gait can simulate almost any type of pronounced paralysis, except during emergencies. The gait is usually bizarre and features exaggerated balancing motions, irregular bobbing movements, lurching, and wild weaving or excessively slow, hesitant steps.

These gaits rarely have a repetitive pattern. It is difficult to match gait signs with neurologic and musculoskeletal findings. Tremor usually appears during observed active exercise, and strength rapidly fades when passive movements are resisted by the patient. Although the motions are gross and unpredictable, falling is rare. If falling occurs, it is well protected. In some chronic cases, the pattern is repetitive. This is usually the result of a "gait habit" that persists long after the cause of malfunction has been eliminated. The clinical picture is often confusing because persistent atrophy, boggy tissues, possible edema, and vasomotor instability may be solely the result of disuse.

Astasia-Abasia

This is a type of hysterical ataxia that features bizarre incoordination to the degree that the patient is unable to stand or walk, yet all movements can be performed normally when the patient is in the sitting or recumbent position.

Gait Apraxia

In this condition, motor power is present but the *memory* of how to use the power is lacking or diminished. Steps are small, slow, and uncertain, and the patient must be urged or assisted to initiate progress. This gait is characteristic of frontal lobe lesions or bilateral lesions of the corticospinal tract in the internal capsule, cerebral peduncles, or high brainstem. It is often seen immediately following prolonged bed confinement; but in this situation, it is soon overcome with practice.

Effects of Spinal Adjustments on Gait

A surface electromyographic study conducted by Hibbard found that significant amplitude changes occurred in the electrical activity of gait muscles following manipulation of the lower extremity articulations to reduce malposition, while the electrical activity of control subjects decreased only slightly. Hibbard cites the work of Rebechini-Zasadny and associates that had earlier found a significant difference in the electrical activity of peripheral muscle following manipulation of just the cervical spine.

REFLEXES

The human body exhibits an astonishingly complex array of neural circuitry. While the study of reflex communication between tissues under "voluntary" control and tissues under "autonomic" control (and their excitatory and inhibitory effect on one another) is still in its infancy, the answers to why so many visceral disorders mimic musculoskeletal disorders and why so many musculoskeletal disorders mimic visceral disorders appear to be on the horizon.

General Types of Reflexes

The reflexes of most concern clinically can be classified into three broad categories.

• *Somatic reflexes:* (1) Reflexes communicating from a site on the body wall, cranium, or limb to another site on the body wall, cranium, or a limb (somatosomatic reflex). (2) Reflexes communicating from a site on the body wall, cranium, or a limb (cutaneous, subcutaneous, musculoskeletal) to an internal organ or gland (somatovisceral reflex).

• *Autonomic reflexes:* (1) Reflexes communicating from an internal organ or gland to a site on the body wall, cranium, or a limb (viscerosomatic reflex). (2) Reflexes communicating from an internal organ or gland to another internal organ or gland (viscerovisceral reflex).

• *Psychic reflexes:* (1) Reflexes communicating from a site within the higher CNS centers to the body wall, cranium, or a limb (psychosomatic reflex). (2) Reflexes communicating from a site on the body wall, cranium, or a limb to the higher CNS centers (somatopsychic reflex).

All three types of reflexes usually have segmental, propriospinal, and/or suprasegmental implications. Autonomic reflexes will be described in Chapter 10.

Inasmuch as many reflexes are modulated within the spinal cord, their potentional interrelationship with a subluxation complex, and vice versa, cannot be ignored when we consider that a vertebral lesion can be a focus for either neuronal hyperexcitability or hypoexcitability. Thus, all afferent fibers entering the IVF and all structures receiving efferent fibers via the IVF are potentially exposed to excessive stimulation or inhibition by some factor producing irritation, pressure, or tension at this vulnerable gateway.

Somatosomatic Reflexes

A somatosomatic reflex develops when a sensory receptor in the skin, subcutaneous tissue, fascia, striated muscle, a tendon, a ligament, or a joint is stimulated to trigger a volley of reflex impulses to another anatomical location of this type via efferent sensory, motor, or autonomic fibers. These reflexes are commonly evoked by gross manipulation, dynamic adjustments, light touch techniques, superficial heat or cold, electrotherapy, meridian therapy, hydrotherapy, traction, compression, vibration, percussion, and massage during case management. See Appendix, Figure A.5.

Korr has shown that muscle spindles in which the "gain" has been turned up by intensified activity in their gamma motor innervation may, with other sensory inputs, account for many motion characteristics and palpatory features of a spinal subluxation complex. "Turning down" the gain seems a common denominator in a variety of manipulative procedures.

Somatovisceral Reflexes

A somatovisceral reflex is initiated when a sensory receptor in the skin, subcutaneous tissue, fascia, striated muscle, a tendon, a ligament, or a joint is stimulated to trigger a volley of reflex impulses to viscera. Body wall stimulation produces both segmental organ responses and suprasegmental responses. Different forms of stimulation may produce similar organ responses and may produce different brain center responses that affect the body. The type of response, prolonged beyond stimulus termination, depends on the state of the organ and the body as a whole (ie, active, resting). These reflexes are commonly evoked therapeutically by manipulation, superficial heat or cold, electrotherapy, meridian therapy (possibly), hydrotherapy, traction, compression, vibration, percussion, and massage. See Appendix, Figure A.6.

Psychosomatic Syndromes

A clinical appreciation of the psychologic factors involved in backache cases is enhanced by recognizing the most pertinent psychiatric syndromes involved in conversion hysteria.

Spinal-Related Psychiatric Syndromes

A large variety of psychologic disturbances may be associated with backache and other musculoskeletal complaints, either as aggravating factors or as a result of their development for reasons commonly seen in practice. For this reason, the term *psychosomatic backache* is the preferred term to use to categorize those cases in which such psychologic disturbance constitutes the dominating feature of the overall clinical picture and in which psychologic investigation and treatment is an essential part of their management.

Psychophysiologic Neuromuscular Reactions

A conditioned reflex in which an emotionally stressful situation refocuses awareness

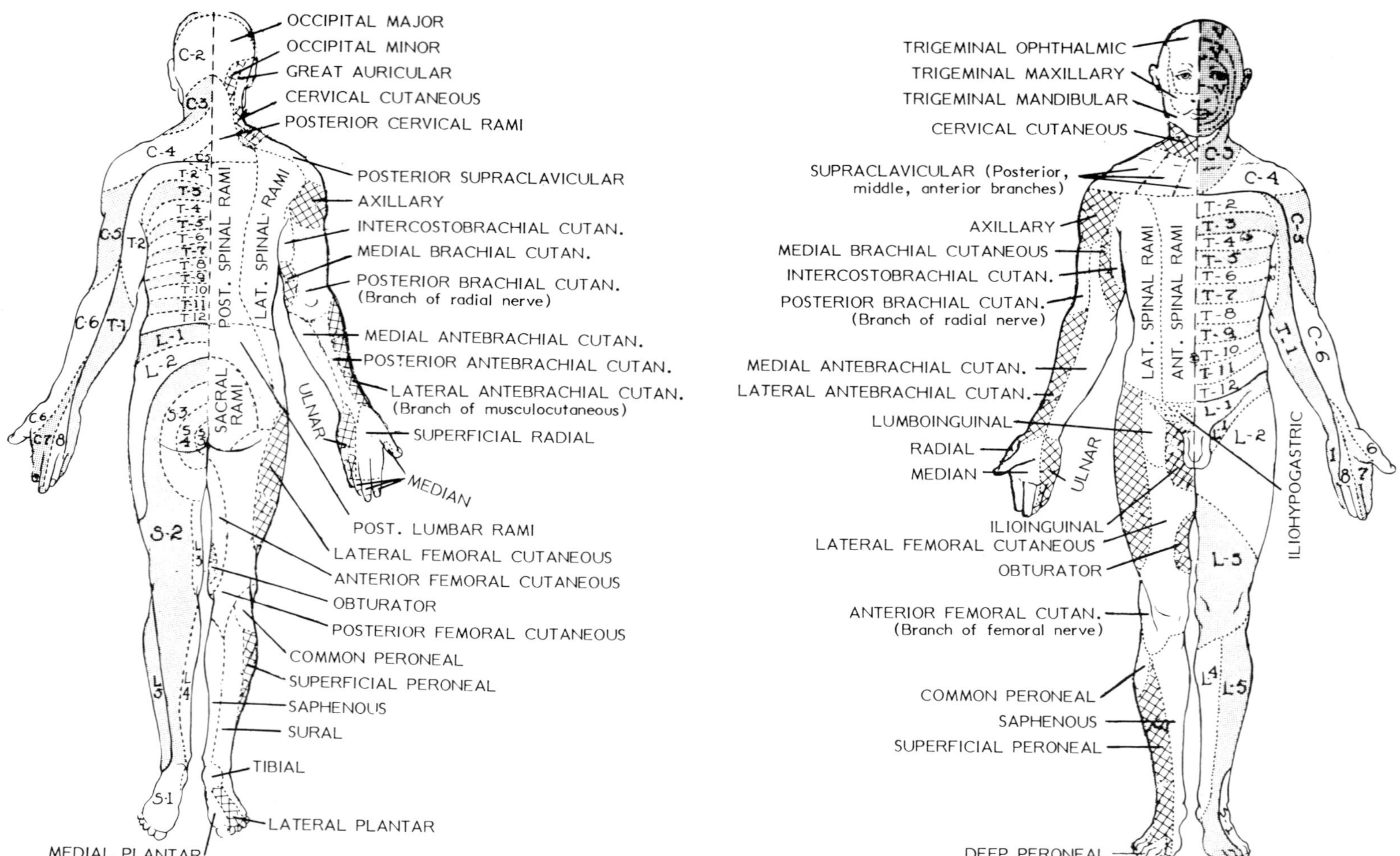

Figure 9.9. Posterior and anterior views of segmental and peripheral nerve distribution of the body. Peripheral distribution is shown on the left of each figure; segmental (radicular) distribution, on the right (adapted from drawings originally attributed to Davis, L.).

on a past physical injury that occurred in a psychologically stressful situation is called a *psychophysiologic neuromuscular reaction*. The new stress stimulates recall of the experience, and this serves as a stimulus for the psychophysiologic responses creating the backache. This renewed attention to the back produces the stimulus for a reflex muscular spasm that, in turn, produces further backache and anxiety and more muscle spasm. Thus, a vicious cycle is established.

Screening Procedures

In evaluating a patient with low back pain, Brown and associates feel strongly that the presence of any four of the below six signs serve as a basis for requesting psychiatric consultation:

- A vague history with irrelevant circumstantiality and poor chronology.
- Dramatization of illness.
- Paranoid attitudes toward the staff.
- Nonanatomical distribution of pain (Fig. 9.9).
- Failure to respond to appropriate therapies.
- Several neurotic symptoms such as acute or chronic anxiety, insomnia, anorexia, irritability, headache, chronic fatigue, crying spells, trembling, sweating, nail biting, hypersensitivity to light and sound, sighing respiration, and patterns of helplessness, failure, and dependency.

EVALUATING THE MOTOR SYSTEM

Any sign of muscle weakness, atrophy, paralysis, and incoordination is a significant clinical finding. The muscular aspect of the motor system should be checked for muscle tone, strength, and volume (mass), and nerve integrity is judged by the deep and superficial reflexes. Motor disorders may be caused by the same processes that cause sensory disturbances; eg, direct nerve injury, pathology, reflexes from visceral organs, and particularly nerve root involvement or upper motor neuron lesions.

Motor nerve root involvement is characterized by deep muscular pain in the muscles innervated. Early hypertonicity or muscular spasm is evident. Later or in chronic conditions, loss of tendon reflexes, muscular weakness, atrophy, and even trophic changes in the overlying skin may be present. Motor disturbances from upper motor lesions may also be a factor (hyperreflexia).

Signs of typical motor abnormalities and their related level in the nervous system are shown in Table 9.7.

Examination Protocol

After nerve trauma, painstaking examination is required as multiple nerve injury, related tendon or other soft-tissue damage, and fractures may complicate the picture. The immediate site of injury should be investigated first, followed by the part's general appearance, voluntary motion, reflexes, and vasomotor changes. Besides sensory and motor loss, the response to electric stimulation should be evaluated whenever the procedure is merited.

Tendon and Periosteal Reflexes

When reflexes are tested, the patient must be relaxed and the part placed in the proper position for each test. As both normal and pathologic reflexes vary widely in people at different times, the examiner should compare reflexes bilaterally when possible and make sure that the same force is used on each side because unilateral differences are common signals of pathology. It should be remembered that abnormal reflexes, particularly if bilateral or similar in other reflexes, may be normal for a particular person. Upper extremity reflexes, especially, are often difficult to evoke even in the healthy. All signs must be correlated.

General Considerations

Muscle movement is the motor response to most reflexes tested. Such tests involve the facilitation or inhibition of the alpha and gamma motor neurons of lamina IX. The

Table 9.7. Common Motor Function Signs Relative to Nervous System Levels*

Tracts	Supratentorial Level	Posterior Fossa	Spinal Level	Peripheral Level
Final common pathway		Atrophy Fasciculations Weakness	Absent abdominal reflexes Atrophy Cramps Fasciculations Hyporeflexia Hypotonia Weakness	Absent abdominal reflexes Atrophy Cramps Fasciculations Hyporeflexia Weakness
Direct activation pathway	Absent abdominal reflexes Apraxia Babinski reflex Hyporeflexia Hypotonia Seizures Weakness	Absent abdominal reflexes Babinski reflex Hyporeflexia Hypotonia Weakness	Absent abdominal reflexes Babinski reflex Weakness	
Indirect activation pathway	Apraxia Clasp-knife reflex Clonus Hyperreflexia Spasticity	Clasp-knife reflex Clonus Decerebrate posture Hyperreflexia Spasticity	Clasp-knife reflex Clonus Decorticate posture Hyperreflexia Spasticity	
Cerebellar control circuit	Ataxia	Ataxia Dysmetria Dyssynergia Hyporeflexia Hypotonia Intention tremor Past-pointing Holmes' rebound phenomenon		
Basal ganglia control circuit	Athetosis Chorea Dystonia Hemiballismus Hyperkinesia Resting tremor Rigidity			

*Adapted from Daube/Sandok with slight modifications.

alpha motor neurons are the largest of the anterior horn cells and can be stimulated monosynaptically through interneurons in response to segmental, intersegmental, and supraspinal reflexes. All descending tracts in the spinal cord are influential.

It should be noted that: (1) In upper motor neuron or pyramidal fiber lesions, the deep tendon reflexes are exaggerated, but the superficial skin reflexes are decreased or absent. (2) In lesions of a lower motor neuron or the motor fibers from the anterior horn cells of the cord, both the deep and the superficial reflexes are decreased or absent.

While a diagnosis of a neurologic disorder cannot be determined by reflexes alone, they are important aids in establishing the type and location of a lesion. Deep reflexes vary in direct proportion to muscle tone, while superficial reflexes apply to any reflex phenomenon that may be induced by a light stimulus such as stroking the skin with a wisp of cotton, resulting in horripilation (gooseflesh) or muscle contraction. The afferent, center, and efferent aspects of the deep tendon reflexes are outlined in Table 9.8.

Testing a tendon reflex segmentally evaluates the integrity of all components of the circuit (from the muscle spindles to the muscle fibers). This includes the sensory receptors, the afferent nerves, the spinal cord segment(s) involved, the alpha motor neurons and their axons, the apparatus at the neuromuscular junction, and the muscle fibers. The speed and magnitude of the reaction also gives clues about adjacent segment and higher control center influence on the efferent neurons (ie, an exaggerated response when the inhibitory influences of the descending tracts are lacking). A grading system for deep reflexes is shown in Table 9.9.

Deep Reflex Techniques

Biceps Reflex. The muscles of the patient's arm are bared and relaxed, and then flexed at the elbow. The examiner places a thumb over the biceps tendon, and then

Table 9.8. Deep Reflexes

Reflex	*Afferent Limb*	*Center*	*Efferent Limb*
Achilles	Tibial	S1—S2	S1—S2
Biceps	Musculocutaneous	C5—C6	C5—C6
Jaw jerk	Trigeminal	Pons	Trigeminal
Patellar	Femoral	L2—L4	L2—L4
Radial	Radial	C6—C8	C6—C8
Triceps	Radial	C6—C7	C6—C7

Table 9.9. Grades of Deep (Tendon) Reflexes

Grade	*Reflex Reaction*
0	Cannot be elicited
-3	Absent except on reinforcement
-2	Markedly decreased
-1	Weak
N	Normal
+1	Slightly hyperactive
+2	Markedly increased and often associated with unsustained clonus
+3	Markedly increased and often associated with sustained clonus.

makes a light blow against the thumb with a percussion hammer (Fig. 9.10). Note if the biceps muscle contracts, how quickly it contracts, and with what force. The biceps reflex, a normal response, tests C5—C6 segments in terms of integrity of the musculocutaneous nerve. It is hyperactive in the same disorders that cause a hyperactive knee jerk.

Triceps Reflex. The patient's arm should be relaxed and flexed at the elbow. Support the elbow and tap the triceps tendon where it crosses the olecranon fossa, observing the same phenomena as in the biceps reflex. The triceps reflex tests C6—C8 afferents, cord segments, and efferents. Both the biceps and triceps reflexes may be diminished in healthy patients.

Radial Reflex. With the patient's arm relaxed, flexed, and well supported, tapping the relaxed forearm over the lower radius results in flexion of the elbow. The response, a periosteal rather than a tendon reflex, tests the C5—C6 levels and has the same significance as the biceps tendon reflex. This reflex, absent in many healthy individuals, is frequently called the *brachioradialis reflex*. In C5—C6 segment lesions, an *inverted radial reflex* may be seen in which the fingers flex but the forearm remains relaxed.

Ulnar Reflex. This refers to tapping of the styloid process of the ulnar that results in pronation of the hand. The ulnar periosteal reflex is a highly unreliable normal reflex.

Patella Reflex. A rolled hard pillow is placed beneath the knees of a supine patient. With the muscles completely relaxed, the patellar tendon is tapped, and contraction of the quadriceps (L2—L4) is noted. Do not rely on the movement of the foot in response to the tapping. Place one hand on the patient's thigh, and use your other hand for the percussion hammer. Test bilaterally, and compare the force of contraction and quickness of response of the two sides. Absence of the reflex is known as *Westphal's sign*. Normal reflex response depends upon the integrity of the femoral nerve and the lumbar segments. Other positions for obtaining the knee reflexes are with the patient sitting on the edge of a bed with muscles relaxed or sitting on a chair with the feet resting on the floor in parallel position (Fig. 9.11). The thighs should be bared and the same methods employed as described previously.

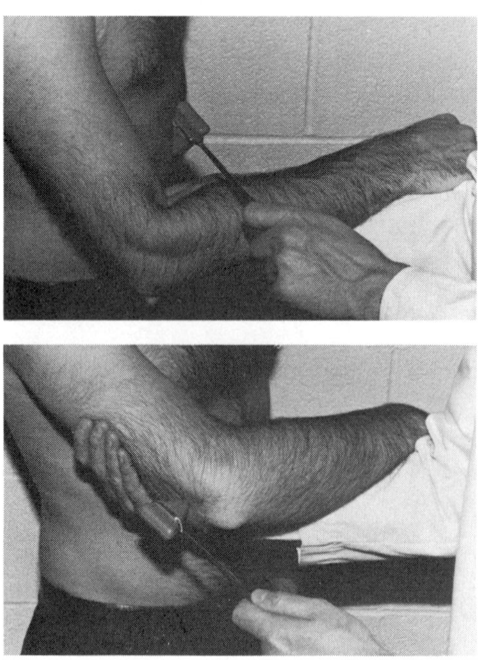

Figure 9.10. *Top,* testing the biceps reflex; *bottom,* testing the triceps reflex.

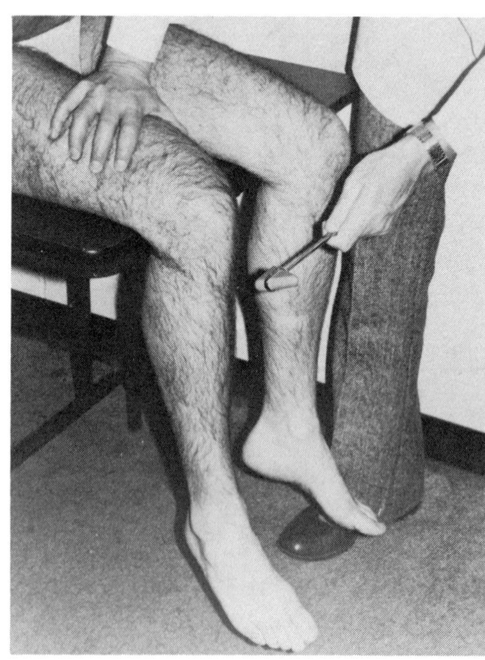

Figure 9.11. Testing the patella reflex in the sitting position.

Absent or diminished knee jerks are found in peripheral nerve lesions, anterior horn cell disease, and posterior column lesions. IVD herniation at the level of L2—L4 will diminish the response. Hyperactive responses will be seen in tense patients, corticospinal tract lesions, general pareses, cord tumor compression or bone compression above L3, multiple sclerosis, and early hemiplegia. The knee jerk is often wanting or feeble in young infants. It varies a great deal in persons of different temperament. In high-strung or oversensitive people, lively knee jerks are often seen without disease.

Achilles Reflex. The ankle jerk is obtained best by having the patient kneel in a padded chair with the feet projecting. The patient is asked to relax the feet, then the Achilles tendon is tapped just below the level of the malleoli, comparing the two sides. Ankle jerks are absent bilaterally in tabes dorsalis and frequently in normal old age. The response is increased in lesions of the pyramidal tract. A reduced or absent reflex may point toward a sciatic IVD herniation between L5 and S1 or L4 and L5. If the patient is in bed, flex and externally rotate the thigh and leg to about 45° until the knee rests on the bed or pillow. Grasp the foot with one hand and hold it easily at right angles to the leg. Then tap the Achilles tendon as previously described. Some examiners test this reflex in the sitting position (Fig. 9.12).

Muscle Strength Testing

The clinical art of muscle testing demands attention to detail and a good working knowledge of anatomy, muscle function, muscle origin and insertion, muscle antagonistic and agonistic action, and their role in joint movement and stabilization. The procedure and its evaluation depend greatly on the skill, knowledge, and experience of the examiner.

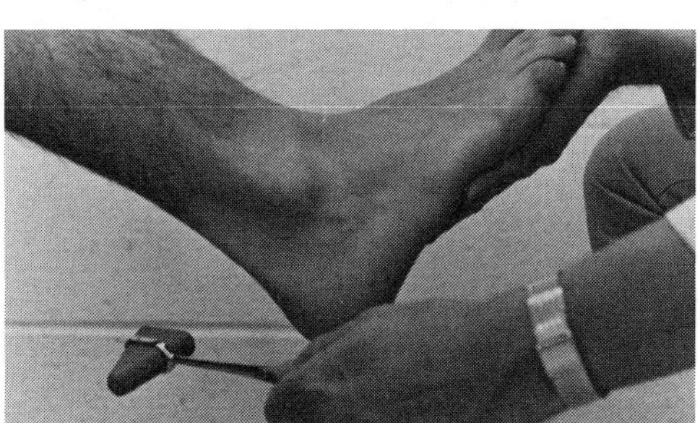

Figure 9.12. Eliciting an Achilles reflex with the patient in the sitting position.

A patient's muscle power should be judged whenever there is a complaint of weakness or incoordination or a need for an aid in subluxation analysis and in evaluating correction. Three techniques are used: (1) active patient motion against an examiner's resistance, (2) examiner resistance against active patient motion, and (3) mechanical resistance against active patient motion.

A large number of neuromuscular and musculoskeletal disorders show evidence of disturbed muscle tone such as weakness or spasm, but weakness is the predominating pattern found in muscle testing. This is often depicted as a compensatory hypertonicity in the antagonistic muscle. Both muscle testing and inspection may disclose a weakness in the absence of palpable or measurable atrophy. This type of relative muscle weakness in comparison to its antagonist is often associated with a palpable trigger point at the origin and/or insertion of affected muscles.

The development of tension against resistance is the most obvious property of muscle. The ability to develop tension and perform mechanical work is greatly influenced by the length of the muscle at the moment of action. The two most common means to measure such tension are the maximum tension readout on a tensiometer (strain gauge) and the amount of load (eg, manual resistance) that can be moved. The customary criteria of grading muscle strength are shown in Table 9.10.

Physical Procedures

Astute gross observation, regional inspection, palpation, bilateral comparison, and correct positioning are essential before manual muscle testing is attempted to assure valid evaluation. When unilateral muscle weakness is suspected, it is always best to test the contralateral muscle first to compare resistance. Pressure against action should be applied in a direction that is opposite to the line of the tested muscle's pull and at the distal aspect of the segment on which it inserts (Fig. 9.13).

The "break" point in muscle testing, when the patient can no longer meet the resistance, is undoubtedly the result of the Golgi tendon organ response. The loss of power is usually abrupt. This suggests that maximum strength depends a great deal on how efficiently an individual can cortically oppose the inhibition of his or her Golgi tendon organ reflex.

The examiner should strive to evaluate one muscle at a time, thus the patient should be requested not to recruit allied muscles during resistance. The testing of individual muscles rather than muscle groups is essential in neuromuscular diagnosis and to determine the neurologic level. It is less important in gross biomechanical evaluation. In either case, extreme caution should be used during resistance to avoid creating cramps, stretch injuries, or excessive fatigue of the patient.

The fault with manual methods is that evaluation rests a great deal upon the subjective skill of the examiner, and some patients are more willing to exert maximum effort than others. Care must be taken that the direction and amount of pressure is controlled and consistent. The degree of strength can be determined only if pressure is applied *gradually* after the patient has "set" the muscle being tested against resistance. Also, the length of lever arms varies with patients and this affects relative strength, as does age, joint angle, bulk of body

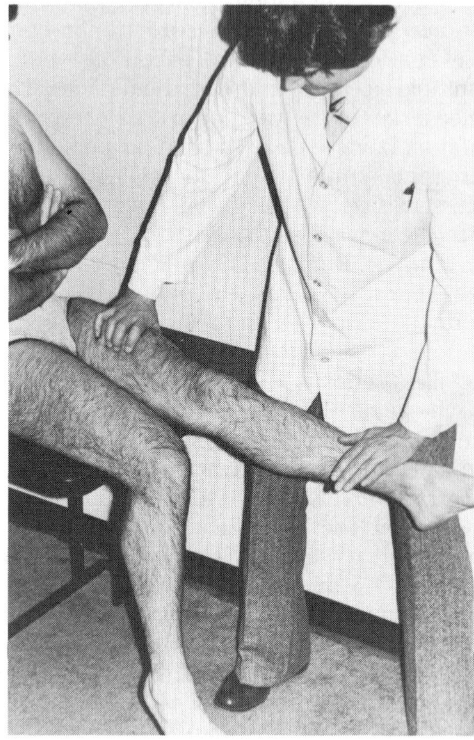

Figure 9.13. Evaluating quadriceps strength against resistance.

Table 9.10. Grades of Muscle Strength

Grade	Degree, Title	Description
Grade 5	100% (Normal)	Complete range of motion against gravity with full resistance.
Grade 4	75% (Good)	Complete range of motion against gravity with some resistance.
Grade 3	50% (Fair)	Complete range of motion against gravity with no resistance.
Grade 2	25% (Poor)	Complete range of motion with gravity eliminated.
Grade 1	10% (Trace)	Evidence of slight contractility, but no joint motion.
Grade 0	0% (Zero)	No evidence of contractility.

parts, and sex differences. Muscles often test differently in various positions such as from prone, supine, to weight bearing. It also is important that the same examiner conduct and record initial and follow-up evaluations of the degree of "resistance."

Stabilization. To obtain maximum contraction, one segment (usually the site of origin) must be stabilized manually if not by muscle tension, body weight, or gravity as a muscle exerts as much pull on its origin as it does its insertion (Fig. 9.14). Poor stabilization results in erroneous conclusions.

Substitution. Possible substitution (eg, in dystrophy) and synergism must be eliminated by careful positioning and stabilization. If a muscle is called into action only in assistance when unusual force is necessary, it is called an *emergency mover* or an *accessory* muscle. When the action of a muscle is to prevent the action of undesired contraction of another muscle, it is called a *neutralizing muscle.* The action of emergency and neutralizing muscles must be carefully considered during clinical muscle testing to avoid erroneous conclusions. In addition, care must be taken that antagonistic muscles are relaxed.

Multiple Innervation. Another point to be considered is that several large muscles such as the pectoralis major, trapezius, deltoid, latissimus dorsi, triceps brachii, and the quadriceps femoris are so constructed and innervated that portions of each muscle may function separately as well as together. The actions of different muscle parts may be palpated during function or recorded with greater accuracy by electromyography.

Mechanical Procedures

The hand dynamometer and electromyograph are the typical objective clinical instruments available to record the force of muscular contraction. In recent years, several sophisticated pieces of equipment that provide objective data, and sometimes a printout, have been placed on the market.

The simple hand dynamometer gives the examiner four measurements: (1) strength of grip muscles, (2) fatigue rate of grip muscles, (3) recovery rate of these muscles, and (4) a bilateral comparison of the muscles of both hands. While initial readings are helpful in diagnosis, subsequent readings are helpful in determining the patient's rate of recovery. In dynamometry, three readings are usually taken on each hand in sequence to show strength, fatigue, and recovery rates.

Electrodiagnosis

The general term *electrodiagnosis* refers to the use of any electrical modality to test the integrity of muscles and nerves. As a common adjunct to the physical examination of the motor system, electrodiagnosis has become a valuable tool in evaluating whether partial degeneration of a motor unit should be suspected.

Electrodiagnostic tests (1) help to determine if disease of the upper or lower motor neuron is being dealt with, (2) help to determine if the nerve is interrupted, and (3) help to determine if the muscles are undergoing degeneration. Low voltage currents are used in the process, and the degree of reaction

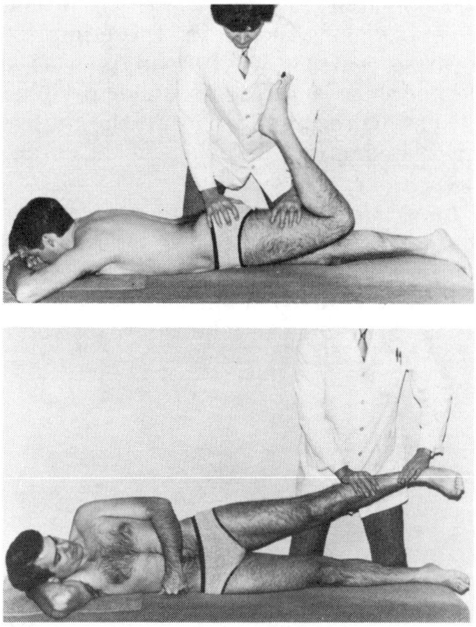

Figure 9.14. *Top,* testing the strength of the hip extensors against resistance with the patient prone; *bottom,* position for testing hip abduction or adduction strength against resistance with the patient in the side position.

gives the practitioner an idea of the extent of disability present. Innervated muscles normally react to electrical stimulation; however, several situations exist where normal responses are not seen.

Nerve Conduction Analyses

Nerve conduction studies are helpful in confirming physical findings of a peripheral nerve disorder, in localizing the site of the lesion, and in assessing the severity of the lesion. Eisen/Hoirch report that there is a 70%—80% correlation among clinical, myelographic, and electrophysiologic findings in cases of spinal root lesions, but only one may be found to be abnormal. They feel that these findings therefore complement each other in the overall evaluation.

When an electrical stimulus is applied to a peripheral nerve, all large myelinated axons can be discharged simultaneously and the resulting action potential can be measured by an oscilloscope (Fig. 9.15). When a stimulus of 20—100 volts are applied for 0.1 millisecond to a mixed peripheral nerve, the action potentials induced will travel in both directions along the nerve. Those impulses traveling centrally will be perceived as an electric shock, but those coursing peripherally can be recorded either in the muscles innervated or on the surface of the cutaneous sensory branches.

Basic Measurements. The *amplitude* of the induced potential spike is determined by the *number* of axons involved in transmitting the stimulus from the point of excitation to the recording site. The *latent period* of the potential is determined by the *rate* (conduction velocity) at which the largest nerve fibers transmit the action potential through the axons involved. *Conduction velocity* can thus be determined by dividing the distance traveled by the time taken from application to recording. This will vary depending on the diameter size and thickness of myelination of the fibers activated.

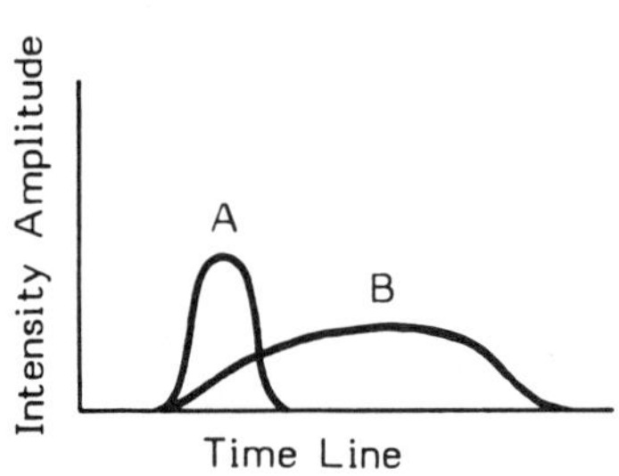

Figure 9.15. Simple graph contrasting the brisk response in normal muscle to a direct current, *A*, and the slow sluggish response to a direct current during degeneration, *B*.

Nerve conduction studies are normal in pure upper motor neuron lesions. Some basic changes occurring in lower motor neuron lesions are briefly described below:

- *Generalized blocks.* Wide-spread demyelinating disorders of the peripheral nervous system feature slowed conduction speeds, amplitude loss (especially distal in axonal dystrophies), or both.
- *Local axonal blocks.* Localized peripheral nerve lesions are characterized by a conduction block or a slowed conduction velocity in the area of the lesion. The response evoked is smaller when applied proximally than when applied distally.
- *Axolemmal lesions.* In axolemmal disorders, impulses are blocked in the region of the lesion. A stimulus applied proximal to the lesion will produce no response or one with an extremely reduced amplitude, but a stimulus applied distal to the lesion will produce a normal response.
- *Axoplasmic lesions.* Axonal narrowing results in slowed conduction, axonal degeneration produces a low-amplitude or an absent response, and demyelinating diseases cause a slowed conduction velocity and a progressive loss of amplitude on more proximal stimulation.
- *Neuromuscular transmission blocks.* In these disorders, there is a progressive loss of amplitude with repetitive stimulation at rates of only 2—5 per second.
- *Primary muscle disease.* Atrophic states are characterized by low-amplitude spikes with normal conduction velocity rates.

Degeneration Reactions

If the conduction of galvanic or faradic current through a peripheral nerve has become impaired because of disease, trauma to the nerve trunks or anterior roots, or a lesion in the spinal cord, changes occur in the electrical reaction of the muscles innervated. Such reactive changes usually occur within 10 days after the initial insult, and they are known as the *reaction of degeneration* (RD). With RD, two responses may be seen: (1) no response to brief impulses of faradic tetanizing current; or (2) a sluggish response to galvanism.

Partial Degeneration. When a muscle is partially denervated or when some of the nerve fibers are normal and others are denervated, greater amounts of current are required to elicit a response. In *partial RD:* (1) the nerve shows a decrease of both tetanic and galvanic responses; and (2) the involved muscles show (a) decreased tetanic excitability, (b) increased galvanic excitability, (c) a slow response, but not as pronounced as in full RD, (d) polar response changes, and possibly, (e) a displacement of the motor point.

Complete Denervation. In *full RD:* (1) the nerve does not respond to either faradic (tetanic) or galvanic stimulation; (2) after about 10 days, the involved muscle tissue does not respond to faradic (tetanic) stimulation; (3) the muscle will respond to galvanic stimuli with a sluggish response but only when greater current intensity is applied; (4) the motor point is displaced toward the periphery where the fibers of the muscle attach to the tendon, and (5) the formula for polar response may change. In full RD, there is absolutely no response to any current in either the nerve or the muscle. Thus, these signs exhibit the final stage of full RD. See Table 9.11. If reinnervation does not occur, destruction of the fibers will eventually take place.

Stages of Degeneration. Three distinct stages are found in the course of RD:

1. *First stage:* 10 days to 2 weeks. After the first week, the nerve loses all response to tetanic stimulation. If the muscle responds at all to tetanic current, it is quite feeble. Galvanic testing elicits only a slow, weak contraction in the muscle(s) involved, rather than the normal brisk contractions. The cathode-closing contraction is greater than the anodal closing contraction—the reverse of the normal response.

2. *Second stage:* the stage of full RD, which lasts from a few weeks to 1 year or more.

3. *Final stage:* In this stage, there is either a gradual return of voluntary function with an electrical response or an absolute irreversible RD develops.

Table 9.11. Electrical Reactions of Muscles and Nerves*

Status	Tissue	Galvanic Stimulation	Tetanizing Faradic
Normal reaction	Muscle	Brisk single contraction	Tetanic contraction
	Nerve	Brisk single contraction	Tetanic contraction
Partial reaction of degeneration	Muscle	Sluggish contraction	Diminished response
	Nerve	Diminished response	Diminished response
Full reaction of degeneration	Muscle	Sluggish response	No response
	Nerve	No response	No response
Complete reaction of degeneration	Muscle	No response	No response
	Nerve	No response	No response

*From Jaskoviak/Schafer: *Applied Physiotherapy.*

Miscellaneous Electrical Muscle Testing Procedures

In cases of peripheral nerve injuries, electrotherapy is indicated to maintain muscle tone and to prevent muscle atrophy. In such cases, electrical muscle testing should become an integral part of therapy to evaluate progress. Accordingly, muscle stimulators should provide features to conduct the following tests along with their therapeutic modes.

Accommodation Test. According to the established principles of electrophysiology, neuromuscular units can accommodate to a gradually increasing current (ie, an *exponentially progressive* current) Totally denervated muscles lose this ability, and this fact permits a simple but reliable test for establishing the degree of denervation.

Faradic Excitability Test. Innervated neuromuscular units should respond by contraction when currents of short duration (eg, 1 ms) are applied. For this test, a simple sine wave would do, but variable frequency generators allow for more precise evaluation.

Galvanic Excitability (Rheobase) Test. In this test where direct current pulses of long duration are used (eg, 500—1000 ms or interrupted dc), the actual amount of current strength (measured in milliamperage) necessary to contract a muscle is measured. Variable frequency generators permit the application of true square wave current and a more precise measurement, but simpler units also can be used for this test.

Chronaxie Test. This test requires a variable frequency generator that incorporates precise timing and current intensity measurements. The chronaxie determines the impulse time necessary for a muscle to contract with double the current strength of the rheobase. Most healthy neuromuscular units have a chronaxie of 1 ms or less.

Strength Duration Curves. This test can be performed with a variable frequency generator, measuring the current intensity in milliamperage, at different impulse settings; eg, 1000 ms (rheobase), 500 ms, 250 ms, 100 ms, 50 ms, 25 ms, 5 ms, 1 ms, 0.1 ms, and 0.05 ms. These measurements can be plotted graphically and provide detailed objective data about the excitability of any selected

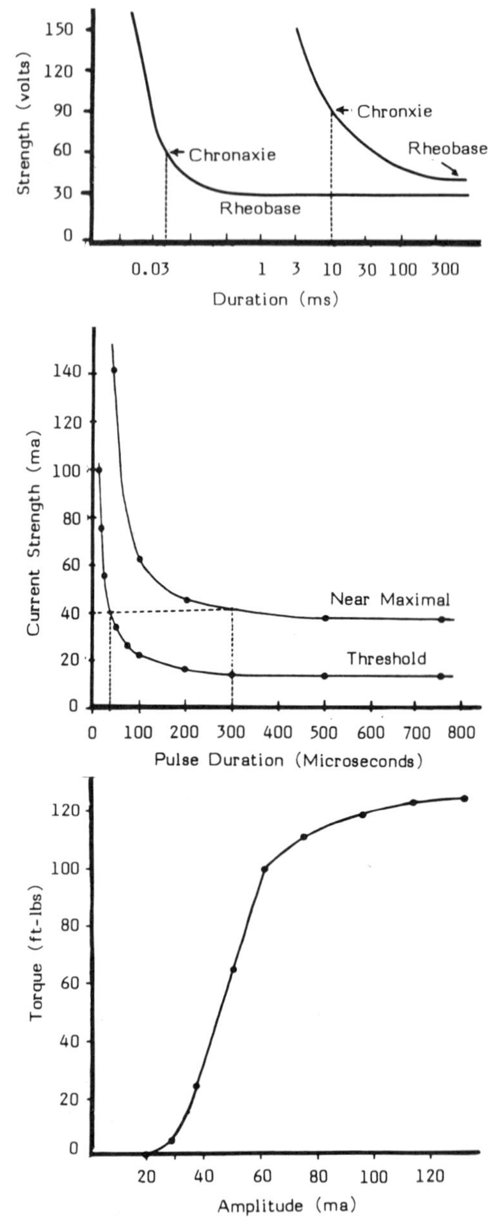

Figure 9.16. *Top,* strength duration curve showing the relationship between pulse duration and amplitude necessary to excite (minimally) muscle tissue. *Middle,* a modified strength duration curve of wrist extensors with an intact neuromuscular unit, showing amplitude and duration characteristics of a threshold contraction and near maximum contraction. *Bottom,* strength amplitude curve of a quadriceps femoris, showing that the force of contraction is dependent on electrical stimulus current amplitude. Note that torque is not produced until a threshold value is reached.

neuromuscular unit (Fig. 9.16). The chronaxie is obtained from this test graphically. With experience, according to Wolf, a physician or therapist can perform the test in less than 5 minutes, particularly when it is used with subsequent treatments.

Because the techniques are similar, nerve conduction studies are usually made at the same time as electromyographic studies.

Electromyography

Electromyography is the study of the electrical impulses arising from muscles during muscle activity. It is based on the fact that a relaxed muscle has no obvious electrical activity, while an active muscle has an action potential that can be measured by electrodes placed within or on the skin over a muscle. The latter is the usual practice. When the electrodes are connected to an oscilloscope, action potentials of muscles and specific parts of muscles may be viewed and tracing can be made.

Rationale

Electromyography (EMG) allows the recording of oscillations in potential variations of skeletal muscles at rest and during activity. It offers a tracing of electrical activity transmitted from muscle to an electrode and then to an oscilloscope. This process allows study of the potential of muscle at rest, the reaction of muscle to contraction, and the response of muscle to external stimulation. Such tracings aid in determining whether a patient's illness is directly affecting the spinal cord, muscles, or peripheral nerves.

Surface electrodes are most frequently used to record myopotentials, but needle electrodes allow the recording of potentials of individual muscle fibers. Surface EMG yields data concerning muscle action or rest but fails to give data about individual fiber potentials.

The purpose of EMG recordings can be placed in several broad categories. EMG is frequently used to evaluate the amount of muscle activity occurring in specific muscles, and it can be used to study kinesiologic function of muscle. The general rule is that there will be less EMG activity in eccentric contractions as compared to concentric contractions. It can be used in pathologies to determine the nature, scope, and prognosis of diseases involving neuromuscular function. It can be used to differentiate between neurogenic and myogenic paralysis and differentiate between organic paralysis and psychogenic reactions. Thus, if muscle weakness is exhibited, an EMG will determine whether the loss of power is caused by a deficit in impulse transmission (eg, myasthenia), myopathy, or neuropathy (Fig. 9.17). The procedure is valuable in determining the affected level of spinal roots, localizing a disorder within the peripheral motor neuron, and differentiating between lesions of the 1st and 2nd neurons. It has also been shown to be effective in differentiating between pyramidal and extrapyramidal hypertonicity, in the analysis of tremor, in assessing myotonic and myasthenic disorders, in evaluating the success of therapy, and in arriving at a prognosis in traumatic and neuritic lesions.

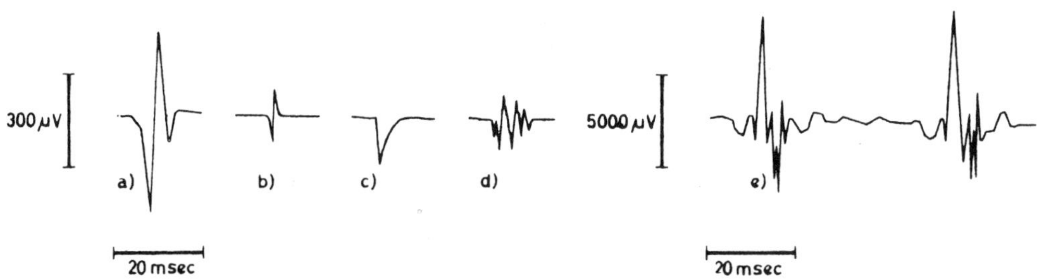

Figure 9.17. Various potentials in electromyography: *a,* normal potential of a motor unit; *b,* fibrillation potential with complete denervation; *c,* sharp positive wave potential in denervation; *d,* polyphasic low potential (eg, as in reinnervation); *e,* giant unit (eg, as in chronic anterior horn disease).

Procedure

The patient should be positioned in a relaxed position while the selected peripheral nerves are stimulated. The electrical activity in muscles and nerves is then recorded. When muscle is at rest, there is normally no electrical activity observed. When muscles are active, the EMG shows a wave-like graph representation of each contraction. Graph lines are amplified with the increase in strength of each contraction. Muscle disease produces a spiked wave pattern, with the shape of the spike often being characteristic of a specific disease. A diminished wave suggests muscle weakness. Waves disappear after a few minutes in myasthenia gravis. Nerve involvement, as opposed to muscle involvement, usually shows a decreased frequency of contractions.

In its common application, EMG provides objective evidence of partial muscle denervation. When test results are positive, it is believed to be of considerable importance in the accurate diagnosis of a herniated IVD. The test will not be positive within 4 days of the onset of root pathology. Thus, tests are helpful in the evaluation of a complex clinical picture in which evidence of radiculopathy is inconsistent or confusing. Abnormal EMG findings can be crucial in the evaluation and management of a patient when compensation, litigation, and psychiatric problems are involved.

The use of EMG recordings helps to establish the scientific basis for both diagnostic conclusions and to monitor the effectiveness of therapy. Spector feels that surface electromyography is one of the best means to assess the reliability of innovative as well as standard methods in the management of musculoskeletal disorders, thus decreasing the possibility of misdiagnosis and/or improper treatment. Accurate analysis, however, is complex and requires special instruction because recordings from different muscles are influenced by electrode configuration, orientation of muscle fibers, the amount of subcutaneous tissue beneath the electrode, and other factors.

Electromyography in Scoliosis

According to a study by Zetterberg and associates, a comparatively higher EMG signal amplitude has been found on the convex side of a scoliosis. This was due to a lower amplitude on the concave side when the scoliosis group was compared to a control group. The amplitude difference was correlated to the degree of scoliosis. A shift in the myoelectric spectrum toward the lower frequencies occurred during loading. There were no differences in this respect between the sides of the scoliosis nor were there differences between the scoliotic patients and the controls. It was concluded that secondary adaptation to the higher load demand by the muscles on the convex side in scoliosis appeared to explain the findings.

A study by Reuber and associates also suggested that the asymmetries in muscle actions shown by myoelectric measurements were the result of scoliosis. According to these investigators, scoliosis progression does not appear to be caused by asymmetry in muscle contractions; rather, it may be caused by a lack of adequate asymmetry.

Electromyographic Studies Following Adjustive Therapy

Widmann defined the advantages of EMG studies in chiropractic research in 1961, but it has only been within the last decade that his advice has been taken seriously. The findings of a few studies are described below.

- In EMG studies of the effects of spinal adjustments on symptomatic patients, Grice found that there was a strong tendency toward decreased action potentials (both in frequency and amplitude) and more symmetry in both static and dynamic muscle potentials as compared with preadjustment imbalances.
- In Thabe's EMG studies of the upper cervical and sacroiliac joints, it was found that manual mobilization techniques have a greater effect in reducing spontaneous segmental muscle activity than if afferent information from a restricted joint is blocked with a local anesthetic.

• Hibbard found that significant EMG amplitude changes occurred in the activity of gait muscles following manipulation of the lower extremity articulations to reduce malposition, while the electrical activity of control subjects decreased only slightly.

• Rebechini-Zasadny and associates found that 12 out of 12 subjects showed increased muscle activity following manipulation of the cervical spine and 9 out 12 subjects showed increased muscle strength.

It was thought for many years that much of the pain in spinal syndromes was due to paravertebral muscle spasm. Recent studies have not confirmed this. For example, Roland points out that EMG studies show increased muscle activity in back-pain patients, but the degree of activity is probably insufficient to produce pain. Current literature tends to view the spasm associated with back pain as a secondary factor in most instances; ie, most back pains originate from the nociceptors of the involved joints.

Table 9.12. Common Causes of Hypotonicity Related to Location and Type

Location	Primary Suspect Disorders	
Anterior horn	Progressive spinal-muscular atrophy	Syringomyelia Poliomyelitis
Cerebellar disease	Oliopontocerebellar diseases	Spinocerebellar diseases Cerebellar ataxia
Muscle	Various myopathies	
Peripheral nerve	Nerve compression	Various neuropathies
Proprioception loss	Pernicious anemia	Tabes dorsalis
Type	**Primary Suspect Disorders**	
Permanent hypotonia	Peripheral defect Anterior horn lesion Myasthenic states Myopathy Myositis (advanced) Peripheral nerve lesion	CNS defect Cerebellar ataxia Cerebellar degeneration Parietal lobe disease Tabes dorsalis
Temporary hypotonia	Cerebral palsy Brain anoxia Kernicterus Degenerative diseases Aminoacidopathy Cerebrohepatorenal syndrome Infantile neuroaxonal dystrophy Krabbe's disease Lipid storage disease Metachromatic leukodystrophy	Drugs Anticonvulsants Muscle relaxants Narcotics Sporifics Tranquilizers Spinal diaschisis (spinal shock) Anoxia Brain or cord trauma Hemorrhage Infarct Sepsis

Evaluating the Cerebellar System

Earlier chapters have described how the lateral lobes of the cerebellum are chiefly concerned with the smooth coordination of striated muscle activity, while the central lobe maintains and controls posture, balance, and a smooth gait. The etiology of myokinetic malcoordination can be found in the sensory receptors, the peripheral nerves, the spinal cord, the brain stem, the cerebral cortex and subcortex, or the cerebellum.

It should be noted that there can be no proprioceptive tract defect, no loss in muscle tone, no muscle weakness, or no gross structural abnormality if coordination and balance are to be properly maintained. Thus, these factors must be eliminated before a disorder can be attributed to the cerebellum itself.

The term *myokinetic coordination* refers to a patient's ability to integrate separate motor abilities into a complex task. Well-coordinated movement, usually involving the large muscles, requires perfect timing between the nervous and muscular systems. Once the cerebral cortex receives an afferent impulse and decides what task must be performed in response, the cerebellum coordinates the reaction so that the act will be carried out smoothly. Thus, once a lower motor neuron lesion has been ruled out, cerebellar function should be evaluated.

Symptomatology

The primary motor signs of a cerebellar lesion are tremor, nystagmus, ataxia, decomposition of movement, dysmetria, dysdiadochokinesia or adiadochokinesia, scanning speech, asthenia, and hypotonia (Table 9.12). Other signs include vertigo, cerebellar fits presenting a rigid convulsion, and vocal dysarthria characterized by an explosive, slurred speech that is peculiar to cerebellar lesions. Any sign of skew deviation of the eyes should be noted; viz, one eyeball deviated up and outward and the other turned down and inward (brachium pontis lesion). Spooning of the hands (hyperextension of the spreadout palms) is also occasionally seen in cerebellar disease.

In time, cerebellar defects are compensated for to a considerable degree by other brain mechanisms. Thus, symptoms are less severe in slowly progressing diseases than those of acute cerebellar disorders.

It should be kept in mind that the left side of the body is under the influence of the left cerebellar hemisphere, and vice versa. Any symptoms that occur unilaterally will then be on the same side as the cerebellar lesion. The opposite is true with cerebral lesions, where the lesion invariably produces contralateral symptoms.

Testing Procedures

General cerebellar function is tested by the evaluation of gait, carriage, and Romberg's station test. Upper extremity coordination is evaluated by the finger-to-nose test, palm pronation and supination, hand patting, and arm extension tests. Lower extremity coordination is judged by gait, heel-to-knee, heel-to-toe, and foot-to-buttock tests.

Upper Extremity Coordination Tests

Finger-to-Nose Tests. If the patient is lying, the patient's arms should be outstretched at the sides; if sitting, the patient's hands should rest on the knees; if standing, the patient's arms should be relaxed at the sides. Direct the patient to touch the tip of the nose with the tip of the forefinger (finger-to-nose test), first with the eyes open, then closed. Note the line between the starting point and the nose to determine if it is straight, curved, or if there is a jerking, irregular motion. Observe whether the finger becomes coarsely tremulous as the nose is touched (intention tremor). If a tremor is present, it indicates a proprioceptive (sensory) defect when the defect is noted primarily when the eyes are closed. Note if the finger goes beyond the nose (*hypermetria*), or fails to reach the nose (*hypometria*). The term *dysmetria* is used to denote if the finger goes beyond the nose or fails to reach it. The action should be smooth, rapid, and the arms should remain in the same plane. Note whether there is a difference when the eyes are closed or if the same degree of incoordination is present with them open. If there is a defect, it is technically called *dysdiadokinesis* and is a part of cerebellar dyssynergia. Failure to perform these tests suggests a lesion of the posterior columns or polyneuritis.

Finger-to-Finger Tests. This is just a variation of the finger-to-nose tests (Fig. 9.18).

Palm Pronation and Supination Tests. The patient should be asked to extend the arms forward on a level with the shoulder and then separate the fingers. Any sign of tremor should be noted. Next, have the patient rapidly pronate and supinate the palms. When the patient is sitting, the patient's hands are first placed on the lower thighs. In these tests, note faulty movements such as (1) tendency to wide movements at the elbow or (2) incomplete supination and pronation. Again, the action should be smooth, rapid, and the arms should remain in the same plane. The presence of changes denotes dyssynergia. The term *adiadokinesia* refers to the inability to perform rapid alternating movements. *Barognosis* means the ability to sense the weight of objects.

Hand Patting Test. In this test, the patient rapidly pats the examiner's hand (Fig. 9.19). Both sides should be checked. This is another method to check for dyssynergia.

Arm Extension Tests. The patient is placed in the erect position with the eyes closed and the arms are extended straight forward with hands parallel and held there actively for 20—30 seconds. The patient's arms are then extended straight up over the patient's head with the palms facing forward and held there actively for 20—30 seconds. It should be noted if there is any drooping of an arm or for a tendency of an arm and hand to flex and rotate internally because this is one of the earliest signs of paresis of the CNS. A drift of the upper extremity down and out suggests a cerebellar disorder. Senile and familial tremors appear most marked in outstretched hands. They disappear at rest and are aggravated by stress.

Holmes' Rebound Phenomenon. A positive sign is noted when the patient flexes his arm against the resistance of the examiner, and when the arm is suddenly released, it strikes the patient's chest. This is a significant finding in ipsilateral cerebellar disease.

Trunk and Lower Extremity Coordination Tests

Coordination of the trunk is judged in relation to carriage, gait, and station, and coordination in the lower extremities is evaluated by the heel-to-knee, heel-to-toe, and foot-to-buttock tests.

Gait. The stability of the trunk is mediated by the cerebellum, and abnormality is reflected by ataxia whether the patient's eyes

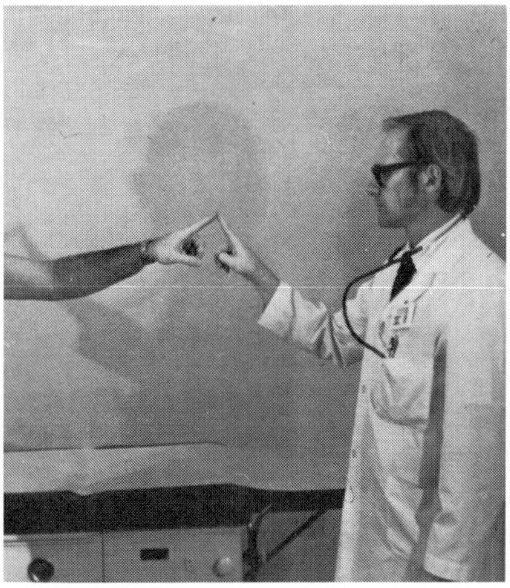

Figure 9.18. Finger-to-finger test (American Chiropractic Association).

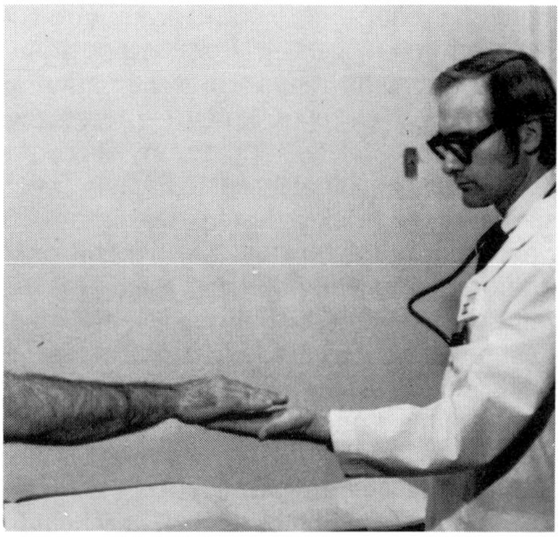

Figure 9.19. Hand patting test (American Chiropractic Association).

are open or not. In screening, the patient is asked to walk a straight line at a normal rate with the eyes opened and then closed. The width of base, unsteadiness in any direction, or tendency to go to one side or the other (dyssynergia) should be noted. If the foot drags (spasticity) or flaps down flatly (ataxia), or if the toes are raised with the heel (foot drop), these signs should be recorded. The patient should then be asked to walk and turn to the right, then to the left, to walk backward, and also to walk on the toes and then on the heels. The examiner should observe the patient's feet, legs, trunk, arms, and shoulders for deviations from the normal gait. Loss of arm swing may indicate basal nucleus disease while exaggeration of arm movements occurs in athetosis. All deviations from the norm should be recorded.

Normal gait features smoothness and ease with little attention required by the patient. The pelvis is fixed and the lower limb is carried straight forward with knee flexion, with the opposite limb swinging forward in harmony. An abnormal gait because of pain may be the result of some form of peripheral neuropathy or irritative radiculopathy. It is characterized by a gingerly walk with slow, short steps. If the pain is unilateral, weight will be thrown to the unaffected side. Besides local and cerebellar causes, gait disturbances also may be reflections of a basal ganglia, subthalamic nuclei, posterior column, or trunk muscle lesion.

Romberg's Station Test. The patient should be requested to stand erect with the heels and toes together (Romberg position) and look straight ahead. Then the patient is asked to close the eyes. Note the presence of any swaying of the body in any direction more than is ordinarily seen. Swaying with the eyes open or closed indicates either dyssynergia or ataxia of the legs or trunk, or of both, depending upon the presence or absence of sensory disturbances. The examiner must be alert to catch the patient if he begins to fall. Although this test may be positive in a normal subject and those with nonneurologic diseases, it is highly indicative of a lesion interrupting the proprioceptive pathways between the lower limbs and the cerebellum.

Heel-to-Knee and Heel-to-Shin Tests. With the patient in the supine position, request that the knee be touched with the heel of the opposite foot (Fig. 9.20). Compare the two sides, and note any curve in the line or irregular movement. Note hypermetria or hypometria. Then have the patient touch the shin with the heel of the opposite foot and make bilateral comparison. Have the tests performed with the eyes opened and closed, noting the same characteristics as in the upper extremities. In cerebellar lesions, the patient will overhit or underhit the mark, and then finally get there. Also observe for a last-minute intention tremor. The patient also may have difficulty from a proprioceptive loss, but this would indicate a defect due to loss of joint sensation rather than a loss of cerebellar coordination. Many examiners also find it advisable to perform these tests with the patient in the standing position (Fig. 9.21).

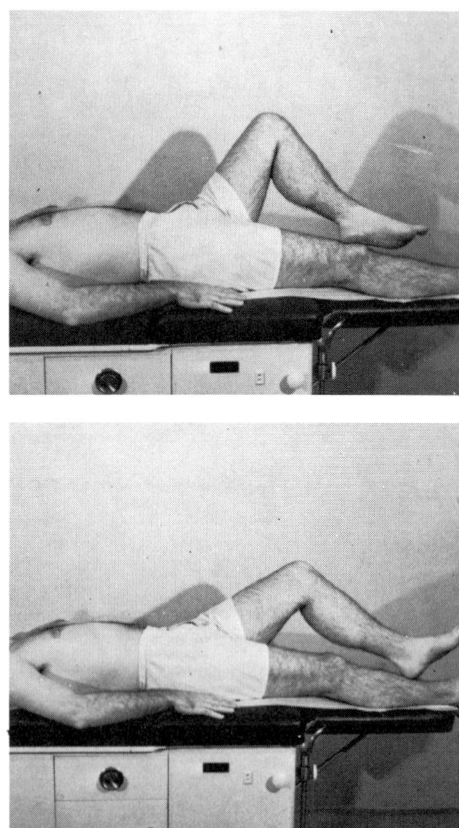

Figure 9.20. *Top,* supine heel-to-knee test; *bottom,* heel-to-shin test (American Chiropractic Association).

Foot-to-Buttock Test. The patient should be asked to flex the thigh and leg, bringing the foot up near the buttock and resting it on the examining table. Note any swaying of the knee from side to side (dyssynergia). Again, many examiners also perform this test with the patient standing.

Evaluating Cranial Nerve Motor Fibers

The Oculomotor System (Cranial III, IV, VI)

Functional defects of cranial nerves III, IV, or VI are frequent but seldom persistent. Lesions of these nerves are commonly noted with various types of strabismus (squint) and pupil dysfunction. Failure to move the eye voluntarily in any given direction indicates muscular incompetence caused by primary muscle disease or a neurogenic factor.

Because of their proximity to one another, cranial nerves III, IV, and VI are usually tested together by examining the eyelids, pupillary changes, and extraocular movements. Each eye should be tested separately and then together.

The Eyelids. It should be noted whether the eyelids droop. Compare the amount of cornea covered by each lid. Ask the patient to look upward. If ptosis exists, the affected lid cannot be raised except by compensatory action of the frontalis muscle, which produces a wrinkling of the forehead on the same side.

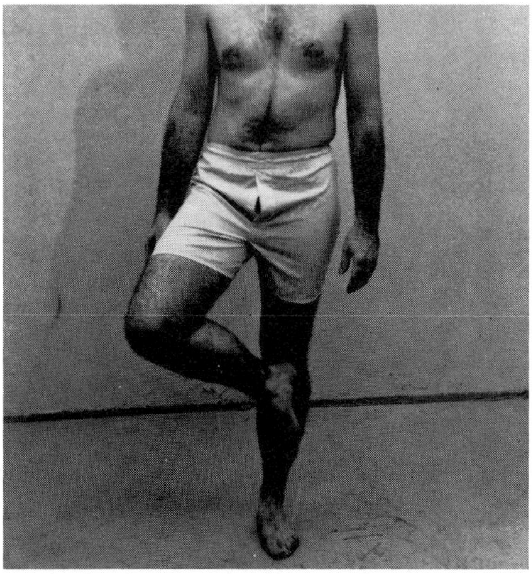

Figure 9.21. Standing (weight-bearing) heel-to-knee test (American Chiropractic Association).

The Pupils. Seek abnormal pupil signs such as of size (miosis, mydriasis, anisocoria), shape (irregularity of margins), position (ectopia), or reactions to light and in accommodation. Place the patient in a position where strong light does not enter the eye; and with a penlight, test each eye separately. Note whether the pupil contracts readily or slowly, whether there is irregularity in the outline of the pupil or any inequality of the pupils. The *light reflex* results in normal constriction of the pupil when light is flashed into the eye. This is a *direct reflex* to light. The *consensual reflex* is tested by flashing light in one eye and noting if the opposite pupil contracts. This is a similar but weaker reaction than with the direct light reflex.

Adie's pupil is a benign disorder featuring a very weak light reflex that is delayed for several seconds, and often confused with an Argyll Robertson pupil. Adie's pupil is larger than normal, reacts slowly to light, and often found in young women with decreased or absent tendon reflexes. An *Argyll Robertson pupil* is an abnormally small pupil that fails to respond to the light reflex but does constrict with accommodation and convergence—a well-established sign of CNS syphilis.

When the eyes are directed to a point close at hand, three different reflexes are brought into cooperative action: (1) *convergence,* (2) *accommodation,* and (3) *pupillary constriction.* All three reactions may be initiated by voluntarily looking at a near object, but an involuntary (reflex) mechanism will accomplish the same end if an object is moved slowly toward the eyes.

Convergence. In this test, the examiner moves a finger or some other object held some distance away toward the patient's eyes, midway between them. The eyes should move inward, and the pupils should contract. The medial recti muscles contract to move the eyes into alignment so that images in each eye focus on the same part of the retina to avoid diplopia. An inability to converge the eyes commonly occurs in encephalitis and vascular diseases of the midbrain.

Accommodation. To test accommodation, the examiner asks the patient to face the light, look at some object about 2 feet or less from the eyes, and then look off at a distant object. When looking at a near object, accommodation should accompany convergence and pupil constriction. During accommodation, the lenses are thickened as a result of tension by the ciliary muscles to maintain a sharply focused image.

Pupillary Constriction. Along with convergence and accommodation, the pupils should contract on looking at a near object. The pupils narrow as an optical aid to regulate the depth of focus. This type of near-object pupil constriction does not depend on any change in illumination and is separate from the direct and consensual light reflexes.

Extraocular Movements

Extraocular neuromuscular integrity is tested by having the patient follow the examiner's finger in all directions. Any difficulty in doing so indicates a weakness of the corresponding muscles (Table 9.13). Note the presence or absence of nystagmus. Impairment of conjugate eye movements indicates a lesion in the midbrain. Certain tests are specific:

- The *oculomotor nerve* supplies all muscles that move the eye except the superior oblique and rectus lateralis. It also supplies the sphincter pupillae and ciliaris muscles. Thus, it is tested by eye movements, particularly medially upward and downward, and by pupillary response to light and accommodation. Lesions of this nerve result in a ptosis of the upper lid and dilation of the pupil with loss of the light reflex.
- The *trochlear nerve* supplies only the superior oblique muscle of the eye. Thus, it is tested for eye movement downward and inward.
- The *abducens nerve* supplies only the rectus lateralis muscle of the eye. Thus, it is tested by the ability to move the eye laterally.

The Visual-Fixation Reflex. This reflex is demonstrated by an auto passenger looking out a side window at the passing scenery. The head and eyes turn slowly in the direction of apparent movement and then jump ahead quickly to fix the gaze on a new approaching site. This is done without conscious effort or awareness that the eyes are moving: a true *optokinetic reflex.* This reflex is also demonstrated and tested as in reading from line to line, which normally exhibits a combination of jerky eye movements interspaced with pauses.

Diplopia. Double vision occurs when the conjugate movements of the eyes are altered so that images do not fall on corresponding areas of the two retinae. The result is that the brain interprets two images that are not exactly superimposed. If only one eye is affected, it will usually show a motion abnormality in the field of the involved muscle.

Trigeminal Nerve (Cranial V Motor Fibers)

The trigeminal nerve (cranial V) is the great sensory nerve to the face and anterior

Table 9.13. Paralysis of Individual Eye Muscles

Nerve	Muscle	Deviation of Eyeball	Diplopia when looking:	Direction of image
III	Inf. oblique	Downward and outward	Upward and inward	Oblique
III	Inf. rectus	Upward and inward	Downward and outward	Oblique
IV	Lat. rectus	Inward (internal squint)	Toward the temple	Vertical
III	Med. rectus	Outward (external squint)	Toward the nose	Vertical
IV	Sup. oblique	Upward and outward	Downward and inward	Oblique
III	Sup. rectus	Downward and inward	Upward and outward	Oblique

scalp. It is also the motor nerve to the muscles of mastication (except the buccinator). The motor division of the trigeminus runs only with the mandibular branch of the sensory division. Thus, weak jaw movements (eg, chewing) are likely to be associated with sensory changes in the chin, lower lip, cheek, upper ear, and lateral scalp.

Motor Function Tests. Motor function of the trigeminal is tested by the examiner placing the hands over the masseter and temporal muscles and asking the patient to make chewing motions with the jaw. Note if the muscles contract unequally. The pterygoids are tested by having the patient open the mouth widely and then close it. Note whether the jaw deviates to one side or the other during this motion. Palpate the masseter and temporalis muscles when the patient is asked to "bite down" on a tongue blade on each side. Jaw strength is tested by trying to extract the blade against the patient's resistance. The motor portion of the trigeminal is commonly impaired in cerebral vascular accidents, basal meningitis, syphilis, and brain tumors. These severe disorders are rarely difficult to differentiate from TMJ dysfunction.

Facial Nerve (Cranial VII Motor Fibers)

There are two components of this nerve: one that carries the motor division and another (the intermediate nerve of Wrisberg) that conveys the sensory and autonomic fibers. The parasympathetic fibers via the pterygopalatine and submandibular ganglions supply the lacrimal glands, the mucosa of the nasal cavity and roof of the mouth, and the sublingual and submandibular glands.

Motor Function Tests. The patient should be asked to raise the eyebrows and wrinkle the forehead, to frown, to close both eyes tightly, and then to close each eye separately. The patient is then asked to show the teeth, open the mouth wide, retract the lips, whistle, and smile. The inability to perform such upper and lower facial muscle tests usually indicates a weakness or paralysis of the nerve.

All facial movements should be equal bilaterally, but some patients habitually talk, smile, and chew more on one side than the other. Weakness of the muscles supplied by the facial nerve may be expressed as drooping of the corner of the mouth, smoothing out of the nasolabial fold, drooping of the lower lid, or inability to close the involved eye such as seen in Bell's palsy where the signs are unilateral. If the frontalis muscle is involved, the forehead is unusually smooth on the affected side (Fig. 9.22). Note the presence or absence of atrophy, abnormal movements, contractures, etc.

In upper motor lesions affecting the face, involuntary movements such as blinking and smiling are far less affected than voluntary movements. The muscles of the forehead are spared in upper motor lesions affecting the face. This latter sign occurs because the muscles of the forehead have bilateral cortical representation. In contrast, all facial muscles are affected in lower motor neuron lesions. Thus, they exhibit paralysis of both voluntary and involuntary muscle groups.

Jaw Jerk. The jaw reflex is manifested by a rapid closure of the mouth that is caused by a downward blow on the lower jaw while it hangs passively open. It is rarely normal and usually considered a pathologic sign (eg, sclerosis of thelateral columns of the cord).

Chvostek's Test. In hypocalcemia, the irritability of the facial nerve is greatly increased and tested by Chvostek's reflex. A positive Chvostek's sign is a frequent but not pathognomonic sign of tetany and sometimes witnessed in tuberculosis. It is positive when tapping the facial nerve along its course (eg, over the parotid gland) induces contraction of muscles on the ipsilateral side of the face.

Glossopharyngeal and Vagus Nerves (Cranial IX and X Motor Fibers)

The *glossopharyngeal nerve* is the sensory nerve to the region of the isthmus faucium and posterior one-third of the tongue and pharynx. It is the motor nerve to the stylopharyngeus muscle and parasympathetic to the parotid gland. Thus, it is tested by the gag reflex (sensory, glossopharyngeal; motor, vagus) and taste sense of the posterior tongue. This nerve may be impaired in skull fractures and diseases affecting the brain stem such as in tumors, syphilis, and tuberculosis. Dysphagia and tachycardia may be associated. An occipital injury may tear through the posterior foramen and paralyze the glossopharyngeal, vagus, and accessory cranial nerves. Multiple cranial nerve signs are also seen in brain stem syndromes.

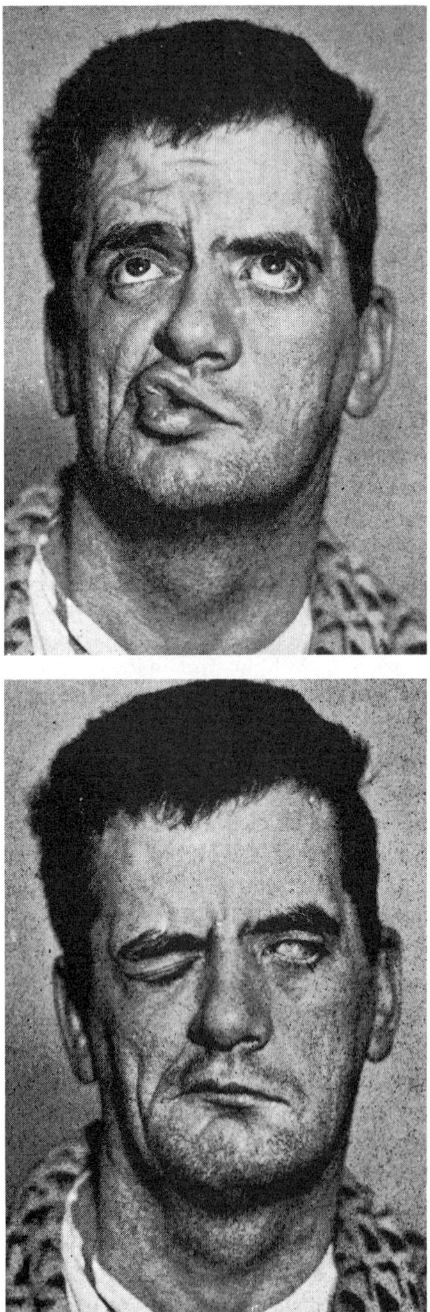

Figure 9.22. A case of left-sided facial palsy; *top,* attempting to wrinkle the forehead and show the teeth; *bottom,* attempting to close the eyes.

The *vagus nerve* is motor to the pharynx, uvula, larynx, and upper part of esophagus. It is sensory to the pharynx, larynx, and upper esophagus; and parasympathetic to the thoracic and upper abdominal viscera. Numerous viscerovisceral and viscerosomatic reflexes course through the vagus nerve. Upper vagal motor integrity is screened by the responses to the gag reflex, the pharyngeal reflex, and movements of the pharyngeal and laryngeal muscles during speech and swallowing.

Nasal speech may be the result of palatal paralysis or paralysis of the vocal cords. Weakness of the oropharynx is suggested by a soft breathy voice associated with nasal escape, while a lesion of the nerve supply to the upper larynx is suggested by a hoarse or husky voice.

Impairment of the vagus nerve may result from diphtheritic paralysis of the pharyngeal branch, injury to the recurrent laryngeal branch by surgery, cervical and mediastinal tumors, aortic aneurysms, or pressure on the nerve from a hypertrophied left atrium. The vagus also may become involved in infectious neuritis, multiple sclerosis, Guillain-Barré syndrome, amyotrophic lateral sclerosis, and bulbar poliomyelitis. In addition, the vagus is sometimes susceptible to trauma because of its long course and its proximity to several important organs. When direct vagal injury is seen, it is usually from damage to the recurrent laryngeal branch following neck trauma.

Motor Function Tests. The glossopharyngeal and vagus nerves are usually considered together as their functions during testing cannot be easily distinguished:

• The patient is asked to open the mouth and say "Ah." The palate will normally rise in the midline. The raphe of the palate is observed and usually deviated to the nonparalyzed side; ie, unilateral palatal weakness will cause the uvula to move toward the intact side. The *pharyngeal reflex* refers to stimulation of the palate, fauces, or posterior pharyngeal wall that results in swallowing. Raising of the uvula (*the uvular reflex*) in phonation or from irritation is absent in disorders of the IX or X cranial nerves. It is important to make this test with the patient's head in the midline and not turned to the side.

• The ability to swallow solids and liquids should be tested. If regurgitation occurs through the nose, its occurrence should be noted.

Spinal Accessory Nerve (Cranial XI)

The spinal accessory nerve provides motor innervation to the sternocleidomastoideus muscles and the upper half of the trapezius muscles. Injury to the spinal accessory nerve may result from subluxation complexes, trauma, IVD lesions, spasmotic torticollis, medulla and cervical cord lesions, and neck tumors and abscesses. Less frequently, multiple sclerosis, certain types of epilepsy, poliomyelitis, amyotrophic lateral sclerosis, and spinal cord tumors and involved. However, singular involvement of this nerve is rare; spinal accessory nerve dysfunction is usually associated with combined disorders of cranial nerves IX, X, and XII.

Motor Function Tests. The patient is asked to elevate the shoulders against resistance (Fig. 9.23) and then to lower the shoulders and thrust the shoulders backward against resistance to test the strength of the trapezius muscles. The patient is then asked to rotate the head from side to side against resistance to test the strength of the sternocleidomastoideus muscles. Note the presence or absence of atrophy, fibrillations, or spasms in the region of the trapezius and sternocleidomastoideus. Strength can be screened bilaterally by having the patient flex the head while the examiner applies resistance to the patient's chin. The strength of the trapezius and sternocleidomastoids should be equal bilaterally unless a unilateral occupation is involved. The strength of lateral flexion against resistance is a helpful indicator. Marked bilateral weakness and atrophy of these muscles are often seen in primary muscle disease (eg, muscular dystrophy).

Hypoglossal Nerve (Cranial XII)

The hypoglossal nerve is the motor nerve to muscles of the tongue. The major signs of a cranial XII lesion are deviation of the tongue and difficult speech. Differentiation should be made from involvement of the carotid artery above its bifurcation or an injury to the recurrent nerve of the high vagus. Positive signs of hypoglossal dysfunction point toward skull fracture, aneurysm of the circle of Willis, and sometimes cervical subluxation. Hemiatrophy of the tongue and fibrillations are seen in bulbar palsy, syringomyelia, and not rarely in poliomyelitis. Coarse tremors are featured in Parkinson's disease and paresis. Fine tremors suggest alcoholism, bromide poisoning, senility, and idiopathic functional disorders. Injury to the

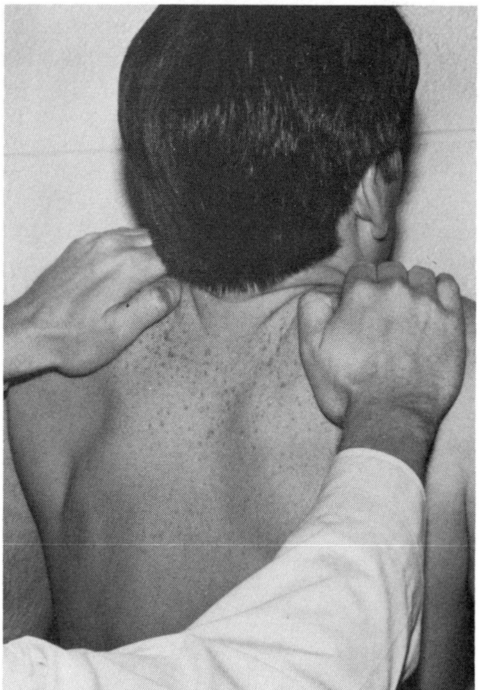

Figure 9.23. Testing the integrity of the spinal accessory nerve and shoulder girdle elevation strength. The patient shrugs his shoulders against the examiner's resistance.

hypoglossal nerve is not infrequently seen from fracture.

When inspecting the tongue, seek signs of atrophy, tremors (an early sign of lower motor neuron disease), wormy fasciculations (amyotrophic lateral sclerosis), and deviation (paralysis). Palpate the tongue if atrophy is seen. Ipsilateral atrophy and fasciculations are characteristic of a unilateral lower motor neuron lesion.

Evaluation of Motor Integrity. The patient is asked to protrude the tongue and rapidly move it from side to side. Rapid movement will be impaired in upper motor neuron lesions. The relaxed tongue will always deviate toward the side of paralysis in lower motor lesions. In bilateral involvement, the tongue may be protruded very slowly or not at all. In central lesions of the nerve, the tongue will be paralyzed on the contralateral side. It will be paralyzed on the homolateral side in peripheral lesions. The strength of the tongue may be estimated by having the patient press the tongue against the inside of the cheek.

Speech Test. Vocal articulation is a complex coordinated function involving the cooperation of muscles supplied by cranial nerves V, VII, IX, and XII. Note whether the patient's speech is clear, distinct, slurring, scanning, or tremulous. Use test phrases such as "truly rural" or "Methodist Episcopal." A vocal dysarthria should be differentiated from an aphasia.

Bibliography

American Orthopaedic Association: *Manual of Orthopaedic Surgery.* Chicago, American Orthopaedic Association, 1972, pp 27-38.

Arbuckle BE: Reflexes. *Journal of the American Osteopathic Association,* 46(7), July 12, 1946.

Balduc HA: Overview of contemporary chiropractic science for the Chiropractic Association of Oklahoma. Northwestern College of Chiropractic, Convention notes, April 24, 1983.

Beardall AG: Additional gait tests. *Digest of Chiropractic Economics,* 19(5), March/April 1977.

Berthold CH: Morphology of normal peripheral axons. In Waxman SG (ed): *Physiology and Pathobiology of Axons.* New York, Raven Press, 1978.

Blacker HM: Evaluating sensory and motor systems. *Patient Care,* 17(16):121-136, 1983.

Brown JR: Diseases of the cerebellum. In Baker AB, Baker LH (eds): *Clinical Neurology.* New York, Harper & Row, 1975, vol 2, chap 29.

Brown T, et al: Psychological factors in low back pain. *New England Journal of Medicine,* 25:4-22, 1954.

Bullock TH: The neuron doctrine and electrophysiology. *Science,* 129:17, 1959.

Burnside JW: *Adams' Physical Diagnosis.* Baltimore, Williams & Wilkins, 1974, pp 200-214.

Cabot RC: *Physical Diagnosis,* ed 7. New York, William Wood, 1919, pp 481-484.

Cailliet R: Disuse syndrome: fibrositic and degenerative changes. In Brena SF, Chapman SL (eds): *Management of Patients with Chronic Pain.* New York, Spectrum Publications, 1983, pp 63-71.

Calbe DB, Eisler T: The pathogenesis and medical treatment of extrapyramidal disease. *Medical Clinics of North America,* 63:715-727, 1979.

Canadian Memorial Chiropractic College: *Segmental Neuropathy.* Toronto, Canadian Memorial Chiropractic College, date of publication not shown, p 29.

Cerny K: Pathomechanics of stance: clinical concepts for analysis. *Physical Therapy,* 64:1851-1859, 1984.

Chusid JG: *Correlative Neuroanatomy & Functional Neurology,* ed 19. Los Altos, CA, Lange Medical, 1985, pp 117-119, 190-199, 205-215, 240, 269-278, 448-460.

Clark RG: *Manter and Gatz's Essentials of Clinical Neuroanatomy and Neurophysiology,* ed 5. Philadelphia, F.A. Davis, 1975, pp 16-23, 31-34, 40-42, 97-103, 127-133, 160-166.

Coers C, Woolf AL: *Innervation of Muscle.* Springfield, IL, Charles C. Thomas, 1959.

Coote JH, et al: Reflex discharges into thoracic white rami elicited by somatic and visceral afferent excitation. *Journal of Physiology,* 202:141-159, 1969.

Cyriax J: *Textbook of Orthopaedic Medicine: Vol One, Diagnosis of Soft Tissue Lesions,* ed 8. London, Bailliere Tindall, 1982, pp 36-53, 453-466.

Daniels L, Worthingham C: *Muscle Testing: Techniques of Manual Examination,* ed 4. Philadelphia, W.B. Saunders, 1980, pp 167-177.

Daube JR, Sandok BA: *Medical Neurosciences.* Boston, Little, Brown, 1978, pp 168, 188-191, 221-222, 287-292, 354-357, 370-371.

Davis L: *Neurological Surgery,* ed 2. Philadelphia, Lea & Febiger, 1942.

Davis NJ, Kovac MP: The command neuron and the organization of movement. *TINS,* 4(3):73-76, 1981.

Debrunner HU: *Orthopaedic Diagnosis,* rev. ed 2. Translated by G Stiasny. Chicago, Year Book Medical, 1982, pp 33-52.

Dee R: Articular neurology. In Sokoloff L (ed): *The Joints and Synovial Fluid.* New York, Academic Press, 1978, p 177.

de Reuck AVS, Knight J (eds): *Myotactic, Kinesthetic, and Vestibular Mechanisms.* Ciba Foundation Symposium. Boston, Little, Brown, 1967.

Ducroquet R, Ducroquet J, Ducroquet P: *Walking and Limping: A Study of Normal and Pathological Walking.* Philadelphia, J.B. Lippincott, 1968.

Eisen A, Hoirch M: The electrodiagnostic evaluation of spinal root lesions. *Spine,* 8(1):98-106, 1983.

Elias SB, Appel SH: Current concepts of pathogenesis and treatment of myasthenia gravis. *Medical Clinics of North America,* 63:745-757, 1979.

Fowler WM Jr, Taylor RG: Differential diagnosis of muscle disease. In D'Ambrosia RD: *Musculoskeletal Disorders: Regional Examination and Differential Diagnosis.* Philadelphia, J.B. Lippincott, 1977, pp 93-95.

Friedman HH: *Problem-Oriented Medical Diagnosis,* ed 2. Boston, Little, Brown, 1979, pp 316-341.

Goldstein M (ed): *The Research Status of Spinal Ma-*

nipulative Therapy. Bethesda, MD, National Institutes of Health, DHEW Publication No. (NIH) 76-998, 1975, p 27.

Goodheart GJ: *Collected Published Articles and Reprints.* Montpellier, OH, Williams County Publishing, 1969, pp 23-24.

Gottschalk L: Psychologic factors in backache. *General Practitioner,* 33:91-94, 1966.

Grice AS: Muscle tonus change following manipulation. *Journal of the Canadian Chiropractic Association,* 18(4):29-31, 1974.

Grieve DW: The assessment of gait. *Physiotherapy,* 55:452-460, 1975.

Guyton AC: *Textbook of Medical Physiology,* ed 6. Philadelphia, W.B. Saunders, 1981, pp 626-670.

Haldeman S: The electrodiagnostic evaluation of nerve root function. *Spine,* 9(1):42-48, 1984.

Heilman KM, Watson RT, Greer M: *Handbook for Differential Diagnosis of Neurologic Signs and Symptoms.* New York, Appleton-Century-Crofts, 1977, pp 105-106.

Hibbard D: Effects of manipulation on gait muscle activity: preliminary electromyographic research. *ACA Journal of Chiropractic,* 17(10):104-106.

Hollingshead WH, Jenkins DB: *Functional Anatomy of the Limbs and Back.* Philadelphia, W.B. Saunders, 1981, pp 17-19, 38-42.

Holmes G: The cerebellum of man. *Brain,* 62:1-30, 1939.

Homewood AE: *The Neurodynamics of the Vertebral Subluxation,* ed 3. Place of publication not shown, published by author, 1981, pp 88-102, 130, 136-139, 284-286.

Hoppenfeld S: *Physical Examination of the Spine and Extremities.* New York, Appleton-Century-Crofts, 1976, pp 134-141.

Inman VT, Ralston HJ, Todd F: *Human Walking.* Baltimore, Williams & Wilkins, 1981, pp 2-21, 103-117.

Inman VT, Saunders JBdeCM: Referred pain from skeletal structures. *Journal of Nervous and Mental Disorders,* 99:660, 1944.

Janda V: Muscle and joint correlations. In Lewit K, Gutmann G (eds): *Rehabitácia. Proceedings of the IVth Congress.* Prague, International Federation of Manual Medicine, 1975, pp 154-157.

Janse J: The integrative purpose and function of the nervous system: A review of classical literature. *Journal of Manipulative and Physiological Therapeutics,* 1(3), September 1978.

Janse J: *Principles and Practice of Chiropractic.* Lombard, IL, National College of Chiropractic, 1976, pp 48-50, 73-74, 310-312.

Jaskoviak PA, Schafer RC: *Applied Physiotherapy: Practical Applications Within Clinical Chiropractic.* Arlington, VA, American Chiropractic Association, 1986, pp 55-58, 87-91, 113-114, 271-273.

Judge RD, Zuidema GD (eds): *Methods of Clinical Examination: A Physiological Approach,* ed 3. Boston, Little, Brown, 1968, pp 341-366.

Karvinen E, Komi PV: Neuromuscular performance. In Larson LA (ed): *Fitness, Health, and Work Capacity.* New York, Macmillan, 1974, pp 73-78, 81-86.

Kellgren JH: Observations on referred pain arising from muscle. *Clinical Science,* 3:175, 1938.

Keesler HH: *Low Back Pain in Industry.* New York, Commerce and Industry Association of New York, 1953.

Kessler RM, Hertling D (eds): *Management of Common Musculoskeletal Disorders.* Philadelphia, Harper & Row, 1983, pp 27-30, 91-98, 202-226.

Korr IM (ed): *The Neurobiologic Mechanisms in Manipulative Therapy.* New York, Plenum Press, 1978, pp 27-40, 61-62, 235-236, 375-390.

Korr IM: Proprioceptors and somatic dysfunction. *Journal of the American Osteopathic Association,* 74(3):638-650, 1975.

Krupp MA, Chatton MJ, Werdegar D: *Current Medical Diagnosis & Treatment—1985.* Los Altos, CA, Lange Medical, 1985, pp 605-610, 613-614.

Krupp MA, Tierney LM Jr, Jawetz E, Roe RL, Camargo CA: *Physician's Handbook,* ed 21. Los Altos, CA, Lange Medical, 1985, pp 34-53.

Landau WM, O'Leary JL: Disturbances of movement. In MacBryde CM, Blacklow RS (eds): *Signs and Symptoms,* ed 5. Philadelphia, J.B. Lippincott, 1970, pp 703-704.

Laporte Y, Emonet-Denand F, Jami L: The skeletal-fusimotor or beta-innervation of mammalian muscle spindles. *TINS,* 4(4):97-99, 1981.

Laufenberg PC: New dimensions in neurologic evaluation. *The Digest of Chiropractic Economics,* pp 10-12, 105-106, May/June 1979.

Luria AR: *Higher Cortical Functions in Man.* New York, Basic Books, 1966, pp 432-439.

MacBryde CM, Blacklow RS: *Signs and Symptoms,* ed 5. Philadelphia, J.B. Lippincott, 1970, pp 655-667.

MacDonald ML, Stanish WD: Neuromuscular system. In Scott WN, Nisonson B, Nicholas JA: *Principles of Sports Medicine.* Baltimore, Williams & Wilkins, 1984, pp 15-24.

Nouwen A, Bush C: The relationship between paraspinal EMG and chronic low back pain. *Pain,* 20(2): 109-123, 1984.

Olson WH, Brumback RA, Gascon G, Christoferson LA: *Practical Neurology for the Primary Care Physician.* Springfield, IL, Charles C Thomas, 1981, pp 1-32, 98-114, 157-178, 236-269.

Pastan RS: Diffuse musculoskeletal pain. *Diagnosis,* 5(3):42-46, 1983.

Penry JK, Porter RJ: Epilepsy: Mechanisms and therapy. *Medical Clinics of North America,* 63:801-812, 1979.

Perry JA: Clinical interpretation of the mechanics of walking. *Physical Therapy,* 47:778-801, 1967.

Pinkenburg C: A basis for the theory of manipulative medicine. *Journal of Manipulative and Physiological Therapeutics,* 3(2):81-85, June 1980.

Pottenger FM: *Symptoms of Visceral Disease,* ed 6. St. Louis, C.V. Mosby, 1949.

Prichard JW: Nerve. In Albright JA, Brand RA (eds): *The Scientific Basis of Orthopaedics.* New York, Appleton-Century-Crofts, 1979, pp 408-412.

Prior JA, Silberstein JS: *Physical Diagnosis,* ed 5. St. Louis, C.V. Mosby, 1977, pp 394-418.

Quigley WH: Self-concept, mental health, and chiropractic. *ACA Journal of Chiropractic,* March 1971.

Rebechini-Zasadny H, Tasharski CC, Heinze WJ: Electromyographic analysis following chiropractic manipulation of the cervical spine: A model to study manipulation-induced peripheral muscle changes. *Journal of Manipulative and Physiological Therapeutics,* 4(2):61-63, 1981.

Reuber M, Schultz A, McNeil T, Spencer D: Trunk muscle myoelectric activities in idiopathic scoliosis. *Spine,* 8:447-456, 1983.

Roland MO: A critical review of the evidence for a pain—spasm—pain cycle in spinal disorders. *Clinical Biomechanics,* 1:102-109, 1986.

Rosse C: Muscle action and its control. In Rosse C, Clawson DK (eds): *The Musculoskeletal System in Health & Disease.* Hagerstown, PA, Harper & Row, 1980, pp 64-65, 70-75.

Rosse C: The vertebral column. In Rosse C, Clawson DK (eds): *The Musculoskeletal System in Health & Disease.* Hagerstown, NJ, Harper & Row, 1980, pp 138, 140.

Sandoz R: Some reflex phenomena associated with spinal derangements and adjustments. *Annals of the Swiss Chiropractic Association,* VII:45, 1981.

Sato A: The somatosympathetic reflexes. In Goldstein M (ed): *The Research Status of Spinal Manipulative Therapy.* NINCDS Monograph No. 15, DHEW Publication No. (NIH) 76-998, Washington, DC, U.S. Government Printing Office, 1975.

Sato A: Spinal and medullary reflex components of the somato-sympathetic reflex discharges evoked by stimulation of the group IV somatic afferents. *Brain Research,* 51:307-318, 1973.

Schafer RC: *Chiropractic Management of Sports and Recreational Injuries.* Baltimore, Williams & Wilkins, 1982, pp 471, 516, 527.

Schafer RC: *Chiropractic Physical and Spinal Diagnosis.* Oklahoma City, Associated Chiropractic Academic Press, 1980, pp I:30-34, II:29-30.

Schafer RC: *Clinical Biomechanics: Musculoskeletal Actions and Reactions.* Baltimore, Williams & Wilkins, 1983, pp 136-137, 148-158, 162-164.

Schafer RC (ed): *Basic Chiropractic Procedural Manual,* ed 4. Arlington, VA, American Chiropractic Association, 1984, pp 39, 517-558.

Schafer RC: *Physical Diagnosis: Procedures and Methodology in Chiropractic Practice.* Arlington, VA, American Chiropractic Association. In preparation, to be released in 1989. Chapter 6, Basic Musculoskeletal Considerations; Chapter 7, Basic Neurologic Considerations.

Schafer RC: *Symptomatology and Differential Diagnosis.* Arlington, VA, American Chiropractic Association, 1986, pp 105-114, 294, 555-556, 939-940, 967-968.

Schwartz HS (ed): *Mental Health and Chiropractic: A Multidisciplinary Approach.* New Hyde Park, NY, Sessions, 1973.

Seliktar R, Susak Z, Najenson T, Solzi P: Dynamic features of standing and their correlation with neurological disorders. *Scandinavian Journal of Rehabilitation Medicine,* 10:59-64, 1978.

Shepherd GM: Microcircuits in the nervous system. *Scientific American,* 238(2): 92, 1978.

Singarajah KV: Neurophysiology evidence for manipulative therapeutic principles: Involvement of synaptic interaction. *Annals of the Swiss Chiropractors' Association,* 6:143-159, 1976.

Skully RL: The nervous system and its disorders. *ACA Journal of Chiropractic,* January and February 1972.

Soderberg GL: *Kinesiology: Application to Pathological Motion.* Baltimore, Williams & Wilkins, 1986, pp 39-43.

Spector B: Surface electromyography as a model for the development of standardized procedures and reliability testing. *Journal of Manipulative and Physiological Therapeutics,* 2:214-222, 1979.

Speransky AD: *A Basis for the Theory of Medicine;* translated by C.P. Dutt. New York, International Publishers, 1943.

Steward SL: An investigation into the effect of chiropractic adjustments on the psychological state of the patient. *Bulletin of the European Chiropractic Union,* 26(2):10-23, 47-59, 1978.

Stolov WC: Normal and pathologic ambulation. In Rosse C, Clawson DK (eds): *The Musculoskeletal System in Health & Disease.* Hagerstown, NJ, Harper & Row, 1980, pp 318-328.

Taylor RG, Fowler WM Jr: Electrodiagonosis of musculoskeletal disorders. In D'Ambrosia RD: *Musculoskeletal Disorders: Regional Examination and Differential Diagnosis.* Philadelphia, J.B. Lippincott, 1977, pp 61, 78-80, 84-85.

Thabe H: Electromyography as a tool to document diagnostic findings and therapeutic results associated with somatic dysfunctions in the upper cervical spinal joints and sacroiliac joints. *Manual Medicine,* 2:53-58, 1986.

Tran TA: Clinical correlations of the pyramidal system. *The Chirogram,* November 1976.

Tran TA: The motor system: A general look at its components and their clinical correlations. *The Chirogram,* October 1976.

Ufberg SH: Muscular nociception. *ACA Journal of Chiropractic,* 14:93-96, September 1980.

Vazuka FA: *Essentials of the Neurological Examination.* Philadelphia, Smith, Kline, & French Laboratories, 1962.

Walker HK, Hall WD, Hurst JW (eds): *Clinical Methods.* Woburn, MA, Butterworth, 1976, pp 796-839.

Walther DS: *Applied Kinesiology; Volume I: Basic Procedures and Muscle Testing.* Pueblo, CO, Systems DC, 1981, pp 220-223, 234-240.

Wayne KM: Disturbances of the nervous system as related to chiropractic. *Journal of the Canadian Chiropractic Association,* 13(2):20-23, 1969.

Widmann BJ: Electromyography for chiropractic. *Annals of the Swiss Chiropractors' Association,* 2: 132-160, 1961.

Williams HG: An anatomical-functional review of selected CNS motor control structures. *The Texas Chiropractor,* April 1977.

Wood KW: Myospasm, myosprain and myalgia. *The Digest of Chiropractic Economics,* pp 126-127, May/June 1985.

Wolf SL (ed): *Clinics in Physical Therapy: Electrotherapy.* New York, Churchhill Livingstone, 1981.

Wyke BD: Articular neurology and manipulative therapy. In *Aspects of Manipulative Therapy.* Proceedings of Multidisciplinary International Conference on Manipulative Therapy. Melbourne, Lincoln Institute of Health Sciences, Carlton, Victoria, Australia, August 1979, pp 67-72.

Zetterberg C, Bjork R, Ortengren R, Anderson GBJ: Electromyography of the paravertebral muscles in idiopathic scoliosis: measurements of amplitude and spectral changes under load. *Acta Orthopaedica Scandinavica,* 55:304-309, 1984.

Chapter 10

Clinical Disorders and the Autonomic Nervous System

This chapter gives an overview of the clinical aspects of autonomic dysfunction, with emphasis on the clinical aspects of sympathetic and parasympathetic disorders. Such topics as stress and the neurodystrophies, the evaluation of visceral function, and reflexology are described. A review of the section titled "The Visceral System" within Chapter 3 will be beneficial to the reader of this chapter.

Wiles has stated that "Visceromotor articles made up 14% of the *ACA Journal of Chiropractic* articles in 1977. They made up 8.9% in 1985. If we wanted to, this could be extrapolated out and this type of article would die out by 1992." If this occurs, a great injustice would be done to the potential of the profession as well as the public it serves. It appears that some in the profession have lost sight of the fact that it was the successful management of visceral and systemic conditions that sustained chiropractic during its early years.

It was the opinion of James Firth, then president of Lincoln Chiropractic College, that chiropractic was a dying profession around the period of World War I. He stated, "There is no question in my mind that it was the successful results of chiropractic during the great influenza epidemic following the war that saved it. Hundreds of thousands of people were dying, and medicine had no solution to the problem. Chiropractors got results, and the word quickly spread throughout the nation. Chiropractic offices that had been nearly empty became filled, and state legislators began to take the chiropractic profession seriously in spite of the opposition of the AMA."

OVERVIEW

Embryologically, the somatic structures appear late in development as compared to the vegetative nervous system, which serves as the chief integrating and correlating system of the visceral structures. The voluntary and vegetative nervous systems are intimately connected and brought into reflex connection so that visceral stimulation has skeletal and somatic expression and skeletal muscle messages are expressed in visceral tissues: *The body is a whole.*

Vegetative action is slow when compared to voluntary action. In addition, human will, at least for normal consciousness without specialized training (eg, biofeedback), has little power to direct visceral effects as one would direct a skeletal muscle because vegetative functions must be conducted whether one is awake or asleep. In certain acts, however, voluntary and vegetative nerves supplement one another such as in swallowing, breathing, defecation, urination, and seminal ejaculation.

Sympathetic Distribution

The sympathetics are widespread in their distribution (Fig. 10.1). Through their innervation of blood vessels, sympathetic fibers reach every tissue of the body. They control blood vessel diameter, subdermal structures, heart muscle, the sphincter system of the gut and urinary apparatus, and parts of the bladder and reproductive organs; they inhibit many structures in the head and chest; and they reach the enteral system's muscles and glands.

While it is widely recognized that the cervical sympathetic chain communicates with the lower cranial nerves, Parkinson and associates have confirmed that the sympathetic nerve running with the carotid artery gives off a multitude of fine branches at irregular intervals as the nerve travels cephally. The largest residual component joins the cranial VI (abducens) and leaves to join the cranial V (trigeminal) nerve. Similar fibers have not been found to join the cranial III (oculomotor) or IV (trochlear) nerves.

Parasympathetic Distribution

The parasympathetics activate the intrinsic eye muscles, glands of the peripheral head, bronchi muscles and glands, entire enteral system, body of the bladder; they inhibit the heart; and they provide vasodilation in many structures (especially the head and penis).

STRESS AND THE NEURODYSTROPHIES

An autonomic efferent nerve has two major functions: (1) impulse conduction and (2) a trophic influence on receptor organ growth, repair, immunity, and cellular alterations in disease. While these conduction and trophic functions are of equal importance and separate actions, trophic functions have unfortunately received secondary interest by most research neurologists. Because interference with trophic function serves an important role within chiropractic concepts, several pertinent findings are described in this section.

Research on nonimpulse initiated communication between the neuron and its end structures has increased in recent years. Singer relates that despite considerable controversy modern consensus accepts the role of neurotrophic and impulse stimulation in the maintenance of muscle tissue. He feels that, experimentally, it has been difficult to report these two mechanisms for individual study because most information has been obtained in model systems.

Autoadaptation and Immunity

Guth, Gutmann, and Gurkalo/Zabezhinski show that there should be no question that the autonomic nervous system regulates directly and indirectly the functions of all organs and tissues and influences even biochemical processes at the cellular and subcellular level.

After observing more than 15,000 patients with infectious diseases and studying the host-parasitic relation in infectious disease, Sato found that the adaptation of the human body to the internal environment is maintained by an autoadaptation mechanism operating upon the biological binary digit. That is, the autoadaptation mechanism has two antagonistic systems (sympathetic and parasympathetic divisions) that are composed of many antagonistic links: (1) the two reciprocal nerves of the autonomic nervous system; (2) two phases (rise and fall) of mitosis of the neurotrophic system in bone marrow; and (3) two defense reactions (the cell-stimulant factor reaction and the antibody-antigen reaction). These binary antagonistic links are interconnected into two systems that are controlled by the two antagonistically functioning nerves (sympathetic and parasympathetic) of the autonomic nervous system.

In a following study, Sato found that the autoadaptation mechanism of the human

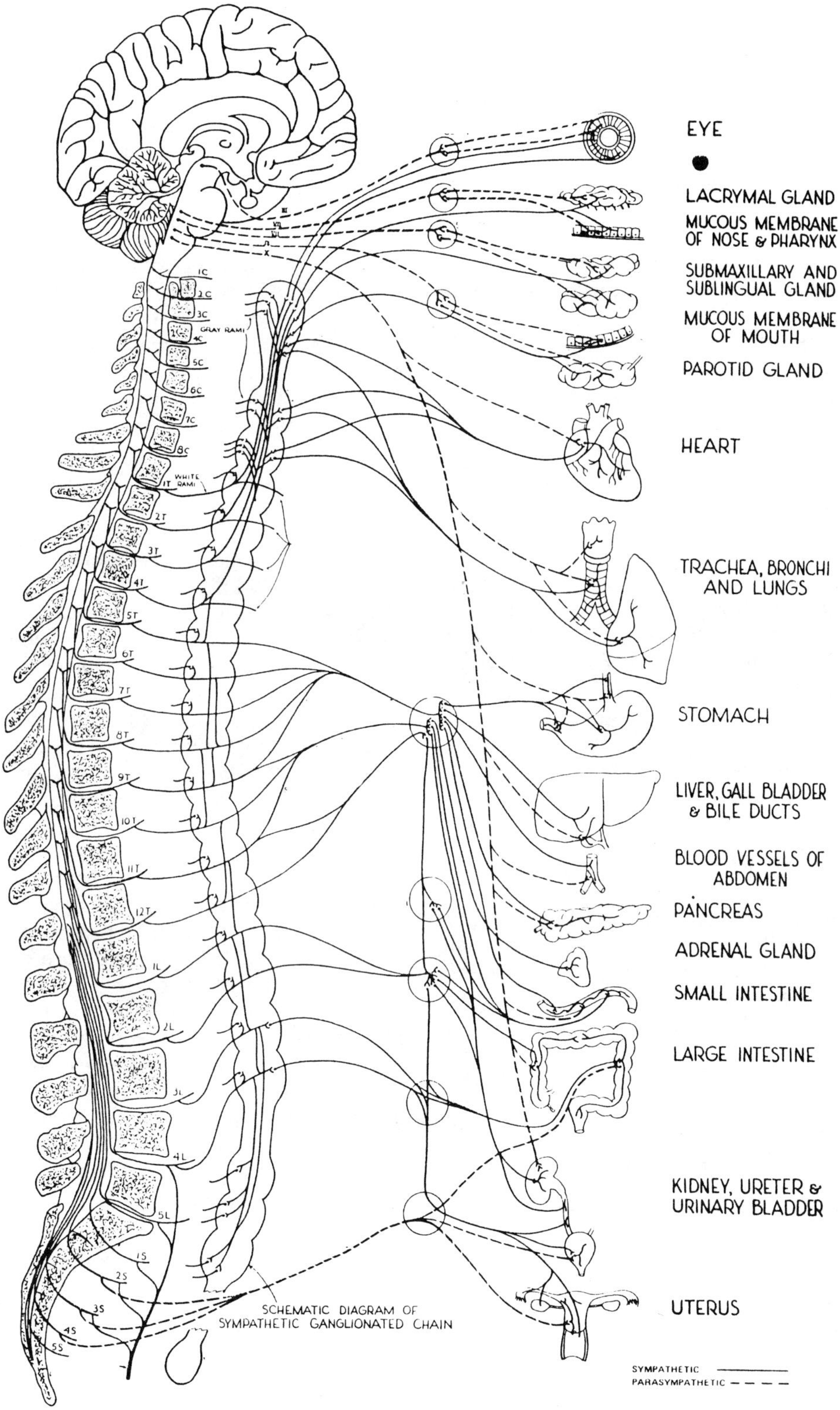

Figure 10.1. Schematic of the autonomic nervous system (from Houser RH: *Visceral Innervation,* 1968).

body loses its rationality and purposefulness by an imbalance of the autonomic nervous system, and the host body falls into adaptational disturbances. He reports that hosts with sympathicotonia often fall into acute adaptational disturbances in the acme to the convalescent stage by stimuli of the second-phase factors (the factors lowering mitosis of the neurotrophic system in the bone marrow), resulting sometimes in death. The disturbances are prominent, particularly in the early stage of stimulation and recognized as shock. Hosts with parasympathicotonia, states Sato, are resistant against the second-phase factors such as typhoid bacilli but weak against the first-phase factors such as cocci. In contrast, hosts with sympathicotonia show strong resistance against the first-phase factors but weak resistance against the second-phase factors.

There are several studies in process investigating the effects of spinal adjustments on the immunologic system. A preliminary study by Vora/Bates demonstrated a significant increase in B-lymphocytes following 4 weeks of semiweekly spinal adjustments in patients exhibiting spinal subluxations radiographically.

Also see Chapter 2, Neurologic Aspects of Immunogenesis.

Tissue Repair

Singer/Schade suggest that one important role of the nervous system is to regulate tissue repair—a projection made by D.D. Palmer before the turn of the century. Several studies have associated this process with neurotubules and axoplasmic mechanisms leading to the formation of vesicles in the terminal buttons that release certain chemical substances which appear to have a distinct influence on trophic activity.

Cellular Alterations

Chronic hyperactivity of the autonomic nervous system is highly detrimental to the tissues and organs innervated and may be related to dysfunction in the spinal area. In this context, Korr explains that the physiologic influence of sympathetic innervation is more varied than previously believed. It extends to (1) skeletal muscle, (2) peripheral sensory mechanisms, (3) the CNS system, (4) collateral circulation, (5) bone growth, (6) adipose tissue, (7) the reticuloendothelial system, and (8) the endocrine system.

Habitual patterns of motor activity can modify bone structure in accordance with *Wolf's law*, and faulty postural habits can produce fibrous deposits within articular cavities that have been chronically overstressed. Feldenkrais reports that the result is contractures within certain muscles and ligaments, hypertrophy of others, and weakening and atrophy of still others. In this context, Homewood postulates that the nervous system, even in its early developmental stages, is in command and remains as the correlating, integrating, and modifying factor that controls the responses of the body to exteroceptive and interoceptive stimuli in both health and disease.

Many postural changes can be attributed to *Davis' law*, which states: "If the origin and insertion of a muscle are moved farther apart for some time, the muscle becomes relaxed and hypotonic. If they are approximated, the muscle contracts, becomes hypertonic, and may become contractured." It can thus be recognized that changes in muscle tone as the effect of chronic tension can result in overt trophic changes.

Il'in and associates report that the similarity between the changes in the isoenzyme composition of muscle, with reversion to the embryonic type, that is found both in muscular dystrophy of neurogenic origin and in primary lesions (myopathies) of the muscle itself is explained on the following grounds: (1) In neurogenic dystrophy, the changes are the result of a disturbance in the conduction of neural impulses to and into the muscle. (2) In myopathy, although the damaged muscle receives the neural impulses, the muscle cells cannot respond adequately.

Diseases Showing Marked Trophic Changes

Trophic changes are marked in various neurogenic, vascular, and some other disorders. Besides lower motor neuron disease,

Chusid lists the neurogenic disorders showing marked trophic changes as causalgia, herpes zoster, neurogenic arthropathy (Charcot's joint), syringomyelia, and tabes dorsalis. Skin changes, ulcers, and gangrene are typical trophic disorders associated with vascular disease. They are especially associated with arteriosclerosis, Buerger's disease, endarteritis obliterans, varicose veins, and Volkmann's ischemic contracture. Trophic changes are also associated with cancer and various endocrine disorders, trophoneuroses, and infections.

EVALUATION OF VEGETATIVE FUNCTION

An understanding of visceral neurology is indispensable to appreciate and explain the possible pathophysiologic processes involved in a patient's condition because (1) the chief purpose of the vegetative nerves is that of correlating and integrating action in the body, and (2) these nerves may be subject to the amount of stimulation necessary to overbalance their normal function whenever an abnormal irritation arises in any organ or its innervation.

Factors Involved in Autonomic Imbalance

Almost all organs are innervated through the functionally antagonistic sympathetic and parasympathetic divisions of the autonomic nervous system. Disturbed activity balance of these two divisions results in some degree of visceral dysfunction. In health, the divisions are tonically stimulated to maintain a physiological balance. For various reasons, however, this balanced harmony may be shifted in favor of one or the other division and create visceral malfunction. Sachs states that every pathologic condition is obviously associated with disturbances in the autonomic nervous system.

Normal vegetative function can usually be maintained if proper nutrition is supplied the cells and their colloidal phases are usual for the structure under consideration provided (1) the necessary electrolytes are supplied in the right proportions, (2) the hormones from the various endocrine glands and vitamins are supplied in normal amounts, and (3) the activating and inhibiting impulses carried to the cells balance each other or at least fail to overbalance each other. If these factors are not provided, deviations from the norm will lead to vegetative imbalance.

For a summary of specific effects of sympathetic and parasympathetic activation, refer to Table 3.13. Systemic effects are shown in Table 3.14.

Pottenger states that a patient need not be sympathicotonic or vagotonic throughout the vegetative structures. Instances of mixed sympathetic and parasympathetic effects include exophthalmic goiter, nausea and vomiting, variations in blood sugar, and anorexia nervosa. Instances of local vegetative imbalance are shown in Table 10.1.

Clinical Signs and Tests

General Screening: The Saliva Test

A convenient way to screen autonomic balance is by determining the pH of saliva. A strip of litmus, nitrazine, or pHydrion paper is moistened with the patient's saliva about a half hour away from food or drink, comparing the resultant color with a standard scale. Normally, saliva has a pH of 7.0, neutral. Normal blood pH is about 7.3 or 7.4, and, at this level, the saliva will be pH 7.0, always a few tenths of a pH more acid than blood serum.

If the test paper indicates a pH below 7.0, it is hyperacidic and the sympathetics will be overactive. The patient will usually present with anxiety, hyperkinesis, tachycardia, a dry mouth and eyes and nose, gooseflesh raised easily, a marked gag reflex, insomnia after excitement, and easy blushing. Rhodifer believes a potassium deficiency will also be present.

If the test paper indicates a pH above 7.0, the saliva is hyperalkaline and the parasympathetics are thought to be overactive. Rhodifer feels that an overactive parasympathetic system is parallel to hyperalkalinity or alkalosis. The normal calcium/phosphorus ratio is distorted in alkalosis. Since phosphorus is needed in alkalosis, it also indicates that the normal calcium/phosphorus ratio of 10 calcium to 4 phosphorus in the blood is distorted, in which condition excess calcium exists for which not enough phosphorus is available to unite with it in this ratio. During rest periods, the calcium may be deposited in joints, muscles, and bursae in the form of calcium carbonate crystals, resulting in stiffness, soreness, bursitis, tendinitis, and cramps. A phosphorus deficiency would thus be indicated.

Tests for Sympathicotonia

Vannerson points out that inasmuch as sympathetic nerves are closely intertwined with blood vessels, any deviation from normal sympathetic function will be first registered in the blood vessels and then other structures will become helplessly vulnerable to the possible harm of an altered blood flow.

Cold Test. This test is used to determine the vasospastic gradient in cases of essential hypertension. It is accomplished by immersing the patient's hand and wrist in ice water with salt added to produce a temperature of approximately 4°C. Blood pressure readings are determined before and at intervals during and after the hand has been immersed from 15 to 30 seconds. When there is no great element of vasospasm or vasomotor activity present, namely, in the normal individual, a rise of 8—10 mm Hg takes place. When vasospastic phenomena take part in the elevation of blood pressure, a marked rise, often as high as 50 mm Hg promptly occurs. If this happens, a large vasomotor element undoubtedly exists.

Finger Wrinkle Test. The functioning of upper extremity sympathetic nerves is tested by placing the patient's hands in warm water for a minimum of 30 minutes and observing if the skin of the fingers wrinkle after the soaking. The skin will normally wrinkle after such soaking, but it will not in diseases of the sympathetic nervous system. Thus, the test is indicated when there is a suspicion of diabetes mellitus, Guillain-Barré syndrome, Raynaud's disease, and other disorders associated with autonomic imbalance.

Table 10.1. Typical Instances of Local Vegetative Imbalance

Allergies
Angiospastic conditions
Bradycardia
Dermographism (Fig. 10.2).
Erythromelalgia
Hypertonia of the pelvic nerve
Ileocecal spasm
Impotence
Immune deficiency diseases (controversial)
Intestinal block (eg, gallbladder reflex)
Pupil disorders
Pylorospasm
Raynaud's disease
Reflex motor effects from viscera
Reflex sensory effects from viscera
Reflex trophic effects from viscera
The neurogenic process in essential hypertension
The pathophysiology involved in gallbladder and biliary tract disease
Trophic changes in dermal tissues
Vasomotor imbalances

Sargent's Sign. This sign is produced by a light stroke drawn in the median line from above downward over the abdominal wall. When a white line appears, it is an indication of increased sympathetic tonus or hyperadrenia. See Figure 10.2.

Pende's Reflex. In subjects who are distinctly sympathicotonic, stroking of the skin (especially of the abdomen) produces a "goose flesh" response; ie, a pilomotor reflex.

Electrical Resistance of the Skin. When cutaneous nerve conduction is disrupted, a loss of sweat secretion occurs because this function is under the control of the sympathetic nervous system. Because moist skin has less resistance to an electric current than dry skin, such tests, utilizing small-diameter probes, are commonly used to aid localization. Minor's iodine-starch reaction and Moberg's ninhydrine test also can be used to demonstrate the presence of sweat.

Thermography. Infrared or liquid crystal thermography may be helpful in locating "cold spots" and areas of subcutaneous hyperemia, suggesting a degree of abnormal vascular tone as the result of increased or decreased sympathetic activity.

Tests for Vagotonia

Oculocardiac Reflex. With the patient in the recumbent position, compression of the eyeball upon closed lids for about 30 seconds and without producing pain may produce slowing of the heart by 5—10 beats. In people who are distinctly vagotonic, it has been found that this slowing may amount to 12 beats or more. Under conditions of excessive stress in marked parasympathicotonics, the heart has often been temporarily inhibited. In people of stable nerve balance, neither inclined to sympathicotonia or parasympathicotonia, the slowing is usually less than 10 beats; in fact, in those who are markedly sympathicotonic, no slowing may occur. The reflex is caused by stimulating the ocular fibers of the trigeminus, through which the impulse is transmitted to the cardiac inhibitory fibers of the vagus. In individuals who are distinctly vagotonic, the reflex may show itself in the gastrointestinal tract as well as in the heart. Pressure over the vagus in the neck will result in a similar manifestation. See Figure 10.3.

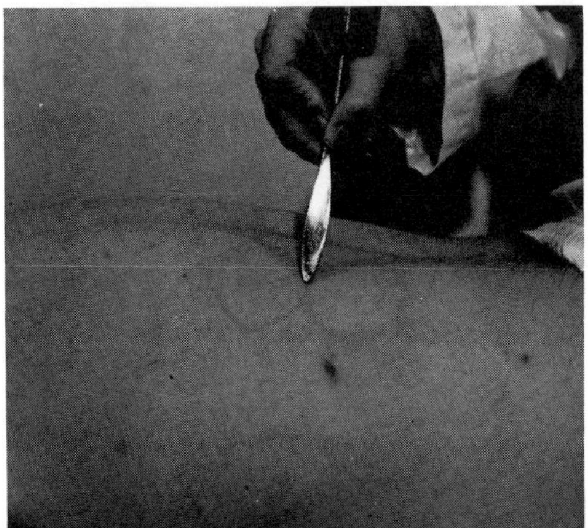

Figure 10.2. Graphesthesia test eliciting a positive sign.

Erben's Reflex. This test consists of a slowing of the pulse when the head is bent strongly forward. It is marked in those who are distinctly vagotonic.

Ruggeri's Sign. This sign shows an acceleration of the pulse, following convergence of the eyeballs, produced by fixing attention upon an object that is brought quite close to the eyes. It is less marked in vagotonics.

Somagyi's Reflex. This response is a manifestation of the instability of the cardiac branch of the vagus. It consists of dilation of the pupils on deep inspiration and contraction on full expiration.

Carotid Sinus Massage. Pressure applied to the carotid area in the neck slows the heart rate and produces a fall in blood pressure. The reflex originates in the wall of the sinus of the internal carotid artery. If heavy prolonged pressure is applied, dizziness or fainting may result. This normal reflex becomes hyperactive during attacks of vasomotor instability and hypoactive in inhibitory lesions of Cranial IX (afferent portion) and Cranial X (efferent portion).

In sinus tachycardia with a normal QRS duration, carotid sinus massage tends to slow the heart gradually but the rate usually reverts to its original rate after the stimulation is released. Carotid sinus massage, states H.H. Friedman, either terminates or has no effect on most paroxysmal atrial or

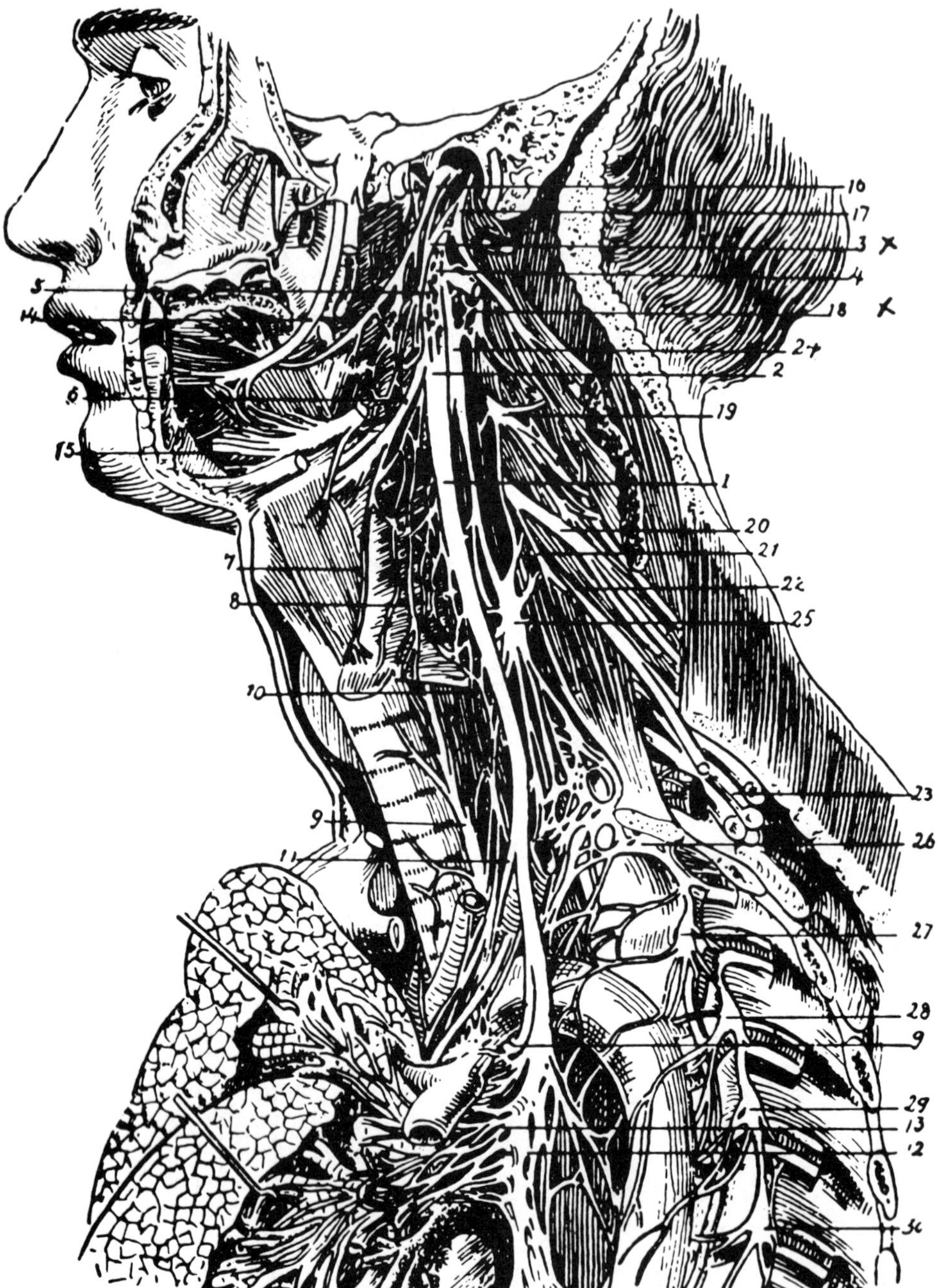

Figure 10.3. Distribution and connection of the vagus nerve and other cervical nerves of the left side of neck and upper part of thorax: *1,* vagus nerve; *2,* ganglion of its trunk; *3,* accessory; *4,* union of vagus with hypoglossal; *5,* pharyngeal branch of vagus; *6,* superior laryngeal; *7,* external laryngeal; *8,* communication of external laryngeal with superior cardiac branch of sympathetic; *9,* recurrent; *10,* superior, and *11,* inferior cervical cardiac branches; *12, 13,* posterior pulmonary plexus; *14,* lingual branch of mandibular; *15,* distal part of hypoglossal nerve; *16,* glossopharyngeal nerve; *17,* accessory nerve; *18,* second cervical nerve; *19—21,* third, fourth, and origin of phrenic nerve; *22, 23,* 5th—8th cervical nerves, forming with the first thoracic nerve; *24,* superior cervical sympathetic ganglion; *25,* middle cervical ganglion; *26,* inferior cervical ganglion; *27—30,* 2nd—5th dorsal ganglia.

AV junctional tachycardias. In atrial flutter, carotid sinus pressure increases the degree of AV block so that fewer flutter impulses are transmitted to the ventricles. The F waves are more clearly revealed with a smaller number of ventricular complexes, making this a useful maneuver when the diagnosis of atrial flutter is uncertain.

Although carotid sinus massage is an excellent evaluative procedure, it should always be conducted with caution, particularly with the elderly, and under ECG control whenever possible. The procedure is contraindicated in heart block and advanced vascular disease.

CLINICAL CONSIDERATIONS

As many patients are inclined to suffer from a particular group of disorders that represent vegetative imbalance, it is often helpful during the examination to classify the patient as sympathicotonic or vagotonic as a guide for future therapeutic applications.

Patient Classifications

The disorders most commonly associated with a *sympathetic predominance* are hyperthyroidism, dryness and paleness of the mucous membrane of the head, deficient salivary secretion, tachycardia, dilatation of the stomach, hypochlorhydria, poor digestion, and atonic constipation.

Common disorders associated with a *parasympathetic predominance* are lacrimation, hay fever, urticaria, angioneurotic edema, intestinal allergies, sinusitis, rhinitis, pharyngitis, excessive salivary secretion, bradycardia, asthma, hyperchlorhydria, peptic ulcer, diarrhea, spastic constipation, mucous colitis, and anaphylaxis. Addison's disease is a classic parasympathetic disorder.

Behavioral Characteristics

It can be generally stated that sympathicotonics tend toward an ectomorphic nature and body type while the parasympathicotonics tend toward an endomorphic nature and body type. In both conditions, structural and behavioral signs and symptoms become the outward manifestation of disturbed autonomic function.

Sympathicotonic individuals tend to be tall and thin, active, impatient, fast talkers, impulsive deciders, mentally alert, nervous, easily angered or fearful, hypersensitive to pain, hungry for excitement and adventure, and sexually aggressive. Strong emotional states are accompanied by dilated pupils, dry throat, peripheral vasoconstriction, raised blood pressure, bulging veins in the neck, increased adrenal secretion, increased blood sugar, erection of hairs, increased heat production, sweating, increased heart and respiratory rates, anorexia, and slowing of the digestive processes so that the body's energy may be massed in the periphery for defense of the organism. Because of this, they are in danger of exhausting the sympathetic nervous system leading to depletion syndromes such as low blood pressure or nervous breakdown. Anxiety syndromes are common. Their defense responses are usually active (eg, quick fever on slight provocation). In minor expressions of imbalance or emotions, the effects are less severe but may be more prolonged with the physiologic disturbances being less acute but more lasting.

Parasympathicotonic individuals, in contrast, tend to build up excessive fat, enjoy good food and comfort, present a slower metabolism, are slow in their actions, are patient in trying situations, need but dislike exercise, are deliberate yet have difficulty in arriving at decisions, and are socially nonassertive. Depression is common. Their defense responses are sluggish, and they tend to acquire chronic diseases and prolonged states of general fatigue.

The above characteristics are general tendencies, not absolutes, that vary greatly in magnitude with specific individuals under specific situations.

Characteristics and Assessment of Autonomic Pain

The pain associated with the autonomic system is not well understood. It does not fit a dermatomal, myotomal, or sclerotomal pattern. Neither does it occur in a distinct location such as a specific joint, muscle, or finger. Gandhavadi and associates give the following examples of the nonspecific pain: (1) pain and burning in the entire lower extremity, (2) pain in the upper extremity with a "raglan sleeve" distribution, and (3) pain in part of a limb not fitting the dermatomal area or peripheral nerve distribution. The major quadrants of the trunks literally supply the quadrants of the body. Thus, the disturbance may be expected to be in the quadrantic distribution.

Gandhavadi recommends that the assessment of the sympathetic system be done: (1) *physically* (orthostatic hypotension, absence of ciliospinal reflex, hypohidrosis); (2) *physiologically* (valsalva maneuver, cold pressor, thermocoupling, plethysmography, sweat test, infrared thermography); and (3) *pharmacologically*, if necessary.

Overgaard agrees with Bennett that the majority of pain sensations in humans are the result of visceral disorders of the thorax, abdomen, or pelvis. They state that autonomic pain may be projected or referred to structures outside the visceral cavity and is often felt in regions distant from the disorder. Overgaard believes that tissue trauma results in the release of agents that trigger nociceptors and produce the sensation of autonomic pain, while Bennett suggests that the initial cause is vasospasm leading to microcirculatory blockage.

Subluxation Effects on Systemic Nutrition

See Appendix, Figures A.9—A.12.

Spinal Therapy in Visceral Dysfunction

In describing the role of spinal treatment in visceral disorders, Beal, an osteopath, summarizes the objectives of manipulative therapy as: (1) to reduce somatic dysfunction, (2) to interrupt the viscerosomatic reflex arcs, (3) to influence the viscus through stimulation of somatovisceral afferents, and (4) to reduce the potential preconditioning effects of somatic dysfunction to body stressors. He also points out several references substantiating that manipulation can reduce recovery time from visceral surgery. As research into the value of adjustive therapy in visceral dysfunction is continued, this list is certainly to expand and be refined.

Background

D.D. Palmer, the founder of chiropractic, believed that a vertebral subluxation could affect tone in either an excitatory or inhibitory manner. However, his son and successor, B.J. Palmer, placed great emphasis on the *blockage* of neural impulses ("pinched nerve") between the higher CNS centers and peripheral tissues at the IVF via inhibiting nerve or root pressure. This concept grew in popularity from the early 1900s through the 1940s primarily because it was helpful in explaining the effects of a vertebral subluxation to the lay public; viz, by the overly simplistic analogy of "a foot (subluxation) on a hose (nerve channel)." Obviously, such an explanation was not acceptable to the scientific community.

Tachycardia, hyperhidrosis, decreased smooth muscle tone and glandular secretion, and increased vascular tone indicate vagal inhibition, and the vagal and sacral parasympathetic nerves have no direct relationship with vertebral IVFs. Thoracic sympathetic inhibition would exhibit opposite functional disturbances. However, clinical evidence gathered over the last 80 years has demonstrated that spinal adjustments are frequently effective in the treatment of disorders manifesting a picture of parasympathetic depression—sympathetic excitation. Thus, a subluxation syndrome is far more complex than can be explained by the "pinched nerve theory," and a segmental chiropractic adjustment has far-reaching effects throughout the nervous system, which cannot be explained with our present knowledge.

According to the "interference in neural transmission concept," any disorder not exhibiting a pattern of inhibition would not be amenable to chiropractic care. There are few practitioners that would not take exception to such a statement. It is a general opinion that any static nerve or root pressure exerted at the IVF that would be strong enough to block autonomic transmission from the cord to peripheral tissues would likely be strong enough to block outflowing motor and inflowing sensory impulses (Fig. 10.4). Such an occurrence would manifest signs of at least partial paralysis. This is rarely seen other than in severe vertebral trauma (eg, fracture-dislocation) or a space-occupying mass.

Much About Autonomic Function and Control Is Still a Mystery

Rare is the chiropractor whose understanding of neuroanatomy has not been put to the test by observations made in clinical practice. A typical example is seen in the female patient who enters the practice following a mild—moderate "whiplash" injury, with the major subluxation determined to be at the C5 level, who reports during treatment that not only has the neck and upper extremity symptoms been relieved but the PMS symptoms and dysmennorhea suffered for many years have suddenly disappeared.

Early in practice, this author's first experience of this nature was with a 73-old female patient whose presenting complaint was a recently arising "nagging ache" in the left lumbar area. Motion tests revealed that the thoracic spine was almost completely immobile in all ranges, and radiographic evidence of osteoarthritis was extensive. Following the second adjustment to L2, she

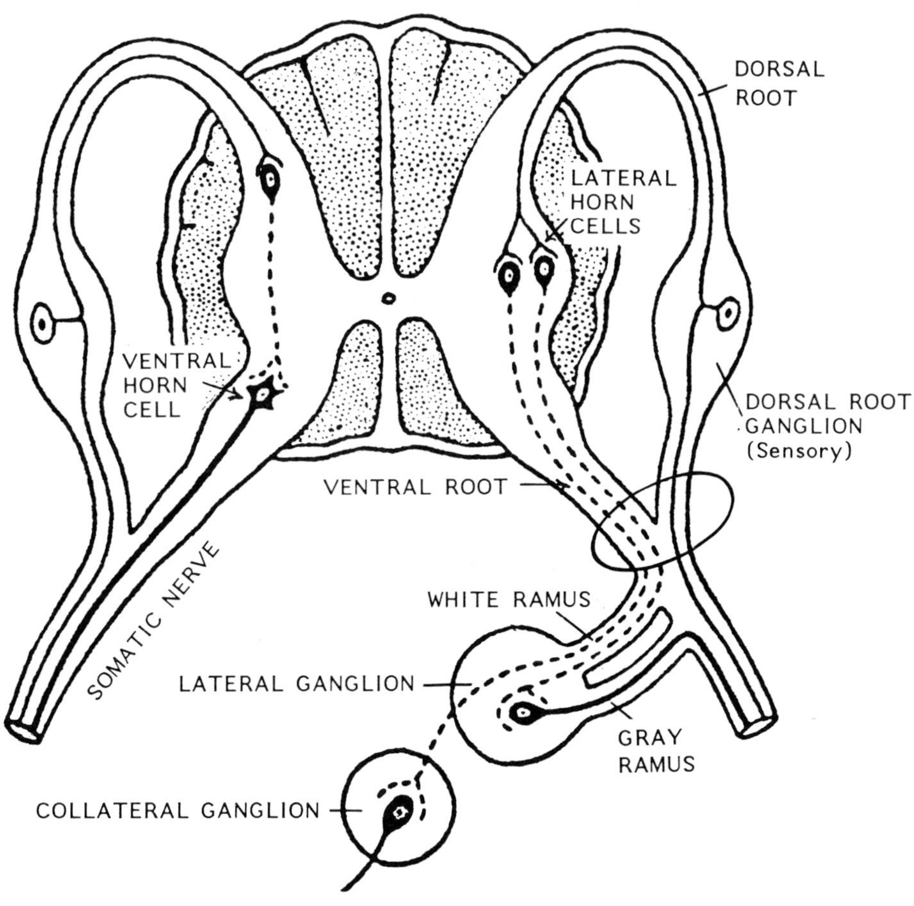

Figure 10.4. Diagram depicting the anterior and posterior roots. *Left,* somatic motor and sensory fibers; *right,* autonomic afferent and efferent pathways in and near the spinal cord.

reported only minor relief of the low-back pain but that she had not had one asthmatic attack, a condition which had caused her distress for the past 60 years. Her asthma remained asymptomatic to her death, 8 years later. Because of its chronicity, treatment for the asthma was not given initial consideration; and why treatment directed to L2 apparently had an effect on the bronchi was bewildering.

Another example of the complexity of neural integration and adaptation is shown in Norman/Whitman's study of vagal contribution to changes to heart rate evoked by stimulation of cutaneous nerves. Their investigation showed that adrenalectomized dogs which have had their sympathetic nerves chemically blocked can have their heart increased by *radial nerve* stimulation. This is caused by a change in the activity of cardioinhibitory fibers in the vagus nerve.

In describing musculoskeletal involvement in chronic lung disease, Hoag shows that involvement of the musculoskeletal system is direct as well as subtle and complex. The bronchopulmonary disturbance may influence the musculoskeletal system, which in turn affects bronchopulmonary function, or else the primary musculoskeletal disturbance alters bronchopulmonary function by adverse somatogenic reflexes. Hoag recommends that the physician should determine whether responses within the musculoskeletal system are excessive or inappropriate. He states that when hypertonicity contributes to hypoventilation of the lungs, adjustive treatment is recommended as well as consideration of the use of muscle-relaxing therapy. The chief aim of spinal therapy is to aid the musculoskeletal system to respond to the pathophysiologic changes.

It is recommended that any somatic dysfunctions producing local or secondary visceral disturbances should be corrected first. Procedures can then be employed to increase mobility of the thoracic cage, improve motions of the diaphragm, lessen bronchospasm, improve ventilation, normalize the amount of bronchial secretions, and improve circulatory function. It should be noted how these procedures differ from the normal allopathic approach of just drugs and bedrest for this condition.

Because of the highly complex, integrated nature of the nervous system, simplistic explanations of causes and effects are difficult to defend. Throughout this book, it has been emphasized that the effects of a vertebral subluxation are widespread and likely to be manifold because of the many neural (local and remote), vascular, CSF, axoplasmic, and hormonal mechanisms that possibly may be involved.

While numerous examples of the complexity of neural integration have been described previously, one more is appropriate here. In a study of cats by Young and associates, it was found that maximal effects on the infraorbital nerve fibers of the *trigeminal nerve* (cranial V) were produced by conditioning stimuli applied to the *lumbar sympathetic chain.* Significantly decreased excitability was observed when the conditioning stimulus was applied to the sciatic or sural nerves.

Spinal-Related Reflex Changes in Internal Dysfunction

In justifying the importance of spinal therapy in cases of splanchnic dysfunction, Rychilková states that four types of reflex changes in vertebrogenic disorders have been differentiated:

- Vertebrogenic and reflex changes imitating internal disease.
- Internal disease caused by a vertebrogenic lesion.
- Reflex changes and vertebrogenic lesions developing during the acute stage of internal disease. This effect is thought to be attributable to paravertebral spasm causing anomalous mobility in the corresponding spinal segment, which leads to blocking. The mechanism is believed to be a viscerosomatic consequence of painful stimuli from the malfunctioning organ.
- Reflex changes occurring during the chronic stage of internal disease. Rychilková states that it is as this stage that manipulation and reflex therapy are most successful. If, however, reflex changes recur in spite of therapy, this points to recurrence of the underlying visceral disease.

Beal makes the point that while somatic dysfunction may not initiate visceral dysfunction, somatic treatment such as spinal manipulation may be helpful for two reasons: (1) visceral disorders may be influenced by reflex facilitation, and breaking this noxious reflex cycle will often allow recovery; (2) reflex somatic pain may persist after the visceral disorder is resolved, mimicking the original problem, and this may resolve with manipulation.

Autonomic Symptoms Associated with Back Pain Syndromes

After studying 250 consecutive back pain subjects, Johnston found that 39% exhibited probable evidence of vertebrogenic autonomic dysfunction. The incidence was distributed as follows: 60%—*cervicogenic cephalgia* (disturbed vision, dysequilibrium, gastrointestional disturbances); 54%—*thoracoalgia* (nausea, flatus); and 31%—*lumbalgia* (constipation, polyuria, menstrual disturbances).

During the analysis of disorders of vasomotor reactions in lumbosacral syndromes, Starý and associates determined that vasomotor nociceptive reflexes are formed more easily and fixed more firmly in patients suffering from painful vertebrogenic syndromes. In arriving at this conclusion, these researchers found that vasodilation was observed especially after nociceptive stimulation and they suspected that the inverse vasodilator responses are mediated by a cholinergic mechanism because the response can be reversed by atropine injection.

Some Documented Effects of Spinal Adjustments on Autonomic Function

Fatigue Index. Busch and associates found that chiropractic adjustments in the C5—T3 area of normal subjects decreased the fatigue ratio considerably, indicating a higher peripheral resistance (ie, increased sympathetic activity). It is theorized that the benefits of such therapy are produced by either a decreased stroke volume of the heart or a lessened pulsatile blood volume through the brachial artery which is caused by direct stimulation of the brachial vasculature.

Vital Capacity. In comparing the results of chiropractic adjustments on respiratory function in patients with and without symptoms of respiratory distress, Hviid's findings suggest a change in peak respiratory flow and vital capacity in response to treatment. In measuring 50 chiropractic patients presenting with musculoskeletal complaints, Masarsky/Weber found that forced expiratory volume was greatly improved after adjustive therapy as compared to pretreatment measurements.

Induced Hypotension and Hypertension. In a study of the effects of upper thoracic adjustments upon the normal physiology of the heart, Tran/Kirby found that adjustments of the T1 and T2 vertebrae, as compared with a control group, appeared to lower blood and pulse pressures within normal physiologic ranges. A similar study of the effects of upper cervical adjustments upon the normal physiology of the heart by Tran/Kirby gave evidence that a chiropractic adjustment, or the stimulation from the thrust alone, can induce increased peripheral tension in which the diastolic pressure and pulse pressure were most affected. ECG patterns showed no significant changes, but some degree of variations in heart rate were noted. Their findings conclude that caution should be given to adjusting nonsubluxated vertebrae.

Spinal Adjustments in Neurodystrophy

In describing chiropractic concepts, such as the role of adjustive spinal therapy in the treatment of infectious diseases, Janse stated that the *neurodystrophic hypothesis of chiropractic*, in its simplest form, may be reduced to D.D. Palmer's concept that "lowered tissue resistance is the cause of disease" and due to "too much or too little energy." During the 1943—1953 period, Olehey, Watkins, Nelson, Keller, and several others emphasized the importance of this concept within chiropractic case management. The concept of "lowered resistance" is, however, not unique to chiropractic, it has been stressed by such medical authorities as Boyd, Dubos, Speransky, Gordienko, Zhigalina, and many others. Several current medical authorities, especially those with a special interest in nutrition, are currently voicing the same principle as if it were something new.

Korr, in writing of the role of spinal manipulation in the treatment of trophic disturbances, reports that mechanical insults or moderate pressure can cause nerve deformation and subsequent neuroischemia. He proposes that the amount of damage is related to the degree of ischemia and that the ischemia affects neuronal protein flow to the spinal cord. He concludes that affected segments are maintained in a hyperirritable state but that this condition can be ameliorated by spinal manipulation.

REFLEXOLOGY

Although the efferent activity of the autonomics had been demonstrated for years, it was not until the 1930s that the existence of afferent fibers was proved. In 1930, H.G. Schwartz reported the finding of some sensory fibers that belonged intrinsically to the autonomic nervous system. Since then, numerous investigators have studied autonomic reflex activity and have attempted to determine their course.

Numerous autonomic and related reflexes have been described previously in this and previous chapters, but a few additional points are worthy of note in this section. Some theoretical patterns of sensation and selection are shown in Figure 10.5.

Autonomic reflexes may be initiated either intrinsically or as a by-product of somatic mechanisms. Concern must be given that the reflex phenomena observed in patients with musculoskeletal disorders are not misjudged as an entity within themselves when they are a by-product of some subclinical primary pathology. In this context, Stiles advises clinicians to remember that a cause and effect relationship within the body will produce a compensatory change in one part of the body as a result of a dysfunction in another. The causes are often multifactorial, including not only the primary problem but also postural stress, anxiety, and microtrauma. The body responds to stress by distributing it in order to maintain homeostasis. This capability allows function through compensation; however, afferent overload from the primary area will eventually require outside help.

Somatosomatic and Somatovisceral Reflexes

Somatosomatic Reflexes

By definition, *somatosomatic reflexes* should not involve the autonomic nervous system; however, it is rare when a spillover effect upon the autonomic supply does not occur. In review, a *somatosomatic reflex* develops whenever a somatic sensory receptor is stimulated to trigger a volley of reflex impulses to another anatomical location of the soma via efferent somatic motor or autonomic fibers.

The projected effects of subluxations on the somatosomatic pathway are shown in the Appendix, Figure A.5.

Pain Control. These reflexes are commonly evoked by cutaneous stimulation, and such reflexes are commonly applied therapeutically to inhibit pain (viz, by counterirritation). It is widely recognized that stimulation of large sensory fibers from the peripheral receptors depress the transmission of pain signs either within the same area of the body or from areas sometimes located many segments away.

Case Management. An understanding of somatosomatic reflexes helps to explain the "stubborn" musculoskeletal case that fails to respond in the time anticipated, requiring frequent and repeated adjustive therapy far beyond average. This occurrence can be due to long-lasting changes in excitability of spinal reflex pathways. Animal studies have shown that if a lesion is induced in the cerebellum, a change in extremity posture is noted. It has been found that the involved limb remains in the abnormal posture if the spinal cord just above the level supplying the extremity is not severed for 45 minutes after the cerebellar lesion was produced; ie, allowing time for the local spinal reflexes to become habituated. In contrast to such a CNS lesion, Patterson/Steinmetz found that long-lasting reflex habituation also could be caused by peripheral stimulation. Their study showed that if an abnormal peripheral stimulus (eg, low-back strain) is produced, the spinal reflexes are habituated for some time after the stimulus is removed and the lesion will spontaneously return with any subthreshold stressor. Thus, more is involved in treating a subluxation complex than simply making a mechanical correction of placement. Repetition is required until the habituation of the spinal reflex center is interrupted. Patterson/Steinmetz state that spinal reflexes should be considered as active participants in the symptoms treated with manipulative therapy, and the role of these reflexes in symptoms should be recognized in the therapy administered.

Somatovisceral Reflexes

In writing of the basic functional aspects of somatosympathetic reflexes, Kuntz states that reflex responses on the viscera (including the splanchnic blood vessels) elicited by stimulation of localized cutaneous areas with the same segmental innervation as the viscera in question are common physiologic phenomena. Sato emphasizes that the functions of the various visceral organs can be influenced by a proper cutaneous stimulation as a result of the somatosympathetic or somatoparasympathetic reflexes.

A *somatovisceral reflex* is initiated when a somatic sensory receptor is stimulated sufficiently to trigger a volley of autonomic reflex impulses to viscera. These reflexes are commonly evoked by cutaneous or musculoskeletal stimulation. They can be initiated therapeutically by vibration, percussion, massage, manipulation, superficial heat or cold, electrotherapy, meridian therapy, hydrotherapy, traction, and compression.

Cutaneovisceral Reflexes. In studying the autonomic and physiologic properties of cutaneovisceral vasomotor reflex arcs in rats, Kuntz found that the receptors through

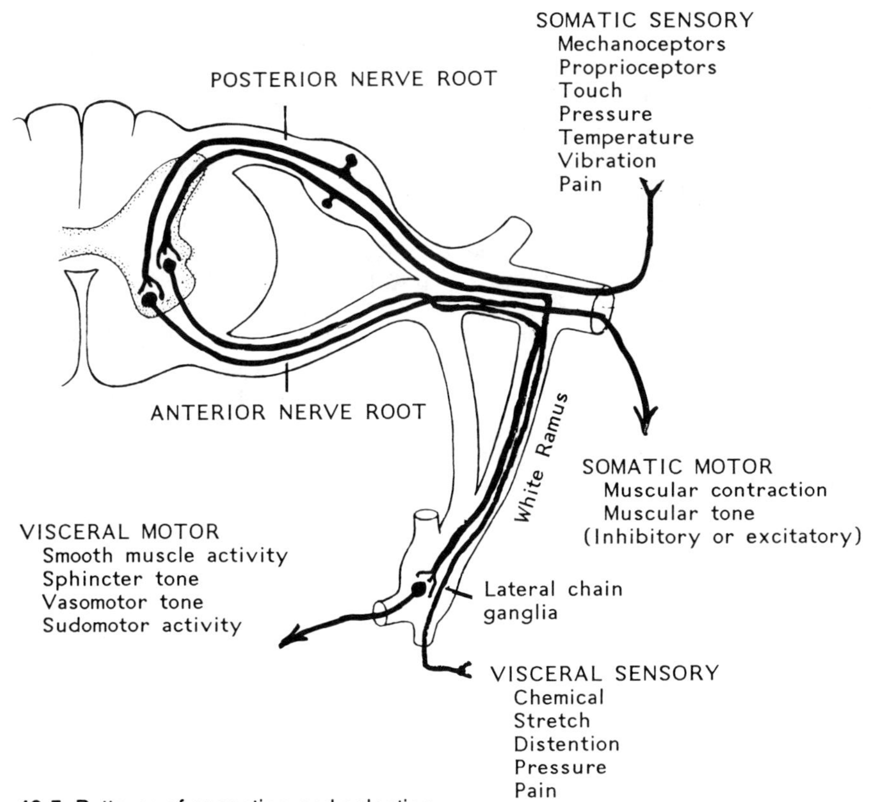

Figure 10.5. Patterns of sensation and selection.

which thermal sensations and reflex reactions in viscera are mediated, elicited by thermal stimulation of the skin, appear to be closely associated with cutaneous blood vessels. Tissue deformation incident to tonic changes in the musculature of these vessels is thought to play an important role in the activation of the receptors in question and, consequently, in sensory adaptation.

In describing the importance of somatoautonomic reflexes in the regulation of visceral function, Sato shows how stimulation of abdominal skin produces a reflex sympathetic change in gastrointestinal tone. Likewise, stimulation of perineal skin causes either a reflex increase in vesical tone through a reflex increase in pelvic discharge activity or a reflex inhibition of the micturation contraction of the bladder through a reflex inhibition of pelvic nerve activity.

Cutaneocardiac Reflexes. Reflex changes in heart rate after mechanical and thermal stimulation of the skin of cats at various segmental levels were studied by Kaufman and associates. They found that there was no doubt that heart rate changes occurred with cutaneous stimulation. In anesthetized cats with the CNS intact, a reflex increase in heart rate was elicited after natural stimuli were applied (eg, rubbing, pinching, warming, cooling) to the neck, chest, abdomen, or perineum. It was shown that this cutaneocardiac acceleration effect was produced mainly by a reflex increase in the discharges of the cardiac sympathetic efferent nerves and partially by a reflex decrease in the discharges of the cardiac vagal efferents. On the other hand, in spinal cats, only stimulation of the chest and abdominal skin produced a reflex increase in heart rate. A possible explanation of the difference between reactions with and without an intact CNS is that a spinal, segmentally organized component of the cutaneocardiac acceleration reflex is dominated by a supraspinal, diffusely distributed component in CNS-intact cats.

Pain Inhibition. Conditioning stimuli to either the caudal sympathetic chain or the lateral femoral cutaneous nerve inhibit the actions of other nerves on dorsal horn interneurons. By recording dorsal root reflexes, reciprocal primary afferent terminal depolarizing actions between visceral and cutaneous afferents have been shown by Selzer/Spencer. The existence of primary afferent terminal depolarization and the close correlation of its time course with that of the mutual inhibition suggest that at least part of this inhibition is of the presynaptic variety. The findings of this study suggest that the pronounced inhibition of visceral afferent action by conditioning cutaneous afferent volleys may underlie the clinical phenomenon of inhibition of visceral pain by cutaneous counterirritation. It is also suggested that the facilitation of cutaneous afferent actions by conditioning visceral afferent volleys might similarly underlie the clinical phenomenon of referred hyperalgesia during states of visceral pathology.

Somatovisceral and Viscerosomatic Reflexes

Somatovisceral Reflexes

Except to mention that cutaneous stimulation has an important influence on visceral function (especially vascular tone), medical authorities rarely discuss somatovisceral reflexes in great detail. However, as Homewood points out, these reflexes form an important aspect of the basic chiropractic contention that a vertebral lesion can produce adverse splanchnic reactions. Most of our contemporary knowledge of these reflexes has come from Pottenger, Speransky, Kuntz, Coote, and Sachs.

A somatovisceral reflex is initiated when a sensory receptor in the skin, subcutaneous tissue, fascia, striated muscle, a tendon, a ligament, or a joint is stimulated to trigger a volley of autonomic reflex impulses to viscera. Body wall stimulation produces both segmental organ responses and suprasegmental responses. See Figures 10.6 and 10.7. Janse postulated that somatosympathetic reflexes to be at least in part responsible for the visceral changes often observed after spinal adjustment, manipulation, trigger point therapy, and spondylotherapy.

After studying the response of some sympathetic neurons to volleys in various af-

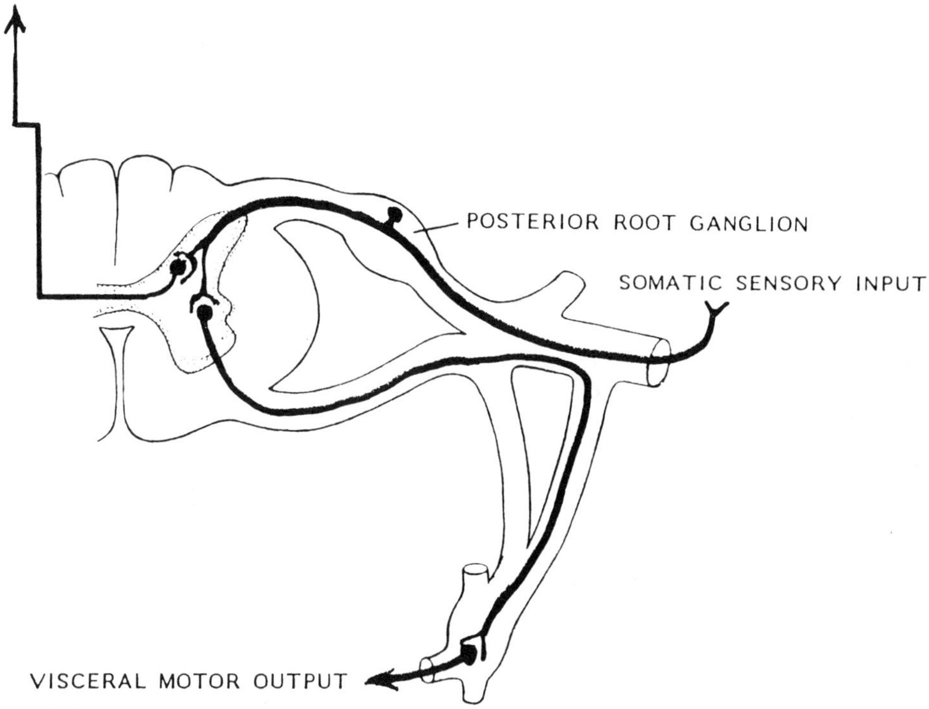

Figure 10.6. A somatosensory to visceromotor reflex.

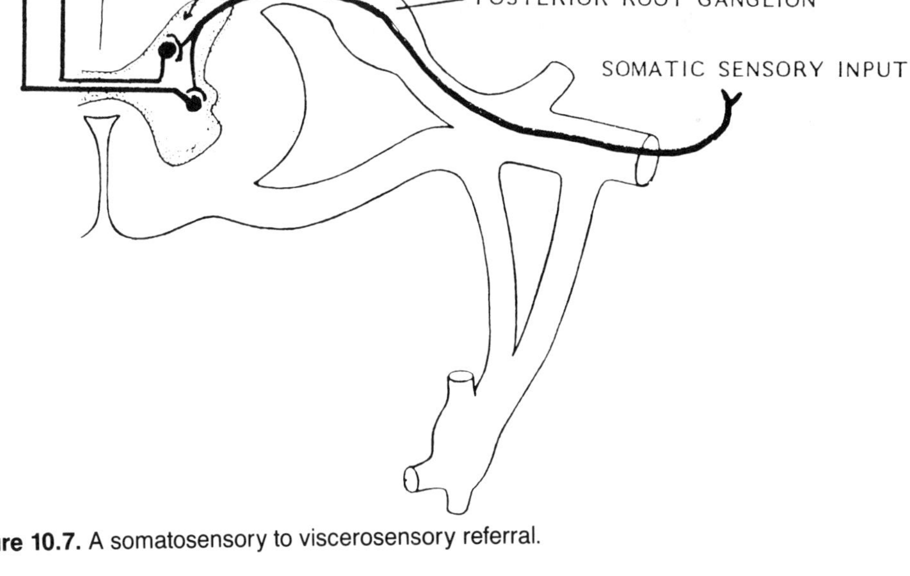

Figure 10.7. A somatosensory to viscerosensory referral.

ferent nerves, Coote/Perez-Gonzales suggest that Group III and IV muscle afferents have a chemoreceptor function and are responsible for mediation of the pressor reflex during muscle exercise.

Koizumi's studies showed that pinching the abdominal skin produced profound inhibition on intestinal motility. The stimuli produce a strong effect on the intestines, which often become completely quiescent. Segmental input strongly affects intestinal movement and nonsegmental input augments intestinal motility. In this mechanism, the control of the effector organ by the sympathetic supply plays a dominant role; ie, the parasympathetic system through vagal innervation of the intestines seems to contribute little to this reflex. To understand spinal adjustive therapy properly, it is Koizumi's opinion that the relationship between cutaneous and other somatic afferents and the autonomic responses must be further clarified.

The projected effects of spinal subluxations on the somatovisceral pathway are shown in the Appendix, Figure A.6.

Different forms of stimulation may produce similar organ responses and may produce different brain center responses affecting the body. The type of response, states Balduc, prolonged beyond stimulus termination, depends on the state of the organ and the body as a whole (ie, active, resting). Therapeutically, these reflexes are commonly evoked by manipulation, superficial heat or cold, electrotherapy, hydrotherapy, traction, compression, vibration, percussion, massage, and meridian therapy.

Viscerosomatic Reflexes

A viscerosomatic reflex develops whenever a sensory receptor of an internal organ, a gland, or a vessel is stimulated enough to trigger a volley of reflex impulses to the skin and subcutaneous tissues or to one or more striated muscles, tendons, ligaments, or joints. Refer to Appendix, Figure A.7. This type of reflex is commonly exhibited in the abdominal spasm overlying peritonitis and the origin of angina pectoris. See Figures 10.8 and 10.9. Therapeutically, these reflexes are commonly evoked remotely by spinal manipulation, spondylotherapy, and spinal trac-

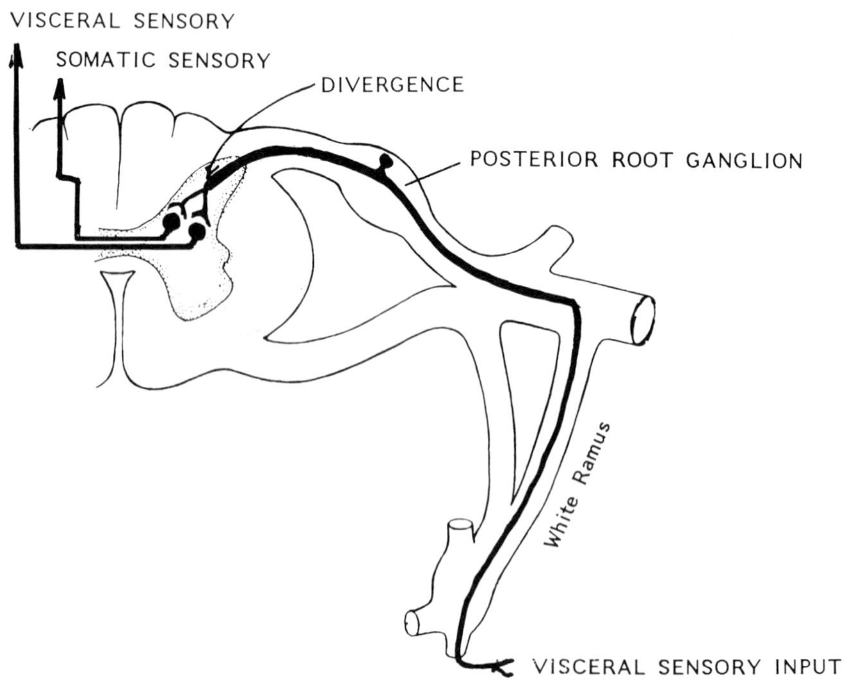

Figure 10.8. A viscerosensory to somatosensory referral (referred pain).

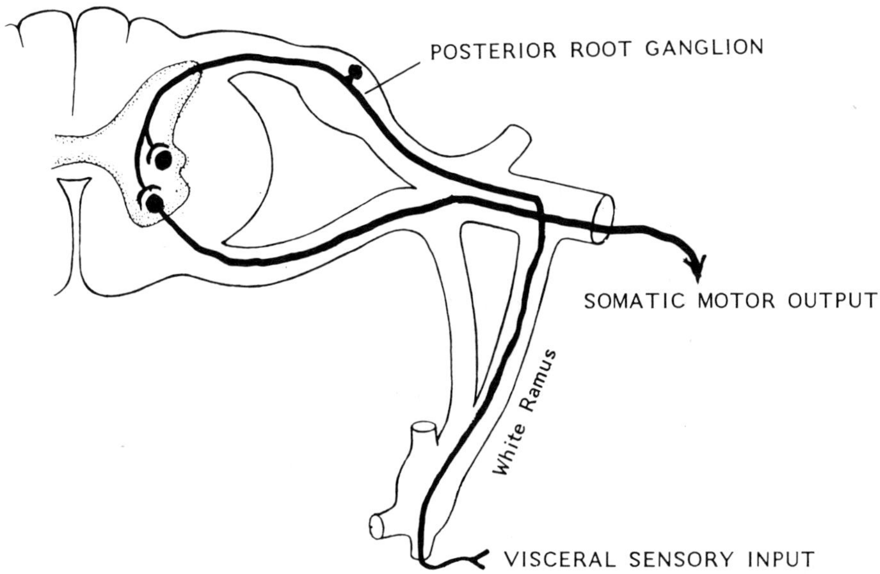

Figure 10.9. A viscerosensory to somatomotor reflex.

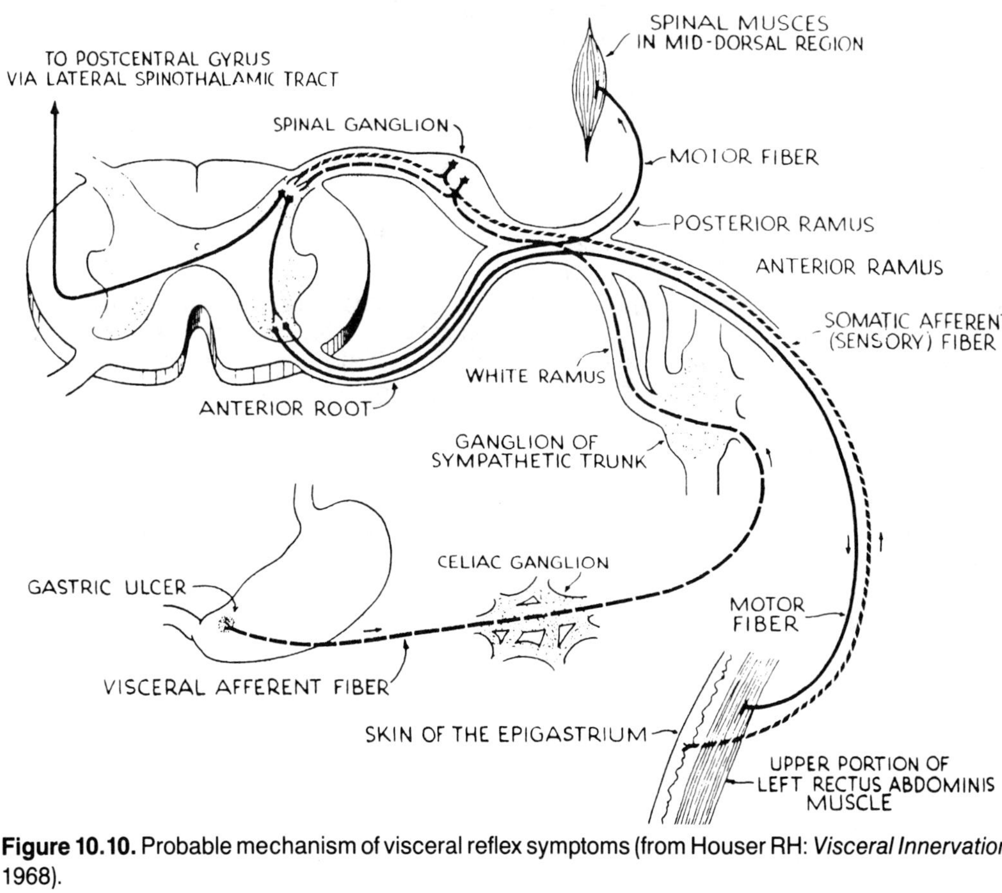

Figure 10.10. Probable mechanism of visceral reflex symptoms (from Houser RH: *Visceral Innervation,* 1968).

tion or compression. Biofeedback training is usually placed in this category.

The *Head-McKenzie sensory zone concept* attempts to explain how visceral pain can radiate to certain parts of the skin (Fig. 10.10). A familiar example, states Hart, is cardiac ischemia with radiating pain to the left arm. According to Gaensler, Wernoe found that a visceral problem can exhibit in a specific dermatomal segment via a viscerocutaneous reflex and that the stimulation of the skin can have a distinct effect on a related visceral area via a cutaneovisceral reflex.

De Sterno and other researchers have attempted to show that visceral problems may refer to the skin or subcutaneous tissues and give rise to trigger points, acupuncture points, and/or other disorders. Diagnostically, certain superficial areas have long been known to relate to an underlying visceral condition such as pain in the right shoulder in gallbladder disease. It is often noted clinically that a disease in an internal organ will produce pain, tenderness, hyperesthesia, or hypesthesia, etc, in some area of the skin. Such a viscerocutaneous reflex is thought by many to be mediated by unknown pathways of the sympathetic chain.

Janse stated that viscerosomatic reflexes have important diagnostic connotations and are frequently reported to be an important cause of referred pain, reflex paravertebral spasm, vertebral subluxations, trigger points, and acupoints.

Most authorities agree that any irritant introduced into a viscus that is adequate to stimulate receptors will send impulses (1) back over splanchnic efferents; (2) produce paravertebral hyperalgesia, hypermyotonia, and frequently spasm; and (3) send pain signals to higher CNS centers (the interpretation of which may be of either a local or referred nature).

The degree of increased muscle tension at the spine will depend upon the strength of the irritation at the receptor site, the functional state of the neurons and synapses involved, and the anatomical location of the lesion. On this latter point, Pottenger found that reflexes initiated at the posterior aspect of a lung manifest somatically at the back, while those initiated at the anterior aspect of a lung will involve the ventral chest muscles. Sachs, however, reports that viscerosensory reflexes cause greater pain posteriorly than anteriorly regardless of origin. This point becomes important in the differential diagnosis of spinal pain.

Balduc points out that viscerosomatic reflexes are intensity-oriented (ie, the reflex response is proportional to the intensity of the visceral input), mediated by gamma fibers (excitation of flexor motor neurons, inhibition of extensor motor neurons), converge on the spine in a spatial gradient, converge on the head and neck or the pelvis, and produce both spinal and extraspinal effects. It is postulated that increased visceral activity influences a neurologic "gate" in the affected spinal cord segment. As the visceral gate opens, the somatic gate closes. The visceral impulses spread from the posterior to the anterior horn of the spinal cord and then to supraspinal centers that control the integrity of the reflex response, which, states Balduc, is prolonged beyond stimulation termination. The difference between somatovisceral and the viscerosomatic reflexes appears to be only quantitative and to be accounted for by the lesser density of the nociceptive receptors in the viscera.

Viscerovisceral Reflexes

A viscerovisceral reflex develops when a sensory receptor in an internal organ, gland, or vessel is stimulated to trigger a volley of reflex impulses to another anatomical location of this type via efferents of the autonomic nervous system. Refer to Appendix, Figure A.8. Rarely, however, does this reflex exist alone; ie, it usually has a segmental somatic component. Therapeutically, similar reflexes are commonly evoked by spinal manipulation, deep heat, and hypnosis or other forms of psychotherapy.

Pottenger stated that viscerovisceral reflexes constitute the basis of normal physiologic integration and form the basis in most, if not all, disease conditions. See Figures 10.11 and 10.12. In disease, exaggerated reflexes can readily confuse the diagnostic process. The classic example is a gallbladder reflex increasing the sympathetic output to the

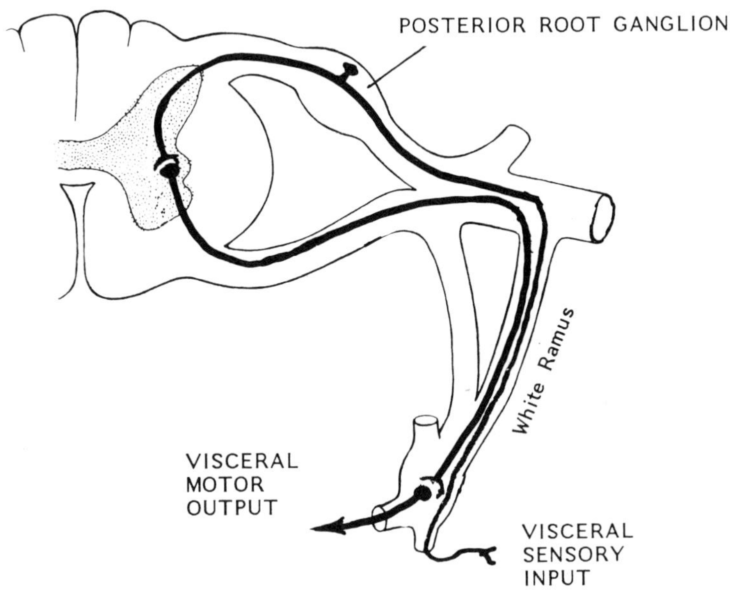

Figure 10.11. A viscerosensory to visceromotor reflex.

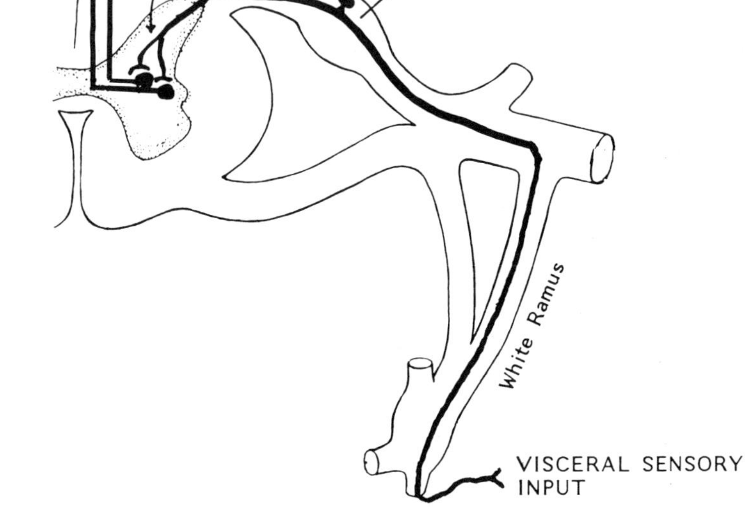

Figure 10.12. A viscerosensory to viscerosensory referral.

stomach, which produces gastric symptoms far greater than the initiating gallbladder lesion. Thus, therapy directed to the stomach would be of minimal benefit.

Visceroviscerel reflexes are not confined to segmentally related regions of the spine. The nausea and vomiting associated with gastrointestinal problems are generally considered visceroviscerel reflexes. Pottenger, Kuntz, and others relate the nausea-vomiting and headaches associated with many genecologic disorders with visceroviscerel reflexes.

In Iggo/Leek's study of reflex regulation of gastric activity, they found that impulses could be recorded from single vagal motor axons in sheep during reflex gastric contrac-

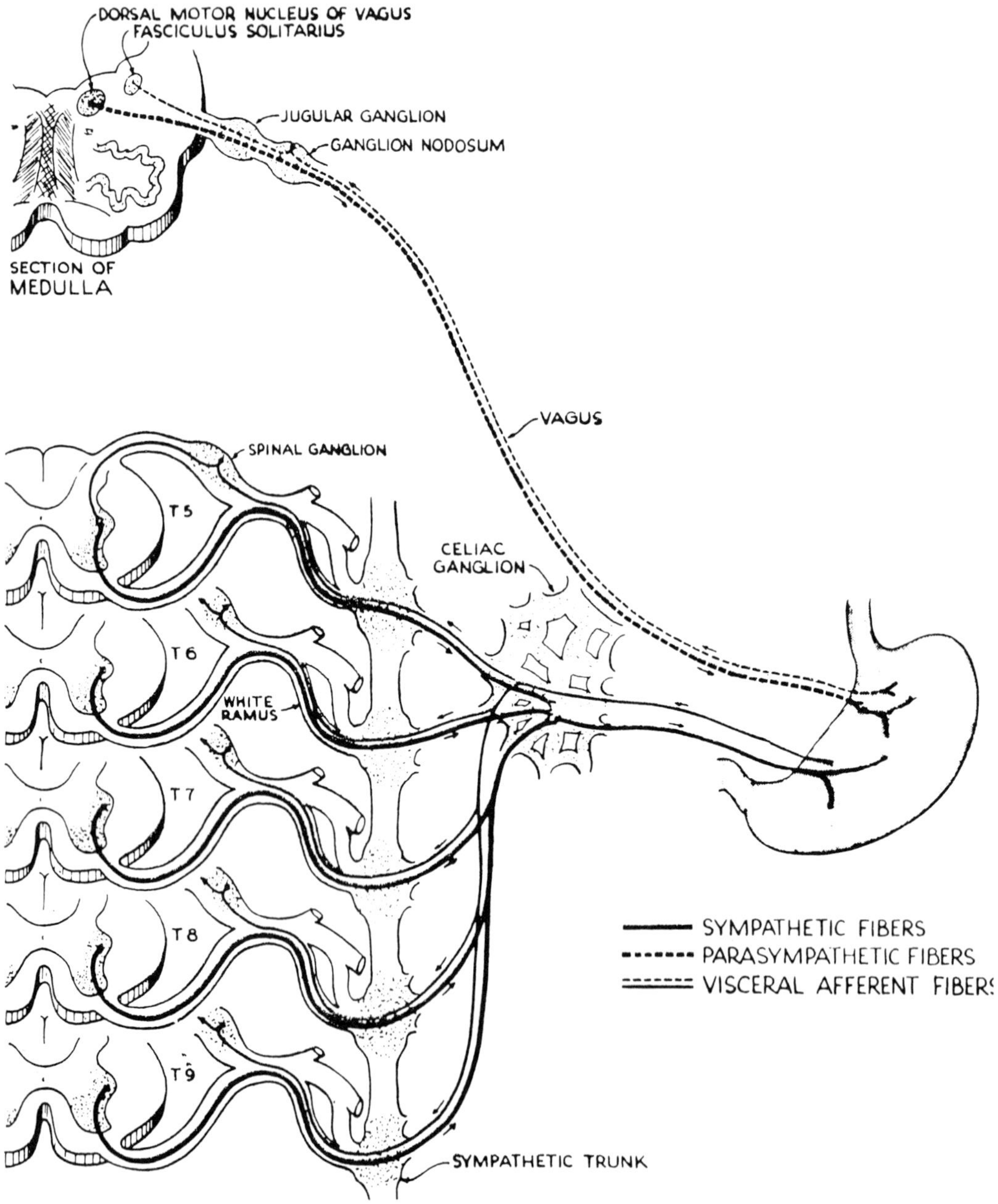

Figure 10.13. Autonomic innervation of the stomach (from Houser RH: *Visceral Innervation,* 1968).

tions. Several different patterns of activity associated with contractions of different parts of the stomach were found. Each unit had a stable and characteristic pattern of discharge, and the discharge of a unit could be modified by a general excitatory stimulus; eg, acidification of the gastric contents or by afferent feedback from the part of the stomach that as contracting.

Psychovisceral and Somatopsychic Reflexes

Psychovisceral Reflexes

Because the body acts and reacts as a whole, some degree of primary or secondary psychosomatic and psychovisceral reflexes are undoubtedly involved in any condition that causes personal distress (mental or physical). The classic example of a psychovisceral reflex is the relationship of chronic worry with gastric hyperacidity leading to the formation of peptic ulcers. In studying this phenomena, Cobb has shown that stimulating the anterior nuclei of the diencephalon produces a barrage of vagal impulses that, in time, results in hemorrhage and ulceration of the lining of the stomach and other functional aberrations. See Figure 10.13.

Freeman, Kuntz, and White/Smithwick state that just about every visceral function has shown to be subject to influence exerted by emotional states through the autonomic nerves, and Sachs suggests that psychic reflexes may produce viscerosensory, visceromotor, and/or viscerovisceral reflexes. Guyton credits the diarrhea associated with emotional stress to hyperparasympathetic activity and emotionally related constipation to hypersympathicotonia.

Somatopsychic and Visceropsychic Reflexes

It also should be kept in mind, because the body is a whole, that the reverse is also true; ie, the role of somatopsychic and visceropsychic reflexes is just as important. Just as the mind can affect somatic and visceral structures, somatic and visceral stimulation can affect mental and emotional processes. Because the nervous system is so highly integrated, distress within the body can never truly have only a localized effect.

While some may not feel that emotional stress is a point for chiropractic treatment, it has been demonstrated by Quigley, Schwartz, Steward, and others that finding and normalizing IVF and apophyseal lesions and reflex foci is a frequently effective method in reducing noxious afferent activity to the psychic centers. A large number of conditions are known to have psychosomatic and psychovisceral relationships. It thus may be assumed that chronic articular fixations may be effective psychologic irritants after nonarticular mechanical, chemical, and thermal irritants have been removed. Janse frequently offered the hypothesis that spinal subluxations have inimical effects upon the ascending pathways of the reticular activating system, which can create numerous stress-producing symptoms, restlessness, and insomnia.

As the effectiveness of case management can be influenced by the psyche, it should be considered when determining diagnosis, scope of therapy, and prognosis. These psychic considerations do not require the scope and depth of clinical psychology, but they should consider the physical, personal, social, and environmental aspects involved in the case before a diagnosis is arrived at if holistic care is the goal.

Homewood points out that chiropractors should not underestimate the potency of their technical armamentarium for normalizing structure as a means of reaching and eliminating a large variety of psychic dysfunctions. This educator believes that the same is true for the normalization of spinal-related somatovisceral reflexes. Unfortunately, there has been a trend in the profession during the past decade or so to quietly restrict chiropractic care to the correction of biomechanical faults and musculoskeletal injuries. While it can be argued that chiropractic care can be readily justified in such "orthopedic" cases, the empiric results obtained by chiropractic therapy directed to visceral and psychic disorders should not be ignored, even if the laboratory means to test the hypothetical mechanisms involved have not as yet been developed. To do so would be an injustice to society.

Some Diagnostic and Therapeutic Procedures Under Investigation

At certain points on the body surface, Janse, Bennett, DeJarnette, Chapman, Goodheart, etc, have shown that there are areas from which the reflexes of muscle relaxation, homeostasis, and postural competence can be initiated. These are called Valleix points. Janse stated that the primary zones appear to be (1) the parasacral areas, (2) the suboccipital zones, and (3) the soles of the feet. Neurolymphatic points and neurovascular points also can be considered in this category, and some authorities place the cranial membranes and various acupoints and auricular points in this general category.

Noxious foci from hypothesized microcirculatory defects have long been thought to be an important consideration in the diagnosis and/or treatment of a wide variety of musculoskeletal and visceral dysfunctions. Because of this, several empiric approaches have been developed. The *acupoints* of meridian therapy might well be an example of such sites. Bennett postulated the concept of *neurovascular reflexes*, and Chapman (as described by Magoun, Mitchell) outlined a similar system of *neurolymphatic reflexes*. De Jarnette describes several topographic reflex sites in his Sacro-Occipital Technique (S.O.T.) manuals that are reported to have far-reaching effects, and Upledger/Vredevoogh have expounded on the studies of Sutherland (as described by Wales) on the effects of cranial subluxations on cerebrospinal circulation and reflexes.

Several empiric concepts frequently used have implications in physical diagnosis and therapy. A few of these are briefly described in this section. The exact interrelationships of the sensory, motor, and autonomic nervous systems, however, have not been determined to the degree they can be described in detail.

The various concepts and clinical approaches described in this section remain in the investigatory stage and may not be appropriate or authorized under state law. The American Chiropractic Association has not adopted specific policy in relation to these concepts or procedures.

Applied Kinesiology

Applied kinesiology is a relatively new branch of clinical chiropractic that utilizes muscle testing as a barometer and monitor of a patient's physiologic, anatomical, and emotional state of health. Analysis (therapy localization and the direction of therapy) is achieved by a complex method of interpreting body language expressing through the muscular system, according to Goodheart and Stoner.

Five basic elements are found within the IVF: nerves, blood vessels, lymph vessels, spinal fluid, and the acupuncture meridian connector. The systemic reflections of these elements are challenged during analysis, then therapy is directed to balancing any one or combination of the five basic elements in addition to adjusting specific vertebrae to relieve the dysfunction of the system(s).

Goodheart, Walther, and others have attempted to correlate the basic neurovascular concepts of Bennett and the neurolymphatic concepts of Chapman with the musculoskeletal system, and Mitchell and Schmitt have related them to the endocrine system. It should be noted that the charts used in applied kinesiology do not correspond in many instances with the original charts of Bennett and Chapman.

Basic Technique

Basic technique is described by Coggins and Gabel as a system of body mechanics that is directed to normalizing body structure to maintain normal function, with emphasis on postural alignment of the spine and pelvis and balancing their associated soft tissues. Certain structural patterns and spinal distortions have been isolated, and their recognition and interpretation guide the direction of therapy.

The primary premise of basic technique states that the body of the lowest freely movable vertebra will rotate to the low side of the sacrum or the vertebral foundation upon which it rests. In other words, the body of the lowest freely movable vertebra will always rotate to the side of least support. This is thought to be indicated by the low side of the sacrum in most but not all instances. Another premise of basic technique is that the sacrum is the mechanical centrum of the body and strategically situated as the foundation of the spinal column. It is considered the key of the mechanical system of spinal levers; viz, the ligaments and muscles that are attached to the spine, pelvis, and rib cage.

Imbalances are treated by a specific cutaneous contact under the sacrotuberous ligament, the gluteal muscles, or other designated areas of the posterior pelvis. These contacts are commonly thought to evoke somatosomatic reflexes, but there is little doubt that somatovisceral reflexes are also associated.

Craniotherapy

Craniotherapy, manipulation of the cranial and facial bones, was developed within pioneer chiropractic by Nephi Cottam and within osteopathy by W.G. Sutherland during the 1920s and 1930s. Interest in this procedure has remained stable within osteopathy, and investigation is currently being spearheaded by Upledger. Few, if any, chiropractic colleges currently teach the technique and rationale, but DeJarnette is developing a group with common interest in this area that appears to be growing within the chiropractic profession.

Craniosacral therapy emphasizes the concept of dynamic activity involving the cranial bones, meningeal membranes, cerebrospinal fluid, the intracranial vascular system, the sacrum, the movement of body fluids, and their effect on the function of all body systems.

Meridian Therapy

Forms of stimulation to specific sites on the skin have been utilized for at least 3000 years. It is only within the last 20 years, however, that comprehensive studies of acupuncture as a legitimate therapy have been seriously undertaken in this country. Acupuncture is founded on the premise that stimulation of certain sites in the skin has an effect on distant functional mechanisms of the body. Various experimental data tend to support the involvement of a *cutaneovisceral* reflex, but the exact mechanism is unknown.

Meridian Point Foci. Meridian therapy with needles, moxa, electrical stimulation, or other modalities most likely works by a neuromechanism; viz, by blocking pain signals in or to the brain by projecting inhibitory impulses to the thalamus and/or cerebral cortex and ultimately to the cord, and finally, by blocking noxious stimuli through the pathophysiologic reflex and thus producing muscular relaxation. Therefore, it should be noted that acupuncture, like the objectives of articular adjustment, is veiled in empiric evidence. Although the Melzack-Wall theory attempted to explain how pain pathways can be blocked, it does not adequately explain any possible localized tissue changes that are known to occur. By extension of this theory, however, local tissue changes may be postulated on the basis of localized vasomotor changes; ie, improvement in the local microcirculation.

Alarm Points. As far as physical diagnosis is concerned, the most important contribution of acupuncture studies recognized in the United States has been the isolation of certain diagnostic "alarm points." Spontaneous pain, pain on pressure, or excessive electropermeability at one of these points is thought by many to indicate that some disorder is present in the associated meridian. For example, it is claimed that spontaneous or induced pain at a specific point on the thorax indicates a problem in the lung meridian; this alarm point is LU-1 (Fig. 10.14). All alarm points are located on the ventral surface of the thorax and the abdomen, and each point is associated with one of the 12 main meridians and its function.

It is thought by Oriental physicians that tenderness or pain elicited by light pressure on or spontaneous pain at any of these points indicates that the meridian has excessive "energy" (Chi). Tenderness only on heavy pressure indicates that there is a deficiency of Chi, according to acupuncturists. Generally, the alarm points are associated with the Yin types of diseases; viz, those diseases associated with cold, depression, and weakness. Table 10.2 lists the alarm points for the 12 meridians and gives the anatomical location of each.

Several journals have developed in recent years that describe case histories, research, and current hypotheses involving meridian therapy. In an independent study, Luciani reports a case history that exemplifies the fact that a pathologic somatic condition may produce an abnormal visceral response and that when the somatic pathology was treated and alleviated by acupuncture, visceral as well as somatic symptoms were relieved.

Neurolymphatic Reflexes

Neurolymphatic receptors are reported to be located singularly or in multiples on the anterior and posterior aspects of the body, varying in size from that of a pea to a bean. Most of the larger muscles have about four drainage points; ie, two anterior and two posterior. It is reported that tender neurolymphatic receptors do not correspond to the sites of lymph glands; rather, they appear to be related to the lymphatic system according to a hypothesis developed by Chapman, an osteopath. See Figure 10.15.

It is believed by many clinicians that neurolymphatic reflexes inhibit lymph flow when the system becomes "overloaded" and that neurolymphatic receptor "blockage" has a similar effect as that of neurovascular blockage; ie, a prohibition of normal dilation and an abnormal local metabolic response. Deep massage on a selected neurolymphatic point is used to break the noxious reflex cycle. In-depth studies are needed to place the empiric results observed on a scientific basis. Some type of somatosomatic and/or somatovisceral reflex is likely involved.

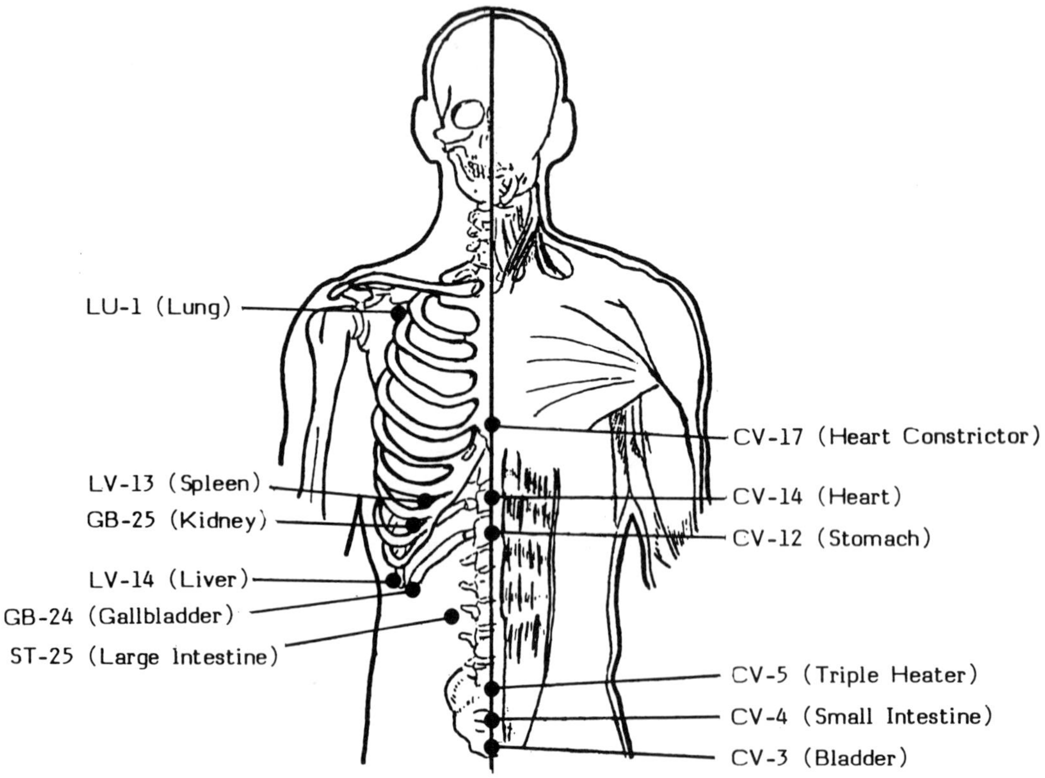

Figure 10.14. Alarm points, according to meridian therapy concepts.

Neurovascular Reflexes

Through observation and personal experimentation, Bennett discovered the neurovascular receptors in the early 1930s, primarily associating these receptors with visceral disturbances. Several neurovascular points were isolated, and they are shown in Figure 10.16. In most instances, one light cutaneous traction contact is taken on a specific distal receptor and another near a specific segment of the spine.

Bennett has attributed specific areas of hypertonicity as indicating specific visceral malfunction. Proponents of the system believe that many somatic problems which resist local and spinal treatment may be cleared by attention to the malfunctioning viscus. In the process, the associated vertebral subluxation (myogenically induced) becomes corrected. Bennett also stressed that the arteriole and capillary bed were the effector mechanism, projecting that it is here that tissue changes occur and function is normalized. Bennett was primarily interested in establishing normal physiology in the vital organs so dependent appendages also would benefit, whereas many others are concerned with normalizing the musculoskeletal system as an end in itself.

Bennett and his associates have based their work in this area on the hypothesis that any blockage (eg, inhibitory reflex) of the neurovascular receptors will prohibit normal metabolic responses from occurring, leading to an accumulation of metabolic debris in the muscles. This, in turn, causes further blood vessel dilation. It is postulated that, as vascular dilation occurs through a vasomotor response, any blockage of a neurovascular receptor prohibits normal function in the capillary bed. Continued research is necessary to verify the abundance of empiric results reported. Some type of somatosomatic and/or somatovisceral reflex is likely involved in the procedure.

Table 10.2. Alarm Points of the Body*

Meridian	Alarm Point	Location
		BILATERAL POINTS
Lung	LU-1	1 cun† below clavicle, lateral 2nd—3rd rib interspace.
Liver	LV-14	On vertical nipple line, between 6th—7th ribs.
Gallbladder	GB-24	On vertical nipple line, between 8th—9th ribs.
Spleen	LV-13	Anterior tip of 11th rib.
Kidney	GB-25	Anterior tip of 12th rib.
Large intestine	ST-25	2 cun lateral to navel.
		MIDLINE POINTS
Heart constrictor	CV-17	Midsternal, nipple level, 3/4ths down from episternal notch.
Heart	CV-14	6 cun above navel, just below xiphoid process.
Stomach	CV-12	4 cun above navel, epigastrium, midway between the sternum and navel.
Triple heater	CV-5	2 cun below navel.
Small intestine	CV-4	3 cun below navel.
Bladder	CV-3	4 cun below navel.

*From Jaskoviak/Schafer: *Applied Physiotherapy.*
†A *cun* is a "human inch," approximately the width of the individual's thumb.

Bibliography

Alpers BJ: *Clinical Neurology.* Philadelphia, F.A. Davis, 1963, p 729.

American Hospital Association: *Stress.* Chicago, American Hospital Association, 1977.

Arbuckle BE: Reflexes. *Journal of the American Osteopathic Association,* 46(7), July 12, 1946.

Armould-Frochot S: Investigation of the effect of chiropractic adjustments on a specific gynecological symptom: dysmenorrhea. *Bulletin of the European Chiropractic Union,* 25(1):17, 1977.

Balduc HA: Overview of contemporary chiropractic science for the chiropractic association of Oklahoma. Northwestern College of Chiropractic, Convention notes, April 24, 1983.

Beal MC: Viscerosomatic reflexes: A review. *Journal of the American Osteopathic Association,* 85:786-801, 1985.

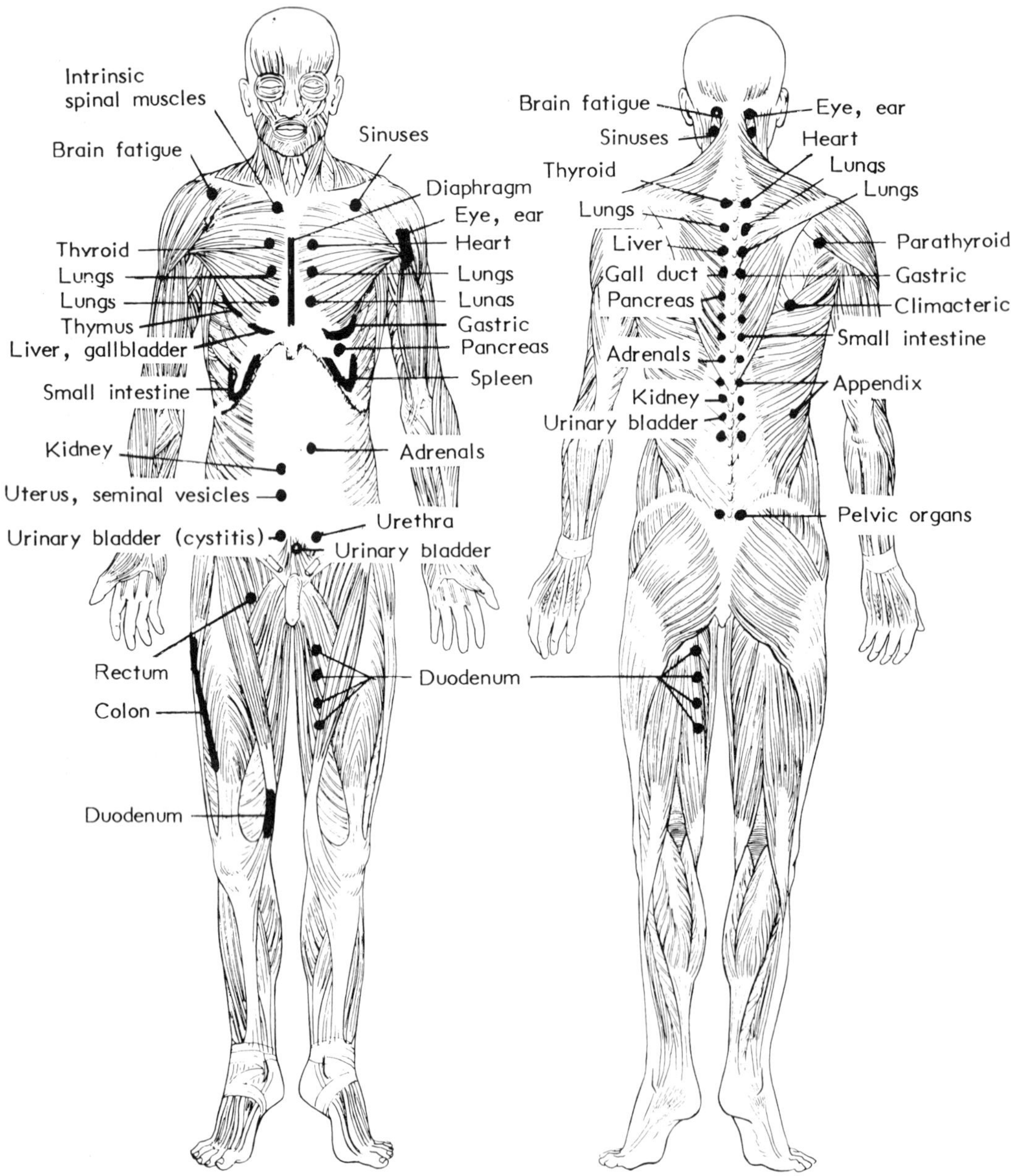

Figure 10.15. Approximate location of some neurolymphatic points. Most points are bilateral except those on or near the sternum, but the points are shown only on one side in the drawings.

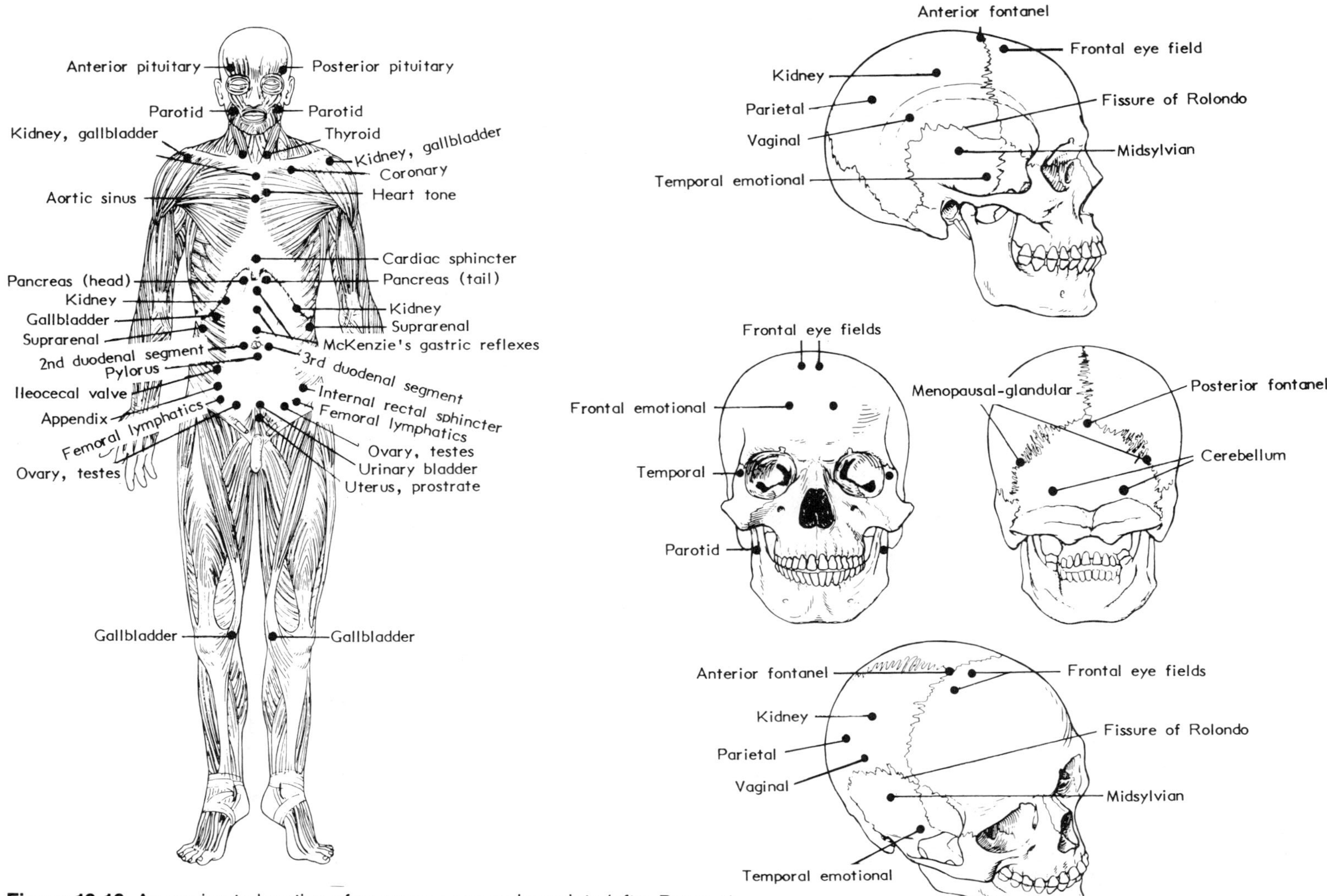

Figure 10.16. Approximate location of some neurovascular points (after Bennett).

Bennett TJ: *A New Clinical Basis for the Correction of Abnormal Physiology* (Formerly, Autonomic Nerve Control). Burlingame, CA, published by author, 1960.

Berger PA: Medical treatment of mental illness. *Science*, 200:974-981, 1978.

Boyd WA: *A Textbook of Pathology*. Philadelphia, Lea & Febiger, 1961.

Brazier MAB: *Electrical Activity of the Nervous System*, ed 4. Baltimore, Williams & Wilkins, 1977, pp 9, 10, 29, 34.

Brown T, et al: Psychological factors in low back pain. *New England Journal of Medicine*, 25:4-22, 1954.

Burns L, Chandler LC, Rice RW: *Pathogenesis of Visceral Disease Following Vertebral Lesions*. Chicago, American Osteopathic Association, 1948.

Busch BW, Danelius BD, Drost SF: Cardiovascular changes after chiropractic: Effects of chiropractic adjustment on selected physiological parameters of the cardiovascular system. *ACA Journal of Chiropractic*, 8(3):S33-S39, 1974.

Cabot RC: *Physical Diagnosis*. New York, William Wood, 1919, pp 270, 490-491.

Canadian Memorial Chiropractic College: *Segmental Neuropathy*. Toronto, Canadian Memorial Chiropractic College, date of publication not shown. Monograph, pp 8-11, 23-28.

Chusid JG: *Correlative Neuroanatomy & Functional Neurology*, ed 19. Los Altos, CA, Lange Medical, 1985, pp 177-179, 241, 250-253.

Clark RG: *Manter and Gatz's Essentials of Clinical Neuroanatomy and Neurophysiology*, ed 5. Philadelphia, F.A. Davis, 1975, pp 120-126.

Cobb S: *Foundations of Neuropsychiatry*. Baltimore, Williams & Wilkins, 1948, pp 18, 100, 108, 117, 180, 235.

Coggins WN: *Basic Technique: A System of Body Mechanics*. Creve Coeur, MO, published by author, 1983.

Coote JH: Central organization of somatosympathetic reflexes. In Haldeman S (ed): *Modern Developments in the Principles and Practice of Chiropractic*. New York, Appleton-Century-Crofts, 1980, pp 107-116.

Coote JH, et al: Reflex discharges into thoracic white rami elicited by somatic and visceral afferent excitation. *Journal of Physiology*, 202:141-159, 1969.

Coote JH: Impulse-based mechanisms: Somatic sources of afferent input as factors in aberrant autonomic, sensory, and motor function. In Korr IM (ed): *The Neurobiologic Mechanisms in Manipulative Therapy*. New York, Plenum Press, 1978, pp 91-127.

Coote JH, Perez-Gonzales JF: The response of some sympathetic neurones to volleys in various afferent nerves. *Journal of Physiology* (British), 208:261-278, 1970.

Cottam C: *Cranial and Facial Adjusting, Illustrated Step-by-Step*. Los Angeles, self-published, 1986.

Daube JR, Sandok BA: *Medical Neurosciences*. Boston, Little, Brown, 1978, pp 226- 227.

Debrunner HU: *Orthopaedic Diagnosis*, rev. ed 2. Translated by G Stiasny. Chicago, Year Book Medical, 1982, p 40.

De Jarnette MB: *Chiropractic Manipulative Technique:* Sacro Occipital Technic; 1975 Seminar Notes. Publication data not shown, privately distributed.

De Jarnette MB: *Sacro Occipital Technic 1977*. Publication data not shown, privately distributed.

De Jarnette MB: *Subluxation Patterns: Sacro Occipital Technic;* 1975 Seminar Notes. Publication data not shown, privately distributed.

de Reuck AVS, Knight J (eds): *Myotactic, Kinesthetic, and Vestibular Mechanisms*. Ciba Foundation Symposium. Boston, Little, Brown, 1967.

De Rusha JL: Upper cervical technic correlated with neurodiagnosis. *ACA Journal of Chiropractic*, September 1961.

De Sterno CV: The pathophysiology of TMJ dysfunction and related pain. In Gelb, H (ed): *Clinical Management of Head, Neck and TMJ Pain and Dysfunction*. Philadelphia, W.B. Saunders, 1977.

Dittmar E: Cutaneo-visceral neural pathways. *Journal of Physical Medicine* (British), 15:208, 1952.

Dubos R: *Biochemical Determination of Microbial Diseases*. Cambridge, MA, Harvard University Press, 1954.

Faulk WP, Demaeyer EM, Davies AJ: Some effects of malnutrition on the immune response in man. *American Journal of Clinical Nutrition*, 27:638-646, 1974.

Feldenkrais M: *Body and Mature Behavior*. New York, International University Press, 1949, pp 5, 15, 20, 69, 119, 128, 130, 152.

Fields HL, Meyer GA, Partridge LD Jr: Convergence of visceral and somatic input on to spinal neurons. *Experimental Neurology*, 26:36-52, 1970.

Freedman BG: The biodynamical aspect of cerebrospinal fluid in disease and health. *Journal of Manipulative and Physiological Therapeutics*, 2:79-84, 1979.

Freeman GL: *Physiological Psychology*. New York, Van Nostrand, 1948, pp 135, 279.

Friedman AP (ed): Symposium on headache and related pain syndromes. *Medical Clinics of North America*, 62:427-623, 1978.

Friedman HH: *Problem-Oriented Medical Diagnosis*, ed 2. Boston, Little, Brown, 1979, p 107.

Gabel RA: Basic technique. In Kfoury PW (ed): *Catalog of Chiropractic Techniques*. Chesterfield, MO, Logan College of Chiropractic, 1977, pp 7-11.

Gandhavadi B, Rosen JS, Addison RG: Autonomic Pain features and methods of assessment. *Postgraduate Medicine*, 7(1):85-90, 1982.

Gaensler EA: in *Journal of Clinical Investigation*, 30:406, 1951.

Giles LG: Spinal fixation and viscera. *Journal of Clinical Chiropractic*, 1(3): 144-145, 1973.

Glasgow EF, Twomey LT, Scull ER, Kleynhans AM, Idczak RM: *Aspects of Manipulative Therapy*, ed 2. New York, Churchill Livingstone, 1985, pp 64-71.

Goodheart GJ: Applied kinesiology. In Kfoury PW (ed): *Catalog of Chiropractic Techniques*. Chesterfield, MO, Logan College of Chiropractic, 1977, pp 117-119.

Goodheart GJ: *Applied Kinesiology (The Neurolymphatic Reflex and Its Relationship to Muscle Balancing)*, ed 3. Published by author, 1965.

Goodheart GJ: *Applied Kinesiology (The Neuro-vascular Reflex and Its Relationship to Muscle Balancing)*, ed 5. Published by author, 1967.

Goodheart GJ: *Applied Kinesiology*, ed 16. Detroit,

published by author, vol I, 1980.

Goodheart GJ: *Collected Published Articles and Reprints.* Montpellier, OH, Williams County Publishing, 1969, pp 23-24.

Gordienko AN (ed): *Control of Immunogenesis by the Nervous System.* Washington, DC, US Department of Commerce, 1958, pp 22-33, 45-52, 53-58.

Green EE, et al: Voluntary control of internal states: psychological and physio logical. *Journal of Transpersonal Psychology,* II, 1970.

Guilliam N: Evolution of the nervous system. *ACA Journal of Chiropractic,* May 1970.

Gurkalo VK, Zabezhinski MA: On participation of the autonomic nervous system in the mechanisms of chemical carcinogenesis. *Neoplasma,* 29:301-307, 1982.

Guth L: "Trophic" influences of nerve on muscle. *Physiological Reviews,* 48:645-687, 1968.

Gutmann E: Neurotrophic relations. *Annual Review of Physiology,* 38:177-216, 1976.

Guyton AC: *Textbook of Medical Physiology,* ed 6. Philadelphia, W.B. Saunders, 1981, pp 707-708, 718-720, 784-835.

Haldeman S: Discussion: The importance of neurophysiological research into the principles of spinal manipulation. In Goldstein M (ed): *The Research Status of Spinal Manipulative Therapy.* Bethesda, MD, National Institutes of Health, DHEW Publication No. (NIH) 76-998, 1975, pp 184-185.

Haldeman S: Referred pain: Extra spinal symptoms of spinal origin. *The Texas Chiropractor,* July 1974.

Hanning JM: The role of the emotions in clinical practice. *The Chirogram,* February 1974.

Hart FD (ed): *The Treatment of Chronic Pain.* Philadelphia, F.A. Davis, 1974, p 8.

Hix EL: Reflex viscerosomatic reference phenomena. *Osteopathic Annals,* 4(12): 496-503, 1976.

Hoag JM: Musculoskeletal involvement in chronic lung disease. *Journal of the American Osteopathic Association,* 7(7): 698-706, 1972.

Homewood AE: *The Neurodynamics of the Vertebral Subluxation,* ed 3. Place of publication not shown, published by author, 1981, pp 40-42, 121-122, 131-132, 278-283, 286-297.

Houser RH: *Visceral Innervation.* Des Moines, IA, Foundation for Chiropractic Education and Research, 1968, pp 9-55.

Hviid C: A comparison of the effect of chiropractic treatment on respiratory function in patients with respiratory distress symptoms and patients without. *Bulletin of the European Chiropractic Union,* 26(1):17-34, 1978.

Iggo A, Leek BF: Reflex regulation of gastric activity. *Acta Neurovegetativa,* 28(4):353-359, 1966.

Il'in VS, Emel'yantsev AM, Komarov GP, Pleskov MV, Razumovskaya NI, Semenova Tyan-Shanskaya VV: Trophic influence of the nervous system: Their biochemical basis and disturbance in skeletal muscle. *Neuroscience and Behavioral Physiology,* 6(2): 175-187, 1973.

Janse J: A concept: The neurological element as it relates to clinical chiropractic. *The Chirogram,* December 1975.

Janse J: History of the development of chiropractic concepts: Chiropractic terminology. In Goldstein M (ed): *The Research Status of Spinal Manipulative Therapy.* Bethesda, MD, National Institutes of Health, DHEW Publication No. (NIH) 76-998, 1975, pp 26-27.

Janse J: The integrative purpose and function of the nervous system: A review of classical literature. *Journal of Manipulative and Physiological Therapeutics,* 1(3), September 1978.

Janse J: Interrelation between psychic disturbances and body balance. *National College Journal of Chiropractic,* 14(4):3-6, December 1941.

Janse J: Nerve reaction—causes of psycho-neurosis are outlined. *Journal of the National Chiropractic Association,* XI:25-27, February 1942.

Janse J: *Principles and Practice of Chiropractic.* Lombard, IL, National College of Chiropractic, 1976, pp 209, 310.

Johnston RJ: Vertebrogrenic autonomic dysfunction—subjective symptoms: A prospective study. *Journal of the Canadian Chiropractic Association,* 25(2): 51-63, 1981.

Judge RD, Zuidema GD (eds): *Methods of Clinical Examination: A Physiological Approach,* ed 3. Boston, Little, Brown, 1968, pp 154, 346, 357-358.

Judovitch B, Bates W: *Segmental Neuralgia in Painful Syndromes.* Philadelphia, F.A. Davis, 1946, pp 3, 6, 221.

Kaufman A, Sato A, Sato Y, Sugimoto H: Reflex changes in heart rate after mechanical and thermal stimulation of the skin at various segmental levels in cats. *Neuroscience,* 2:102-109, 1977.

Keller RM: Consideration of the electronic factor in irritation. *Journal of the National Chiropractic Association,* XXIII:13-14, February 1953.

Kellgren JH: Observations on referred pain arising from muscle. *Clinical Science,* 3:175, 1938.

Kfoury PW (ed): *Catalog of Chiropractic Techniques.* Chesterfield, MO, Logan College of Chiropractic, 1977.

Koizumi K: Autonomic system reaction caused by excitation of somatic afferents: Study of cutaneo-intestinal reflex. In Korr IM (ed): *The Neurobiologic Mechanisms in Manipulative Therapy.* New York, Plenum Press, 1978, pp 219-227.

Korr IM (ed): *The Neurobiologic Mechanisms in Manipulative Therapy.* New York, Plenum Press, 1978, pp 11-16, 58-60, 179-217, 295-301.

Korr IM: Neurochemical and neurotrophic consequences of nerve deformation: Clinical implications in relation to spinal manipulation. *Journal of the American Osteopathic Association,* 75(12):409-414, 1975.

Korr IM: Trophic functions of nerves and their mechanisms. *Journal of the American Osteopathic Association,* 72(2):163-171, 1972.

Kunert W: Functional disorders of internal organs due to vertebral lesions. *Ciba Symposium,* 13(3), 1965.

Kuntz A: Autonomic and physiologic properties of cutaneovisceral vasomotor reflex arcs. *Journal of Neurophysiology,* 8:421-429, 1945.

Kuntz A: *The Autonomic Nervous System,* ed 4. Philadelphia, Lea & Febiger, 1949, pp 21-22, 36-37, 43-86, 151-157, 205, 248-255, 270, 289-304, 427-429, 457, 492.

Leach RA: *The Chiropractic Theories,* ed 2. Baltimore,

Williams & Wilkins, 1986, pp 132-150, 153-185, 193-202.

Luciani R: The somatic-visceral autonomic reflex: One mechanism in acupuncture therapeutics. *Osteopathic Annals*, 2(12):34-41, 1974.

Magoun HI: *Osteopathy in the Cranial Field*, ed 2. Kirksville, MO, Journal Printing Company, 1966.

Magoun HI: *Practical Osteopathic Procedures*. Kirksville, MO, Journal Printing Company, 1978.

Masarsky C, Weber M: Chiropractic and lung volumes—A retrospective study. *ACA Journal of Chiropractic*, 23(9):65-68, September 1986.

Matsumoto T, Hayes MF: Acupuncture, electric phenomena of the skin, and postvagotomy gastrointestinal atony. *American Journal of Surgery*, 125:176-180, 1973.

Miller WD: The treatment of visceral disorders by manipulative therapy. In Goldstein M (ed): *The Research Status of Spinal Manipulative Therapy*. Bethesda, MD, National Institutes of Health, DHEW Publication No. (NIH) 76-998, 1975, pp 295-299.

Mitchell FL, et al: *An Evaluation and Treatment Manual of Osteopathic Manipulative Procedure*. Kansas City, The Institute for Continuing Education in Osteopathic Principles, 1973.

Mitchell FL: The influence of Chapman's reflexes and the immune reactions. In Stark EH (ed): *Osteopathic Medicine*. Acton, MA, Publishing Sciences Group, 1975, pp 179-182.

Morgan WP: Selected psychological considerations. *Research Quarterly*, 45:374, 1974.

Mumenthaler M: *Neurology*, ed 2; translated by EH Burrows. New York, Thieme Stratton, 1983, p 266.

Nelson GE: A study of chiropractic and the neurodystrophic process. *Journal of the National Chiropractic Association*, XVIII:30-33, December 1948.

Norman J, Whitman JG: The vagal contribution to changes to heart rate evoked by stimulation of cutaneous nerves. *Journal of Physiology* (British), 234:89-90, 1973.

Olehey IH, Parker AM: Our basis for chiropractic survival. *Journal of the National Chiropractic Association*, XII:21-23, December 1943.

Olson WH, Brumback RA, Gascon G, Christoferson LA: *Practical Neurology for the Primary Care Physician*. Springfield, IL, Charles C Thomas, 1981, pp 122, 220.

Overgaard J: The autonomic nervous system and pain. In Beks JW (ed): *The Management of Pain*. Amsterdam, Elsevier, North-Holland, 1979, pp 306-316.

Palmer DD: *Textbook of the Science, Art and Philosophy of Chiropractic*. Portland, OR, Portland Printing House, 1910, p 7.

Parke WW: Applied anatomy of the spine. In Rothman RH, Simeone FA (eds): *The Spine*. Philadelphia, W.B. Saunders, 1975, vol I, pp 33-35.

Parkinson D, Johnston D, Chaudhuri A: Sympathetic connections to the fifth and sixth cranial nerves. *Anatomical Record*, 19(2):221-226, 1978.

Patterson MM, Steinmetz JE: Long-lasting alterations of spinal reflexes: A potential basis for somatic dysfunction. *Manual Medicine*, 2:38-42, 1986.

Paulson GW, Gottlieb G: Developmental reflexes: The reappearance of fetal and neoplastic reflexes in aged patients. *Brain*, 91:37, 1968.

Pottenger FM: *Symptoms of Visceral Disease*, ed 6. St. Louis, C.V. Mosby, 1949, pp 21, 31-32, 76-78, 134-135, 143, 160, 166, 169, 171, 174, 180, 183, 191, 199, 202, 225, 330, 355, 412.

Prior JA, Silberstein JS: *Physical Diagnosis*, ed 5. St. Louis, C.V. Mosby, 1977, pp 394, 417.

Quigley WH: Self-concept, mental health, and chiropractic. *ACA Journal of Chiropractic*, March 1971.

Rasmussen AT: *The Principal Nervous Pathways*, ed 3. New York, MacMillan, pp 39, 140.

Roddie JC: Autonomic nervous system. *Practitioner*, 205:828-835, 1970.

Rychilková E: Vertebrogenic disorders in internal affections, their importance in therapy. In Lewit K, Gutmann G (eds): *Rehabilitácia, Proceedings of the IVth Congress*. Prague, International Federation of Manual Medicine, 1975.

Sachs W: *The Vegetative Nervous System*. London, England, Cassell and Company, 1936, pp 138-140.

Sandoz R: Some reflex phenomena associated with spinal derangements and adjustments. *Annals of the Swiss Chiropractic Association*, VII:45, 1981.

Sato A: Acute adaptional disturbances due to the imbalance of the autonomic nervous system. *Tohoku Journal of Experimental Medicine*, 103:71-92, 1971.

Sato A: Autoadaptation mechanism of the human body. *Tohoku Journal of Experimental Medicine*, 102: 289-312, 1970.

Sato A: The importance of the somato-autonomic reflexes in the regulation of visceral organ function. *Journal of the Canadian Chiropractic Association*, 20(4):32-38, 1976.

Sato A: Physiological studies of the somatoautonomic reflexes. In Haldeman S (ed): *Modern Developments in the Principles and Practice of Chiropractic*. New York, Appleton-Century-Crofts, 1980, pp 93-104.

Sato A: Somatosympathetic reflexes: afferent fibers, central pathways, discharge characteristics. *Physiological Reviews*, 53(4):916-947, 1973.

Sato A: The somatosympathetic reflexes. In Goldstein M (ed): *The Research Status of Spinal Manipulative Therapy*. NINCDS Monograph No. 15, DHEW Publication No. (NIH) 76-998, Stock No. 017-049-00060-7, Washington, DC, U.S. Government Printing Office, 1975, pp 163-171.

Sato A: Spinal and medullary reflex components of the somato-sympathetic reflex discharges evoked by stimulation of the group IV somatic afferents. *Brain Research*, 51:307-318, 1973.

Schafer RC: *Chiropractic Physical and Spinal Diagnosis*. Oklahoma City, Associated Chiropractic Academic Press, 1980, pp V:32-39.

Schafer RC: *Physical Diagnosis: Procedures and Methodology in Chiropractic Practice*. Arlington, VA, American Chiropractic Association. In preparation, to be released in 1989. Chapter 7, Basic Neurologic Considerations.

Schafer RC: *Symptomatology and Differential Diagnosis*. Arlington, VA, American Chiropractic Association, 1986, pp 88-90, 132, 295-297.

Schmitt WH: *Common Glandular Dysfunctions in the General Practice*. Chapel Hill, NC, published by author, 1981.

Schwartz HS (ed): *Mental Health and Chiropractic: A Multidisciplinary Approach.* New Hyde Park, NY, Sessions, 1973.

Schwartz HS: *Home Care for the Emotionally Ill.* Elmhurst, NY, Sessions, 1957, pp 40-52, 139-148, 175-187.

Schwartz HG: Reflex activity within the sympathetic nervous system. *American Journal of Physiology,* 109(4):593-604, 1934.

Selye H: *Stress and Disease.* New York, McGraw-Hill, 1956.

Selye H: *The Stress of Life.* New York, Longmans, 1957.

Selzer M, Spencer WA: Interactions between visceral and cutaneous afferents in the spinal cord: Reciprocal primary efferent fiber depolarization. *Brain Research,* 14:349-366, 1969.

Sherrington C: *The Integrative Action of the Nervous System.* Cambridge, England, Cambridge University Press, 1947, pp 80, 101, 148, 156, 160, 230.

Singer M: Discussion of the trophic function of nerves and their mechanisms in relation to manipulative therapy. In Korr IM (ed): *The Neurobiologic Mechanisms in Manipulative Therapy.* New York, Plenum Press, 1978, pp 411-422.

Singer M, Schade JP (eds): Degeneration patterns in the nervous system. *Progress in Brain Research.* New York, Elsevier, 1965, vol 14.

Speransky AD: *A Basis for the Theory of Medicine;* translated by C.P. Dutt. New York, International Publishers, 1943.

Starý O, Figar S, Andelová E, Hladká V, Janský M, Kalvodova E: The analysis of disorders of vasomotor reactions in lumbosacral syndromes. *Acta Universitatis Carolinac: Medica,* supplement 21:70-72, 1965.

Steward SL: An investigation into the effect of chiropractic adjustments on the psychological state of the patient. Anglo-European Chiropractic College. Thesis, date unknown.

Stiles EG: Reflexology: An osteopathic perspective. *Osteopathic Annals,* 4(9): 376-379, 1976.

Stoddard A: *Manual of Osteopathic Practice.* New York, Harper & Row, 1969, pp 3, 14, 18, 19, 55.

Stoner F: *The Eclectic Approach to Chiropractic.* Las Vegas, F.L.S. Publishing, 1975, pp 16-20, 67-71,

Stoner F: Kinesiology. In Kfoury PW (ed): *Catalog of Chiropractic Techniques.* Chesterfield, MO, Logan College of Chiropractic, 1977.

Strang VV: *Essential Principles of Chiropractic.* Davenport, IA, Palmer College of Chiropractic, 1984, pp 106-109.

Sutherland WG: *The Cranial Bowl.* Mankato, MN, Free Press, 1939.

Tran TA, Kirby JD: The effects of upper cervical adjustment upon the normal physiology of the heart. *ACA Journal of Chiropractic,* 14(6):S58-S62, 1977.

Tran TA, Kirby JD: The effects of upper thoracic adjustment upon the normal physiology of the heart. *ACA Journal of Chiropractic,* 14(3):S25-S28, 1977.

Travell J, Bigelow NH: Referred somatic pain does not follow a simple segmental pattern. *Federation Proceedings,* 5:106, 1946.

Upledger JE, Vredevoogd JD: *Craniosacral Therapy,* Seattle, Eastland Press, 1983.

Vannerson JF: Sympathetic vascular functions in health: Sympathetic vascular malfunction in disease. *Digest of Chiropractic Economics,* 20(1):24-26, 99-100, 1977.

Vazuka FA: *Essentials of the Neurological Examination.* Philadelphia, Smith, Kline, & French Laboratories, 1962.

Vora GS, Bates HA: The effects of spinal manipulation on the immune system (a preliminary report). *ACA Journal of Chiropractic,* 14:S103-S105, 1980.

Wales AL: The Work of William Garner Sutherland. *Journal of the American Osteopathic Association,* 71:788-793, 1972.

Walker HK, Hall WD, Hurst JW (eds): *Clinical Methods.* Woburn, MA, Butterworth, 1976, vol II, pp 789-792.

Walther DS: *Applied Kinesiology; Volume I: Basic Procedures and Muscle Testing.* Pueblo, CO, Systems DC, 1981, pp 42, 110, 220-223, 234-240.

Wang GH, Brown VW: Suprasegmental inhibition of the autonomic reflex. *Journal of Physiology,* 19:564-572, 1956.

Watkins CO: Interference with nerve function. *Journal of the National Chiropractic Association,* XV:19-20, April 1945.

Watkins RJ: A study of typical neurodystrophies under chiropractic treatment. *Journal of the National Chiropractic Association,* XXI:16, June 1951.

White JC, Smithwick R: *The Autonomic Nervous System,* ed 2. New York, MacMillan, p 65.

Wiles M: Footnote. *Spinal Manipulation,* 2(2):5, July 1986.

Young RF, Yu YJ, King RB: Hyperpolarization of trigeminal primary afferents evoked by stimulation of lumbar sympathetic trunk and peripheral nerves. *Experimental Neurology,* 38:64-69, 1973.

Zhigalina LI: The role of non-specific stimulation of the nervous system in cer tain immunological reactions. In Gordienko AN (ed): *Control of Immunogenesis by the Nervous System.* Washington, DC, US Department of Commerce, 1958, pp 110-124.

EPILOGUE

The general purpose I had in mind when setting out to develop this book was to design a manual, directed to the doctor and student of chiropractic, that would serve as a companion to standard texts on clinical neurology and its subdivisions by (1) delineating the essential neurologic principles that I believe form the basis of chiropractic health care and (2) describing how the chiropractic profession has contributed to the core knowledge of clinical neurology.

Among the many excellent suggestions received from the distinguished members of the Editorial Board of Review for this book was the frequent request that descriptions for certain topics be greatly expanded. As can be anticipated, no two reviewers agreed on their selections. If all suggestions were followed, this book could easily have been at least double in size. Such requests, however, are logical because they come from chiropractic educators who wish to impart as much information as possible to chiropractic students and practitioners. Thus, all suggestions were carefully considered, and many were accepted.

An author must face the reality of certain practicalities. For example, an agreement is made between author and publisher prior to book development regarding the general size and scope of a proposed manuscript. While there is usually some latitude for deviation to this initial agreement, an author is obligated to strive to the best of his or her ability to deliver a completed manuscript that is near to its original projection. This means that a decision of priority must often be made during research and creative development of how much space should be allotted for a certain topic and what information should be condensed or deleted to allow for expanded descriptions and explanations. The size and number of tables and figures also enter this equation.

Two other considerations must be made: first, a book's cost quite closely parallels its size. If it becomes too large and expensive to meet a mass audience's approval, its distribution will be sharply limited despite its quality. This would not meet either author's or publisher's communication objectives. Second, a book that becomes too large is more often than not consciously or unconsciously relegated to the bookcase to serve as an occasional reference rather than to a spot near one's favorite reading chair to serve as a practical clinical reference and review of basic principles. It is my hope that the latter will be true for this book.

My intention was to describe the basic principles that comprise the neuroscience foundation of clinical chiropractic, yet I realized that any one topic of the literally hundreds listed could easily be expanded into a full-size text. For example, the subject of neural embryology, which is summarized in about 10 pages in this book, has been the sole subject of many books of comparable size as this. Thus, my task was to describe concisely the vast neurologic implications involved with each topic that would be of *practical value* to the field practitioner and advanced student so that the reader would be encouraged to seek more explicit details from other sources if the need should arise.

As an aid to those who have such an interest in literature documentation, bibliographies have been included at the end of each chapter that will serve as a formative starting point for a comprehensive literature search. Again, because of physical parameters, the bibliographies included in this book represent only about half the number used. Excellent sources for additional titles are the three volume set: *Chiropractic Research Archives Collection (CRAC)*, published by Canadian Memorial Chiropractic College; *Medical Books and Serials in Print*, published by R.R. Bowker Company (New York); and the resources of your nearest reference library. In addition, some chiropractic college libraries provide literature search and abstract services and/or other aids for the field. If you are a "computer buff," you will find CompuServe's "Paperchase" an invaluable aid, and new data bases are being developed by numerous networks at a rapid rate.

I also hope that this and other books of this nature will encourage in-depth applied research into the various chiropractic concepts and neurologic models that have been described in this book and so often debated in the field. We know that chiropractic health care has achieved positive benefits in literally millions of cases that suffered little or no results under traditional medical care. It is for this reason that chiropractic has established itself as a profession. But many questions about *how* and *why* these results have been achieved still remain hypothetical. To recite a random example, what is the primary focal site of functional fault at the IVF area in a typical vertebral *subluxation complex?* In answer to this question, I have frequently taken the liberty to coin the term subluxation complex in this book, as well as others that I have authored, for the following reasons:

- Is it the noxious effect upon the paravertebral ganglia, the nerve root and its contents, the meninges, CSF circulation, or the ultimate effect in the spinal cord?
- Is it the harmful effect on normal somatosomatic, somatovisceral, somatopsychic, viscerosomatic, or viscerovisceral reflexes, or the establishment of self-sustaining pathologic spinosomatic and spinovisceral reflexes?
- Is it the noxious effect of impaired circulation in the dural sleeve, the local accumulation of edema and metabolic debris, the irritating or fatiguing CNS upper-center bombardment by mechanoreceptor input that is out of time, phase, or need, or simply interference with normal axoplasmic flow?
- Is it a unique combination of several of these factors that may explain the dramatic results so often seen with cases exhibiting signs of advanced dysfunction and the sometimes unsatisfying results witnessed with cases that appear (according to experience) to be relatively simple to correct.

Much evidence has been gathered to support each of the above listed impulse-related, nonimpulse-related, and biochemical theories, but few of the data gathered to date lead to undisputed conclusions. These and many other rational theories have been described in this manual, but specific direction to which concern(s) should take clinical priority must be left to the findings of further clinical and laboratory research. If this book is well received by the field, I will do my best to keep abreast of and report such findings in subsequent editions.

—RCS

APPENDIX
Projected Effects of Vertebral Subluxations

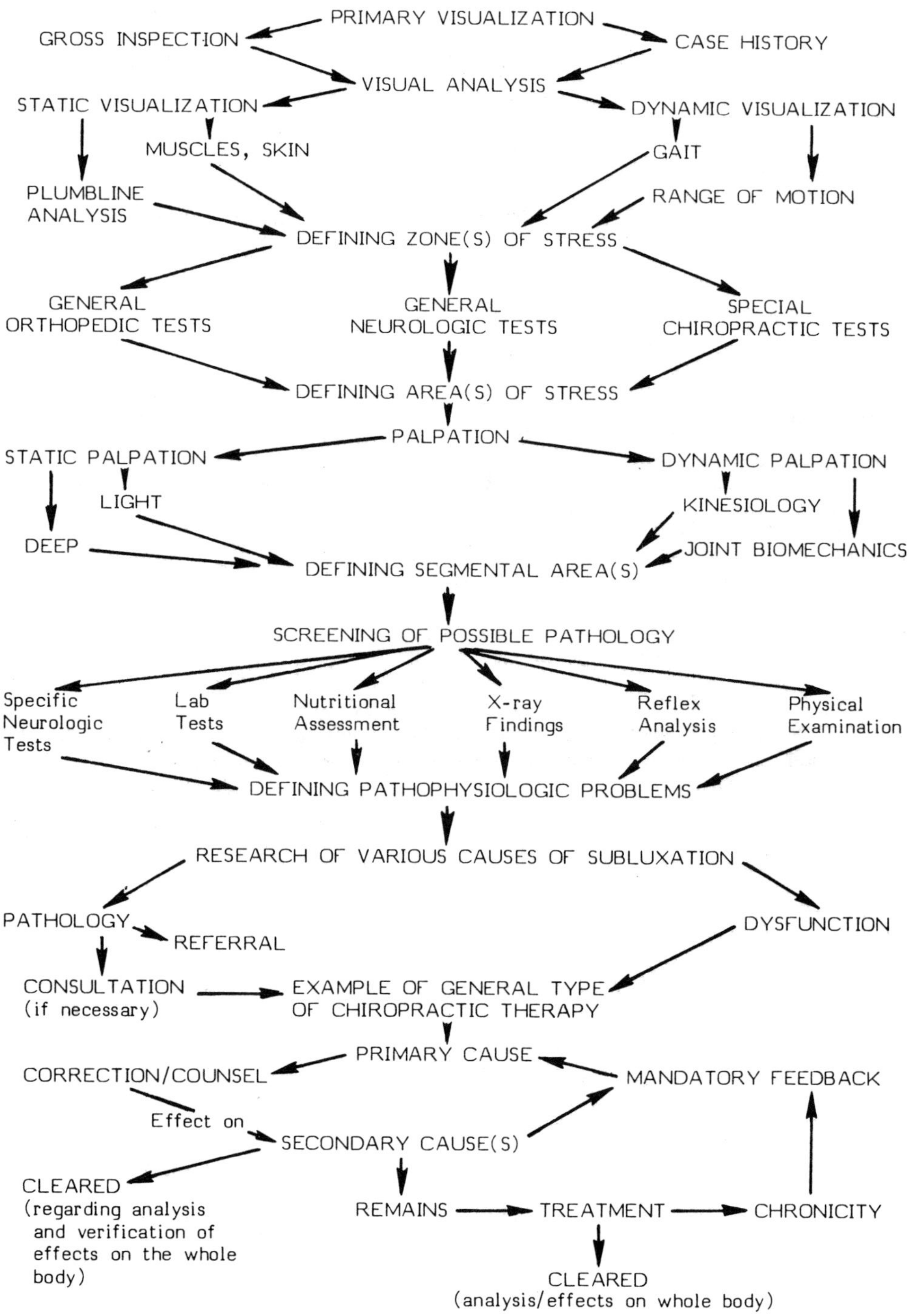

Figure A.1. Determination of subluxations by chiropractic procedures. Based on charts prepared by B. Faucret, et al (reprinted with permission of the Los Angeles College of Chiropractic).

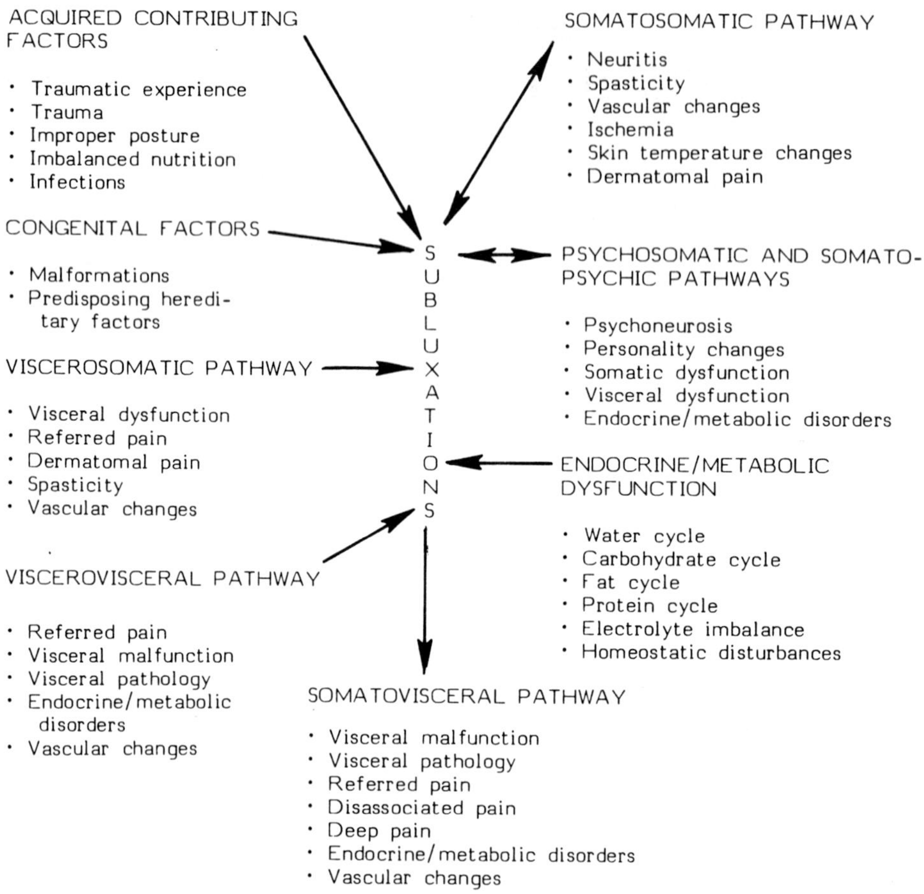

Figure A.2. General overview of cause-and-effect relationships involved in subluxation complexes. Based on charts prepared by B. Faucret, et al (reprinted with permission of the Los Angeles College of Chiropractic).

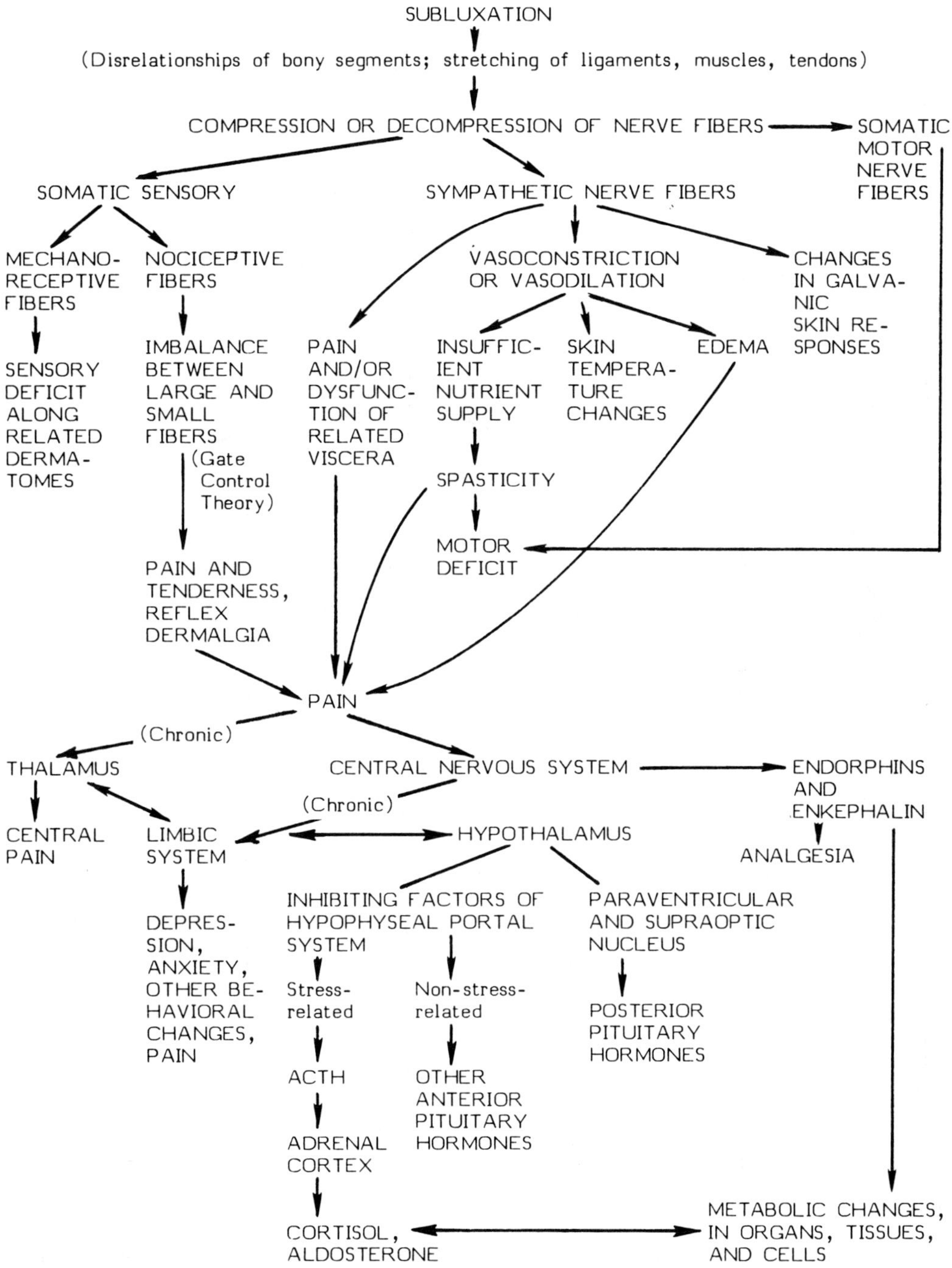

Figure A.3. Neurophysiologic pathways of subluxation complexes. Based on charts prepared by B. Faucret, et al (reprinted with permission of the Los Angeles College of Chiropractic).

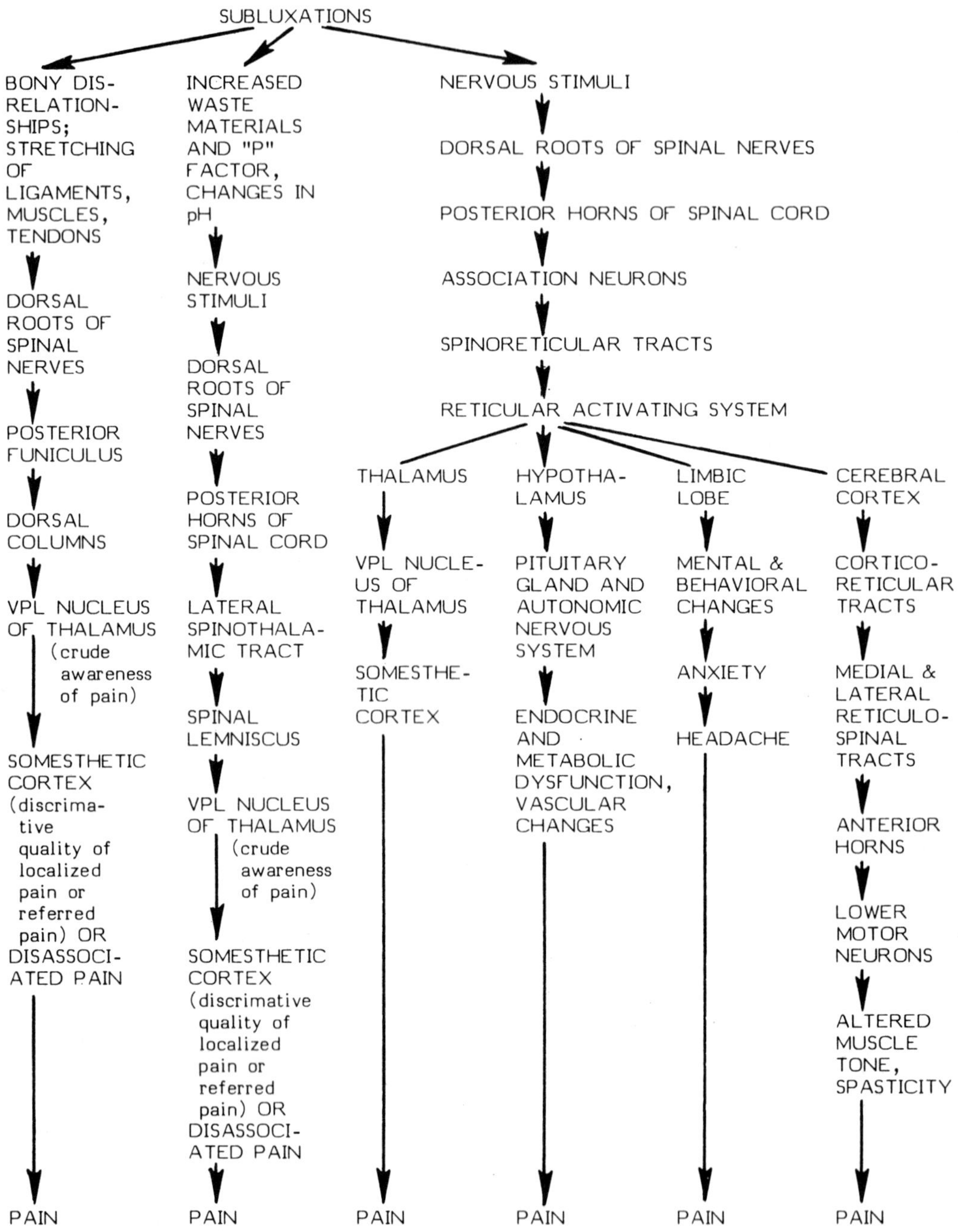

Figure A.4. Pain pathways of subluxations. Based on charts prepared by B. Faucret, et al (reprinted with permission of the Los Angeles College of Chiropractic).

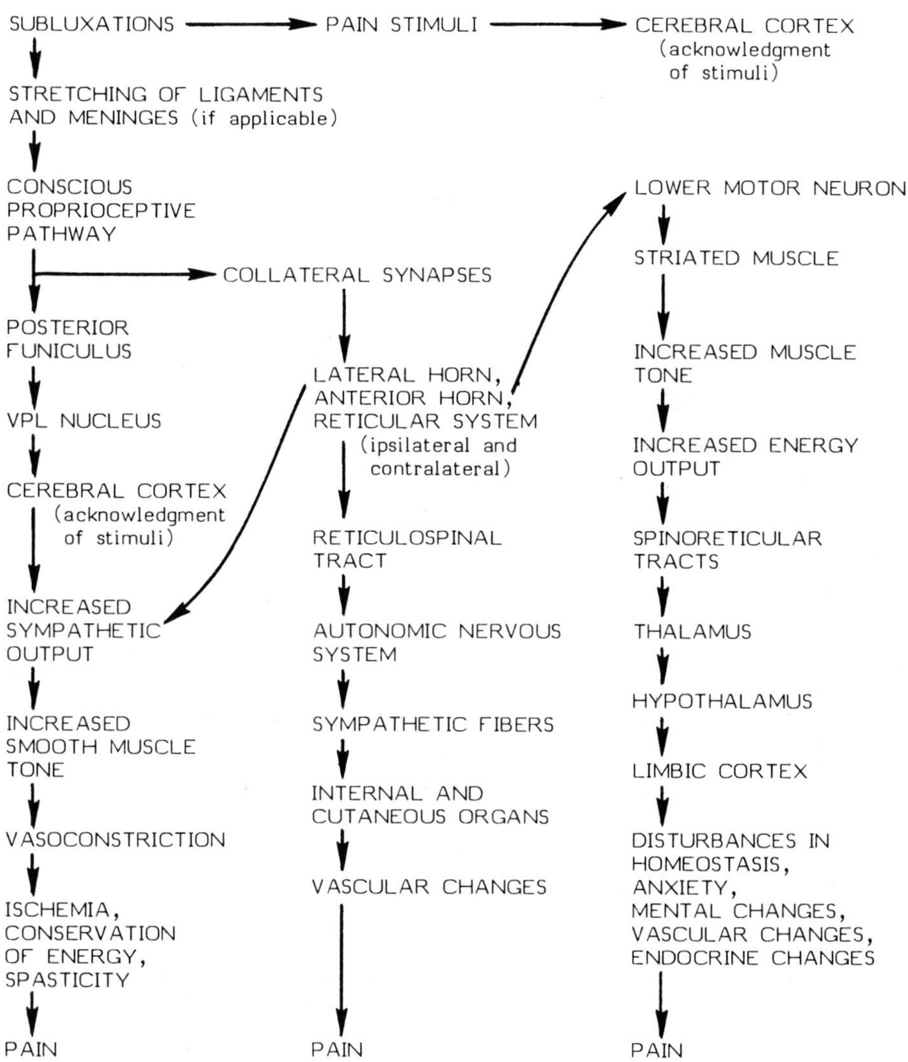

Figure A.5. Projected effects of subluxations on the somatosomatic pathway. Based on charts prepared by B. Faucret, et al (reprinted with permission of the Los Angeles College of Chiropractic).

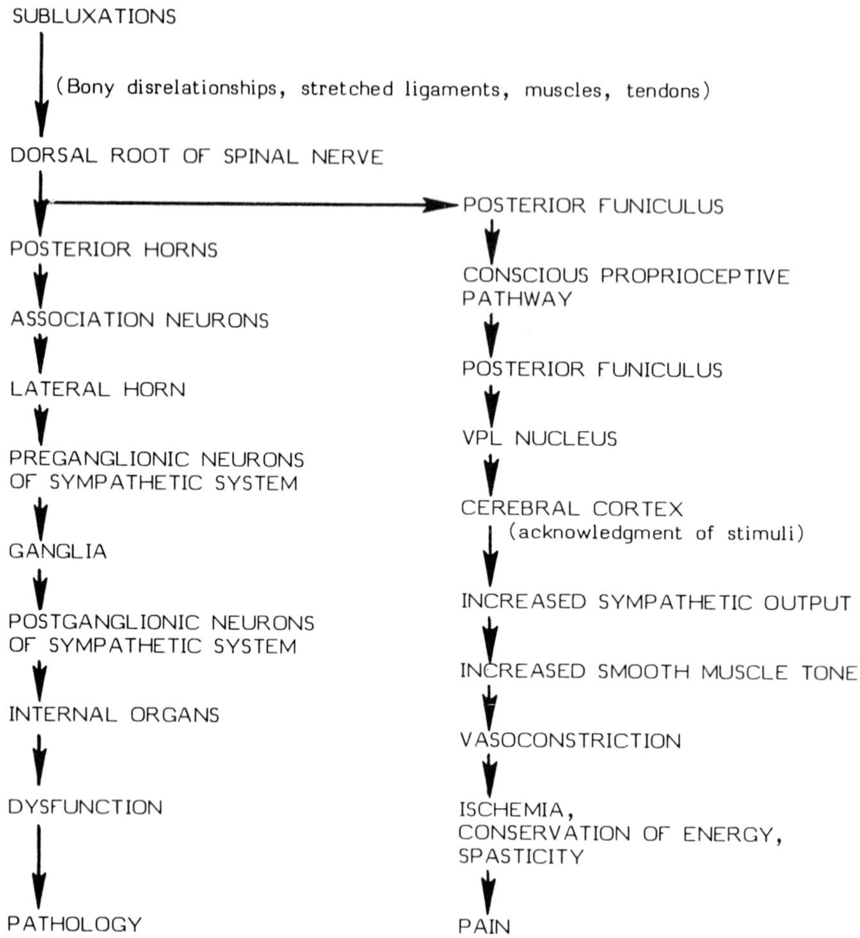

Figure A.6. Projected effects of subluxations on the somatovisceral pathway. Based on charts prepared by B. Faucret, et al (reprinted with permission of the Los Angeles College of Chiropractic).

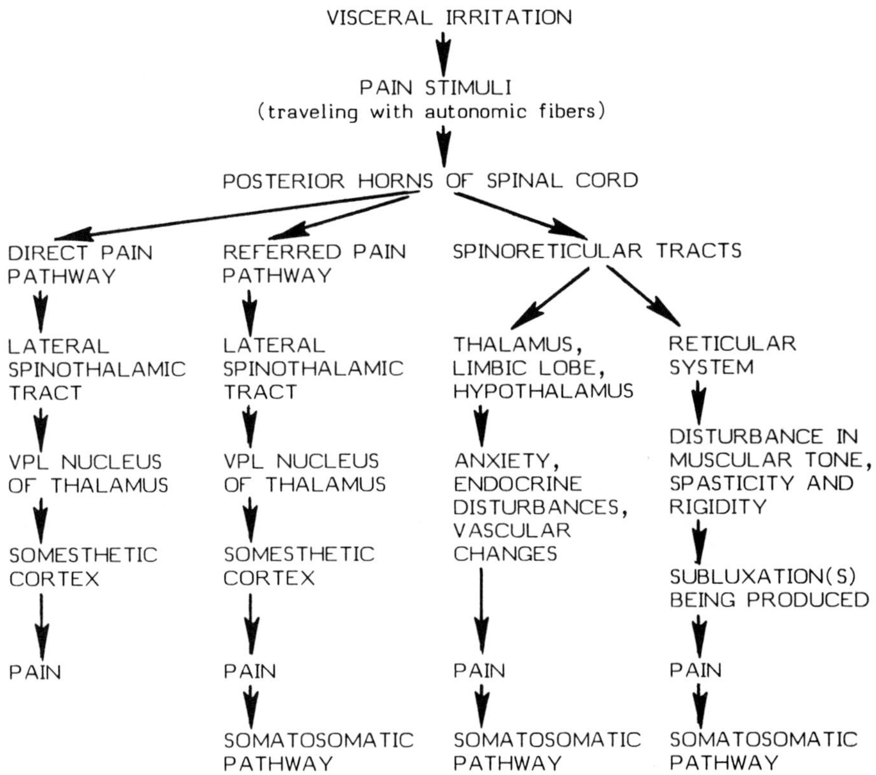

Figure A.7. Viscerosomatic pathway, showing how visceral irritation leads to pain and the development of subluxations. Based on charts prepared by B. Faucret, et al (reprinted with permission of the Los Angeles College of Chiropractic).

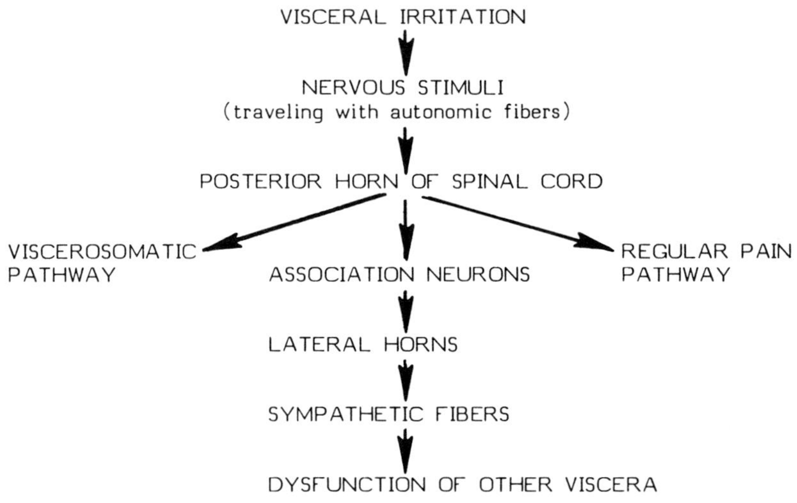

Figure A.8. Viscerovisceral pathway, showing how visceral irritation leads to viscerosomatic syndromes and regular pain. Based on charts prepared by B. Faucret, et al (reprinted with permission of the Los Angeles College of Chiropractic).

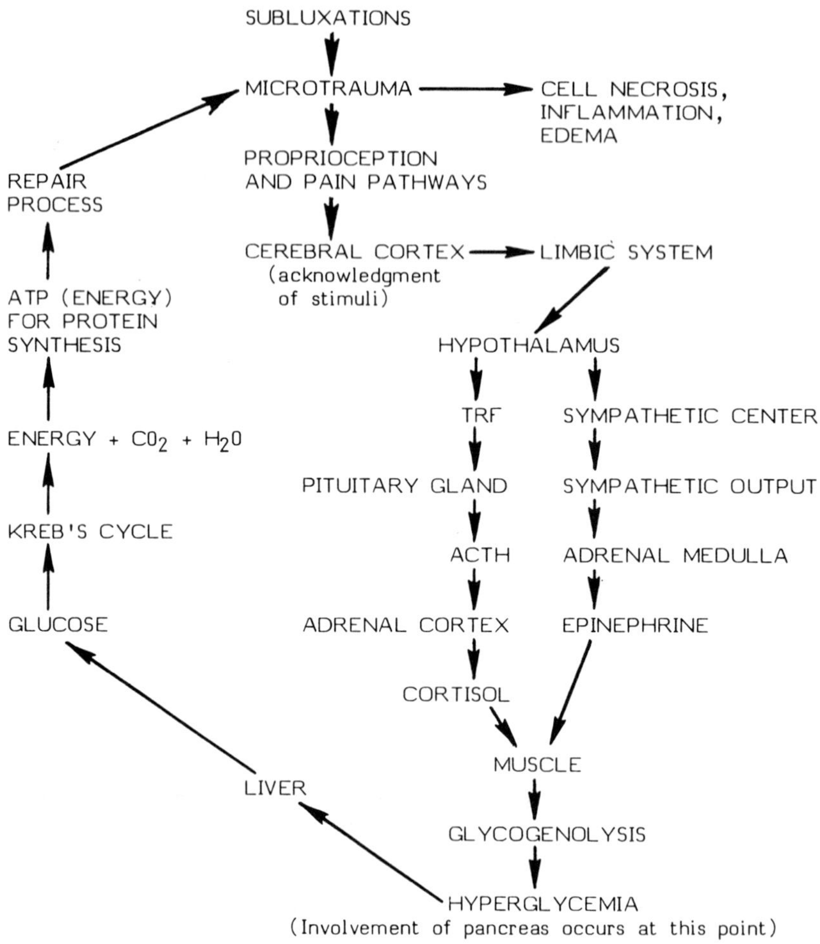

Figure A.9. Projected effects of subluxations on the carbohydrate cycle (carbohydrate metabolism). Based on charts prepared by B. Faucret, et al (reprinted with permission of the Los Angeles College of Chiropractic).

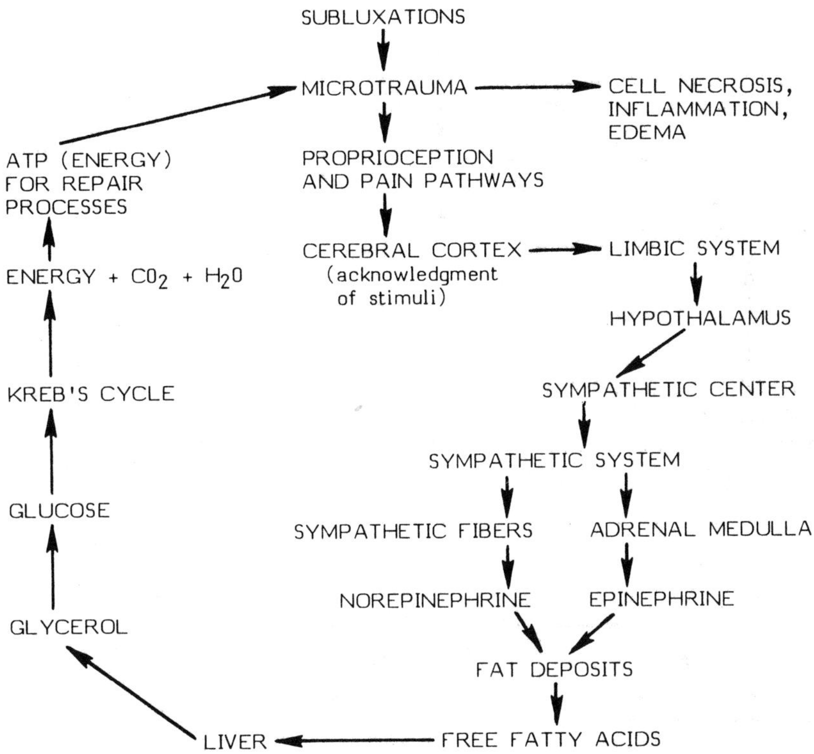

Figure A.10. Projected effects of subluxations on the fat cycle (fat metabolism). Based on charts prepared by B. Faucret, et al (reprinted with permission of the Los Angeles College of Chiropractic).

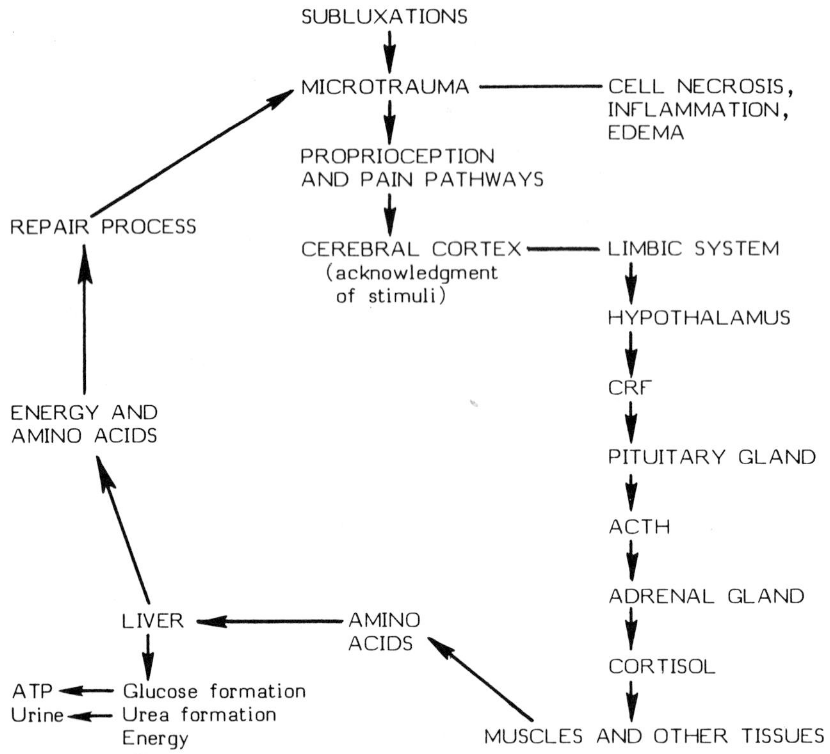

Figure A.11. Projected effects of subluxations on the protein cycle (protein metabolism). Based on charts prepared by B. Faucret, et al (reprinted with permission of the Los Angeles College of Chiropractic).

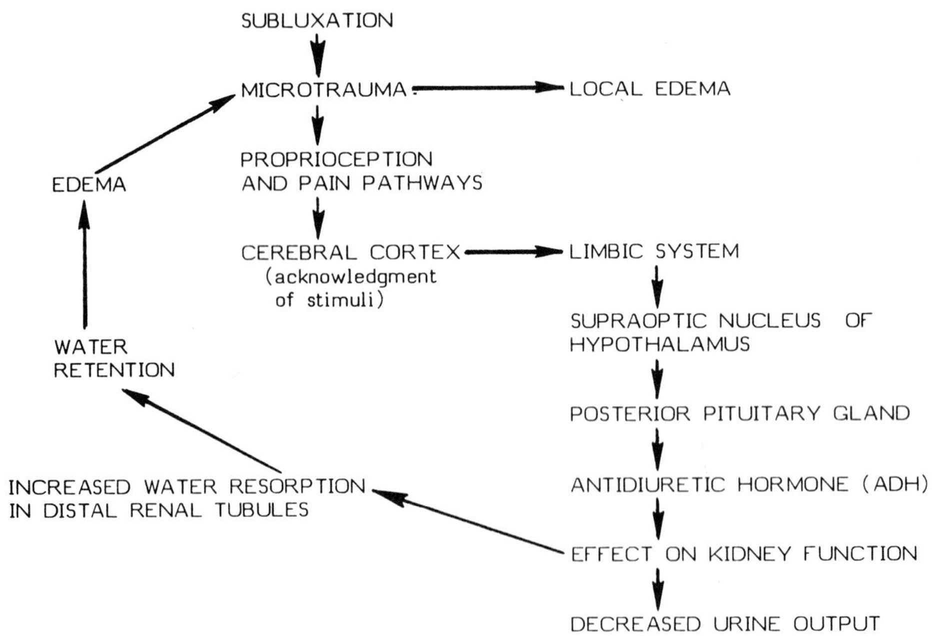

Figure A.12. Projected effects of subluxations on the water cycle (water metabolism). Based on charts prepared by B. Faucret, et al (reprinted with permission of the Los Angeles College of Chiropractic).

Index

-D-

-E-

-F-

-N-

-R-

-T-

-U-

-V-

-W-